Handbook of
Nutraceuticals
and
Functional Foods
Second Edition

Handbook of

Nutraceuticals and Functional Foods

Second Edition

EDITED BY
ROBERT E. C. WILDMAN

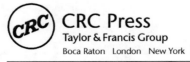

CRC Press
Taylor & Francis Group
Boca Raton   London   New York

CRC Press is an imprint of the
Taylor & Francis Group, an informa business

CRC Press
Taylor & Francis Group
6000 Broken Sound Parkway NW, Suite 300
Boca Raton, FL 33487-2742

International Standard Book Number-10: 0-8493-6409-4 (Hardcover)
International Standard Book Number-13: 978-0-8493-6409-9 (Hardcover)

Library of Congress Cataloging-in-Publication Data

Handbook of nutraceuticals and functional foods / edited by Robert E.C. Wildman. -- 2nd ed.
    p. cm.
  Includes bibliographical references and index.
  ISBN 0-8493-6409-4 (alk. paper)
  1. Functional foods--Handbooks, manuals, etc. I. Wildman, Robert E. C., 1964-

QP144.F85H36 2006
613.2--dc22   2006045563

Visit the Taylor & Francis Web site at
http://www.taylorandfrancis.com

and the CRC Press Web site at
http://www.crcpress.com

To Dawn, Gage, and Bryn

Preface

It may be difficult to imagine a more exciting time than today to be involved in nutrition research, education, and general health promotion. The investigative opportunities seem to be limitless and research tools range from large-scale epidemiology survey assessment to focused assessment of cellular gene expression using molecular biology technique. Furthermore, scientific information can be shared rapidly and globally via a variety of channels including scientific journals, magazines, and Internet Web sites. The advent of many of the probing investigative techniques occurred in the latter half of the 20th century and has evolved to the current state of the art. These advances have allowed scientists to objectively investigate some of the most ancient concepts in the application of foods as well as epidemiological relationships related to optimizing health and performance and the prevention and/or the treatment of diseases.

Throughout the bulk of the twentieth century nutrition recommendations seemed to focus more upon "what not to eat" on a foundation consisting of the adequate provision of essential nutrients such as essential amino and fatty acids, vitamins, minerals, and water. For instance, recommendations were to limit dietary substances such as saturated fatty acids, cholesterol, and sodium. Today scientists are recognizing that the other side of the nutrition coin, or "what to eat," may be just as important, if not more so. We have known for some time now that people who eat a diet rich in more natural foods, such as fruits, vegetables, nuts, whole grains, and fish, tend to lead a more disease-free life. The incidences of certain cancers and heart disease are noticeably lower than in populations that eat considerably lower amounts of these foods. For a while many nutritionists believed that this observation was more of an association rather than cause and effect. This is to say that the higher incidence of disease was more the result of higher calories, fat and processed foods in conjunction with lower physical activity typically associated with the lower consumption of fruits, vegetables, etc., rather than the lack of these foods. Thus, recommendations focused on limiting many of the "bad" food items by substituting them with foods that were not associated with the degenerative diseases, deemed "good" foods somewhat by default. With time scientists were able to better understand the composition of the "good" foods. Evidence quickly mounted to support earlier beliefs that many natural foods are seemingly prophylactic and medicinal.

Today we find ourselves at what seems to be an epoch in understanding humanity's relationship with nature. Nutraceutical concepts remind us of our vast reliance upon other life forms on this planet. For it is these entities that not only provide us with our dietary essentials but also factors that yield protection against the environment in which we exist and the potentially pathological events we internally create. Food was an environmental tool used in the sculpting of the human genome. It is only logical to think then that eating more natural foods such as fruits and vegetables would lead to a healthier existence.

The advancement of scientific techniques has not only allowed us to better understand the diet we are supposed to eat, but it has also opened the door to one of the most interesting events in commerce. Food companies are now able to market foods with approved health claims touting the nutraceutical or functional properties of the food. Food companies are also able to fortify existing foods with nutraceutical substances and/or create new foods designed to include one or more nutraceutical substances in their recipes. The opportunity afforded to food companies involved in functional foods appears without limitations at this time.

Despite the fact that this book reviews numerous nutraceuticals and functional foods, the field is still very young and surely there is much more to be learned and applied to a healthier existence.

It is hard to imagine that nutrition science would ever be more exciting than this. But perhaps some scientist wrote that very same thought less than a century ago during the vitamin and mineral boom. I truly hope you enjoy this book and welcome your comments and thoughts for future editions.

The Editor

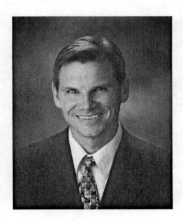

Robert E.C. Wildman is a native of Philadelphia, Pennsylvania, and attended the University of Pittsburgh (B.S.), Florida State University (M.S.), and Ohio State University (Ph.D.). He is coauthor of the textbooks *Advanced Human Nutrition* and *Exercise and Sport Nutrition* and author of *The Nutritionist: Food, Nutrition, and Optimal Health.*

Contributors

D. Lee Alekel
Department of Food Science and Human
  Nutrition
Iowa State University
Ames, Iowa, USA

Jose Antonio
International Society of Sports Nutrition
www.theissn.org

Leonard N. Bell
Department of Nutrition and Food Science
Auburn University
Auburn, Alabama, USA

Richard S. Bruno
Department of Nutritional Sciences
University of Connecticut
Storrs, Connecticut, USA

Robin Callister
School of Biomedical Sciences
University of Newcastle
Callaghan, New South Wales, Australia

Claude P. Champagne
Food Research and Development Centre
Agriculture Canada
Saint Hyacinthe, Quebec, Canada

Pratibha Chaturvedi
KGK Synergize Inc.
London, Ontario, Canada

Nancy M. Childs
Department of Food Marketing
Saint Joseph's University
Philadelphia, Pennsylvania, USA

Michael A. Dubick
Institute of Surgical Research
U.S. Army
Fort Sam Houston, Texas, USA

Edward R. Farnworth
Food Research and Development Centre
Agriculture Canada
Saint Hyacinthe, Quebec, Canada

Manohar L. Garg
School of Biomedical Sciences
University of Newcastle
Callaghan, New South Wales, Australia

Najla Guthrie
KGK Synergize Inc.
London, Ontario, Canada

Meghan Hampton
Department of Human Nutrtion
Kansas State University
Manhattan, Kansas, USA

Suzanne Hendrich
Department of Food Science and Human
  Nutrition
Iowa State University
Ames, Iowa, USA

Luke R. Howard
Department of Food Science
University of Arkansas
Fayetteville, Arkansas, USA

Thunder Jalili
Division of Nutrition
University of Utah
Salt Lake City, Utah, USA

Sidika E. Kasim-Karakas
Department of Internal Medicine
University of California–Davis
Davis, California, USA

Mike Kelley
Melaleuca Inc.
Idaho Falls, Idaho, USA

Donald K. Layman
Department of Food Science and Human
  Nutrition
University of Illinois
Urbana, Illinois, USA

Peony Lee
School of Molecular and Microbial Biosciences
University of Sydney
Sydney, New South Wales, Australia

Yong Li
Department of Food Science
Lipid Chemistry and Molecular Biology
  Laboratory
Purdue University
West Lafayette, Indiana, USA

Denis M. Medeiros
Department of Human Nutrtion
Kansas State University
Manhattan, Kansas, USA

John A. Milner
Nutritional Science Research Group
National Cancer Institute
National Institutes of Health
Rockville, Maryland, USA

Patricia A. Murphy
Food Science and Human Nutrition
Iowa State University
Ames, Iowa, USA

Jade Ng
Goodman Fielder
Macquarie Park
New South Wales, Australia

Stanley T. Omaye
Department of Nutrition
University of Nevada
Reno, Nevada, USA

Susan S. Percival
Food Science and Human Nutrition Department
University of Florida
Gainesville, Florida, USA

Brendan Plunkett
School of Biomedical Sciences
University of Newcastle
Callaghan, New South Wales, Australia

Sharon A. Ross
Nutritional Science Research Group
National Cancer Institute
National Institutes of Health
Rockville, Maryland, USA

Steven J. Schwartz
Department of Food Science and Technology
The Ohio State University
Columbus, Ohio, USA

Jennifer E. Seyler
Bally Total Fitness Corporation
Chicago, Illinois, USA

Lem Taylor
Exercise and Biochemical Nutrition Laboratory
Baylor University
Waco, Texas, USA

R. Elaine Turner
Food Science and Human Nutrition Department
University of Florida
Gainesville, Florida, USA

Darrell Vachon
KGK Synergize Inc.
London, Ontario, Canada

Marie-Rose Van Calsteren
Food Research and Development Centre
Agriculture and Agri-Food Canada
Saint Hyacinthe, Quebec, Canada

Dianne H. Volker
Department of Psychology
University of Sydney
Sydney, New South Wales, Australia

Bruce A. Watkins
Department of Food Science
Purdue University
West Lafayette, Indiana, USA

Trent A. Watson
School of Biomedical Sciences
University of Newcastle
Callaghan, New South Wales, Australia

Robert E.C. Wildman
Melaleuca Inc.
Idaho Falls, Idaho, USA

Diah Yunianingtias
School of Molecular and Microbial Biosciences
University of Sydney
Sydney, New South Wales, Australia

Contents

1 Nutraceuticals and Functional Foods

Robert E.C. Wildman and Mike Kelley

CONTENTS

I. INTRODUCTION

The interest in nutraceuticals and functional foods continues to grow, powered by progressive research efforts to identify properties and potential applications of nutraceutical substances, and coupled with public interest and consumer demand. The principal reasons for the growth of the functional food market are current population and health trends. Across the globe, populations are aging. Life expectancy continues to rise, as does the contribution made by older individuals to the total population. Also, obesity is now recognized as a global issue as its incidence continues to climb in countries throughout the world. In the U.S., approximately 62% of the adult population is classified as overweight (based on body mass index (BMI)), and more than half of those adults are classified as obese. Heart disease continues to be a primary cause of death, responsible for 32% of deaths in the U.S., and cancer, osteoporosis, and arthritis remain highly prevalent. As of this writing, the International Obesity Task Force reports that the incidence of obesity in the majority of European countries has increased by 10 to 50% in the last 10 years.[1]

Although genetics play a major role in the development of the diseases mentioned above, by and large most are considered preventable or could be minimized by a proper diet and physical activity, weight management, and a healthier lifestyle including environment. Additionally, people can optimize the health-promoting capabilities of their diet by way of supplementation and by consuming foods that have been formulated or fortified to include health-promoting factors.

1

Another reason for the growing trend in functional foods is public education. People today are more nutrition-savvy than ever before, their interest in health-related information being met by many courses of information. Each year more and more newspaper and magazine articles are devoted to the relationship between diet and health, and more specifically, to nutraceutical concepts. Furthermore, more health-related magazines and books are appearing on bookstore shelves than ever before. More television programs address topics of disease and prevention/treatment than ever. But perhaps one of the most significant events to influence public awareness was the advent of the Internet (World Wide Web). The Internet provides a wealth of information regarding the etiology, prevention, and treatment of various diseases. Numerous Web sites have been developed by government agencies such as the U.S. Department of Agriculture (USDA; www.nal.usda.gov) and organizations such as the American Heart Association (www.americanheart.org) and the American Cancer Society (www.cancer.org). Other information-based businesses such as CNN have information Web sites (i.e., www.WebMD.com) and Internet search engines exist for perusing medical abstracts (e.g., www.nlm.nih.gov/medlineplus).

II. DEFINING NUTRACEUTICALS AND FUNCTIONAL FOODS

The term *nutraceutical* is a hybrid or contraction of *nutrition* and *pharmaceutical*. Reportedly, it was coined in 1989 by DeFelice and the Foundation for Innovation in Medicine.[2] Restated and clarified in a press release in 1994, its definition was "any substance that may be considered a food or part of a food and provides medical or health benefits, including the prevention and treatment of disease. Such products may range from isolated nutrients, dietary, supplements and diets to genetically engineered 'designer' foods, herbal products, and processed foods such as cereals, soups, and beverages."[3] At present there are no universally accepted definitions for nutraceuticals and functional foods, although commonality clearly exists between the definitions offered by different health-oriented professional organizations.

According to the International Food Information Council (IFIC), functional foods are "foods or dietary components that may provide a health benefit beyond basic nutrition."[4] The International Life Sciences Institute of North America (ILSI) has defined functional foods as "foods that by virtue of physiologically active food components provide health benefits beyond basic nutrition."[5] Health Canada defines functional foods as "similar in appearance to a conventional food, consumed as part of the usual diet, with demonstrated physiological benefits, and/or to reduce the risk of chronic disease beyond basic nutritional functions." The *Nutrition Business Journal* classified functional food as "food fortified with added or concentrated ingredients to functional levels, which improves health or performance.[6] Functional foods include enriched cereals, breads, sport drinks, bars, fortified snack foods, baby foods, prepared meals, and more."

As noted by the American Dietetics Association in a position paper dedicated to functional foods, the term "functional" implies that the food has some identified value leading to health benefits, including reduced risk of disease, for the person consuming it.[7] One could easily argue that functional foods include everything from natural foods, such as fruits and vegetables endowed with antioxidants and fiber, to fortified and enriched foods, such as orange juice with added calcium or additional carotenoids, to formulated ready-to-drink beverages containing antioxidants and immune-supporting factors.

The *Nutrition Business Journal* states that it uses the term nutraceutical for anything that is consumed primarily or particularly for health reasons. Based on that definition, a functional food would be a kind of nutraceutical.[8] On the other hand, Health Canada states that nutraceuticals are a product that is "prepared from foods, but sold in the form of pills or powders (potions), or in other medicinal forms not usually associated with foods. A nutraceutical is demonstrated to have a physiological benefit or provide protection against chronic disease."[6] Based on this definition and how functional foods are characterized, as noted previously, nutraceuticals would be distinct from functional foods.

TABLE 1.1
Food Label Claim Guidelines

Claim	Purpose	Example
Nutrient content claim	Describe content of certain nutrients.	"Fat-free," "low sodium."
Qualified health claim	Describe the relationship between food, food component, or dietary supplement and reduced risk of a disease or health related condition. This claim uses qualifying language because the evidence for this relationship is emerging and is not yet strong enough to meet the standard of significant scientific advancement set by the FDA.	"Some scientific evidence suggests that consumption of antioxidant vitamins may reduce the risk of certain forms of cancer. However, FDA has determined that this evidence is limited and not conclusive."
NLEA authorized health claims	Characterize a relationship between a food, a food component, dietary ingredient, or dietary supplement and risk of a disease.	"Diets high in calcium may reduce the risk of osteoporosis."
Structure/function claim	Describes role of nutrient or ingredient intended to affect normal structure or function in humans. May characterize the means by which the nutrient or ingredient affects the structure or function. May describe a benefit related to a deficiency. Must be accompanied by a disclaimer stating that FDA has not reviewed the claim and that the product is not intended to "diagnose, treat, cure, or prevent any disease."	"Calcium builds strong bones."

Source: Adapted from International Life Sciences Institute of North America Web site, http://www.ilsi.org/, 2006.

The potential functions of nutraceutical/functional food ingredients are so often related to the maintenance or improvement of health that it is necessary to distinguish between a food ingredient that has function and a drug. The core definition of a drug is any article that is "intended for use in the diagnosis, cure, mitigation, treatment, or prevention of disease in man or other animals."(21 U.S.C. 321(g)(1)(B)). At the same time, certain health claims can be made for foods and ingredients that are associated with health conditions. In the U.S., such health claims are defined and regulated by the U.S. Food and Drug Administration (USFDA). Health claims related to foods and ingredients include an implied or explicit statement about the relationship of a food substance to a disease or health-related condition (21 U.S.C.343(r)(1)(B) and 21 C.F.R.101.14(a)(1)). The major categories of health claims are listed in Table 1.1 with examples of each.

III. CLASSIFYING NUTRACEUTICAL FACTORS

The number of purported nutraceutical substances is in the hundreds, and some of the more recognizable substances include isoflavones, tocotrienols, allyl sulfur compounds, fiber, and carotenoids. In light of a long and growing list of nutraceutical substances, organization systems are needed to allow for easier understanding and application. This is particularly true for academic instruction, as well as product formulation by food companies.

Depending upon one's interest and/or background, the appropriate organizational scheme for nutraceuticals can vary. For example, cardiologists may be most interested in those nutraceutical substances that are associated with reducing the risk factors of heart disease. Specifically, their interest may lie in substances purported to positively influence hypertension and hypercholester-olemia and to reduce free radical- or platelet-dependent thrombotic activity. Nutraceutical factors such as n-3 fatty acids, phytosterols, quercetin, and grape flavonoids would be of particular interest. Meanwhile, oncologists may be more interested in those substances that target anticarcinogenic activities. These substances may be associated with augmentations of microsomal detoxification systems and antioxidant defenses, or they may slow the progression of existing cancer. Thus, their interest may lie in both chemoprevention or potential adjunctive therapy.

On the other hand, the nutraceutical interest of food scientists working on the development of a functional food product will not only include physiological properties, but also stability and sensory properties, as well as issues of cost efficiency. To demonstrate this point, the anticarcino-genic triterpene limonin is lipid-soluble and intensely bitter, somewhat limiting its commercial use as a functional food ingredient.[10] However, the glucoside derivative of limonin, which shares some of the anticarcinogenic activity of limonin, is water soluble and virtually tasteless, thereby enhancing its potential use as an ingredient.[11]

Whether it is for academic instruction, clinical trial design, functional food development, or dietary recommendations, nutraceutical factors can be organized in several ways. Cited below are a few ways of organizing nutraceuticals based upon food source, mechanism of action, and chemical nature.

IV. FOOD AND NONFOOD SOURCES OF NUTRACEUTICAL FACTORS

One of the broader models of organization for nutraceuticals is based upon their potential as a food source to humans. Here nutraceuticals may be separated into plant, animal, and microbial (i.e., bacteria and yeast) groups. Grouping nutraceutical factors in this manner has numerous merits and can be a valuable tool for diet planning, as well as classroom and seminar instruction.

One interesting consideration with this organization system is that the food source may not necessarily be the point of origin for one or more substances. An obvious example is conjugated linoleic acid (CLA), which is part of the human diet, mostly as a component of beef and dairy foods. However, it is actually made by bacteria in the rumen of the cow. Therefore, issues involving the food chain or symbiotic relationships may have to be considered for some individuals working with this organization scheme.

Because of fairly conserved biochemical aspects across species, many nutraceutical substances are found in both plants and animals, and sometimes in microbes. For example, microbes, plants, and animals contain choline and phosphotidylcholine. This is also true for sphingolipids; however, plants and animals are better sources. Also, linolenic acid (18:3 ω-3 fatty acid) can be found in a variety of food resources including animal flesh, despite the fact that it is primarily synthesized in plants and other lower members of the food chain. Table 1.2 presents some of the more recognizable nutraceutical substances grouped according to food-source providers.

Nonfood sources of nutraceutical factors have been sourced by the development of modern fermentation methods. For example, amino acids and their derivatives have been produced by bacteria grown in fermentation systems. The emergence of recombinant-genetic techniques have enabled new avenues for obtaining nutraceutical compounds. These techniques and their products are being evaluated in the arenas of the marketplace and regulatory concerns around the world. An example is the production of eicosapentaenoic acid (EPA) by bacteria. This fatty acid is produced by some algae and bacteria. The EPA derived from salmon are produced by algae and are later incorporated in the salmon that consume the algae. EPA can now be produced by non-EPA producing bacteria by importing the appropriate DNA through recombinant methods.[12] The ability to transfer the production of nutraceutical molecules into organisms that allows for economically feasible production is cause for both optimism and discussion concerning regulatory and popular acceptance.

TABLE 1.2
Examples of Nutraceutical Substances Grouped by Food Source

Plants	Animal	Microbial
β-Glucan	Conjugated Linoleic Acid (CLA)	*Saccharomyces boulardii* (yeast)
Ascorbic acid	Eicosapentaenoic acid (EPA)	*Bifidobacterium bifidum*
γ-Tocotrienol	Docosahexenoic acid (DHA)	*B. longum*
Quercetin	Spingolipids	*B. infantis*
Luteolin	Choline	*Lactobacillus acidophilus* (LC1)
Cellulose	Lecithin	*L. acidophilus* (NCFB 1748)
Lutein	Calcium	*Streptococcus salvarius* (subs. Thermophilus)
Gallic acid	Coenzyme Q_{10}	
Perillyl alcohol	Selenium	
Indole-3-carbonol	Zinc	
Pectin	Creatine	
Daidzein	Minerals	
Glutathione		
Potassium		
Allicin		
δ-Limonene		
Genestein		
Lycopene		
Hemicellulose		
Lignin		
Capsaicin		
Geraniol		
β-Ionone		
α-Tocopherol		
β-Carotene		
Nordihydrocapsaicin		
Selenium		
Zeaxanthin		
Minerals		
MUFA		

Note: The substances listed in this table include those that are either accepted or purported nutraceutical substances.

V. NUTRACEUTICAL FACTORS IN SPECIFIC FOODS

In an organization model related to the one above, nutraceuticals can be grouped based upon relatively concentrated foods. This model is more appropriate when there is interest in a particular nutraceutical compound or related compounds, or when there is interest in a specific food for agricultural/geographic reasons or functional food-development purposes. For example, the interest may be in the nutraceutical qualities of a local crop or a traditionally consumed food in a geographic region, such as pepper fruits in the southwestern United States, olive oil in Mediterranian regions, and red wine in western Europe and Northern California.

There are several nutraceutical substances that are found in higher concentrations in specific foods or food families. These include capsaicinoids, which are found primarily in pepper fruit, and allyl sulfur (organosulfur) compounds, which are particularly concentrated in onions and garlic. Table 1.3 provides a listing of certain nutraceuticals that are considered unique to certain foods or food families. One consideration for this model is that for several substances, such as those just

TABLE 1.3
Examples of Foods with Higher Content of Specific Nutraceutical Substances

Nutraceutical Substance/Family	Foods of Remarkably High Content
Allyl sulfur compounds	Onions, garlic
Isoflavones (e.g., genestein, daidzein)	Soybeans and other legumes, apios
Quercetin	Onion, red grapes, citrus fruit, broccoli, Italian yellow squash
Capsaicinoids	Pepper fruit
EPA and DHA	Fish oils
Lycopene	Tomatoes and tomato products
Isothiocyanates	Cruciferous vegetables
β-Glucan	Oat bran
CLA	Beef and dairy
Resveratrol	Grapes (skin), red wine
β-Carotene	Citrus fruit, carrots, squash, pumpkin
Carnosol	Rosemary
Catechins	Teas, berries
Adenosine	Garlic, onion
Indoles	Cabbage, broccoli, cauliflower, kale, brussels sprouts
Curcumin	Tumeric
Ellagic acid	Grapes, strawberries, raspberries, walnuts
Anthocyanates	Red wine
3-n-Butyl phthalide	Celery
Cellulose	Most plants (component of cell walls)
Lutein, zeaxanthin	Kale, collards, spinach, corn, eggs, citrus
Psyllium	Psyllium husk
Monounsaturated fatty acids	Tree nuts, olive oil
Inulin, Fructooligosaccharides (FOS)	Whole grains, onions, garlic
Lactobacilli, Bifidobacteria	Yogurt and other dairy
Catechins	Tea, cocoa, apples, grapes
Lignans	Flax, rye

Note: The substances listed in this table include those that are either accepted or purported nutraceutical substances.

named, there is a relatively short list of foods that are concentrated sources. However, the list of food sources for other nutraceutical substances can be much longer and can include numerous seemingly unrelated foods. For instance, citrus fruit contain the isoflavone quercetin, as do onions, a plant food seemingly unrelated. Citrus fruit grow on trees, whereas the edible bulb of the onion plant (an herb) develops at ground level. Other plant foods with higher quercetin content are red grapes — but not white grapes, broccoli (which is a cruciferous vegetable), and the Italian yellow squash. Again, these foods appear to bear very little resemblance to citrus fruit or onions for that matter. On the other hand, there are no guarantees that closely related or seemingly similar foods contain the same nutraceutical compounds. For example, both the onion plant and the garlic plant are perennial herbs arising from a rooted bulb and are also cousins in the lily family. However, although onions are loaded with quercetin, with some varieties containing up to 10% of their dry weight of this flavonoid, garlic is quercetin-void.

VI. MECHANISM OF ACTION

Another means of classifying nutraceuticals is by their mechanism of action. This system groups nutraceutical factors together, regardless of food source, based upon their proven or purported

TABLE 1.4
Examples of Nutraceuticals Grouped by Mechanisms of Action

Anticancer	Positive Influence on Blood Lipid Profile	Antioxidant Activity	Antiinflammatory	Osteogenetic or Bone Protective
Capsaicin	β-Glucan	CLA	Linolenic acid	CLA
Genestein	γ-Tocotrienol	Ascorbic acid	EPA	Soy protein
Daidzein	δ-Tocotrienol	β-Carotene	DHA	Genestein
α-Tocotrienol	MUFA	Polyphenolics	GLA	Daidzein
γ-Tocotrienol	Quercetin	Tocopherols	(gamma-linolenic	Calcium
CLA	ω-3 PUFAs	Tocotrienols	acid)	Casein phosphopeptides
Lactobacillus acidophilus	Resveratrol	Indole-3-carbonol	Capsaicin	FOS
Sphingolipids	Tannins	α-Tocopherol	Quercetin	(fructooligosaccharides)
Limonene	β-Sitosterol	Ellagic acid	Curcumin	Inulin
Diallyl sulfide	Saponins	Lycopene		
Ajoene	Guar	Lutein		
α-Tocopherol	Pectin	Glutathione		
Enterolactone		Hydroxytyrosol		
Glycyrrhizin		Luteolin		
Equol		Oleuropein		
Curcumin		Catechins		
Ellagic acid		Gingerol		
Lutein		Chlorogenic acid		
Carnosol		Tannins		
L. bulgaricus				

Note: The substances listed in this table include those that are either accepted or purported nutraceutical substances.

physiological properties. Among the classes would be antioxidant, antibacterial, antihypertensive, antihypercholesterolemic, antiaggregate, anti-inflammatory, anticarcinogenic, osteoprotective, and so on. Similar to the scheme just discussed, credible Internet resources may prove invaluable to this approach. Examples are presented in Table 1.4. This model would also be helpful to an individual who is genetically predisposed to a particular medical condition or to scientists trying to develop powerful functional foods for just such a person. The information in this model would then be helpful in diet planning in conjunction with the organization scheme just discussed and presented in Table 1.3. It would also be helpful to a product developer trying to develop a new functional food, perhaps for heart health. This developer might consider the ingredients listed in several categories to develop a product that would reduce blood pressure, LDL cholesterol level, and inflammation. However, as mentioned numerous times in this book, many issues related to toxicity, synergism, and competition associated with nutraceutical factors and their foods are not yet known.

It is worth considering that nutraceuticals occupy poorly defined research and regulatory positions that lie somewhere between those of pharmaceuticals and foods. In recent times, it is not uncommon for a successfully introduced pharmaceutical to incur $800 million in research costs throughout a research and approval path that can easily span 10 years or more.[13,14] Candidate compounds must move through a range of animal studies that assess their toxicity in acute, chronic, and multigenerational situations. The absorption, metabolism, and excretion of candidate compounds are also studied in animal models, along with studies on their potential efficacy. Compounds that exhibit acceptable characteristics in these early studies proceed through a total of four phases of human studies, including a postmarketing phase. It is not unusual for a compound to have been studied in thousands of subjects before it is first marketed. By contrast, only a very few ingredients classed as nutraceuticals even approach this level of study, and there is no codified requirement that this should be done. The beta-glucan from oats, now extended to include barley, was the first substance to achieve an FDA-approved health claim for labeling purposes, following the evaluation of numerous animal and clinical studies that demonstrated a hypocholesterolemic effect. Plant sterols and sterol esters have been the topic of more than 50 clinical studies and are also the subject of an approved health claim. However, many other nutraceutical compounds have been the topic of few or no clinical studies. A number of ingredients have been classified as "Generally Regarded as Safe" (GRAS), based upon documentation submitted to the FDA, on the presence and safety of the ingredients in the human diet. The GRAS designation allows an ingredient to be introduced as a food-product ingredient. However, the comparison between the introduction of new pharmaceuticals and nutraceuticals indicates the substantial difference between the developmental and safety hurdles that compounds in each category must surmount.

Some nutraceutical ingredients or mixtures are marketed on the basis that they have been used for many years in the practice of traditional or cultural medicine, i.e., treatments for medical ills that have developed in cultural tradition as a result of trial and error. This rationale for use is at the same time both superficially compelling and a cause for concern. The plant and animal kingdoms contain many compounds that offer therapeutic benefit or danger; often the same compound offers both, with the difference being dependent upon the dose. In addition, there has been no systematic follow-up of side effects and fatalities that may possibly have arisen from the use of traditional medicines. A 5-year study that followed over 1,000 cases reported a possible or confirmed association between use and toxicity in nearly 61% of the cases.[15] Thus, whereas a statement regarding traditional use seems to offer a sense of safety by virtue of use by many individuals over time, there has been no systematic regulatory effort to determine safety and little documentation to confirm safety in this category of nutraceuticals.

What may be of interest is that there are several nutraceuticals that can be listed as having more than one mechanism of action. One of the seemingly most versatile nutraceutical families is the ω-3 PUFAs. Their nutraceutical properties can be related to direct effects as well as to some indirect effects. For example, these fatty acids are used as precursors for eicosanoid substances that locally vasodilate, bronchodilate, and deter platelet aggregation and clot formation. These roles can be prophylactic for asthma and heart disease. Omega-3 PUFA may also reduce the activities of protein kinase C and tyrosine kinase, both of which are involved in a cell-growth-signaling mechanism. Here, the direct effects of these fatty acids may reduce cardiac hypertrophy and cancer-cell proliferation. Omega-3 PUFA also appears to inhibit the synthesis of fatty acid synthase (FAS), which is a principal enzyme complex involved in *de novo* fatty acid synthesis. Here the nutraceutical effect may be considered indirect, as chronic consumption of these PUFAs may theoretically lead to decreased quantities of body fat over time and the development of obesity. The obesity might then lead to the development of hyperinsulinemia and related physiological aberrations such as hypertension and hyperlipidemia.

VII. CLASSIFYING NUTRACEUTICAL FACTORS BASED ON CHEMICAL NATURE

Another method of grouping nutraceuticals is based upon their chemical nature. This approach allows nutraceuticals to be categorized under molecular/elemental groups. This preliminary model includes several large groups, which then provide a basis for subclassification or subgroups, and so on. One way to group nutraceuticals grossly is as follows:

- Isoprenoid derivatives
- Phenolic substances
- Fatty acids and structural lipids
- Carbohydrates and derivatives

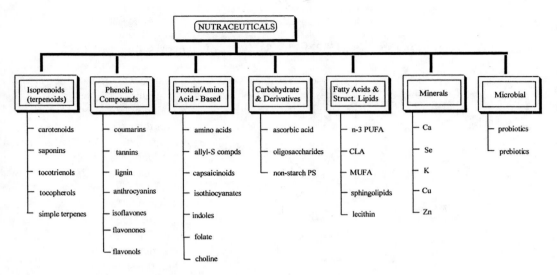

FIGURE 1.1 Organizational scheme for nutraceuticals.

- Amino acid-based substances
- Microbes
- Minerals

As scientific investigation continues, several hundred substances will probably be deemed nutraceuticals. As many of these nutraceutical compounds appear to be related in synthetic origin or molecular nature, there is the potential to broadly group many of the substances together (Figure 1.1). This scheme is by no means perfect, and it is offered "in pencil," as opposed to being "etched in stone." It is expected that scientists will ponder this organization system, find flaws, and suggest ways to evolve the scheme, or disregard it completely in favor of a better concept. Even at this point several "gray" areas are apparent. For instance, mixtures of different classes can exist, such as mixed isoprenoids, prenylated coumarins, and flavonoids. Also, phenolic compounds could arguably be grouped under a very large "amino acid and derivatives" category. Although most phenolic molecules arise from phenylalanine as part of the shikimic acid metabolic pathway, other phenolic compounds are formed via the malonic acid pathway, thereby circumventing phenylalanine as an intermediate. Thus, phenolics stand alone in their own group, whose most salient characteristic is chemical structure, not necessarily synthetic pathway.

A. ISOPRENOID DERIVATIVES (TERPENOIDS)

Isoprenoids and *terpenoids* are terms used to refer to the same class of molecules. These substances are without question one of the largest groups of plant secondary metabolites. In accordance with this ranking, they are also the basis of many plant-derived nutraceuticals. Under this large umbrella are many popular nutraceutical families such as carotenoids, tocopherols, tocotrienols, and saponins. This group is also referred to as isoprenoid derivatives because the principal building block molecule is isoprene (Figure 1.2). Isoprene itself is synthesized from acetyl coenzyme A (CoA), in the well-

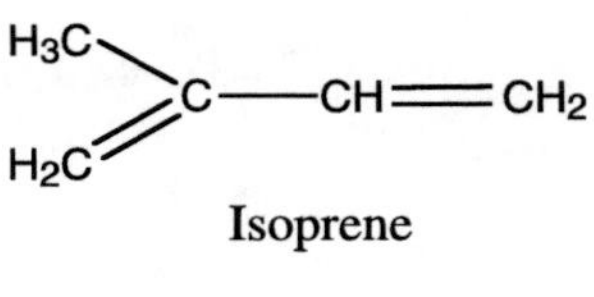

$$H_3C{-}\underset{H_2C}{\overset{}{\diagup}}C{-}CH{=}CH_2$$

Isoprene

FIGURE 1.2 Isoprene.

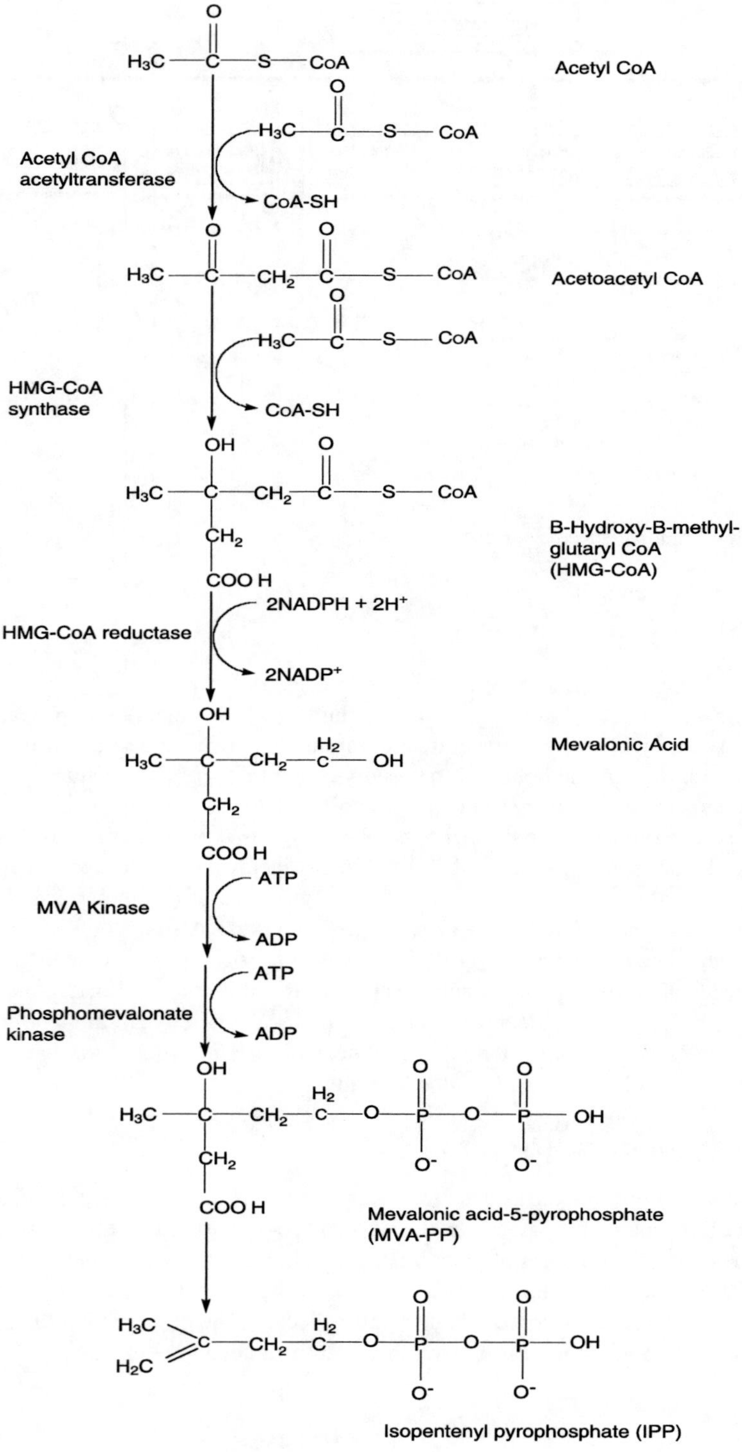

FIGURE 1.3 The mevalonic acid pathway.

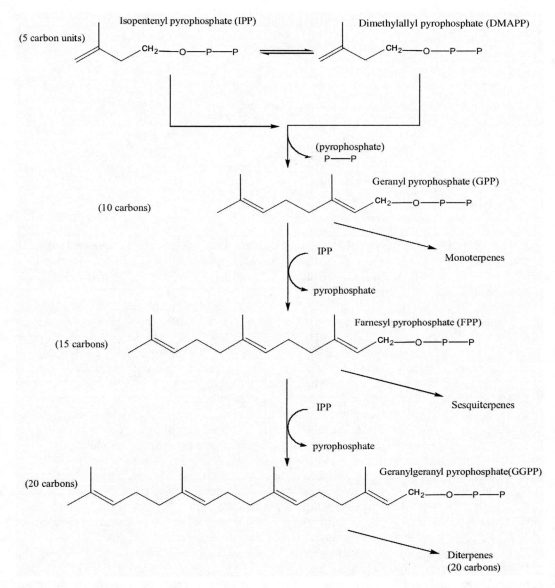

FIGURE 1.4 Formation of terpene structures. In addition: (1) FPP + FPP produces squalene (30 carbons) which yields triterpenes and steroids, and (2) GGPP + GGPP produces phytoene (40 carbons) which yields tetraterpenes.

researched mevalonic acid pathway (Figure 1.3), and the glycolysis-associated molecules pyruvate and 3-phosphoglycerate in a lesser-understood metabolic pathway.[16] In both pathways the end product is isopentenyl phosphate (IPP), and IPP is often regarded as the pivotal molecule in the formation of larger isoprenoid structures. Once IPP is formed, it can reversibly isomerize to dimethylallyl pyrophosphate (DMAPP) as presented in Figure 1.4. Both of these five-carbon structures are then used to form geranyl pyrophosphate (GPP), which can give rise to monoterpenes. Among the monoterpenes are limonene and perillyl alcohol.

GPP can also react with IPP to form the 15-carbon structure farnesyl pyrophosphate (FPP), which then can give rise to the sesquiterpenes. FPP can react with IPP or another FPP to produce

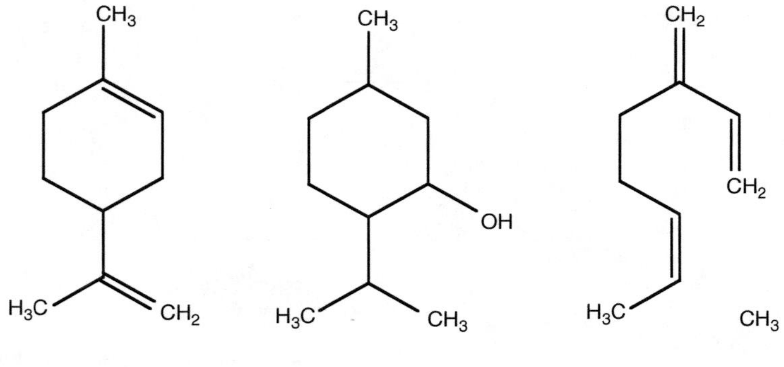

Limonene   Menthol   Myrcene

FIGURE 1.5 Structure of select monoterpenes.

either the 20-carbon geranylgeranyl pyrophosphate (GGPP) or the 30-carbon squalene molecule, respectively. GGPP can give rise to diterpenes while squalene can give rise to triterpenes and steroids. Lastly, GGPP and GPP can condense to form the 40-carbon phytoene structure which then can give rise to tetraterpenes.

Most plants contain so-called essential oils, which contain a mixture of volatile monterpenes and sesquiterpenes. Limonene is found in the essential oils of citrus peels, whereas menthol is the chief monoterpene in peppermint essential oil (Figure 1.5). Two potentially nutraceutical diterpenes in coffee beans are kahweol and cafestol.[17,18] Both of these diterpenes contain a furan ring. As discussed by Miller and colleagues,[19] the furan-ring component might be very important in yielding some of the potential antineoplastic activity of these compounds.

Several triterpenes (examples in Figure 1.6) have been reported to have nutraceutical properties. These compounds include plant sterols; however, some of these structures may have been modified to contain fewer than 30 carbons. One of the most recognizable triterpene families is the limonoids. These triterpenes are found in citrus fruit and impart most of their bitter flavor. Limonin and nomilin are two triterpenoids that may have nutraceutical application, limonin more so than nomilin.[19] Both of these molecules contain a furan component. In citrus fruit limonoids can also be found with an attached glucose, forming a limonoid glycoside.[20] As discussed above, the addition of the sugar group reduces the bitter taste tremendously and makes the molecule more water soluble. These properties may make it more attractive as a functional food ingredient. Saponins are also triterpene derivatives, and their nutraceutical potential is attracting interest.[21–24]

The carotenoids (carotenes and xanthrophils), whose name is derived from carrots (*Daucus carota*), are perhaps the most recognizable form of coloring pigment within the isoprenoid class. Carotenes and xanthrophils differ only slightly, in that true carotenes are purely hydrocarbon molecules (i.e., lycopene, α-carotene, β-carotene, γ-carotene); the xanthrophils (i.e., lutein, capsanthin, cryptoxanthin, zeaxanthin, astaxanthin) contain oxygen in the form of hydroxyl, methoxyl, carboxyl, keto, and epoxy groups. With the exception of crocetin and bixin, naturally occurring carotenoids are tetraterpenoids, and thus have a basic structure of 40 carbons with unique modifications. The carotenoids are pigments that generally produce colors of yellow, orange, and red. Carotenoids are also very important in photosynthesis and photoprotection.

Different foods have different kinds and relative amounts of carotenoids. Also the carotenoid content can vary seasonally and during the ripening process. For example, peaches contain violaxanthin, cryptoxanthin, β-carotene, persicaxanthin, neoxanthin, and as many as 25 other carotenoids;[25] apricots contain mostly β-carotene, γ-carotene, and lycopene; and carrots contain about 50 to 55 parts per million of carotene in total, mostly α-carotene, β-carotene, and γ-carotene, as well as lycopene. Many vegetable oils also contain carotenoids, with palm oil containing the most. For example, crude palm oil contains up to 0.2% carotenoids.

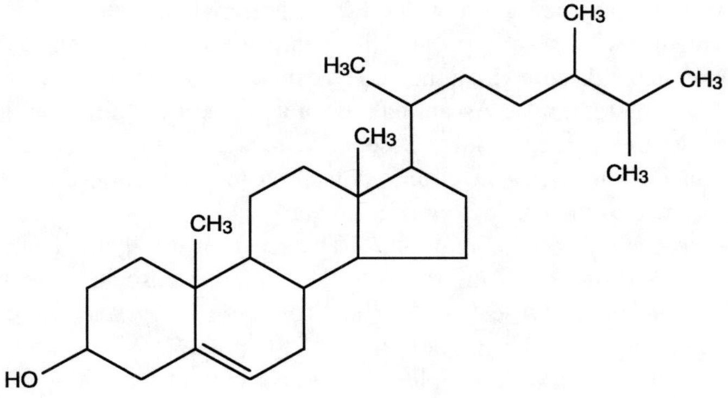

Sitosterol (a plant sterol)

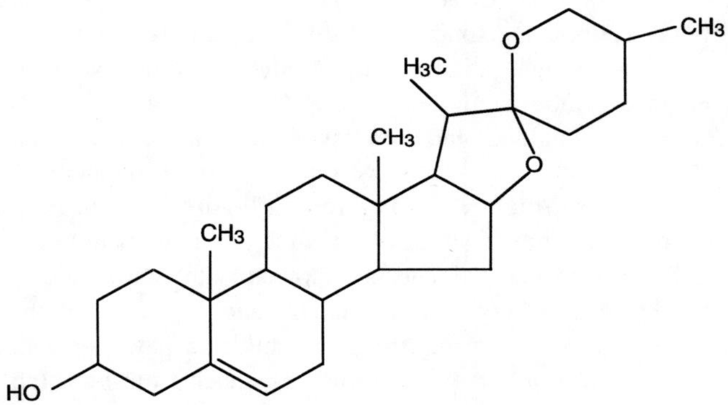

Yamogenin (a saponin)

FIGURE 1.6 Examples of triterpenes.

There are a few synthetic carotenoids, including β-apo-8′-carotenal (apocarotenal), and canthaxanthin. Beta-Apo-8′-carotenal (apocarotenal) imparts a light reddish orange color, and canthaxanthin imparts an orange-red to red color.

B. PHENOLIC COMPOUNDS

Like the terpenoids, phenolic compounds are also considered secondary metabolites. The base for this very diverse family of molecules is a phenol structure, which is a hydroxyl group on an aromatic ring. From this structure, larger and interesting molecules are formed such as anthocyanins, coumarins, phenylpropamides flavonoids, tannins, and lignin. Phenolic compounds perform a variety of functions for plants including defending against herbivores and pathogens, absorbing light, attracting pollinators, reducing the growth of competitive plants, and promoting symbiotic relationships with nitrogen-fixing bacteria.

There are a couple of biosynthetic pathways that form phenolic compounds. The predominant pathways are the shikimic acid pathway and the malonic acid pathway. The shikimic pathway is more significant in higher plants; although the malonic acid pathway is also present.[16] Actually, the malonic pathway is the predominant source of secondary metabolites in lower plants, fungi, and bacteria. The shikimic pathway is so named because an intermediate of the pathway is shikimic acid. Inhibition of this pathway is the purpose of a commercially available herbicide (Roundup).

The malonic acid pathway begins with acetyl CoA. Meanwhile, in the shikimic pathway, simple carbohydrate intermediates of glycolysis and the pentose phosphate pathway (PPP) are used to form the aromatic amino acids phenylalanine and tyrosine. A third aromatic amino acid, tryptophan, is also a derivative of this pathway. As animals do not possess the shikimic acid pathway, these aromatic amino acids are diet essentials. Obviously, these amino acids are considered primary metabolites or products. Thus, it is the reactions beyond the formation of these amino acids that are of greater importance to the production of secondary metabolites. Once formed, phenylalanine can be used to generate flavonoids (Figure 1.7). The reaction that generates cinnamic acid from phenylalanine is catalyzed by one of the most-studied enzymes associated with secondary metabolites, phenylalanine ammonia lyase (PAL). The expression of PAL is increased during fungal infestation and other stimuli which may be critical to the plant.

From *trans*-cinnamic acid several simple phenolic compounds can be made. These include the benzoic acid derivatives vanillin and salicylic acid (Figure 1.8). Also, *trans*-cinnamic acid can be converted to *para*-coumaric acid. Simple phenolic derivatives of *para*-coumaric acid include caffeic acid and ferulic acid. CoA can be attached to *para*-coumaric acid to form *para*-coumaryl CoA. Both *para*-coumaric acid and *para*-coumaryl CoA can also be used to form lignin-building blocks, *para*-coumaryl alcohol, coniferyl alcohol, and sinapyl alcohol. After cellulose, lignin is the most abundant organic molecule in plants. To continue the formation of other phenolic classes, *para*-coumaryl CoA can undergo further enzymatic modification, involving three malonyl CoA molecules, to create polyphenolic molecules such as chalcones and then flavonones. The basic flavonone structure is then the precursor for the flavones, isoflavones, and flavonols. Also flavonones can be used to make anthocyanins and tannins via dihydroflavonols (Figure 1.7, Figure 1.9, and Figure 1.10).

The flavonoids are one of the largest classes of phenolic compounds in plants. The basic carbon structure of flavonoids contains 15 carbons and is endowed with 2 aromatic rings linked by a 3-carbon bridge (Figure 1.11).[16] The rings are labeled A and B. Whereas the simpler phenolic compounds and lignin-building blocks result from the shikimic pathway and are phenylalanine derivatives, formation of the flavonoids requires some assistance from both the shikimic pathway and the malonic acid pathway. Ring A is derived from acetic acid (acetyl CoA) and the malonic acid pathway (see the use of 3 malonyl CoA to form chalcones in Figure 1.7). Meanwhile, ring B and the 3-carbon bridge are derived from the shikimic acid pathway.[16] The flavonoids are subclassified based primarily on the degree of oxidation of the 3-carbon bridge. Also, hydroxyl groups are typically found at carbon positions 4, 5, and 7 as well as other locations. The majority of naturally occurring flavonoids are actually glycosides, meaning a sugar moiety is attached. The attachment of hydroxyl groups and sugars will increase the hydrophilic properties of the flavonoid molecule, while attachment of methyl esters or modified isopentyl units will increase the lipophilic character.

Anthocyanins and anthocyanidins (Figure 1.9) are produced by plants and function largely as coloring pigments. Basically, anthocyanins are anthocyanidins with sugar moieties attached at position 3 of the 3-carbon bridge between ring A and B.[16] These molecules help attract animals for pollination and seed dispersal. They are responsible for the red, pink, blue, and violet coloring of many fruits and vegetables, including blueberries, apples, red cabbage, cherries, grapes, oranges, peaches, plums, radishes, raspberries, and strawberries. Only about 16 anthocyanidins have been identified in plants and include pelargonidin, cyanidin, delphinidin, peonidin, malvidin, and petunidin.

Although the flavonols and flavones are structurally similar to their close cousin anthocyanidins and the anthocyanidin-glycoside derivatives anthocynanins, they absorb light at shorter wavelengths and thus are not perceived as color to the human eye. However, they may be detected by insects and help direct them to areas of pollination. Because flavones and flavonols do absorb UV–B light energy (280 to 320 nm), they are believed to serve a protective role in plants. Also as discussed in more detail in the first chapter, certain flavonoids promote the formation of a symbiotic relationship between plant roots and nitrogen-fixing bacteria. The primary structural feature that separates the isoflavones from the other flavonoids is a shift in the position of the B ring. Perhaps the most ubiquitous flavonoid is quercetin. Hesperidin is also a common flavonoid especially in citrus fruit.

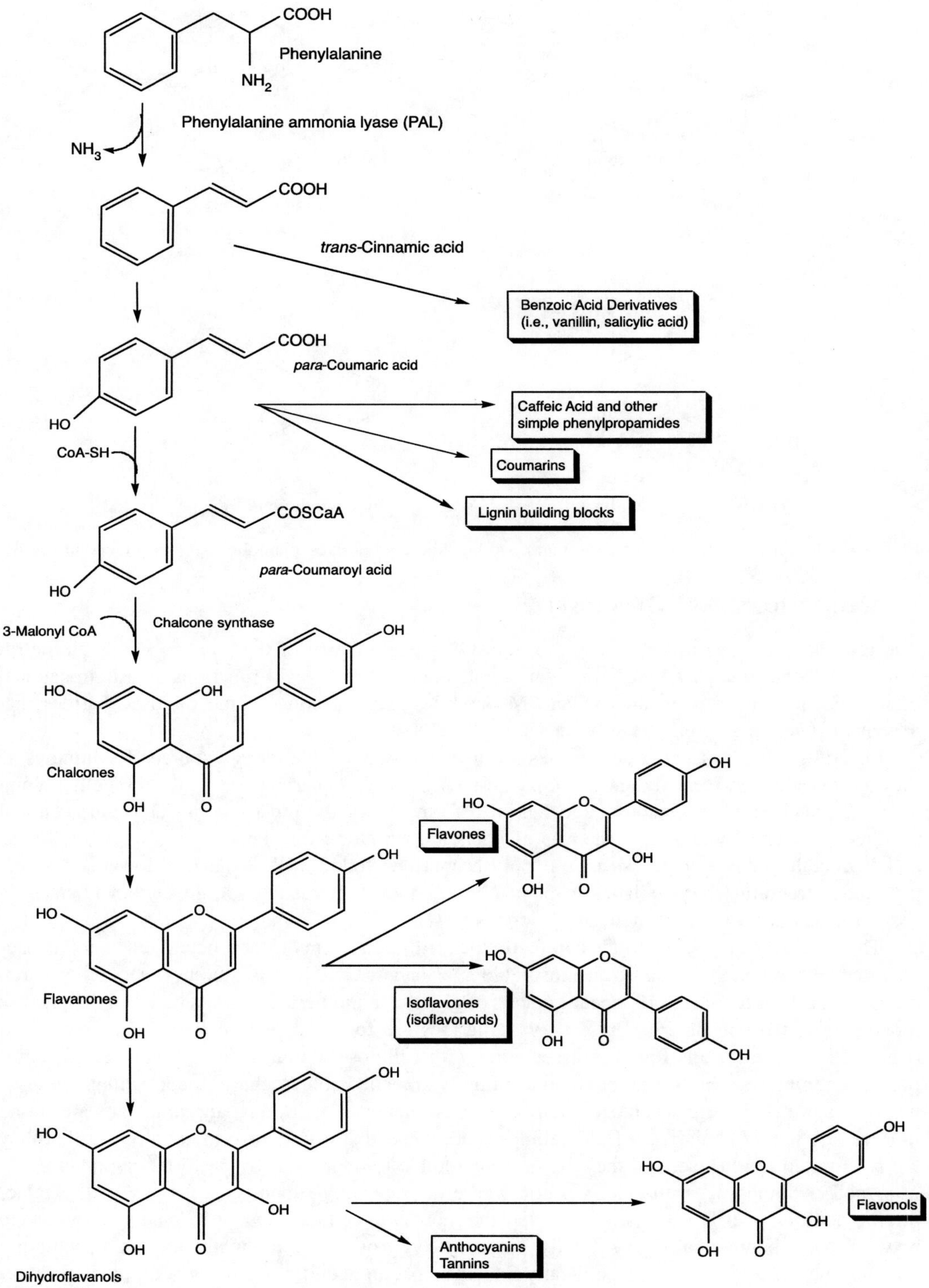

FIGURE 1.7 Production of plant phenolic molecules via phenylalanine.

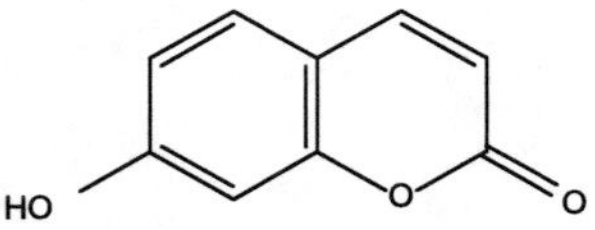

Umbelliferone
(a simple coumarin)

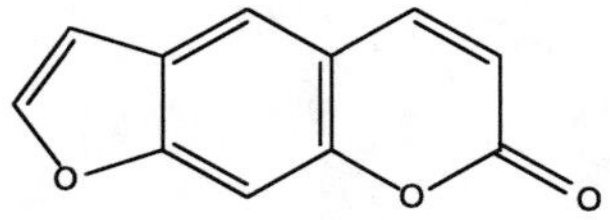

Psoralen
(a furanocoumarin)

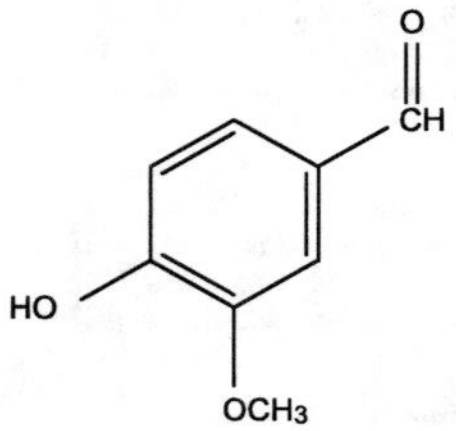

Vanillin

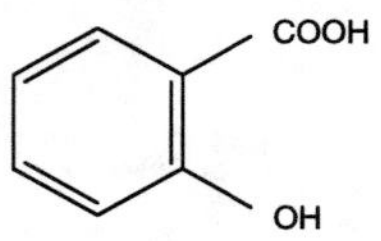

Salicylic acid

FIGURE 1.8 Select coumarins (first row) and two benzoic-acid-derived phenolic molecules (second row).

C. CARBOHYDRATES AND DERIVATIVES

The glucose derivative ascorbic acid (vitamin C) is perhaps one of the most recognizable nutraceutical substances and is a very popular supplement. Ascorbic acid functions as a nutraceutical compound, primarily as an antioxidant. Meanwhile, plants produce some oligosaccharides that appear to function as prebiotic substances.

Several plant polysaccharide families are not readily available energy sources for humans as they are resistant to secreted digestive enzymes. These polysaccharides are grouped together along with the phenolic polymer compound lignin to form one of the most recognizable nutraceutical families — fibers. By and large the role of fibers are structural for plants. For example, cellulose and hemicellulose are major structural polysaccharides found within plant cell walls. Beyond providing structural characteristics to plant tissue, another interesting role of certain fibers is in tissue repair after trauma, somewhat analogous to scar tissue in animals.

The nonstarch polysaccharides can be divided into homogeneous and heterogeneous polysaccharides, as well as into soluble and insoluble substances. Cellulose is a homegeneous nonstarch polysaccharide as it consists of repeating units of glucose monomers. The links between the glucose monomers is β1-4 in nature. These polysaccharides are found in plant cell walls as microfibril bundles. Hemicellulose is found in association with cellulose within plant-cell walls and is composed of a mixture of both straight-chain and highly branched polysaccharides containing pentoses, hexoses, and uronic acids. Pentoses such as xylans, mannans, galactans, and arabicans are found in relatively higher abundance. Hemicelluloses are somewhat different from cellulose in that they are not limited to glucose, and they are also vulnerable to hydrolysis by bacterial degradation.

Another homopolysaccharide is pectin where the repeating subunits are largely methylgalacturonic acid units. It is a jelly-like material that acts as a cellular cement in plants. The linkage between the subunits is also β1-4 bonds. The carboxyl groups become methylated in a seemingly random manner as fruit ripen. Chemically related to pectin is chitin. Chitin is not a plant polysaccharide but is found within the animal kingdom, although not necessarily in humans. It is a β1-4 homopolymer of N-acetyl-glucosamine found in shells or exoskeletons of insects and crustacea.[26] Chitin has recently surfaced as a dietary supplement for weight loss.

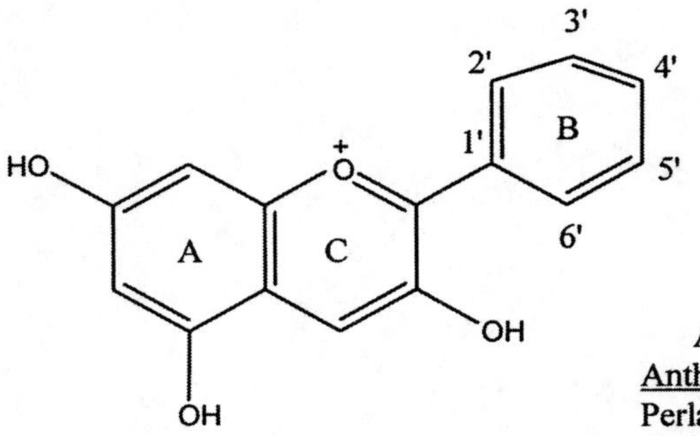

Anthocyanidin Structures and Pigment Properties

Anthocyanidin	Substitutes	Color
Perlargonidin	4'-OH	Orange Red
Cyanidin	3'-OH, 4'-OH	Purplish red
Delphinidin	3'-OH, 4'-OH, 5'OH	Blue-Purple
Peonidin	3'-OCH3, 4-OH	Rose Red
Petunidin	3'-OCH$_3$, 4'-OH, 5'-OCH$_3$	Purple

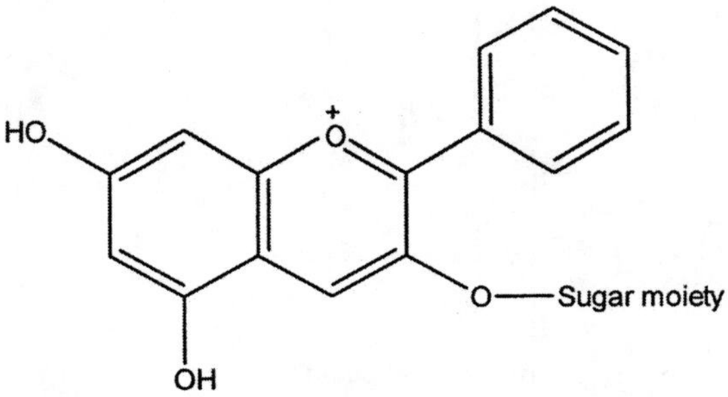

A   Anthocyanidin

B   Anthocyanin

FIGURE 1.9 Anthocyanidin (A) and molecular derivatives including anthocyanin (B).

Another family of polysaccharides that is worthy of discussion is glycosaminoglycans (GAGs). While these compounds are found in animal connective tissue, they are important to this discussion as they are potential components of functional foods. At present, GAG and chondroitin sulfate are popular nutrition supplements being used by individuals recovering from joint injuries and suffering joint inflammatory disorders. Glycosaminoglycans are often referred to as mucopolysaccharides. They are characterized by their content of amino sugars and uronic acids, which occur in combination with proteins in secretions and structures. These polysaccharides are responsible for the viscosity of body-mucus secretions and are components of extracellular amorphous ground substances surrounding collagen and elastin fibers, and cells of connective tissues and bone. Some examples of glycosaminoglycans are hyaluronic acid and chondroitin sulfate. Hyaluronic acid is a component of the ground substance found in most connective tissue including the synovial fluid of joints. It is a jelly-like substance composed of repeating disaccharides of β-glucuronic acid and N-acetyl-D-glucosamine. Hyaluronic acid can contain several thousand disaccharide residues and is unique from the other glycosaminoglycans in that it will not interact with proteins to form proteoglycans.

Chondroitin sulfate is composed of β-glucuronic acid and N-acetylgalactosamine sulfate. This molecule has a relatively high viscosity and ability to bind water. It is the major organic component of the ground substance of cartilage and bone. Both of these polysaccharides have β1-3 linkage between uronic acid and acetylated amino sugars but are linked by β1-4 covalent

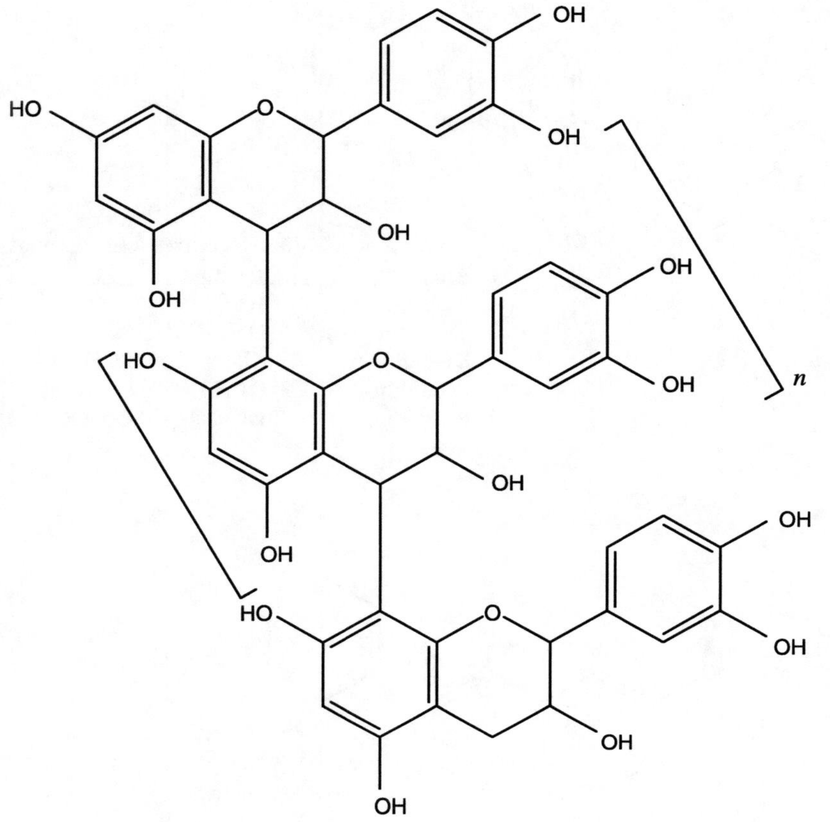

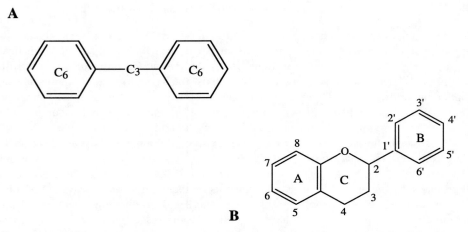

FIGURE 1.10 Basic tannin structure formed from phenolic units.

FIGURE 1.11 (A) Basic flavonoid carbon structure and (B) Flavonoid structure production: Carbons 5 to 8 are derived from the malonate pathway and 2 to 4 and 1′ to 6′ are derived from the shikimic acid pathway via the amino acid phenylalanine. Carbons 2 to 4 comprise the 3-carbon bridge.

bonds to other polysaccharide units. Unlike hyaluronic acid, chondroitin sulfate will bind to proteins to form proteoglycans.

D. FATTY ACIDS AND STRUCTURAL LIPIDS

At present, there are several fatty acids and/or their derivatives that have piqued the interests of researchers for their functional potential. These include the ω-3 PUFA found in higher concentrations in plants, fish, and other marine animals, and conjugated linoleic acid (CLA) produced by bacteria in the rumen of grazing animals such as cattle. The formation of CLA probably serves to help control the vitality of the released bacterial population in the rumen, whereas plants and fish use ω-3 fatty acids for their properties in membranes. Some plants also use ω-3 PUFA in a second-messenger system to form jasmonic acid when plant tissue is under attack (i.e., by insect feeding).

The CLA precursor, linoleic acid, and ω-3 PUFA are produced largely in plants. In processes very similar to those found in humans, plants construct fatty acids using two-carbon units derived from acetyl CoA. In humans and other animals, the reactions involved in fatty-acid synthesis occur in the cytosol, whereas in plants they occur in the plastids. In both situations, FAS, acetyl CoA carboxylase enzymes, and acyl carrier protein (ACP) are major players. Plants primarily produce fatty acids to become components of triglycerides in energy stores (oils) as well as components of cell membrane glycerophospholipids and glyceroglycolipids, which serve roles similar to the phopholipids in humans. In fact, several of the plant glycerophospholipids are generally the same as phospholipids. Some of the major fatty acids produced include palmitic acid (16:0), oleic acid (18:1 ω-9), linoleic acid (18:2 ω-6), and linolenic acid (18:3 ω-3). Grazing animals ingest linoleic acid which is then metabolized to CLA by rumen bacteria. Herbivorous fish also ingest these fatty acids when they consume algae and other seaweeds and phytoplankton. Carnivorous fish and marine animals then acquire these PUFA and derivatives from the tissue of other fish and marine life. Fish will further metabolize the PUFA to produce longer and more unsaturated fatty acids such as DHA (docosahexaenoic acid, 22:6 ω-3) and EPA (eicosapentaenoic acid, 20:5 ω-3). The elongation and further unsaturation yields cell-membrane fatty acids more appropriately suited for colder temperatures and higher hydrostatic pressures, usually associated with deeper water environments.

CLA is distinct from typical linoleic acid in that CLA is not necessarily a single structure. There seem to be as many as nine different isomers of CLA. However, the primary forms are mainly 9-*cis*, 11-*trans*, and 10-*trans*, 12-*cis* From these positions it is clear that the locations of the double bonds are unique. The double bonds are conjugated and not interrupted by methylene. Said another way, the double bonds are not separated by a saturated carbon but are adjacent. CLA is found mostly in the fat and milk of ruminant animals, which indicates that beef, dairy foods, and lamb are major dietary sources.

Two other types of lipids in food products are structured lipids and diglycerides. Structured lipids are triglycerides that have undergone hydrolysis and reesterification under conditions that resulted in triglycerides with new combinations of fatty acids.[27] For example, a mixture of medium-chain triglycerides and fish oil taken through this process results in triglycerides that can contain medium-chain fatty acids and EPA, and DHA. The basic process results in the free fatty acids being randomly reesterified to the glycerol backbones. However, the process can be manipulated to place specific fatty acids in preferred positions on the glycerol molecule. This option is quite expensive and thus has not been adopted by the food industry to any degree. However, the random reesterification process has been used to produce structured triglycerides designed to facilitate the absorption of both medium-chain and long-chain omega-3 fatty acids.[28]

Diglycerides have been used as emulsifying agents in manufactured food products for many years. More recently, more specialized diglycerides, termed *diacylglycerols* (DAG) have been produced by limited hydrolysis of triglycerides. This process results in a mixture of 1,2-diglycerides and 1,3-diglycerides. These diglycerides have absorption and metabolism characteristics similar to those of medium-chain triglycerides, i.e., some of the fatty acids escape reesterification within the cells of the small intestine and subsequent delivery to adipose tissue via the lymphatic system. Instead, they are delivered to the liver where they are oxidized to produce energy and possibly, to produce ketones. The result is an apparent caloric content that is somewhat less than the 9 kcal/g associated with most fats.[29]

E. Amino Acid-Based

This group has the potential to include intact protein (i.e., soy protein), polypeptides, amino acids, and nitrogenous and sulfur amino acid derivatives. Today, a few amino acids are also being investigated for their nutraceutical potential. Among these amino acids is arginine, ornithine, taurine, and aspartic acid. Arginine has been speculated to be cardioprotective in that it is a precursor molecule for the vasodilating substance nitric oxide (NO).[30] Also, arginine may reduce atherogenesis. Meanwhile, the nonprotein amino acid taurine may also have blood pressure-lowering properties as well as antioxidant roles. However, the research in these areas is still inconclusive, and the effects of supplementation of these amino acids on other aspects of human physiology is unclear. Several plant molecules are formed via amino acids. A few of the most striking examples are isothiocyanates, indole-3-carbinol, allyl sulfur compounds, and capsaicinoids. Another nutraceutical amino acid-derived molecule is folic acid, which is believed to be cardioprotective in its role of minimizing homocysteine levels.[31] Other members of this group would include the tripeptide glutathione and choline.

F. Microbes (Probiotics)

Where the other groupings of nutraceuticals involve molecules or elements, probiotics involves intact microorganisms. This group largely includes bacteria, and its criteria are that a microbe must be resistant to: acid conditions of the stomach, bile, and digestive enzymes normally found in the human gastrointestinal tract; able to colonize the human intestine; be safe for human consumption; and, lastly, have scientifically proven efficacy. Among the bacterial species recognized as having functional food potential are *Lactobacillus acidophilus, L. plantarum, L. casei, Bifidobacterium bifidum, B. infantis*, and *Streptococcus salvarius* subspecies *thermophilus*. Some yeasts have been noted as well, including *Saccharomyces boulardii*.

G. Minerals

Several minerals have been recognized for their nutraceutical potential and thus become candidates for functional food recipes. Among the most obvious is calcium with relation to bone health, colon cancer, and perhaps hypertension and cardiovascular disease. Potassium has also been purported to reduce hypertension and thus improve cardiovascular health. A couple of trace mineral have also been found to have nutraceutical potential. These include copper, selenium, manganese, and zinc. Their nutraceutical potential is usually discussed in relation to antioxidation. Copper, zinc, and manganese are components of superoxide dismutase (SOD) enzymes, whereas selenium is a component of glutathione peroxidase. Certainly more investigation is required in the area of trace elements in light of their metabolic relationships to other nutrients and the potential for toxicity.

REFERENCES

1. http://www.obesity.chair.ulaval.ca/index.htm.
2. Kalra, E.K. Nutraceutical — Definition and Introduction. AAPS PharmSci 2003; 5: Article 25 (found at http://www.aapsj.org/).
3. DeFelice, S.L. What is a true nutraceutical? And what is the nature and size of the U.S. Market? 1994 http://www.fimdefelice.org/archives/arc.whatisnut.html.

4. International Food Information Council Web site, http://ific.org/nutrition/functional/index.cfm, 2006.
5. International Life Sciences Institute of North America Web site, http://www.ilsi.org/, 2006.
6. Health Canada Web site, http://www.hc-sc.gc.ca, 2006.
7. American Dietetics Association. Position of the American Dietetic Association: functional foods position statement. *J. Am. Diet. Assoc.*, 104: 814–826, 2004.
8. *Nutrition Business Journal.* Weight Loss and Sport Nutrition Review 2005.
9. U.S. Food and Drug Administration, Center for Food Safety and Applied Nutrition, A Food Labeling Guide, September 1994, http://www.cfsan.fda.gov.
10. Miller, E.G., Gonzales-Sanders, A.P., Couvillon, A.M., Binnie, W.H., Hasegawa, S., and Lam, L.K.T., Citrus liminoids as inhibitors of oral carcinogenesis, *Food Technol.*, 110–114, 1994.
11. Fong, C.H., Hasegawa, S., Herman, Z., and Ou, P., Liminoid glucosides in commercial citrus juices, *J. Food Sci.*, 54: 1505–1506, 1990.
12. Yu, R., Yamada, A., Watanabe, K., Yazawa, K., Takeyama, H., Matsunaga, T., and Kurane, R., *Lipids*, 35(10): 1061–4, 2000.
13. Wierenga, D.E. and Eaton, C.R., Phases of Drug Development, found at http://www.allp.com/drug_dev.htm.
14. Novartis Institutes for Biomedical Research, The Drug Development Process at Novartis, found at http://www.nibr.novartis.com/OurScience/drug_development.shtml.
15. Shaw, D., Leon, C., Kolev, S., and Murray V., Traditional remedies and food supplements: a 5-year toxicological study (1991–1995), *Drug Saf.* 17: 342–56, 1997.
16. Taiz, L. and Zeiger, E., Plant defenses, in *Plant Physiology*, 2nd ed., Sinauer Associates, Sunderland, MA, 1998.
17. Wattenberg, L.W. and Lam, L.K.T., Protective effects of coffee constituents on carcinogenesis in experimental animals, *Banbury Rep.*, 17: 137–145, 1984.
18. Miller, E.G., McWhorter, K., Rivera-Hidalgo, F., Wright, J.M., Hirsbrunner, P., and Sunahara, G.I., Kahweol and cafestol: inhibitors of hampster buccal pouch carcinogenesis, *Nutr. Cancer*, 15: 41–46, 1991.
19. Miller, E.G., Gonzalez-Sanders, A.P., Couvillon, A.M., Binnie, W.H., Hasegawa, S, and Lam, L.K.T., Citrus limonoids as inhibitors of oral carcinogenesis, *Food Technol.*, 110–114, 1994.
20. Hasegawa, S., Bennet, R.D., Herman, Z., Fong, C.H., and Ou, P., Limonoids glucosides in citrus, *Phytochemistry*, 28: 1717–1720, 1989.
21. Chang, M.S., Lee, S.G., and Rho, H.M., Transcriptional activation of Cu/Zn superoxide dismutase and catalase genes by panaxadiol ginsenosides extracted from Panax ginseng, *Phytother. Res.*, 13(8): 641–644, 1999.
22. Lee, S.J., Sung, J.H., Lee, S.J., Moon, C.K., and Lee, B.H., Antitumor activity of a novel ginseng saponin metabolite in human pulmonary adenocarcinoma cells resistant to cisplatin, *Cancer Lett.*, 144(1): 39–43, 1999.
23. Craig, W.J., Health-promoting properties of common herbs, *Am. J. Clin. Nutr.*, 70(3 Suppl.): 491S–499S, 1999.
24. Wattenberg, L.W., Inhibition of neoplasia by minor dietary constituents, *Cancer Res.*, 43: 2448s–2453s, 1994.
25. Wildman, R.E.C. and Medeiros, D.M., Food in relation to the human body, in *Advanced Human Nutrition*, CRC Press, Boca Raton, FL, 2000.
26. Wildman, R.E.C. and Medeiros, D.M., Carbohydrates, in *Advanced Human Nutrition*, CRC Press, Boca Raton, FL, 1999.
27. Babayan, V.K., Medium chain triglycerides and structured lipids, *Lipids*, 22(6): 417–20, 1987.
28. Tso, P., Lee, T., Demichele, S.J., Lymphatic absorption of structured triglycerides vs. physical mix in a rat model of fat malabsorption, *Am. J. Physiol.*, 277(2 Pt. 1): G333–40, 1999.
29. Rudkowska, I., Roynette, C.E., Demonty, I., Vanstone, C.A., Jew, S., Jones, P.J., Diacylglycerol: efficacy and mechanism of action of an anti-obesity agent. *Obes Res.* 13(11): 1864–76, 2005.
30. Nittynen, L., Nurminen, M.L., Korpela, R., and Vapaatalo, H., Role of arginine, taurine and homocysteine in cardiovascular diseases, *Ann. Med.*, 31(5): 318–326, 1999.
31. Wildman, R.E.C. and Medeiros, D.M., Nutrition and cardiovascular disease, in *Advanced Human Nutrition*, CRC Press, Boca Raton, FL, 2000.

2 Isoflavones: Source and Metabolism

Suzanne Hendrich and Patricia A. Murphy

CONTENTS

Isoflavones (Figure 2.1) continue to be a topic of great current interest due to their potentially significant beneficial health effects in lowering cardiovascular disease, cancer, and osteoporosis risk, as well as in reducing menopausal symptoms. Their potential for toxicity is also under intensive investigation, as dietary and environmental substances with estrogenic activity have been linked with endocrine disruption under some circumstances. The design of novel foods, food ingredients, and dietary supplements with enhanced health properties has targeted isoflavones as a component class. Increasing numbers of such isoflavone-containing products raises both awareness and concern regarding efficacy and safety. To this end, understanding isoflavone sources, analysis, food processing interactions, bioavailability, and metabolism remain important interests of the research and regulatory communities.

I. FOOD CHEMISTRY OF ISOFLAVONES

Murphy recently reviewed the analytical and food chemistry of soybean isoflavones.[1] Therefore, this chapter will focus on literature published since the 2004 review. Earlier reviews by Murphy[1–3] have expressed concern that authors are not reporting their isoflavone analysis data in appropriate scientific units such as µmoles per g food or as total aglucon (µg/g food). Fortunately, the situation

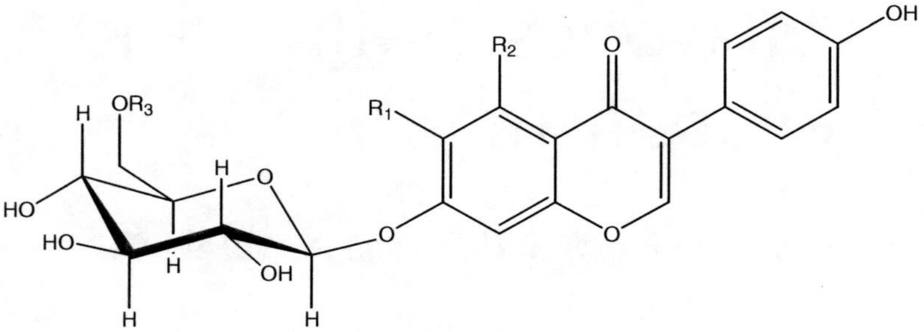

Isoflavone	R_1	R_2	R_3
G	H	OH	H
GI	OCH_3	H	H
D	H	H	H
MG	H	OH	$OCCH_2COOH$
MG I	OCH_3	H	$OCCH_2COOH$
MD	H	H	$OCCH_2COOH$
AG	HO	H	$COCH_3$
AGI	OCH_3	H	$COCH_3$
AD	H	H	$COCH_3$

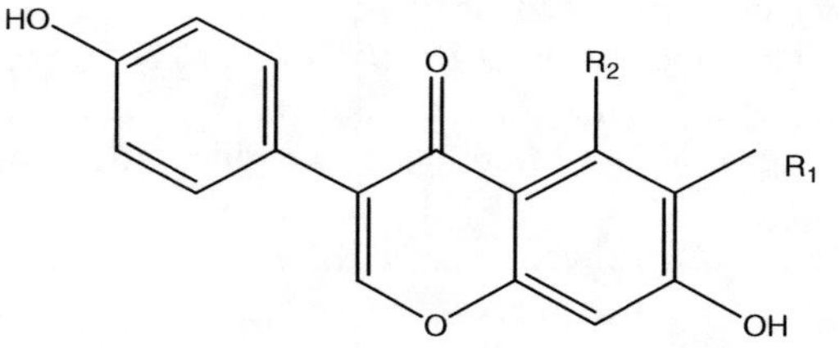

Isoflavone	R_1	R_2
Daidzein	H	H
Genistein	H	OH
Glycitein	OCH3	H

FIGURE 2.1 Isoflavone glucoside and aglucon structures.

in the literature is improving as more authors are using the correct nomenclature in presenting their isoflavone data. A summary of method reports in Table 2.1 reveal 34% of the reports used μmole per g food and 6% reported isoflavones as aglucon totals. However, 60% of the papers cited in this table are still using confusing and incorrect concentration units to express their data. Thus, authors, reviewers and journal editors still need to rectify the problems and misinterpretation in the scientific literature.

One of the reasons for the problems in accurate reporting of isoflavone data in the literature results from the methodology used to analyze isoflavones in food matrices. Unfortunately, the analytical quality control used by laboratories evaluating isoflavones is not even. Not all researchers account for all 12 of the isoflavone forms found in most foods. Too many authors use only aglucon standards to quantify all 12 forms. The extraction protocols reported in the literature continue to use solvents that have been demonstrated to underestimate several of the isoflavone forms. Table

TABLE 2.1
Food Analysis of Isoflavones

Method	Isoflavones Reported[a]	Sample Extraction	Standards Used	Internal Standard[b]	Recovery (%)	Data Reported As	Source
ELISA	Dein, Gein	Glucuronidase hydrolysis	Dein, Gein			mg/tablet, µg/m	4
HPLC-UV DAD C_{18}, 250 × 4.5 mm Gradient	Dein, Gein, Glein, D, G, Gl, MD, MG, MGl	80% ACN or 80% MeOH or 80% EtOH	Dein, Gein, Glein, D, G, Gl	FL		µg/g individual forms no MW adj	5
HPLC-UV DAD C_{18}, 250 × 4.5 mm Gradient	Dein, Gein, Glein, D, G, Gl, MD, MG, MGl	80% MeOH	Dein, Gein, Glein, D, G, Gl	E		mg/l as aglucons	6
HPLC-UV DAD and ESI-MS C_{18}, 100 × 4.6 mm Gradient, 4 mL/min	None reported	20% DMSO in MeOH sonication, time unknown	Dein, Gein, D, G	E	101	%	7
HPLC-UV DAD and tandem-MS C_{18}, 250 × 4.5 mm Gradient	None reported	80% MeOH glucosides by alkaline hydrolysis	Dein, Gein		101	µg/g? MW adj unknown	8
HPLC-UV 254 nm C_{18}, 250 × 4.5 mm Step Gradient	Dein, Gein	acid hydrolysis	unknown			µg/g	9
HPLC-UV DAD C_{18}, 250 × 4.5 mm Gradient	Dein, Gein, Glein, D, G, Gl	80% hot MeOH	Gein			mg/100g	10

Continued.

TABLE 2.1 (Continued)
Food Analysis of Isoflavones

Method	Isoflavones Reported[a]	Sample Extraction	Standards Used	Internal Standard[b]	Recovery (%)	Data Reported As	Source
HPLC-UV DAD and ESI-MS C$_{18}$, 250 × 4.6 mm Gradient	Dein, Gein D, G	90% MeOH	Dein, Gein, D, G	FL added to extract	103-106	µg/g no MW adj	11, 12, 20
HPLC-UV C$_{18}$, 250 × 5 mm Gradient	Dein, Gein, Glein, D, G, Gl	80% MeOH	G, D, Gein, Dein	FL		µmol/mL	13
HPLC-UV C$_{18}$, 250 × 5 mm Gradient	Dein, Gein, Glein, D, G, Gl MD, MG, MGl, AD, AG, AGl	80% MeOH	G, D Gein, Dein			µmol/g	14
HPLC-UV C$_{18}$, 250 × 5 mm Gradient	Dein, Gein, Glein, D, G, Gl MD, MG, MGl, AD, AG, AGl	80% MeOH	G, D, Gein, Dein			µmol/g	15
CE-ampermetric Detector	Dein, Gein	70% EtOH	Dein, Gein	Dein, Gein	96	µg/g	16
HPLC-UV CEAD C$_{18}$, 250 × 4.5 mm Gradient	Dein, Gein, Glein, D, G, Gl	83% MeOH or 80% EtOH 2M NaOH 65°C	Dein, Gein, D, G, Gl MD, MG, MGl, AD, AG, AGl	Dein, Gein, Glein, D, G, Gl	100	µg/g individual forms µg/g adj MW totals	17, 31
HPLC-MS-MS C$_{18}$, 250 × 5 mm Gradient	Dein, Gein	Dein, Gein	80% MeOH			µg/l aglucons	18

Method	Forms detected	Extraction	Forms reported / Notes	Recovery (%)	Units	Ref
HPLC-UV C18, 250 × 5 mm Gradient	Gein, G, MG, AG	80% MeOH	G, AG, MG Gein		μg/ml	19
HPLC-UV DAD C18, 250 × 4.5 mm Gradient	Dein, Gein, Glein, D, G, Gl, MD, MG, MGl	80% MeOH	Dein, Gein, Glein, D, G, Gl		μmol/g	21
HPLC-UV DAD C18, 250 × 4.5 mm Gradient	Dein, Gein, Glein, D, G, Gl, MD, MG, MGl, AD, AG, AGl	83% ACN	D, G, Gl	81–98	μg/g individual forms μg/g no MW adj totals	22
HPLC-UV DAD C18, 250 × 4.5 mm Gradient	Dein, Gein, Glein, D, G, Gl, MD, MG, MGl, AD, AG, AGl	80% MeOH	unclear	81–98	μg/g individual forms μg/g no MW adj totals	23
HPLC-UV DAD C18, 250 × 4.5 mm Gradient	Dein, Gein, Glein, D, G, Gl, MD, MG, MGl, AD, AG, AGl	83% ACN	D, G, Gl, THB	75–100	μmol/g	24, 36, 40
HPLC-UV DAD C18, 250 × 3 mm Gradient	Dein, Gein, Glein, D, G, Gl, MD, MG, MGl, AD, AG, AGl	50% ACN			no data	25
HPLC-UV DAD Column not specified Gradient	Dein, Gein, Glein, D, G, Gl, MD, MG, MGl, AD, AG, AGl	50% acetone 0.1 N HCl	FO added to extract; all 12 isoflavones added to food	65–92	μg/g individual forms μg/g no MW adj totals	26
HPLC-UV DAD C18, 250 × 4.6 mm Gradient	Dein, Gein, Glein, D, G, Gl	83% MeOH 2M NaOH 65°C	Dein, Gein, D, G, Gl		μmol/g	27

Continued.

TABLE 2.1 *(Continued)*
Food Analysis of Isoflavones

Method	Isoflavones Reported[a]	Sample Extraction	Standards Used	Internal Standard[b]	Recovery (%)	Data Reported As	Source
HPLC-UV DAD C$_{18}$, 250 × 4.5 mm Gradient	Dein, Gein, D, G	80% MeOH	D, G, Gein Dein			µg/g individual forms µg/g no MW adj totals	28
HPLC-UV DAD ESI-MS C$_{18}$, 250 × 405 mm Gradient	Dein, Gein, Glein	80% MeOH & acid hydrolysis	Dein, Gein Glein	FL		µg/g individual forms µg/g no MW adj totals	29
HPLC-UV DAD C$_{18}$, 150 × 3.9 mm Gradient	Dein, Gein, Glein, D, G, Gl, MD, MG, MGl, AD, AG, AGl	83% ACN	Dein, Gein, D, G, Gl, MD, MG, MGl, AD, AG	FL, Glein	98, 97	µmol/g	30
HPLC-UV DAD C$_{18}$ 250 × 4 mm Gradient	Dein, Gein, Glein, D, G, Gl, AD, AG, AGl, MD, MG MGl	80% MeOH	Dein, Gein, Glein, G, D Gl	equilenin added to extract	72-94	µg/g individual µg/g total no MW adj	32
HPLC-UV DAD C$_{18}$, 250 × 5 mm Gradient	Gein, G	80% MeOH 60°C	Gein, G		91	µg/g, no MW adj	33
HPLC-UV DAD C$_{18}$ 150 × 3.9 mm Gradient	Dein, Gein, Glein, D, G, Gl, AD, AG, AGl, MD, MG, MGl	83% ACN + acid	specifics not described			nmol/g	34

HPLC-UV DAD C$_{18}$ 250 × 4 mm Gradient	Dein, Gein, Glein, D, G	80% MeOH	Dein, Gein,	mg/g individual mg/g total no MW adj	35
HPLC-UV DAD C$_{18}$ 150 × 4 mm Gradient	Dein, Gein, Glein	80% MeOH	Dein, Gein, Glein, D, G, Gl	μg/g individual μg/g total no MW adj	37
HPLC-UV DAD C$_{18}$ 250 × 4.5 mm Gradient	Dein, Gein, Glein, D, G, Gl	83% MeOH 2M NaOH 65°C	Dein, Gein, D, G, Gl	μmol/g μg/g total no MW adj	37
HPLC-UV DAD C$_{18}$ 150 × 4.5 mm Gradient	Dein, Gein, Glein, D, G, Gl	80% MeOH ASE	Gein, D, G, Gl, FO, B	μmol/g individual na total	38
HPLC-UV DAD C$_{18}$ 250 × 4 mm Gradient	aglucons, β-glucosides, malonyls, acetyls	70% EtOH reported	none	% ? MW adj	39
HPLC-UV DAD & MS C$_{18}$ 250 × 3.2 Gradient	Dein, Gein, Glein, D, G, Gl, AD, AG, AGl, MD, MG, MGl	80% EtOH	Gein, Dein, Glein D, G, Gl, FO, B, C	mg/kg individual mg/kg MW adj	41
HPLC-UV DAD C$_{18}$ 250 × 4.5 mm Gradient	Dein, Gein, Glein, D, G, Gl, MD, MG, MGI, AD, AG, AGl	90% MeOH	c Dein, Gein, D, G, Gl, MD, MG, MGI, AD, AG, AGI	mole%	42
HPLC-UV DAD C$_{18}$ 150 × 4.5 mm Gradient	Dein, Gein, Glein, D, G, Gl	75% EtOH	Dein, Gein, Glein D, G, Gl T	unknown	43

Continued.

TABLE 2.1 (*Continued*)
Food Analysis of Isoflavones

Method	Isoflavones Reported[a]	Sample Extraction	Standards Used	Internal Standard[b]	Recovery (%)	Data Reported As	Source
HPLC-UV DAD ESI-MS C$_{18}$, 150 × 4.5 mm Gradient	Dein, Gein, G	SPE of waste H$_2$O	Dein, Gein Glein	Dein, Gein, G	87, 62 52 in H$_2$O	µg/l individual forms	44
HPLC-UV DAD C$_{18}$, 100 × 4.6 mm Gradient	Dein, Gein, Glein, D, G, Gl, MD, MG, MGl, AD, AG, AGl	50% EtOH 60°C	Dein, Gein, D, G, Gl, MD, MG, MGl, AD, AG, AGl	Dein, Gein, D, G, Gl, MD, MG, MGl, AD, AG, AGl	99	µg/g individual forms and %	45
HPLC-UV ESI-MS C$_{18}$, 150 × 4.5 mm Gradient	Dein and glucosylated products	solvent	Dein			nM	46
HPLC-UV DAD C$_{18}$ Gradient	Dein, Gein, Glein, D, G, Gl, AD, AG, AGl, MD, MG, MGl	diff% MeOH or ACN + H$^+$	Gein, G D, AG	FL, Gein, G D, AG	not added to sample	µmol/g	47

Method	Isoflavones	Solvent	Internal standard	Spike	Units	Ref.
HPLC-UV C$_{18}$, 250 × 4.5 mm Gradient	Dein, Gein, Glein, D, G, Gl, MD, MG, MGl	53% ACN	none listed	BA, added to extract	µmol/g	48
HPLC-UV DAD EPI-MS C$_{18}$, 100 × 4.6 mm Gradient	Dein, Gein, Glein, D, G, Gl, MD, MG, MGl	50% EtOH 60°C	Dein, Gein, D, G, Gl, MD, MG, MGl		µ*M*	49
HPLC-UV C$_{18}$, 300 × 4.6 mm Gradient	Dein, Gein, Glein, D, G, Gl MD, MG, MGl	80% MeOH	Dein, Gein, Glein, D, G, Gl		mg aglucon/100 g mole%	50
HPLC-UV 365 nm C$_{18}$, 300 × 4.6 mm Gradient	Gein, G, D	80% ACN or acid hydrolysis	none listed		µg/ml	51

[a] Dein = daidzein, Gein = genistein, Glein = glycitein, D = daidzin, G = genistin, Gl = glycitin, MD = 6″-O-malonyldaidzin, MG = 6″-O-malonylgenistin, MGl = 6″-O-malonylglycitein, AD = 6″-O-acetyldaidzin, AG = 6″-O-acetylgenistin, AGl = 6″-O-acetylglycitin, F = fluorescein, THB = 2,4,4′-trihydroxydeoxybenzoin, FL = flavone, FO = formononetin, B = biochanin A; C = coumesterol, T = theophylline, BA = benzoic acid, adj MW = weight data adjusted for molecular weight differences of isoflavone glucosides and aglucons, DAD = photodiode array detection, MS-SIM = mass spectrum-single ion monitoring, EC = electrochemical, CE = capillary electrophoresis, CEAD = coulometric electron array detector, ASE = accelerated solvent extractor, na = not applicable.

[b] Internal standard and/or recovery spike added to dry food matrix before extraction solvents unless noted otherwise.

[c] MDin and MGin not available from reported supplier (Fisher Scientific).

2.1 tabulates the analytical quality control used by 47 isoflavone analysis reports in the literature since Murphy (2004).[1]

The current USDA-Iowa State University Isoflavone Database 1.3 contains data on 128 foods and is currently undergoing an update by the USDA Food Composition Laboratory.[4] These data are derived for the peer-reviewed literature.

II. ANALYSIS METHODS

The methodology for HPLC isoflavone analysis continues to be refined. Bennetau-Pelissero et al. reported an ELISA method for the aglucons.[5] Food and supplement extracts were analyzed after enzymatic hydrolysis with glucoronidase/sulfatase, apparently, although no data were presented on the efficacy of these enzymes hydrolyzing glucosides. Antonelli et al. reported total isoflavones after alkaline hydrolysis of glucosides.[6] Peng et al. reported using capillary electrophoresis with electrochemical detection for only genistein and daidzein from 70% ethanol sonicated extracts of foods.[7] Several "fast" HPLC procedures have been reported with flow rates > 2 ml/min and short columns (10 cm).[8–10] Apers et al. report good analytical quality control (QC) data but give no data on concentrations in food or other biological samples.[8] Klejdus et al. report on accelerated solvent extraction (ACE) protocols for isoflavones from soy.[9–11] Klejdus et al. compared sonication at room temperature, Soxhlet extraction at solvent boiling point and ACE at solvent boiling point, all in 90% aqueous methanol.[11] Very low yields of extraction amounts (by a factor of 10) were reported compared to their room temperature extractions. Klejdus et al. report some of the same data.[9] Klejdus et al. report using ACE conditions of 140°C and 140 bar for a few food samples.[10] Malonyl-β-glucosides concentrations are not reported but are clearly apparent in their chromatograms. Rostango et al. reported on a solid phase extraction technique for soy isoflavone analysis using initial 50% ethanol extraction at 60°C for 30 min and data reported in μg/g for all 12 forms.[12] Rostango et al. evaluated the stability of isoflavone extracts and reported data in μM.[12] Sample extracts stored in ethanol between –20 and 10°C were stable for one week. Lin and Guisti thoroughly evaluated 83% acetonitrile vs. 53% acetonitrile ± acid for isoflavone extraction but only for soybeans, not other foods.[13] Kawanishi et al. measured the isoflavone levels in waste water effluent in Osaka and reported averages of 143 μg/l genistein and 43 μg/l daidzein.[14]

A. Isoflavones in Soy Ingredients (including Soybeans)

There are about 24 reports documenting the isoflavone levels in soy ingredients. These ingredients, which consumers rarely have direct access to, are soybeans, defatted soy flours, soy protein concentrates, soy protein isolates, and texturized vegetable protein. Most of these reports extracted the isoflavones with 80% methanol, report their data in μg isoflavone/g ingredient, do not adjust for the difference in molecular weight of the different isoflavone forms, and use a limited number of authentic isoflavone standards for quantification. However, there have been a few reports that give us accurate insight into isoflavone levels in ingredients since the 2004 review.

Achouri et al. reported isoflavone levels in defatted soy flours and soy protein isolates that were lower than literature values.[15] The solvent volume to sample weight ratio was 5 or less and was probably the reason for the low analytical values. Although isoflavones are soluble in alcoholic solvents, their solubility is limited, even in the best solvents. A minimum of 10:1 solvent to weight is needed with an even larger ratio for samples very concentrated in isoflavones such as soy germ.

Park et al. reported on isoflavone levels in the anticarcinogenic protein lunasin but provided no details on how analysis was performed.[16] These authors stated that isoflavones levels in mature soybeans were lower than immature beans in contrast to all other reports comparing maturity.[17] Hubert et al. compared isoflavone with soyasaponin μmole levels in soybean seeds, soy germ, and soy supplements.[18] The isoflavone/saponin were 1 to 3 for soybeans and soy germ but ranged from

2–17 in soy supplements. Lee et al. report levels of isoflavones in 2002 Ohio-grown soybeans using good analytical QC.[19] The isoflavone contents ranged from 4.2 to 11.8 µmole/g.

Yu et al. attempted altering the synthetic pathway of isoflavone synthesis in soybeans to alter distribution of genistein and daidzein forms as well as total isoflavone synthesis.[20] Two analytical methods were used for different soybean generations. All 12 isoflavones were reported to be analyzed in F1 and F2 generations, whereas the AOAC method, which yields results for 6 isoflavone forms (the other six are converted to β-glucosides), was used for the F3 generation.[21] Samples were all extracted with 80% methanol that under-extracts total isoflavones in this type of matrix.[22] Duke et al. evaluated isoflavone levels in glyphosate-treated glyphosate-resistant soybeans using an unusual combination of analytical methods.[23] Soy flours were extracted using accelerated solvent extraction technology with 80% methanol, but no validation data were provided to compare with conventional extract procedures. The β-glucosides and genistein were quantified by HPLC and daidzein and glycitein were quantified by gas chromatography. The concentrations reported the aglucons are very high compared to other reports in literature for control as well as experimental treatments. Li et al. describe a procedure to glucosylate daidzein on multiple hydroxyl groups using *Thermotoga maritima* maltosyltransferase.[24] They created daidzein forms that were very hydrophilic. The authors quantified their products by HPLC using a daidzein standard curve, which was reasonable because they were using pure daidzein in this model system.

Variyov et al. reported the dose effect of irradiation on isoflavones in soybeans.[25] When isoflavone contents are recalculated on a µmol/g basis, the glucoside content decreases markedly with irradiation dose from 3.4 µmol/g to 1.8 µmol/g; however, the aglucon contents remained unchanged averaging 0.26 ± 0.03 µmol/g. Unfortunately, the authors used a hot methanol extraction method, thus giving a very limited picture of the processing effects.

Barbosa et al. reported the distribution of isoflavones in soy protein isolate manufacture on a laboratory scale.[26] These authors use an unusual polyamide column preparation of the hot 80% methanol extracts. They report acidified water washing compared to water washing resulted in soy protein isolates with higher isoflavone concentrations. Fukui et al. described a chromatography process using a hydrophobic Diaion HP20 column to produce an isoflavone-free soy protein isolate.[27] This isoflavone-free protein isolate reduced serum cholesterol in a rat feeding study.

Rickert et al. reported mass balance distributions of isoflavones and saponins during pilot plant manufacture of the isolated soy proteins, glycinin and β-conglycinin, as well as an intermediate protein product.[28] At the laboratory scale, increased temperature of protein extraction, and to a limited extent, solvent to flake ratio, resulted in more isoflavones in the intermediate protein fraction, a more denatured protein than either the glycinin or β-conglycinin fractions. However, these altered distributions did not translate to 10 kg defatted soy flake pilot plant scale extraction.

Rickert et al. demonstrated that increasing temperature and pH significantly increases saponin and isoflavone concentrations during soy protein isolate manufacture.[29] These authors show that initial pH neutralization in analytical extraction of isoflavones and saponins from soy protein isolates increased recovery rate and normalized the mass balance discrepancies observed without pH adjustment.

Xu et al. report a carefully performed study to determine effectiveness in using reverse-osmosis and ultrafiltration to fractionate isoflavones from soymilk and to further concentrate the isoflavone permeate.[30] The mass balance analysis revealed about 50% of mole mass of isoflavones could be recovered in retentate for other uses such as supplements or food additives. These authors suggest that additional optimization would increase yield.

Penalvo et al. evaluated commercial soy supplements and reported all but one had isoflavone levels 1–76% lower than label claim.[31] Penalvo et al.[32] reported on the analytical quality control of their modification of the Klump et al. method[21] by using an electrochemical detector. Chua et al. examined 13 reportedly isoflavone-containing supplements.[33] Unfortunately, the authors extracted their samples in 75% ethanol at room temperature for 24 h, conditions that under-extract isoflavones from most matrices.[22] The authors seem totally unaware of the acetyl- and malonyl-isoflavone forms and report these as impurities in their chromatograms.

Pinto et al. conducted isoflavone distribution storage studies at −18 to 42°C and at several water activities at 40°C for defatted soy flour and soy protein isolates.[34] The temperature storage study revealed no change in total mole mass of isoflavone at all temperatures. However, at 42°C, 10–20% of the malonyl-glucosides were converted to their β-glucosides. These conversions were attributed to the effects of temperature. Under controlled water activity conditions, major conversions of glucosides to aglucons occurred in soy flours, but not soy protein isolates, at Aw = 0.87 but not at lower water activities. These conversions were attributed to the effect of native glucosidases in soy flour. Kim et al. compared isoflavone levels for 8 Korean soybean varieties after 3 y storage without adjusting for molecular weight differences of the isoflavone forms.[35] Under room temperature storage, malonyl-β-glucosides decreased by a factor of 3 on mole basis but other isoflavone forms remained unchanged. At −30°C, extractable malonyl-β-glucosides decreased and β-glucosides increased but not on an equimolar basis. The authors do not indicate if data are on an "as is" or dry weight basis.

Ismail and Hayes investigated the effects of β-glucosidase action on the different isoflavone glucoside standards.[36] The authors report using all 12 isoflavone standards but cited Fisher Scientific as a source for malonyl-genistin and malonyl-daidzin, which cannot be correct. The data are reported in mole%. These authors report no change in the concentrations of acetyl-genistein and malonyl-genistin incubated 2 h at 37°C at pH 2, which seems unusual. The β-glucosides showed mixed specificity for the isoflavone forms. Mixtures of isoflavone glucosides were hydrolyzed faster than single glucosides. Almond β-glucoside hydrolyzed less than *E. coli* β-glucosidase. The *E. coli* β-glucosidase preferentially hydrolyzed the β-glucosides with far less activity for the malonyl-β-glucosides and acetyl-β-glucoside in the order of 90:6:5 mole% and these activities were consistent for daidzein, genistein and glycitein forms. Whether this specificity holds for food matrices containing isoflavones remains to be examined.

Choi et al. examined the effect of several strains of lactic acid bacteria's β-glucosidases to hydrolyze isoflavone glucosides.[37] Yields of 70–80% for genistin and 25–40% for daidzin were reported. However, some lactic acid bacteria strains did not hydrolyze any isoflavone glucosides. Isoflavones were analyzed as aglucons and amount hydrolysis was calculated by difference.

B. ISOFLAVONES IN SOY FOODS

Isoflavones in soy foods were reported in about 14 citations. The same analytical and data reporting problems cited above for soy protein ingredients are still a problem in interpreting the soy food literature.

Chien et al. conducted a critical study on the kinetics of genistein and its glucosides interconversions in a model system with kinetic estimates for this apparent first order reaction under dry and moist heat treatments.[38] Malonyl-genistin had the highest rate constant conversion to genistin in both dry and moist systems; however, the magnitude of the rate constants were about ten times faster in moist systems compared to dry. The rate constants for degradation in dry systems were: MG to G > MG to AG >AG to G > MG to Gein ~ G to Gein ~ AG to Gein. The rate constants for degradation in moist systems were: MG → G > MG → AG > AG → D$_2$ > Gein → D$_4$ > G → D$_3$ > AG → G >MG → D$_1$ where D$_x$ represents degradation products. The energies of activation for moist heat conversions were in the following order: MG → G > G → D$_3$ > Gein → D$_4$ > MG → AG > AG → G > AG → D$_2$. The energies of activation for dry heat conversions were in the following order: G → D$_3$ > MG → D$_1$ > Gein → D$_4$ > MG → AG >MG → G > AG → G. This is the first report to give thermodynamic interpretation of isoflavone redistribution resulting from thermal processing. These results mimic what has been observed in soy food systems for all 3 isoflavone forms.[22]

Setchell and Cole report isoflavone levels in 85 samples of soymilk and 2 types of soy protein isolate produced commercially over a 3-year period.[39] The data are not presented as individual isoflavone forms but as total isoflavones or total malonyl, total β-glucoside, total acetylglucoside and total aglucons, all adjusted for molecular weight differences. Soy milks were made from soybeans or soy protein isolates. Most soybean-based soy milks had higher isoflavone levels than soy protein isolate-based soy milks. Traditionally produced soymilks, from soybeans, had the highest variability in isoflavone content.

Zhang et al. examined the isoflavone distribution in wheat breads made with soy flour comparing distributions between crumb and crust.[40] These authors monitored the temperature exposure to each site, 100°C for crumb and 165°C for crust. The authors reported their data on a nmole isoflavone/g sample basis. Crumb and crust have very different distributions of isoflavone forms as expected from the different heat treatments. In crumb, the glucoside:malonyl-glucoside:acetyl-glucoside:aglucon mole% were 33:36:7:24 whereas in crust, the mole% were 44:9:23:25. The authors tested the biological activity of these food forms of isoflavones in cell systems, although the aglucon and β-glucosides would not be what cells in intact organisms would ever be exposed to. Hydrolysis and glucuronidation in the intestinal mucosa occur in isoflavone absorption and cells would be exposed to glucuronides.

Hu et al. compared the total mole concentration of isoflavones with Group B soyasaponin in several soy foods and soy ingredients.[41] Soybeans, soymilk, tofus and ethanol-washed soy protein concentrates had relatively equal mole concentrations of saponins and isoflavones. Tempeh and textured vegetable (soy) protein (made from unknown starting soy ingredients) had about two times the mole mass of isoflavones to soyasaponins. In contrast, soy protein isolates had 25 to 100 mole% more soyasaponins to isoflavones. Acid-washed soy protein concentrates had 4–5X the mole mass of soyasaponins to isoflavones. Two concentrated sources of isoflavones, soy germ and Nova Soy, had 20 and 9 times greater mole% isoflavones to saponins. Clearly, processing has very different effects on these two types of soy phytochemicals.

Kao et al. attempted to monitor the change in isoflavone form distribution during soaking and cooking times for soymilk and coagulant for tofu production.[42] Although the authors used all 12 isoflavone standards to accurately estimate the concentrations, they report their data in μg isoflavone form/g sample rather than convert data to moles so direct comparisons can be made. As the data was not reported in a mass balance form, we cannot account for masses in each fraction but rather we can infer the trend based on isoflavone concentrations. When the authors' data are converted to μmole/g sample, there does not appear to be an equimole conversion between the isoflavone forms. Soaked soybeans at 45°C for 12 h show decreases of 2.90 μmol/g malonyl-genistin and 1.35 μmol/g genistin with a 2.89 μmol/g increase in genistein. The mass balance does not match. Similar lack of agreement in trends were observed in the soymilk cooking data with malonyl-genistin decreasing 0.89 μmol/g and genistin increasing by 0.25 μmole/g with no change in aglucons. Comparisons within the same sample should predict the mass balance trend.

Tsangalis et al. reported effects of *Bifidobacteria* fermentation on the distribution of 12 isoflavones using 6 standards and 80% methanol extraction of the samples.[43] The data are reported as mg isoflavone/100 ml soymilk, although the "soymilk" was actually soy protein isolate or soy germ flour dispersed in water. When the data are converted to moles, the authors have fair mass balance accounting. However, the authors' data show a 49.6 nmole/mL increase in genistein with a 41.0 nmol/ml decrease in the glucoside forms for their "soymilk." The total mole concentration of all isoflavones revealed a similar small lack of mass accounting. In a subsequent paper, Tsangalis et al. report on isoflavone levels in artificial soy milks made with soy protein isolates.[44] The analytical method was the same as reported in Tsangalis et al.[43] that had many anomalies.[1] The authors concluded that the bioavailability of the aglucons was no different from the glucoside isoflavone forms.

Kao et al. attempted to quantify 6 isoflavone forms, genistin, malonyl-genistin, genistein, daidzin, malonyl-daidzin, and daidzein, in tofu production although no source of standards was reported nor chromatogram reported for the analyses.[45] Only data for the β-glucosides and aglucons were compared among the soy milk and tofu processing conditions although the authors report the initial concentrations of all 6 forms, including the malonylglucosides, in the benchmark soybean,

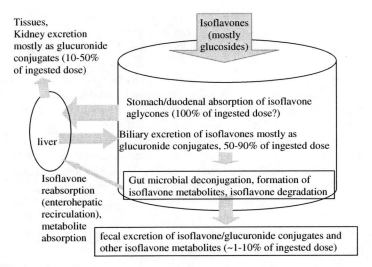

FIGURE 2.2 A current picture of isoflavone bioavailability.

soymilk, and tofu. As the malonyl-glucosides accounted for a significant proportion of the isoflavones in each food, it is not clear why the authors ignored them in their processing effects analysis.

Antignac et al. examined cow's milk for dietary phytoestrogens and report isoflavone levels from 0.1 to 5 µg/l by LC/MS/MS.[46] The isoflavone levels were 10 to 200 times lower than equol and enterolactone in these dairy milks. Wu et al. used a koji extract containing glucosidases to potentially produce higher yields of isoflavone aglucons from glucosides during tofu production.[47] A 9 mole% increase in aglucons in the tofu was observed.

Wu et al. reported analytical quality control data for HPLC-electrochemical and mass spectrometry measurements of isoflavones.[17] However, the data reported for edamame and mature soybeans were the results of acid hydrolyzed samples; thus, only aglucon concentrations were reported. Mature soybeans contained twice the mole mass of isoflavones compared to edamame, although the authors do not report if data are on a dry weight or "as is" weight basis.

Wiseman et al. reported the isoflavone content and distribution of 39 different soy containing foods using HPLC-MS to quantify the isoflavones.[48] The authors classified 24 foods as "high" isoflavone foods that would yield between 0.8 and 80 mg aglucons isoflavones per serving.

Thirty-three patents[49–81] involving isoflavone contents or processing effects in foods have been disclosed since the Murphy review.[1] In contrast to those reviewed in 2004, most of the patents cited here report on methods to recover or alter isoflavone composition in food or food ingredients. A significant number of the patents cited here are modifications of previous patents in making concentrated soy isoflavone extracts and recovering isoflavones in soy protein isolate production.

C. SOY ISOFLAVONE BIOAVAILABILITY

A major determinant of the safety and efficacy of isoflavones is their bioavailability. A few reviews of isoflavone bioavailability have been published recently.[82,83] Bioavailability is the access of a compound to its sites of action. The solubility, absorption mechanisms, metabolism by mammalian and microbial biotransformation, and interaction of the compounds with other dietary components and host factors all determine isoflavone bioavailability (see Figure 2.2).[84]

D. MAJOR SITES OF ACTION OF ISOFLAVONES

Several recent reviews have described the actions of isoflavones, both potentially beneficial and detrimental.[3, 85–88] Isoflavones may benefit health by protecting bone mineralization,[89] lowering blood LDL-cholesterol,[90] improving arterial dilation,[91] suppressing mammary[92] and other cancers, and inhibiting menopausal symptoms.[93] Isoflavones have shown no apparent long-term toxicity in humans exposed to soy-based infant formula[94] nor in single doses of up to 16 mg/kg body weight,[95] but immunotoxicity in mice[96] and reports of isoflavone genotoxicity *in vitro*[97] suggest that certain toxicological issues regarding isoflavones remain to be resolved.

1. Health Beneficial Potential of Isoflavones

A recent review of clinical trials and epidemiology related to isoflavones and osteoporosis indicated that a dose of 80 mg isoflavones/d may protect bone mineral in younger postmenopausal women.[89] Soy protein containing 80 mg isoflavones/d improved bone mineral density (BMD) of the lumbar spine in 24 perimenopausal women compared with women fed a whey-based control product after a 24 w trial.[98] Mei et al. showed that in 357 postmenopausal women, those in the highest tertile of phytoestrogen intake (mean isoflavone intake 26 mg/d) had greater lumbar spine BMD than did those in the lowest tertile of phytoestrogen intake (mean isoflavone intake of 3 mg/d).[99] Premenopausal women sorted by phytoestrogen intake did not differ in BMD. But 38 postmenopausal women given 118 mg isoflavones/d in soy protein for 3 months did not differ from 40 controls given a placebo in indices of bone resorption.[100] Ovariectomized 12-week-old Sprague-Dawley rats given 45 mg genistein/kg b.w. per day for 12 weeks showed decreased bone resorption and increased markers of bone formation (osteocalcin).[101] It is not known if this estrogen-like mechanism of action would hold true for lesser (and more human-relevant) doses of isoflavones. The data so far provide limited support for bone protective effects of isoflavones, and suggest sites of action in osteoclasts and osteoblasts.

Reviews of the role of isoflavones in protection from cardiovascular disease showed some support for their preventive effects.[102–105] Among 939 postmenopausal women from the Framingham study, those in the highest quartile of isoflavone intake had a significantly lower cardiovascular risk factor metabolic score (blood pressure, waist-hip ratio and lipoprotein status) than did women in the lowest quartile of isoflavone intake.[106] The role of isoflavones in cholesterol-lowering effects of soy protein was shown in a group of 31 hypercholesterolemic subjects fed 62 mg isoflavones/d; in subjects in the top half of the population with respect to LDL cholesterol, 37 mg isoflavones/d was also effective in cholesterol-lowering after the 9-week treatment.[90] The treatment diets did not control for soyasaponin content, which may also be cholesterol-lowering. Hamsters (n = 10 males and 10 females) fed 300 mg daidzein/kg diet (~20 mg/kg body weight) for 10 weeks showed significantly lesser plasma total and non-HDL cholesterol than did casein-fed controls. This effect was similar to that in hamsters fed 25% soy protein either containing the same total amount of isoflavones or soy protein that had almost all of the isoflavones removed.[107] In rabbits fed 1% cholesterol, cholesterol peroxides and extent of atherosclerotic lesions were suppressed after feeding 1% isoflavones for 8 weeks, compared with a control group fed the high cholesterol diet, but the isoflavone extracts did not affect serum lipids in the rabbits.[108] Isoflavone composition may affect cholesterol-lowering efficacy. In 10 hypercholesterolemic humans, 25 g soy protein containing equal amounts of genistein, daidzein and glycitein did not lower LDL cholesterol, whereas in a previous study of similar subjects, soy protein high in genistein and low in glycitein did lower LDL cholesterol.[109] Feeding ovariectomized cynomolgus monkeys an isoflavone extract (360 mg isoflavones/kg diet) for 20 w did not lower blood lipids, but soy protein containing isoflavones did.[110] The effects of isoflavones on cholesterol status vary with the model used, which could be related to differences in isoflavone bioavailability. This remains to be determined. Effects of isoflavones on cardiovascular disease other than cholesterol-lowering may be significant. Postmenopausal women (n = 28) fed 25 g soy protein containing isoflavones for 6 weeks showed a vasodilatory effect not seen when the women were fed soy protein with isoflavones removed or milk protein.[91] Arterial stiffness was lessened in 80 subjects fed 80 mg isoflavones/d for 6 weeks compared with placebo treatment in a randomized, crossover study.[111] Isoflavones may be protective against some aspects of cardiovascular disease, but the mechanisms remain to be discovered, and results are equivocal as yet regarding cholesterol-lowering by these compounds. With respect to cardiovascular diseases, isoflavone sites of action may include arterial smooth muscle and sympathetic nervous system, and LDL receptor or other cholesterol regulatory gene expression.

Human epidemiology of the role of isoflavones in reducing cancer risk has shown a significant association between urinary excretion of these compounds and reduced risk of mammary cancer,[92,112] but the causal link is not established because most of these studies measured isoflavones in subjects who already had cancer, compared with subjects who did not have cancer. Genistein or daidzein (250 mg/kg diet) fed for up to 27 weeks to mouse mammary tumor virus-neu mice increased the length of time for development of spontaneous mammary tumors.[113] But daidzein (250 mg/kg diet) given just after birth for 21 d to litters of Sprague-Dawley rats did not protect against dimethylbenz[a]anthracene-induced mammary tumors.[114]

Moyad[115] and Messina[116] reviewed evidence regarding soy and isoflavones and prostate cancer, concluding that these compounds showed promise in reducing this disease risk. A prospective study of 12,395 Seventh Day Adventist men showed that drinking soy milk at least once per day was associated with significantly reduced prostate cancer risk.[117] Fifteen men with benign prostate hyperplasia showed significantly less prostatic genistein, but not other isoflavones, than did 25 control subjects.[118] 34 men fed soy with and without isoflavones for 6 weeks in a randomized crossover design showed no difference in prostate specific antigen.[119] In the human prostate cancer cell lines, LNCaP and PC-3, genistein and daidzein (10 μM) inhibited cell growth; only genistein caused DNA damage to the cells.[120] Prostates from rats fed 1000 mg genistein.kg diet for 2 weeks postweaning showed somewhat reduced growth but normal expression of 2 prostate-specific proteins.[121] Mentor-Marcel et al.[122] showed that genistein at 250 and 500 mg/kg diet suppressed the incidence of poorly differentiated prostate adenocarcinomas in the transgenic mouse prostate adenocarcinoma (TRAMP) model. Possible beneficial effects of isoflavones against human prostate cancer are suggested but far from proven.

Other types of cancer may be prevented by isoflavones based on neoplastic cell culture, animal model, and limited human studies.[123] For example, genistein at 6 and 20 mg/kg body weight given for 28 d decreased melanoma lung tumor nodules in B6C3F1 female mice and enhanced indicators of innate immune defense.[124] The mechanisms of action of isoflavones as anticancer agents, both to prevent and treat this host of diseases are under very active investigation. Dose, model, and metabolic relevance remain key issues. Numerous cell growth regulatory factors and their expression could be sites of action for isoflavones, mediated by interaction with estrogen receptors or inhibition of tyrosine phosphorylation by genistein.[125] Treatment of cancer by genistein might be mediated by its effects on DNA topoisomerase II, which induce DNA strand breaks that can lead to cancer cell apoptosis.[126]

Messina and Hughes reviewed 13 clinical trials of isoflavones used in treatment of hot flushes.[93] Women experiencing greater numbers of hot flushes/d (>5) experienced moderate relief from 35–100 mg isoflavones/day. Whereas this conclusion needs much more supporting evidence, isoflavones may act on neuromuscular signals involved in the vasodilation of hot flushes. Postmenopausal women who took 110 mg isoflavones/d showed improved cognitive function, especially verbal memory after 6 mos in a randomized, double-blind placebo-controlled trial involving 53 subjects in total.[127] Isoflavones seem promising for improved mental function in aging populations, suggesting neuronal sites of action.

2. Toxicology of Isoflavones

Concerns about the toxicology of environmental estrogens have prompted investigation of isoflavones, known weak estrogens. The few human studies show a lack of adverse effects on endocrine function and reproduction from exposure to soy infant formulas during infancy in 248 adults ages 20–34 compared with 563 subjects fed cow's milk formula as infants. Women fed soy as infants showed greater discomfort during menstruation than those fed cow's milk formula.[94] Infant development was shown not to be adversely affected by soy formula in several clinical trials recently reviewed, but no data exist on early indicators of reproductive development.[128] Single doses of up to 16 mg purified isoflavone mixtures/kg body weight fed to postmenopausal women showed a few instances of nausea, edema, and breast tenderness, but otherwise no signs of toxicity from measurements of vital signs or clinical chemistry were observed.[95] Takimoto et al. gave single doses of up to 8 mg genistein/kg body weight to 13 cancer patients.[129] One patient developed a rash and no other toxicities were seen; peripheral blood mononuclear cells showed increased tyrosine phosphorylation of proteins as genistein dose increased.

Animal models indicate a few toxicological concerns for genistein. C57Bl/6 ovariectomized mice (5 w old) fed 1000 mg (n = 20) or 1500 mg genistein/kg diet (n = 10) had significantly less thymic weight than did controls (n = 18) fed an AIN-93G diet after 12 d.[96] Ovariectomy was thought to create a model more similar to human infants in estrogen status. The circulating genistein concentration (1 μM) was less than that measured in soy-fed human infants. A subsequent study feeding 1000 mg equol/kg diet in a similar model showed that this isoflavone did not affect thymus weight.[130] Interactions among isoflavones have not been studied, but genistein was shown to alter expression of numerous mouse thymic genes, suggesting sites of action.[131] Thyroid peroxidase activity was decreased significantly in Sprague-Dawley rats fed as little as 5 mg genistein/kg diet throughout the lifespan until 140 days of age.[132] Thyroid hormone levels were unaffected, but this suggests another site of action. Huang et al. showed that rats fed soy protein isolate but not isoflavones (50 mg/kg diet) for 90 d had increased hepatic thyroid hormone receptor $\beta 1$, a key regulator of cholesterol metabolism, so this was not a site of action for isoflavones in this model.[133] Postmenopausal women given soy protein with 118 mg isoflavones/d for 90 d did not differ from placebo controls in a randomized double blind study (n = 25/group) in hepatic protein synthesis, or in thyroid or sex hormone binding proteins or sex hormones in plasma.[134] When 817 female thyroid cancer patients and 793 case controls were assessed for phytoestrogen intake, this cancer risk was significantly less in the highest quintile of daidzein and genistein intake than for the lowest quintile (~8 mg/d v. < 1 mg/d).[135] Animal models suggest additional sites of action that should be investigated in humans; thyroid may be a target of isoflavones in humans, but perhaps not for toxic effects of these compounds.

Ovariectomized adult Long Evans rats fed isoflavones (13 mg genistein and 33 mg daidzein/kg diet) for 6 d showed decreased sexual receptivity and decreased oxytocin receptor in ventromedial hypothalamus compared with estrogen treatment alone.[136] The isoflavones also increased estrogen receptor β (ERβ) mRNA in the same tissue, but not in the presence of estrogen. Male rats, n = 12, combined from 2 generations fed 500 mg genistein/kg diet throughout life until 12 weeks of age showed significantly increased dopamine release from amphetamine-stimulated striatum compared with controls (n = 13).[137] This was not seen in females. When 420 mg isoflavones/kg diet was fed to male and female Long-Evans rats until 120 d of age, the sexually dimorphic nucleus of the preoptic area of the brain was significantly larger in males but not females compared with controls. Similar phytoestrogen-fed male and female rats showed decreased anxiety as measured by time spent in open areas of a maze compared with controls. Visual/spatial memory measured by maze learning was enhanced in phytoestrogen-fed females, but diminished in phytoestrogen-fed males compared with their controls within each sex.[138] Opposite changes in anteroventricular periventricular nucleus (decreased size in male, increased in female) were seen in adult Long-Evans rats switched to a diet containing 420 mg isoflavones/kg from an isoflavone-free diet from d 75–120 of age.[139] But young adult (8 weeks old) male Lister rats fed 150 mg isoflavones/kg for 14 days showed increased anxiety (less time spent in open arms of a maze) and stress-induced vasopressin release.[140] Possible neurotoxic effects of isoflavones should be explored further; which animal models and isoflavone doses are issues to be resolved.

Genotoxic effects of isoflavones have also been shown to occur. Human peripheral blood lymphocytes exposed to 25 μM genistein, but not 100 μM daidzein, showed chromosomal abnormalities by microscopic examination of Giemsa-stained metaphase spreads.[141] Syrian hamster embryo cells showed chromosomal aberrations by similar microscopic examination after treatment with 50 μM genistein, but not 200 μM daidzein. ^{32}P-post labeling revealed DNA adducts formed in these cells by 50 μM daidzein and 12.5 μM genistein.[142] Ishikawa (human endometrial carcinoma) cell cultures exposed to 5 μM equol and 10 μM 3'-OH-daidzein, two possible daidzein metabolites in humans, showed increased micronuclei, another indicator of chromosomal damage.[143] These isoflavone doses may be pharmacologically but not nutritionally relevant, and suggest both cancer treatment efficacy (killing neoplastic cells by deranging their genetic information) and adverse side effects of such treatments (genetic damage to normal or neoplastic cells that are not killed).

3.   Interactions of Isoflavones with Estrogen Receptors — Key Sites of Action?

Because isoflavones are weakly estrogenic, their fundamental sites of potential benefit or toxicity may be estrogen receptors (ERs), especially ER-β. Genistein showed an IC_{50} (50% inhibitory concentration) of 8.4 nM competing against 17β-estradiol for binding to human recombinant ER-β, and 145 nM with ER-α, whereas daidzein showed IC50 of 100 nM for ER-β and 420 nM for ER-α. Genistein was ~150-fold less active than estradiol for ER-α binding but only 8-fold less active for ER-β binding.[144] Genistein was about 100-fold less active than estradiol for binding to solubilized extract of human ER-α but only 10-fold less active than estradiol in binding to ER-β whereas 5-O-methyl- and 7-O-methyl-genistein were much less active than genistein.[145] Human fetal osteoblasts responded in a manner similar to estrogen to 0.1-1 μM genistein, mediated through both ER-α and β.[146] Genistein was ~70-fold less potent than diethylstilbestrol (DES, a synthetic estrogen) in binding to ERα but similar in potency to DES for ERβ binding in Ishikawa cells.[147] ERβ is widely distributed in human tissues, so this may be an important site of action for isoflavones, especially genistein. Genistein was also shown to interact with human sex hormone binding globulin in nutritionally relevant concentrations (~1.5 μM), with an ability to displace estradiol significantly at genistein concentrations of ~10 μM.[148] Kurzer reviewed hormonal effects of soy isoflavones during studies of human isoflavone intake; slightly lengthened menstrual cycles, and decreased blood concentrations of estradiol, progesterone, and sex hormone binding globulin were suggested in women, but few effects were seen in men.[149] Isoflavone sites of action mediated by ER binding deserve more investigation; at least some of these effects are likely to occur in nutritionally relevant isoflavone concentrations.

Isoflavones have also been identified to interact with numerous other proteins (e.g., protein tyrosine kinases, DNA topoisomerase II, thyroid peroxidase), but the link between these effects and ER binding has been examined rarely, if at all. The ability of isoflavones to suppress human natural killer (NK) activity *in vitro*[150] is probably related to this inhibition, because tyrosine kinases are crucial activators of NK cells.[151] It is possible that this presumed effect on tyrosine kinases is an indirect effect, mediated by ER binding; this remains to be determined. Because ERs are expressed in numerous cell types,[152] isoflavone sites of action, either possibly detrimental or beneficial, occur throughout the body. Thus, general indicators of isoflavone bioavailability such as plasma concentrations, or direct cellular measurements of isoflavone contents or the extent of isoflavone binding to ERs would be appropriate measurements of these compounds. To our knowledge, methods for measurement of ER binding by isoflavones *in vivo* have not been developed as of yet. But both plasma and cellular isoflavone contents have been measured, the latter only in animal models (see below). A recent novel technique for detecting metabolomic changes associated with isoflavone intake in humans used ^{1}H-NMR to detect urinary compounds during a period in which healthy women were fed texturized vegetable protein (45 mg isoflavone glucosides) or miso (25 mg isoflavone aglucons) daily for one month. Trimethylamine-N-oxide excretion was significantly increased by either treatment, but it was not clear if this was solely attributable to isoflavone intake.[153] In any case, this method holds great promise for more detailed assessment of isoflavone sites of action. When specific isoflavone metabolites or endogenous metabolites that are characteristically associated with isoflavone intake are identified to be important, these would become crucial to the assessment of isoflavone bioavailability.

E. APPARENT ABSORPTION AND RELATIVE PHARMACOKINETICS OF ISOFLAVONES

Physicochemical interactions of the isoflavones with the gastrointestinal mucosa seem to depend partly on the relative hydrophobicity/hydrophilicity of the compounds. The isoflavone aglucon molecular weights (~250 g/mol) permit their diffusion. Although isoflavones are predominantly in glucosidic form in foods, isoflavone glucosides have not been detected in human blood plasma or urine. Thus, either human intestinal or gut microbial glucosidases must act before the isoflavones are absorbed. Due to the time course of apparent absorption of isoflavones in which these compounds appear quite rapidly in plasma, with peak concentrations achieved at 5–8 h, small intestinal deglucosylation must be involved. Human lactase phlorizin hydrolase (LPH) cleaves isoflavone glucosides.[154] Isoflavone glucosides may also be absorbed intact by glucose transporters in the gastrointestinal mucosa, and immediately deglucosylated by the transporter, such that no isoflavone glucoside reaches circulation.[155] Based on research on quercetin, it seems likely that flavonoids in general, including isoflavones, are mainly deglucosylated by LPH in humans.[156] Dietary isoflavone aglucons are absorbed more rapidly than are glucosides (e.g., Zheng et al.[157]). Although the aglucon isoflavones are absorbed more rapidly, all of the studies published so far except one[158] show that their overall bioavailability (overall plasma area under curve (AUC) or total urinary excretion) is the same as for isoflavone glucosides, so that human isoflavone bioavailability is not limited appreciably by mucosal absorption mechanism, in most subjects. Izumi et al.[158] was the only study performed with subjects from Japan. In this study 4 men and 4 women were fed a single isoflavone dose and plasma isoflavone contents measured at 0, 2, 4, 6, and 24 h after dosing. Consuming a product rich in isoflavone aglucons produced nearly tenfold greater plasma concentrations than did a product rich in isoflavone glucosides. It is possible that later time points would have revealed greater isoflavone concentrations from the isoflavone glucosides. Asian subjects are typically lactase deficient, so this might explain the difference in result between this study and others.[45, 157, 159, 160] In a randomized crossover design, for 14 d per treatment, 16 postmenopausal women in Australia were given soymilk fermented with bifidobacteria (aglucon content 36–69% depending on isoflavone dose fed) compared with unfermented soymilk (7–10% aglucons). Total urinary excretion was similar across all treatments measured as 31% of ingested dose from analysis of four 24-h urine samples per treatment.[13] In a randomized, double-blind study of 15 middle aged women in the U.S. given isoflavone aglucon or glucoside tablets in a single dose, plasma AUCs did not differ for the isoflavone forms, based on plasma samples collected at 0, 1, 2, 4, 8, 12, and 24 h after dosing.[159] In a randomized study of groups of 8 to 9 women fed fermented or unfermented soygerm flour (~85% aglucon v. ~7% aglucon, respectively) for 7-d, 24-h urinary isoflavone excretion (mean of day 1 and day 7 combined) did not differ with the type of isoflavone fed, although plasma daidzein at 3 h after dosing was greater in women fed fermented soygerm. So, although there may be short-term differences in pattern of absorption between isoflavone glucons and aglucons, the apparent absorption of the two forms did not differ overall.[157] The question of comparative absorption of isoflavone aglucons vs. glucosides could be of health significance if there are important health effects that depend on more rapid absorption of isoflavones. This could be worth further study.

The relative absorbability and bioavailability of genistein, daidzein, and glycitein have been studied; glycitein comparatively less so. Plasma and urinary isoflavone contents do not always agree in the pattern of absorption reflected. Studies of urinary isoflavone excretion show a greater percentage of ingested dose of daidzein excreted than of genistein, reflecting apparent absorption (postmenopausal women,[95] men,[161, 162] premenopausal women[163, 164]). Urinary glycitein excretion was similar to that of daidzein as a proportion of ingested dose.[165] Xu et al. showed that 2 female subjects who were high excreters of isoflavones, excreting ~10–30 times greater amounts of isoflavones in feces than did 5 low excreters, excreted similar amounts of daidzein and genistein in urine and had similar plasma contents of the 2 isoflavones at 6.5 and 24 h after the initial isoflavone dose during a day in which subjects were fed soymilk at 7am, 12pm, and 5 pm.[166] Low isoflavone excreters showed significantly greater plasma daidzein than genistein. At 24 h after initial isoflavone dose, high excreters showed greater plasma genistein contents than did low isoflavone excreters. When similar doses of genistein and daidzein (~2 mg/kg body weight) were compared in the study of single-dose pharmacokinetics in 24 postmenopausal women,[95] based on AUC over 24 h, daidzein showed ~67% greater bioavailability than did genistein. Setchell et al.[163] in a study of 4 single doses of isoflavones given to 16 premenopausal women showed 20% greater plasma AUC for genistein than for daidzein. Interindividual differences in isoflavone metabolism between subjects in these different studies might account for the differing results, perhaps due to gut microbes (see below).

F. ENDOGENOUS BIOTRANSFORMATION OF ISOFLAVONES

Isoflavones seem to be rapidly and predominately glucuronidated in the gastrointestinal mucosa, if genistein can be considered to be a model for all of the isoflavones.[167] A recent study in CaCO2 cells confirmed this, in that glucuronide conjugates were the main isoflavone metabolites produced in this human colon carcinoma-derived cell line. Isoflavone glucuronides were secreted to the basolateral side of the cell membrane, whereas isoflavone sulfate conjugates tended to be secreted more into the luminal side, but not for genistein or glycitein sulfates.[168] Further glucuronidation and sulfation occur in the liver. It seems that biliary excretion is a major fate of the isoflavones, with more than 70% of a dose recovered in bile within 4 h after dosing in rats. This seems to be a general characteristic of flavonoids.[156]

Genistein and daidzein glucuronides accounted for 72% of total isoflavones excreted in urine of women fed soy in single meals on single days or during 6 d of soy feeding; daidzein and genistein glucuronides constituted ~60% of total isoflavones in plasma at 3 h after daily dosing with aglucons accounting for ~25% of total plasma isoflavones. Sulfate conjugates, measured by difference after glucuronide-specific hydrolysis accounted for ~20% of urine and plasma isoflavone contents.[169] Rats fed genistein showed ~90% isoflavone glucuronides in plasma, with 1–3% aglucons and 0.3–7% sulfate conjugates detected.[170] But another study showed 52% of isoflavones in rat urine as aglucons, with 26% as sulfate conjugates.[171] An earlier study had shown about 4% of total genistein dose excreted as sulfate conjugate and 2% of dose excreted as glucuronide conjugate.[172] These studies used the same rat strain (Sprague Dawley) and similar isoflavone doses. Sulfation of isoflavones was increased by fasting in Wistar male rats.[173] The rat studies do not correspond well with the limited human data available. Rats may not be appropriate models for human disease studies of isoflavones if endogenous biotransformation is accounted for, as it should be. The endogenous metabolites of isoflavones deserve additional study, as they are not inert and are less toxic than the parent isoflavones.

Peterson et al. identified sulfate and hydroxylated and methylated metabolites of genistein in breast cancer cell lines.[174] The production of hydroxylated and methylated genistein metabolites correlated with inhibition of cancer cell proliferation, but the sulfates were not associated with antiproliferative effects of genistein. Genistein sulfate was less potent than genistein at inhibiting platelet aggregation *in vitro* by about fivefold, although this metabolite showed antioxidant activity similar to genistein in ferric reducing ability of plasma and less potent than genistein in Trolox®-equivalent antioxidant capacity.[175] Isoflavone sulfates were ineffective at preventing copper-induced LDL oxidation *in vitro*.[176] But in HeLa human cervical carcinoid cell line transfected with an estrogen-response element, 0.1 μM daidzein-7-sulfate induced this response element and 1.0 mM daidzein-7-sulfate significantly suppressed the proliferation of this cell line.[177] This isoflavone metabolite may exert some anticarcinogenic effects *in vivo*, but likely concentrations *in vivo* may be less than those shown to be effective *in vitro*. Additional studies should be expected on isoflavone sulfates.

Zhang et al.[150] showed that genistein and daidzein glucuronides were about an order of magnitude less estrogenic than their respective isoflavone aglycones, as measured by *in vitro* binding with mouse uterine cytosolic estrogen receptor. The glucuronides also possessed modest ability to enhance human natural killer cell activity *in vitro*, comparable in magnitude to genistein, but effective and nontoxic over a wider concentration range than genistein. As little as 0.1 μM–0.5 μM isoflavone or isoflavone glucuronide concentrations affected NK activity, which constitute readily achievable plasma levels after consumption of soy foods.[162, 164, 166]

In vitro studies of isoflavone effects might be misleading unless isoflavone metabolism and metabolites are considered. Isoflavone metabolism seemingly has importance to bioavailability and efficacy of these compounds. Characterization of physiologically relevant metabolite levels and patterns is likely to be necessary to determine the mechanisms of isoflavone action.

III. MICROBIAL BIOTRANSFORMATION AND APPARENT DEGRADATION OF ISOFLAVONES

A. EQUOL

Isoflavone activity may be altered by microbial biotransformation. The phytoestrogens equol and O-desmethylangolensin (ODMA) are produced from daidzein by gut microbes.[178] Both of these metabolites are more estrogenic than is daidzein, with about one-third to one-half of human subjects producing equol and at least four-fifths of subjects producing ODMA. Human cancer epidemiology comparing equol and/or ODMA production with cancer risk, mostly in case-control studies, have tended to show reduced cancer risk with increased production of these metabolites. ODMA has been much less studied than has equol. Cardiovascular disease risk has shown similar weak but possibly beneficial effects of equol production (disease risk and daidzein metabolites reviewed by Atkinson et al.[178]). 0.5 μM equol, a relatively high concentration in comparison to that measured in human plasma after soy challenge, inhibited LDL-oxidation *in vitro* by inhibiting superoxide production and enhancing free nitric oxide in the J774A.1 mouse macrophage cell line.[179] High producers of equol showed a putative benefit of consuming soy not found in equol non-producers, that of greater urinary 2-hydroyxestrogen: 16-hydroxyestrone ratio, associated with decreased breast cancer risk, in a study of 20 breast cancer survivors and 20 matched control postmenopausal women fed soy protein for 6 week intervals.[180] The quantitative relationships between these metabolites and health effects are not yet clearly established, but a prescreening protocol providing a 3-d soy challenge and analyzing urinary excretion of these compounds is probably needed to most reliably identify this seemingly quite stable gut microbial activity.[178] Such screenings in human clinical trials of soy efficacy and safety are highly desirable in helping to clarify findings.

Equol production may be influenced by dietary factors. Allred et al.[181] showed that soy flour and molasses containing similar or somewhat less daidzein than Novasoy® or mixed pure isoflavones caused significantly greater peak equol concentrations in ovariectomized 6-week-old BALB/c mice fed these isoflavone sources for 10 days, suggesting that purer isoflavone sources are not as effective as substrates for equol production. In 30 women given a 3-day soy challenge, 35% were equol producers. The equol producers consumed ~15% more dietary carbohydrate than did non-producers and about 30% more total dietary fiber. These dietary differences were not observed among 30 men who were sorted by their equol producing ability.[182] Among 24 subjects fed soy for 17 d, 36% of subjects who were equol producers consumed 17% more carbohydrate as percentage of energy and 26% less fat.[183] In a study of 45 men, 20 subjects who consumed >30 mg soy isoflavones/day for more than 2 y showed a fivefold greater probability of producing equol; regular meat consumers had about a fivefold greater probability of producing equol; equol producer showed high concentrations of this metabolite in prostatic fluid, which could be protective against prostate cancer.[184]

1. General Significance of Gut Microbial Metabolism of Isoflavones

Kelly et al.[185] also identified several other urinary isoflavone metabolites likely to have been derived from gut microbial fermentation including 6-hydroxy-ODMA, dehydro-ODMA, dihydrogenistein, two isomers of tetrahydrodaidzein, and confirmed the presence of dihydrodaidzein. In addition to these metabolites, cis-4-OH-equol was identified in human urine.[186] Other gut microbial metabolites of isoflavones identified in human urine include 3″-OH-ODMA, 3′,4′,7-trihydroxyisoflavanone, 4′,7, 8-trihydroxy-isoflavanone and 4′,6, 7-trihydroxyisoflavanone.[187] Simons et al.[188] incubated glycitein anaerobically with feces from 12 human subjects; dihydroglycitein, dihydro-6,7,4′-trihy-droxyisoflavone, and 5′-O-methyl-ODMA were identified as the main glycitein metabolites. Two subjects produced a metabolite tentatively identified as 6-O-methyl-equol, a glycitein analog of equol. The health significance of these isoflavone metabolites deserves further study.

Interindividual variation in isoflavone metabolism and degradation by gut microorganisms seems to follow certain patterns. In a study of bioavailability of isoflavones from three soymilk meals over a day, 2 women consistently showed 10–20 fold greater fecal excretion of isoflavones in feces compared with the other 5 women. This paralleled 2–3 fold greater urinary and plasma levels of isoflavones in the "high excretors" compared with the other 5 subjects.[166] In vitro isoflavone degradation by human fecal samples was shown to occur rapidly for both genistein and daidzein (degradation half-lives of 3.3 and 7.5 h respectively). A study of in vitro human fecal isoflavone degradation with 20 men and women showed that subjects sorted into three distinct degradation phenotypes, with degradation rate constants for genistein of 0.023 (high degrader, n = 5), 0.163 (moderate degrader, n = 10), and 0.299 (low degrader, n = 5).[189] These phenotypes seemed to be relatively constant when reexamined 10 months later with degradation rate constants of 0.049 (high degrader, n = 5), 0.233 (moderate, n = 4), and 0.400 (high, n = 5). Twelve of 14 subjects who remained in the study after 10 months maintained their initial isoflavone degradation phenotype (data not shown). When 8 men of varying degradation phenotypes were fed soymilk, plasma isoflavone contents correlated negatively and significantly ($p < 0.05$) with degradation rate constant, $r = -0.88$ for daidzein and $r = -0.74$ for daidzein.[190] These data suggest that part of the interindividual variability in isoflavone disposition might be accounted for by variation in gut microbial isoflavone degradation rate. In 68 women, 35 recent Chinese immigrants to Iowa, and 33 Caucasian Iowans, women sorted into high, moderate, and low fecal isoflavone degradation rates, with a significantly greater proportion of Chinese subjects as high isoflavone degraders. Dietary habits, physical activity and gut transit time (GTT) were assessed by questionnaire, physical test, and bead marker, respectively. Subjects with significantly more rapid GTT (mean of 40 hours) and low isoflavone degradation rate showed significantly greater apparent absorption of genistein than did other subjects with longer GTT (mean > 60 hours), regardless of in vitro fecal isoflavone degradation rate. Neither dietary habits nor physical activity were associated with in vitro fecal isoflavone degradation rate.[191] In 25 women prescreened for anaerobic fecal daidzein degradation rate and GTT, 12 women with low daidzein degradation rate (< 0.2 h^{-1}) and more rapid GTT (mean of 71 h) showed about 50% greater apparent isoflavone absorption (urinary excretion) compared with 13 women of high daidzein degradation rate (>0.3 h^{-1}) and long GTT (mean of 106 h), measured after day 1 and 7 of a week of soy feeding.[157] Thus, fecal isoflavone degradation rate and GTT may be useful predictors of isoflavone bioavailability. This remains to be done in human clinical trials of the health effects of isoflavones, but might be helpful, especially coupled with equol and ODMA production screening, in sorting out the effects of isoflavones.

Isoflavone degrading microorganisms remain to be identified. Some *Clostridia* strains may cleave the C-ring of flavonoids, including isoflavones.[193] *Clostridia* are absent from the gastrointestinal tracts of some individuals and may be introduced during meat consumption.[193] Isoflavones can be broken down into other compounds that possess biological activity, especially monophenolics. For example, p-ethylphenol is a nonestrogenic metabolite of genistein identified in ruminants.[194] Methyl p-hydroxyphenyllactate is a flavonoid metabolite that blocks nuclear estrogen receptor binding and inhibits the growth of MCF-7 breast cancer cells *in vitro*.[195] Characterization of their metabolism by gut microorganisms may yield insights into the mechanisms of action of isoflavones. Identification of human gut microbes causing the disappearance of isoflavones from *in vitro* fecal incubations is ongoing in our laboratory, using genomic techniques to characterize gut microbial ecology based on variable regions within the 16S ribosomal RNA gene.[196]

IV. SUMMARY

Isoflavones continue to be of great interest, especially for their estrogen-like effects. The design of foods that contain these phytochemicals is ongoing, but the health protective efficacy of these compounds remains uncertain. Better control of clinical trials to account for the great extent of interindividual variation in bioavailability of these compounds should facilitate understanding. Best practices in screening for such trials are emerging, with a combination of examination of equol and ODMA production, and analysis of isoflavone fecal degradation phenotypes and gut transit time likely to be quite useful in clarifying the picture of isoflavones and human health.

ACKNOWLEDGMENTS

This work was supported in part by the U.S. Army Medical Branch and Material Command under DAMD17-MM 4529EVM and by the Iowa Agricultural and Home Economic Experiments Station, project 3375, the Center for Designing Foods to Improve Nutrition, and the USDA Fund for Rural America.

REFERENCES

1. Murphy, P.A. Isoflavones in soybean processing, in *Nutritionally Enhanced Edible Oil and Oilseed Processing*, Eds., N.T. Dunford and H.B. Dunford, AOCS Press, Champaign, IL, 2004, pp. 38–70, chap. 3.
2. Hendrich, S. and Murphy, P.A. Soybean isoflavones: source and metabolism. Ed., R. Wildman, *Handbook of Nutraceuticals and Functional Foods*, CRC Press, Boca Raton, FL, 2000, pp. 55–75.
3. Murphy, P.A. and Hendrich, S. Phytoestrogens in foods. *Adv. Food Nutr. Res.*, 44: 195–246, 2002.
4. USDA-Iowa State University Database on Isoflavone Content of Food, Release 1.3, 2002. http://www.nal.usda.gov/fnic/foodcomp/Data/isoflav/isoflav.html.
5. Bennetau-Pelissero, C., Arnal-Schnebelen, B., Lamothe, V., Sauvant, P., Sagne, J.L., Verbruggen, M.A., Mathey, J., and Lavialle, O. ELISA as a new method to measure genistein and daidzein in food and human fluids. *Food Chem.* 82: 645–658, 2003.
6. Antonelli, M.L., Faberi, A., Pastorini, E., Samperi, R., and Lagan, A. Simultaneous quantitation of free and conjugated phytoestrogens in Leguminosae by liquid chromatography–tandem mass spectrometry. *Talanta* 66: 1025–1033, 2005.
7. Peng, Y., Chu, Q., Liu, F., and Ye, J. Determination of isoflavones in soy products by capillary electrophoresis with electrochemical detection. *Food Chem.* 87: 135–139, 2004.
8. Apers, S., Naessens, T., Van Den Steen, K., Cuyckens, F., Claeys, M., Pieters, L., and Vlietinck, A. Fast high-performance liquid chromatography method for quality control of soy extracts. *J. Chromatogr. A*, 1038: 107–112, 2004.
9. Klejdus, B., Mikelová, R., Petrlova, J., Potesil, D., Adam, V., Stiborov´, M., Hodekc, P., Vacek, J., Kizek, R., and Kuban, V. Determination of isoflavones in soy bits by fast column high-performance liquid chromatography coupled with UV-visible diode-array detection. *J. Chromatogr. A*, 1084: 71–79, 2005.
10. Klejdus, B., Mikelova, R., Petrlova, J., Potesil, D., Adam, V., Stiborova, M., Hodek, P., Vacek, J., Kizek, R., and Kuban, V. Evaluation of isoflavone aglycon and glycoside distribution in soy plants and soybeans by fast column high-performance liquid chromatography coupled with a diode-array detector. *J. Agric. Food Chem.* 53: 5848–5852, 2005.

11. Klejdus, B., Mikelová, R., Adam, V., Zehnálek, J., Vacek, J., Kizek, R., and Kubán, V. Liquid chromatographic–mass spectrometric determination of genistin and daidzin in soybean food samples after accelerated solvent extraction with modified content of extraction cell. *Anal. Chim. Acta* 517: 1–11, 2004.

12. Rostango M.A., Palma, M., and Barr, C.G. Short-term stability of soy isoflavones extracts: sample conservation aspects. *Food Chem.* 93: 557–564, 2005.

13. Lin, F. and Giusti, M.M. Effects of solvent polarity and acidity on the extraction efficiency of isoflavones from soybeans (Glycine max). *J. Agric. Food Chem.* 53: 3795–3800, 2005.

14. Kawanishi, M., Takamura, E.T., Ermawati, R., Shimohara, C., Sakamoto, M., Matsukawa, K., Matsuda, T., Murahashi, T., Matsui, S., Wakabayashi, K., Watanabe, T., Tashiro, H.Y., and Yagi, T. Detection of genistein as an estrogenic contaminant of river water in Osaka. *Environ. Sci. Technol.* 38: 6424–6429, 2004.

15. Achouri, A., Boye, J.I., and Belanger, D., Soybean isoflavones: efficacy of extraction conditions and effect of food type on extractability. *Food Res. Int.* 38: 1199–1204, 2005.

16. Park J., Park, H., Jeong, H.J., and De Lumen, B.O. Contents and bioactivities of lunasin, Bowman-Birk inhibitor, and isoflavones in soybean seed. *J. Agric. Food Chem.* 53: 7686–7690, 2005.

17. Wu, Q., Wang, M., Sciarappa, W.J., and Simon, J.E. LC/UV/ESI-MS analysis of isoflavones in edamame and tofu soybeans. *J. Agric. Food Chem.* 52: 2763–2769, 2004.

18. Hubert, J., Berger, M. and Dayde, J. Use of simplified HPLC-UV analysis for soyasaponin B determination: study of saponin and isoflavone variability in soybean cultivars and soy-based health food products. *J. Agric. Food Chem.* 53: 3923–3930, 2005.

19. Lee, J.H., Renita, M., Fioritto, R.J., St. Martin, S.K., Schwartz, S.J., and Vodovotz, Y. Isoflavone characterization and antioxidant activity of Ohio soybeans. *J. Agric. Food Chem.* 52: 2647–2651, 2004.

20. Yu, O., Shi, J., Hession, A.O., Maxwell, C.A., McGonigle, B., and Odell, J.T. Metabolic engineering to increase isoflavone biosynthesis in soybean seed. *Phytochemistry* 63: 753–763, 2003.

21. Klump, M.C., Allured, J.L., MacDonald, J., and Balaam, M.M. Determination of isoflavones in soy and selected foods containing soy by extraction, specification, and liquid chromatography: collaborative study. *J. Assoc. Off. Anal. Chem. Int.* 84: 1865–1883, 2001.

22. Murphy, P.A., Barua, K., and Hauck, C.C. Solvent extraction selection in analysis of isoflavones in soy foods. *J. Chromatogr. B*, 777: 129–138, 2002.

23. Duke, S.O., Rimando, A.M., Pace, P.F., Reddy, K.N., and Smeda, R.J. Isoflavone, glyphosate, and aminomethylphosphonic acid levels in seeds of glyphosate-treated, glyphosate-resistant soybean. *J. Agric. Food Chem.* 51: 340–344, 2003.

24. Li, D., Park, J., Park, J.T., Park, C.S., and Park, K.H. Biotechnological Production of Highly soluble daidzein glycosides using thermotoga maritima maltosyltransferase. *J. Agric. Food Chem.* 52: 2561–2567, 2004.

25. Variyov, P.S., Limaye, A. and Sharma, A. Radiation-induced enhancement of antioxidant contents of soybean (Glycine max Merrill). *J. Agric. Food Chem.* 52: 3385–3388, 2004.

26. Barbosa, A.C.L., Lajolo, F.M., and Genovese, M.I. Influence of temperature, pH and ionic strength on the production of isoflavone-rich soy protein isolates. *Food Chem.* doi:10.1016/j.foodchem.2005.07.014, 2006.

27. Fukui, K., Tachibana, N., Wanezaki, S., Tsuzaki, S., Takamatsu, K., Yamamoto, T., Hashimoto, Y., and Shimoda, T. Isoflavone-free soy protein prepared by column chromatography reduces plasma cholesterol in rats. *J. Agric. Food Chem.* 50: 5717–5721, 2002.

28. Rickert, D.A., Johnson, L.A., and Murphy, P.A. Improved fractionation of glycinin and β-conglycinin and partitioning of phytochemicals. *J. Agric. Food Chem.* 52: 1726–1734, 2004.

29. Rickert, D.A., Meyer, M.A., Hu, J., and Murphy, P.A. Effect of extraction pH and temperature on isoflavone and saponin partitioning and profile during soy protein isolate production. *J. Food Sci.* 69: C623–C631, 2004.

30. Xu, L., Lamb, K., Layton, L., and Kumar, A. A membrane-based process for recovering isoflavones from a waste stream of soy processing. *Food Res. Int.* 37: 867–874, 2004.

31. Penalvo, J.L., Nurmi, T., and Adlercreutz, H. A simplified HPLC method for total isoflavones in soy products. *Food Chem.* 87: 297–305, 2004.

32. Penalvo, J.L., Heinonen, S.M., Nurmi, T., Deyama, T., Nishibe, S., and Adlercreutz, H. Plant lignans in soy-based health supplements. *J. Agric. Food Chem.* 52: 4133–4138, 2004.

33. Chua, R., Anderson, K., Chen, J., and Hu, M. Quality, labeling accuracy, and cost comparison of purified soy isoflavonoid products. *J. Altern. Complement. Med.* 10: 1053–1060, 2004.
34. Pinto, M.S., Lajolo, F.M., and Genovese, M.I. Effect of storage temperature and water activity on the content and profile of isoflavones, antioxidant activity and in vitro protein digestibility of soy protein isolates and defatted soy flours. *J. Agric. Food Chem.* 53: 6340–6346, 2005.
35. Kim, J.J., Kim, S.H., Hahn, S.J., and Chung, I.M., Changing soybean isoflavone composition and concentrations under two different storage conditions over three years. *Food Res. Int.* 38: 435–444, 2005.
36. Ismail, B. and Hayes, K., Beta-glycosidase activity toward different glycosidic forms of isoflavones. *J. Agric. Food. Chem.* 53: 4918–4924, 2005.
37. Choi, Y.B., Kim, K.S., and Rhee, J.S. Hydrolysis of soybean isoflavone glucosides by lactic acid bacteria. *Biotechnol. Lett.* 24; 2113–2116, 2002.
38. Chien, J.T., Hsieh, H.C., Kao, T.H., and Chen, B.H. Kinetic model for studying the conversion and degradation of isoflavones during heating. *Food Chem.* 91: 425–434, 2005.
39. Setchell, K.D.R. and Cole, S.J. Variations in isoflavone levels in soy foods and soy protein isolates and issues related to isoflavone databases and food labeling. *J. Agric. Food Chem.* 51: 4146–4155, 2003.
40. Zhang, Y.C., Albrecht, D., Bomser, J., Schwartz, S.J., and Vodovotz, Y. Isoflavone profile and biological activity of soy bread. *J. Agric. Food Chem.* 51: 7611–7616, 2003.
41. Hu, J., Lee, S.O., Hendrich, S., and Murphy, P.A. Quantification of the group B soyasaponins by high-performance liquid chromatography. *J. Agric Food Chem.* 50: 2587–2594, 2002.
42. Kao, T.H., Lu, Y.F., Hsieh, H.C., and Chen, B.H. Stability of isoflavone glucosides during processing of soymilk and tofu. *Food Res. Int.* 37: 891–900, 2004.
43. Tsangalis, D., Ashton, J.F., McGill, A.E.J., and Shah, N.P. Enzymic transformation of isoflavone phytoestrogens in soymilk by β-glucosidase-producing Bifidobacteria. *J. Food Sci.* 67: 3104–3113, 2002.
44. Tsangalis, D., Wilcox, G., Shah, N.P., and Stojanovska, L. Bioavailability of isoflavone phytoestrogens in postmenopausal women consuming soya milk fermented with probiotic bifidobacteria. *Brit. J. Nutr.* 93: 867–877, 2005.
45. Kao F.-J., Su, N.W., and Lee, M.H. Effect of water-to-bean ratio on the contents and compositions of isoflavones in tofu. *J. Agric. Food Chem.* 52: 2277–2281, 2004.
46. Antignac, J.P., Cariou, R., Le Bizec, B., and Andr, F. New data regarding phytoestrogens content in bovine milk. *Food Chem.* 87: 275–281, 2004.
47. Wu, M.L., Chang, J.C., Lai, Y.H., Cheng, S.L., and Chiou, R.Y.Y. Enhancement of tofu isoflavone recovery by pretreatment of soy milk and koji enzyme extract. *J. Agric. Food Chem.* 52: 4785–4790, 2004.
48. Wiseman, H., Casey, K., Clarke, D.B., Barnes, K.A., and Bowey, E. Isoflavone aglycon and gluco-conjugate content of high- and low-soy U.K. foods used in nutritional studies. *J. Agric. Food Chem.* 50: 1404–1410, 2002.
49. Banz, W.J., Peluso, M.R., Winters, T.A., and Shanahan, M.F. Methods of Treating Clinical Diseases with Isoflavones. U.S. Patent 6,592,910, 2003.
50. Bates, G.A. and Bryan, B.A. Process for Separating and Recovering Protein and Isoflavones from a Plant Material. U.S. Patent 6,703,051, 2004.
51. Blatt, Y., Arad, O., Kimelman, E., Cohen, D., Pinto, R., and Rotman, A. Microencapsulated and Controlled-Release Formulations of Isoflavone from Enriched Fractions of Soy and Other Plants. U.S. Patent 6,890,561, 2005.
52. Bombardelli, E. and Gabetta, B. Soya Extract, Process for its Preparation and Pharmaceutical Composition. U.S. Patent 6,607,757, 2003.
53. Bringe, N.A. High Beta-Conglycinin Products and Their Use. U.S. Patent 6,566,134, 2003.
54. Bryan, B.A. and Allred, M.C. Aglucone Isoflavone Enriched Vegetable Flour and Vegetable Grit and Process for Making the Same from a Vegetable Material Containing Isoflavone. U.S. Patent 6,579,561, 2003.
55. Daicho, T. Health Food Products. U.S. Patent 6,793,943, 2004.
56. Empie, M. and Gugger, E. Method of Preparing and using Compositions Extracted from Vegetable Matter for the Treatment of Cancer. U.S. Patent 6,900,240, 2005.

57. Forusz, S.L., Liu, H., and Muatine, R.M. Composition for Increasing Bone Density. U.S. Patent 6,761,912, 2004.
58. Green, M.R., Hailes, A., Tasker, M.C., and Yates, P.R. Blends of Isoflavones and Flavones. U.S. Patent 6,617,349, 2003.
59. Gugger, E. and Grabiel, R. Production of Isoflavone Enriched Fractions from Soy Protein Extracts. U.S. Patent 6,565,912, 2003.
60. He, M.M., Liu, F.Y., Fix, J.A., Link, M., Kang, M.L., and Bombardelli, E. Tablets Incorporating Isoflavone Plant Extracts and Methods of Manufacturing Them. U.S. Patent 6,669,956, 2003.
61. Lars, H. Composition Comprising Soy Protein, Dietary Fibres and a Phytoestrogen Compound and Use Thereof in the Prevention and/or Treatment of Cardiovascular Diseases. U.S. Patent 6,630,178, 2003.
62. Kelly, G.E. Methods for Treating or Reducing Prediposition to Breast Cancer, Pre-Menstrual Syndrome or Symptoms Associated with Menopause by Administration of Phytoestrogen. U.S. Patent 6,562,380, 2003.
63. Kelly, G.E. and Husband, A.J. Therapy of Estrogen-Associated Disorders. U.S. Patent 6,599,536, 2003.
64. Kelly, G.E. Health Supplements Containing Phytoestrogens, Analogues or Metabolites Thereof. U.S. Patent 6,642,212, 2003.
65. Khare, A.B. Soluble Isoflavone Compositions. U.S. Patent 6,855,359, 2005.
66. Lu, K.M. Methods for Inhibiting Cancer Growth, Reducing Infection and Promoting General Health with a Fermented Soy Extract. U.S. Patent 6,855,350, 2005.
67. Meijer, G.W., Franke, W.C., and Reddy, P.R. Composition for Lowering Blood Cholesterol. U.S. Patent 6,787,151, 2004.
68. Monagle, C.W. Soy Protein Product and Process for Its Manufacture. U.S. Patent 6,797,309, 2004.
69. Monagle, C.W. Method for Manufacturing a Soy Protein Product. U.S. Patent 6,811,798, 2004.
70. Ono, M., Koya, K., Tatsuta, N., Yamaguchi, N., and Chen, L.B. Water-Soluble Bean-Based Extracts. U.S. Patent 6,616,959, 2003.
71. Patel, G.C., Cipollo, K.L., and Strozier, D.C. Juice and Soy Protein Beverage and Uses Thereof. U.S. Patent 6,811,804, 2004.
72. Peters, S.E. and Woods, D.H. Stable Aqueous Dispersion of Nutrients. U.S. Patent 6,617,305, 2003.
73. Singh, N. Soy Protein Concentrate Having High Isoflavone Content and Process for Its Manufacture. U.S. Patent 6,818,246, 2004.
74. Uchiyama, S., Ueno, T., Kumemura, M., Imaizumi, K., Masaki, K., and Shimizu, S. Streptococcus and Isoflavone-Containing Composition. U.S. Patent 6,716,424, 2004.
75. Uckun, F.M., Trieu, V.N., and Liu, X.P. Estrogens for Treating ALS. U.S. Patent 6,592,845, 2003.
76. Waggle, D.H., Potter, S.M., and Henley, E.C. Administering a Composition Containing Plant Sterol, Soy Protein and Isoflavone for Reducing LDL-Cholesterol. U.S. Patent 6,572,876, 2003.
77. Waggle, D.H., Potter, S.M., and Henley, E.C. Composition Containing Soy Hypocotyl Material and Plant Sterol for Reducing LDL-Cholesterol. U.S. Patent 6,579,534, 2003.
78. Waggle, D.H. and Bryan, B.A. Recovery of Isoflavones from Soy Molasses. U.S. Patent 6,664,382, 2003.
79. Waggle, D.H., Potter; S.M., and Henley, E.C. Composition Containing Isoflavone Material and Plant Sterol for Reducing LDL-Cholesterol. U.S. Patent 6,669,952, 2003.
80. Waggle, D.H. and Bryan, B.A., Recovery of Isoflavones from Soy Molasses. U.S. Patent 6,680,381, 2004.
81. Waggle, D.H. and Bryan, B.A., Recovery of Isoflavones from Soy Molasses. U.S. Patent 6,706,292, 2004.
82. Hendrich, S. Bioavailability of isoflavones. *J. Chromatogr. B* 777: 203–210, 2002.
83. Barnes, S., D'Alessandro, T., Kirk, M.C., Patel, R.K.P., Boersma, B.J., and Darley-Usmar, V.M., The importance of in vivo metabolism of polyphenols and their biological actions. Eds., Meskin, M.S., Bidlack, W.R., Davies, A.J., Lewis, D.S., and Randolph, R.K. In *Phytochemicals: Mechanisms of Action.* CRC Press, Boca Raton, FL, 2004, pp. 51–60.
84. Hendrich, S., Wang, G.-J., Lin, H.-K., Xu, X., Tew, B.-Y., Wang, H.-J., and Murphy, P.A. Isoflavone metabolism and bioavailability. In *Antioxidant Status, Diet, Nutrition and Health,* Ed., Papas, A.M. CRC Press, Boca Raton, FL, 1998, pp. 211–230.

85. Birt, D.F., Hendrich, S., and Wang, W. Dietary agents in cancer prevention: flavonoids and isoflavonoids. *Pharmacol. Ther.* 90: 157-177, 2001.

86. Fitzpatrick, L.A. Soy isoflavones: hope or hype? *Maturitas* 44: S21–S29, 2003.

87. Hendrich, S. Dietary estrogens. In *Pesticides, Veterinary and Other Chemical Residues in Foods.* Woodhead Publ. Ltd., Cambridge, U.K., pp. 436-472, 2004.

88. Birt, D.F., Hendrich, S., Anthony, M., and Alekel, D.L. Human health benefits of soybeans. Soy Monograph, Agronomy Monograph No. 16, 4th ed. American Society of Agronomy, Madison, WI. pp. 1047–1117, 2004.

89. Messina, M., Ho, S., and Alekel, D.L. Skeletal benefits of soy isoflavones: a review of the clinical trial and epidemiologic data. *Curr. Opin. Clin. Nutr. Metab. Care* 7: 649–658, 2004.

90. Crouse, J.R., III, Morgan, T., Terry, J.G., Ellis, J., Vitolins, M., and Burke, G.L. A randomized trial comparing the effect of casein with that of soy protein containing varying amounts of isoflavones on plasma concentrations of lipids and lipoproteins. *Arch. Intern. Med.* 159: 2070–2076, 1999.

91. Steinberg, F.M., Guthrie, N.L., Villablanca, A.C., Kumar, K., and Murray, M.J. Soy protein with isoflavones has favorable effects on endothelial function that are independent of lipid and antioxidant effects in healthy postmenopausal women. *Am. J. Clin. Nutr.* 78: 123–130, 2003.

92. Yan, L. and Spitznagel, E., A meta-analysis of soyfoods and risk of breast cancer in women. *Int. J. Cancer Prev.* 1: 281–293, 2004.

93. Messina, M. and Hughes, C., Efficacy of soyfoods and soybean isoflavone supplements for alleviating menopausal symptoms is positively related to initial hot flush frequency. *J. Med. Foods* 6: 1–11, 2003.

94. Strom, B.L., Schinnar, R., Ziegler, E.E., Barnhart, K.T., Sammel, M.D., Macones, G.A., Stallings, V.A., Drulis, J.M., Nelson, S.E., and Hanson, S.A. Exposure to soy-based formula in infancy and endocrinological and reproductive outcomes in young adulthood. *J. Am. Med. Assoc.* 286: 807–814, 2001.

95. Bloeden, L.T., Jeffcoat, A.R., Lopaczynski, W., Schell, M.J., Black, T.M., Dix, K.J., Thomas, B.F., Albright, C., Busby, M.G., Crowell, J.A., and Zeisel, S.H. Safety and pharmacokinetics of purified soy isoflavones: single-dose administration to postmenopausal women. *Am. J. Clin. Nutr.* 76: 1126–1137, 2002.

96. Yellayi, S., Naaz, A., Szewczykowski, M.A., Sato, T., Woods, J.A., Chang, J., Segre, M., Allred, C.D., Helferich, W.G., and Cooke, P.S. The phytoestrogen genistein induces thymic and immune changes: a human health concern? *Proc. Natl. Acad. Sci.* 99: 7616–7621, 2002.

97. Lehmann, L., Esch, H.L., Wagner, J., Rohnstock, L., and Metzler, M. Estrogenic and genotoxic potential of equol and two hydroxylated metabolites of daidzein in cultured human Ishikawa cells. *Toxicol. Lett.* 158: 72–86, 2005.

98. Alekel, D.L., St. Germain, A., Peterson, C.T., Hanson, K.B., Stewart, J.W., and Toda, T. Isoflavone-rich soy protein isolate attenuates bone loss in the lumbar spine of perimenopausal women. *Am. J. Clin. Nutr.* 72: 844–852, 2000.

99. Mei, J., Yeung, S.S.C., and Kung, A.W.C. High dietary phytoestrogen intake is associated with higher bone mineral density in postmenopausal but not premenopausal women. *J. Clin. Endocrin. Metab.* 86: 5217–5221, 2001.

100. Dalais, F.S., Ebeling, P.R., Kotsopoulos, D., McGrath, B.P., and Teede, H.J. The effects of soy protein containing isoflavones on lipids and indices of bone resorption in postmenopausal women. *Clin. Endocrinol.* 58: 704–709, 2003.

101. Li, B. and Yu, S. Genistein prevents bone resorption diseases by inhibiting bone resorption and stimulating bone formation. *Biol. Pharm. Bull.* 26: 780–786, 2003.

102. Park, D., Huang, T., and Frishman, W.H. Phytoestrogens as cardioprotective agents. *Cardiol. Rev.* 13: 13–17, 2005.

103. Clarkson, T. Soy, soy phytoestrogens and cardiovascular disease. *J. Nutr.* 132: 566S–569S, 2002.

104. van der Schouw, Y.T., de Kleijn, M.J.J., Peeters, P.H.M., and Grobbee, D.E. Phyto-estrogens and cardiovascular disease risk. *Nutr. Metab. Cardiovas. Dis.* 10: 154–167, 2000.

105. Lichtenstein, A.H., Soy protein, isoflavones and cardiovascular disease risk. *J. Nutr.* 128: 1589–1592, 1998.

106. de Kleijn, M.J.J., van der Schouw, Y.T., Wilson, P.W.F., Grobbee, D.E., and Jacques, P.F. Dietary intake of phytoestrogens is associated with a favorable metabolic cardiovascular risk profile on postmenopausal U.S. women: The Framingham study. *J. Nutr.* 132: 276–282, 2002.

107. Song, T.T., Lee, S.O., Murphy, P.A., and Hendrich, S. Soy protein with or without isoflavones, soy germ and soy germ extract, and daidzein lessen plasma cholesterol levels in golden Syrian hamsters. *Exp. Biol. Med.* 228: 1063–1068, 2003.

108. Yamakoshi, J., Piskula, M.K., Izumi, T., Tobe, K., Saito, M. Kataoka, S., Obata, A., and Kikuchi, M. Isoflavone aglycone-rich extract with soy protein attenuates atherosclerosis development in cholesterol-fed rabbits. *J. Nutr.* 130: 1887–1893, 2000.

109. Sirtori, C.R., Bosisio, R., Pazzucconi, F., Bondioli, A., Gatti, E., Lovati, M.R., and Murphy, P. Soy milk with a high glycitein content does not reduce low-density lipoprotein cholesterolemia in Type II hypercholesterolemic patients. *Ann. Nutr. Metab.* 46: 88–92, 2002.

110. Greaves, K.A., Wilson, M.D., Rudel, L.L., Williams, K.J., and Wagner, J.D., Consumption of soy protein reduces cholesterol absorption compared to casein protein alone or supplemented with an isoflavone extract or conjugated equine estrogen in ovariectomized cynomolgus monkeys. *J. Nutr.* 130: 820–826, 2000.

111. Teede, H., McGrath, B.P., DeSilva, L., Cehun, M., Fassoulakis, A., and Nestel, P.J. Isoflavones reduce arterial stiffness: a placebo-controlled study in men and postmenopausal women. *Arterioscler. Thromb. Vasc. Biol.* 23: 1066–1071, 2003.

112. Peeters, P.H.M., Keinan-Boker, L., van der Schouw, Y.T., and Grobbee, D.E. Phytoestrogens and breast cancer risk. *Breast Cancer Res. Treat.* 77: 171–183, 2003.

113. Jin, Z. and MacDonald, R.S. Soy isoflavones increase latency of spontaneous mammary tumors in mice. *J. Nutr.* 132: 3186–3190, 2002.

114. Lamartiniere, C.A., Wang, J., Smith-Johnson, M., and Eltoum, I.-E. Daidzein: bioavailability, potential for reproductive toxicity, and breast cancer chemoprevention in female rats. *Toxicol. Sci.* 65: 228–238, 2002.

115. Moyad, M.A., Soy, disease prevention, and prostate cancer. *Sem. Urin. Oncol.* 17: 97–102, 1999.

116. Messina, M.J. Emerging evidence on the role of soy in reducing prostate cancer risk. *Nutr. Rev.* 61: 117–131, 2003.

117. Jacobsen, B.K., Knutsen, S.F., and Fraser, G.E. Does high soy milk intake reduce prostate cancer incidence? The Adventist Health Study (U.S.). *Cancer Causes Control* 9: 553–557, 1998.

118. Hong, S.J., Kim, S.I., Kwon, S.M., Lee, J.R., and Chung, B.C. Comparative study of concentration of isoflavones and lignans in plasma and prostatic tissue of normal control and benign prostatic hyperplasia. *Yonsei Med. J.* 43: 236–241, 2002.

119. Urban D., Irwin, W., Kirk, M., Markiewicz, M.A., Myers, R., Smith, M., Weiss, H., Grizzle, W.E., and Barnes, S. The effect of isolated soy protein on plasma biomarkers in elderly men with elevated serum prostate specific antigen. *J. Urol.* 165: 294–300, 2001.

120. Mitchell, J.H., Duthie, S.J., and Collins, A.R. Effects of phytoestrogens on growth and DNA integrity in human prostate tumor cell lines: PC-3 and LNCaP. *Nutr. Cancer* 38: 223–228, 2000.

121. Fritz, W.A., Eltoum, I.-E., Cotroneo, M.S., and Lamartiniere, C.A. Genistein alters growth but is not toxic to the rat prostate. *J. Nutr.* 132: 3007–3011, 2002.

122. Mentor-Marcel, R., Lamartiniere, C.A., Eltoum, I.E., Greenberg, N.M., and Elgavish, A. Genistein in the diet reduces the incidence of prostate tumors in a transgenic mouse (TRAMP). *Cancer Res.* 61: 6777–6782, 2001.

123. Omoni, A.O., and Aluko, R.E. Soybean foods and their benefits: potential mechanisms of action. *Nutr. Rev.* 63: 272–283, 2005.

124. Guo, T.L., McCay, J.A., Zhang, L.X., Brown, R.D., You, L., Karrow, N.A., Germolec, D.R., and White, K.L. Jr. Genistein modulates immune responses and increases host resistance to B61F10 tumor in adult female B6C3F1 mice. *J. Nutr.* 131: 3251–3258, 2001.

125. Akiyama, T., Ishida, J., Nakagawa, S., Ogawara, H., Watanabe, S., Itoh, N., Shibuya, M., and Fukami, Y. Genistein, a specific inhibitor of tyrosine-specific protein kinases. *J. Biol. Chem.* 262: 5592–5595, 1987.

126. Markovits, J., Linassier, C., Fosse, P., Couprie, J., Pierre, J., Jacquemin-Sablon, A., Saucier, J.M., Le Pecq, J.B., and Larsen, A.K. Inhibitory effects of the tyrosine kinase inhibitor genistein on mammalian DNA topoisomerase II. *Cancer Res.* 49: 5111–5117, 1989.

127. Kritz-Silverstein, D., Von Mühlen, D., Barrett-Connor, E., and Bressel, M.A.B., Isoflavones and cognitive function in older women: the SOy and postmenopausal health in aging (SOPHIA) study. *Menopause* 10: 196–202, 2003.

128. Mendez, M.A., Anthony, M.S., and Arab, L. Soy-based formula and infant growth and development: a review. *J. Nutr.* 132: 2127–2130, 2002.

129. Takimoto, C.H., Glover, K., Huang, X., Hayes, S.A., Gallot, L., Quinn, M., Jovanovic, B.D., Shapiro, A., Hernandez, L., Goetz, A., Llorens, V., Lieberman, R., Crowell, J.A., Poisson, B.A., and Bergan, R.C. Phase I pharmacokinetic and pharmacodynamic analysis of unconjugated soy isoflavones administered to individuals with cancer. *Cancer Epidemiol. Biomarkers Prev.* 12: 1213–1221, 2003.

130. Selvaraj, V., Zakroczymski, M.A., Naaz, A., Mukai, M., Ju, Y.H., Doerge, D.R., Katzenellenbogen, J.A., Helferich, W.G., and Cooke, P.S. Estrogenicity of the isoflavone metabolite equol on reproductive and non-reproductive organs in mice. *Biol. Reprod.* 71: 966–972, 2004.

131. Selvaraj, V., Bunick, D., Finnigan-Bunick, C., Johnson, R.W., Wang, H., Liu, L., and Cooke, P.S. Gene expression profiling of 17beta-estradiol and genistein effects on mouse thymus. *Toxicol. Sci.* 87: 97–112, 2005.

132. Doerge, D. and Sheehan, D.M. Goitrogenic and estrogenic activity of soy isoflavones. *Environ. Health Perspect.* 110(Suppl. 3): 349–353, 2002.

133. Huang, W., Wood, C., L'Abbé, M., Gilani, G.S., Cockell, K.A., and Xiao, C.W., Soy protein isolate increases hepatic thyroid hormone receptor content and inhibits its binding to target genes in rats. *J. Nutr.* 135: 1631–1635, 2005.

134. Teede, H.J., Dalais, F.S., and McGrath, B.P. Dietary soy containing phytoestrogens does not have detectable estrogenic effects on hepatic protein synthesis in postmenopausal women. *Am. J. Clin. Nutr.* 79: 396–401, 2004.

135. Horn-Ross, P.L., Hoggatt, K.J., and Lee, M.M. Phytoestrogens and thyroid cancer risk: the San Francisco Bay Area thyroid cancer study. *Cancer Epidemiol. Biomark. Prev.* 11: 43–49, 2002.

136. Patisaul, H.B., Dindo, M., Whitten, P.L., and Young, L.J., Soy isoflavone supplements antagonize reproductive behavior and estrogen receptor α- and β-dependent gene expression in the brain. *Endocrinology* 142: 2946–2952, 2001.

137. Ferguson, S.A., Flynn, K.M., Delclos, K.B., Newbold, R.R., and Gough, B.J. Effects of lifelong dietary exposure to genistein or nonylphenol on amphetamine-stimulated striatal dopamine release in male and female rats. *Neurotoxicol. Teratol.* 24: 37–45, 2002.

138. Lephart, E.D., West, T.W, Weber, K.S., Rhees, R.W., Setchell, K.D.R., Adlercreutz, H., and Lund, T.D. Neurobehavioral effects of dietary soy phytoestrogens. *Neurotoxicol. Teratol.* 24: 5–16, 2002.

139. Lephart, E.D., Rhees, R.W., Setchell, K.D.R., Bu, L.H., and Lund, T.D. Estrogens and phytoestrogens: brain plasticity of sexually dimorphic brain volumes. *J. Steroid Biochem. Mol. Biol.* 85: 299-309, 2003.

140. Hartley, D.E., Edwards, J.E., Spiller, C.E., Alom, N., Tucci, S., Seth, P., Forsling, M.L., and File, S.E., The soya isoflavone content of rat diet can increase anxiety and stress hormone release in male rats. *Psychopharmacology* 167: 46–53, 2003.

141. Kulling, S.E., Rosenberg, B., Jacobs, E., and Metzler, M. The phytoestrogens coumestrol and genistein induce structural chromosomal aberrations in cultured human peripheral blood lymphocytes. *Arch. Toxicol.* 73: 50–54, 1999.

142. Tsutsui, T., Tamura, Y., Yagi, E., Hori, H., Hori, I., Metzler, M., and Barrett, J.C. Cell-transforming activity and mutagenicity of 5 phytoestrogens in cultured mammalian cells. *Int. J. Cancer* 105: 312–320, 2003.

143. Lehmann, L., Esch, H.L., Wagner, J., Rohnstock, L., Metzler, M. Estrogenic and genotoxic potential of equol and two hydroxylated metabolites of daidzein in cultured human Ishikawa cells. *Toxicol. Lett.* 158: 72–86, 2005.

144. Kuiper, G.J.M., Lemmen, J.G., Carlsson, B., Corton, J.C., Safe, S.H., van der Saag, P.T., van der Burg, B., and Gustafsson, J.-Å., Interaction of estrogenic chemicals and phytoestrogens with estrogen receptor β. *Endocrinology* 139: 4252–4263, 1998.

145. Morito, K., Aomori, T., Hirose, T., Kinjo, J., Hasegawa, J., Ogawa, S., Inoue, S., Muramatsu, M., Masamune, Y. Interaction of phytoestrogens with estrogen receptors α and β. *Biol. Pharm. Bull.* 25: 48–52, 2002.

146. Rickard, D.J., Monroe, D.G., Ruesink, T.J., Khosla, S., Riggs, B.L., and Spelsberg, T.C. Phytoestrogen genistein acts as an estrogen agonist on human osteoblastic cells through estrogen receptors α and β. *J. Cell. Biochem.* 89: 633–646, 2003.

147. Mueller, S.O., Kling, M., Firzani, P.A., Mecky, A., Duranti, E., Shields-Botella, J., Delansorne, R., Broschard, T., Kramer, P.-J. Activation of estrogen receptor α and ERβ by 4-methylbenzylidene-camphor in human and rat cells: comparison with phyto- and xenoestrogens. *Toxicol. Lett.* 142: 89–101, 2003.

148. Dechaud, H., Ravard, C., Claustrat, F., Brac de la Perriere, A., and Pugeat, M. Xenoestrogen interaction with human sex hormone-binding globulin (hSHGB). *Steroids* 64: 328–334, 1999.

149. Kurzer, M. Hormonal effects of soy in premenopausal women and men. *J. Nutr.* 132: 570S–573S, 2002.

150. Zhang, Y., Song, T.T., Cunnick, J.E., Murphy, P.A., and Hendrich, S. Daidzein and genistein glucuronides in vitro are weakly estrogenic and activate human natural killer cells in nutritionally relevant concentrations. *J. Nutr.* 129: 399–405, 1999.

151. Vivier, E., Nunës, J.A., and Vèly, F., Natural killer cell signaling pathways. *Science* 306: 1517–1519, 2004.

152. Kuiper, G.G.J.M., Enmark, E., Pelto-Huikko, M., Nilsson, S., and Gustafsson, J.-Å. Cloning of a novel estrogen receptor expressed in rat prostate and ovary. *Proc. Natl. Acad. Sci. USA* 93: 5925–5930, 1996.

153. Solanky, K.S., Bailey, N.J., Beckwith-Hall, B.M., Bingham, S., Davis, A., Holmes, E., Nicholson, J.K., Cassidy, A. Biofluid ^{1}H NMR-based metabonomic techniques in nutrition research — metabolic effects of dietary isoflavones in humans. *J. Nutr. Biochem.* 16: 236–244, 2005.

154. Day, A.J., Cañada, F.J., Díaz, J.C., Kroon, P.A., Mclauchlan, R., Faulds, C.B., Plumb, G.W., Morgan, M.R.A., and Williamson, G. Dietary flavonoid and isoflavone glycosides are hydrolyzed by the lactase site of lactase phlorizin hydrolase. *FEBS Lett.* 468: 166–170, 2000.

155. Setchell, K.D., Brown, N.M., Zimmer-Nechemias, L., Brashear, W.T., Wolfe, B.E., Kirschner, A.S., and Heubi, J.E. Evidence for lack of absorption of soy isoflavone glycosides in humans, supporting the crucial role of intestinal metabolism for bioavailability. *Am. J. Clin. Nutr.* 76: 447–453, 2002.

156. Williamson G. Common features in the pathways of absorption and metabolism of flavonoids. Eds., Meskin, M.S., Bidlack, W.R., Davies, A.J., Lewis, D.S., and Randolph, R.K. In *Phytochemicals: Mechanisms of Action*, CRC Press, Boca Raton, FL, 2004, pp. 21–33.

157. Zheng, Y., Lee, S.-O., Verbruggen, M.A., Murphy, P.A., and Hendrich, S. Apparent absorption of isoflavone glucosides and aglucons is similar in women and increased with rapid gut transit time and low fecal isoflavone degradation. *J. Nutr.* 134: 2534–2539, 2004.

158. Izumi, T., Piskula, M., Osawa, S., Obata, A., Tobe, K., Saito, M., Kataoka, S., Kubota, Y., and Kikuchi, M., Soy isoflavone aglycones are absorbed faster and in higher amounts than their glucosides in humans. *J. Nutr.* 130: 1695–1699, 2000.

159. Zubik, L. and Meydani, M., Bioavailability of soybean isoflavones from aglycone and glucoside forms in American women. *Am. J. Clin. Nutr.* 77: 1459–1465, 2003.

160. Setchell, K.D.R., Brown, N.M., Desai, P., Zimmer-Nechemias, L., Wolfe, B.E., Brashear, W.T., Kirschner, A.S., Cassidy, A., and Heubi, J.E., Bioavailability of pure isoflavones in healthy humans and analysis of commercial soy isoflavone supplements. *J. Nutr.*, 131: 1362S–1375S, 2001.

161. Busby, M., Jeffcoat, A.R., Bloedon, L.T., Koch, M.A., Black, T., Dix, K.J., Heizer, W.D., Thomas, B.F., Hill, J.M., Crowell, J.A, and Zeisel, S.H. Clinical characteristics and pharmacokinetics of purified soy isoflavones: single-dose administration to healthy men. *Am. J. Clin. Nutr.* 75: 126–136, 2002.

162. King, R.A. and Bursill, D.B. Plasma and urinary kinetics of the isoflavones daidzein and genistein after a single soy meal in humans. *Am. J. Clin. Nutr.* 67, 867–872, 1998.

163. Setchell, K.D.R., Faughnan, M.S., Avades, T., Zemmer-Nechemias, Brown, N.M., Wolfe, B.E., Brashear, W.T., Desai, P., Oldfield, M.F., Botting, N.P., and Cassidy, A. Comparing the pharmacokinetics of daidzein and genistein with the use of ^{13}C-labeled tracers in premenopausal women. *Am. J. Clin. Nutr.* 77: 411–419, 2003.

164. Xu, X., Wang, H.-J., Cook, L.R., Murphy, P.A., and Hendrich, S. Daidzein is a more bioavailable soymilk isoflavone to young adult women than is genistein. *J. Nutr.* 124, 825–832, 1994.

165. Zhang, Y., Wang, G.-J., Song, T.T., Murphy, P.A., and Hendrich, S. Differences in disposition of the soybean isoflavones, glycitein, daidzein and genistein in humans with moderate fecal isoflavone degradation activity. *J. Nutr.* 129: 957–962, 1999. *Erratum J. Nutr.* 131: 147–148, 2001.

166. Xu, X., Harris, K., Wang, H.-J., Murphy, P., and Hendrich, S. Bioavailability of soybean isoflavones depends upon gut microflora in women. *J. Nutr.* 125: 2307–2315, 1995.

167. Sfakianos, J., Coward, L., Kirk, M., and Barnes, S., Intestinal uptake and biliary excretion of the isoflavone genistein in rats. *J. Nutr.* 127: 1260–1268, 1997.

168. Chen, J., Lin, H., and Hu, M. Absorption and metabolism of genistein and its five isoflavone analogs in the human intestinal Caco-2 model. *Cancer Chemother. Pharmacol.* 55: 159–169, 2005.

169. Zhang, Y., Murphy, P.A., and Hendrich, S. Glucuronides are the main isoflavone metabolites in women. *J. Nutr.* 133: 399–4004, 2003.

170. Holder, C.L., Churchwell, M.I., and Doerge, D.R. Quantification of soy isoflavones, genistein and daidzein, and conjugates in rat blood using LC/ES-MS. *J. Agric. Food Chem.* 47: 3764–3770, 1999.

171. Cimino, C., Shelnutt, S.R., Ronis, M.J.J., and Badger, T.M. An LC-MS method to determine concentrations of isoflavones and sulfate and glucuronide conjugates in urine. *Clin. Chim. Acta* 287: 69–82, 1999.

172. Yasuda, T., Mizunuma, S., Kano, Y., Saito, K., and Ohsawa, K. Urinary and biliary metabolites of genistein in rats. *Biol. Pharm. Bull.* 19: 413-417, 1996.

173. Piskula, M. Soy isoflavone conjugation differs in fed and food-deprived rats. *J. Nutr.* 130: 1766–1771, 2000.

174. Peterson, T.G., Ji, G.P., Kirk, M., Coward, L., Falany, C.N., and Barnes, S. Metabolism of the isoflavones genistein and biochanin A in human breast cancer cell lines. *Am. J. Clin. Nutr.* 68(6 Suppl.), 1505S–1511S, 1998.

175. Rimbach, G., Weinberg, P.D., de Pascual-Teresa, S., Alonso, M.G., Ewins, B.A., Turner, R., Minihane, A.M., Botting, N., Fairley, B., Matsugo, S., Uchida, Y., and Cassidy, A., Sulfation of genistein alters its antioxidant properties and its effect on platelet aggregation and monocyte and endothelial function. *Biochim. Biophys. Acta* 1670: 229–237, 2004.

176. Turner, R., Baron, T., Wolffram, S., Minihane, A.M., Cassidy, A., Rimbach, G., and Weinberg, P.D. Effect of circulating forms of soy isoflavones on the oxidation of low density lipoprotein. *Free Radic. Res.* 38: 209-216, 2004.

177. Totta, P., Acconcia, F., Virgili, F., Cassidy, A., Weinberg, P.D., Rimbach, G., and Marino, M. Daidzein-sulfate metabolites affect transcriptional and antiproliferative activities of estrogen receptor-{beta} in cultured human cancer cells. *J. Nutr.* 135: 2687–2693, 2005.

178. Atkinson, C., Frankenfeld, C.L., and Lampe, J.W. Gut bacterial metabolism of the soy isoflavone daidzein: exploring the relevance to human health. *Exp. Biol. Med.* 230: 155–170, 2005.

179. Hwang, J., Wang, J., Morazzoni, P., Hodis, H.N., and Sevanian, A. The phytoestrogen equol increases nitric oxide availability by inhibiting superoxide production: an antioxidant mechanism for cell-mediated LDL modification. *Free Radic. Biol. Med.* 34: 1271–1282, 2003.

180. Nettleton, J.A., Greany, K.A., Thomas, W., Wangen, K.E., Adlercreutz, H., and Kurzer, M.S. The effect of soy consumption of the urinary 2:16-hydroxyestrone ratio in postmenopausal women depends on equol production status but is not influenced by probiotic consumption. *J. Nutr.* 135: 603–608, 2005.

181. Allred, C.D., Twaddle, N.C., Allred, K.F., Goeppinger, T.S., Churchwell, M.I., Ju, Y.H., Helferich, W.G., and Doerge, D.R. Soy processing affects metabolism and disposition of dietary isoflavones in ovariectomized BALB/c mice. *J. Agric. Food Chem.* 53: 8542–8550, 2005.

182. Lampe, J.W., Karr, S.C., Hutchins, A.M., and Slavin, J.L. Urinary equol excretion with a soy challenge: influence of habitual diet. *Proc. Soc. Exp. Biol. Med.* 217: 335–339, 1998.

183. Rowland, I.R., Wiseman, H., Sanders, T.A.B., Adlercreutz, H., and Bowey, E.A. Interindividual variation in metabolism of soy isoflavones and lignans: influence of habitual diet on equol production by the gut microflora. *Nutr. Cancer* 36: 27–32, 2000.

184. Hedlund, T.E., Maroni, P.D., Ferucci, P.G., Dayton, R., Barnes, S., Jones, K., Moore, R., Ogden, L.G., Wähälä, K., Sackett, H.M., and Gray, K.J. Long-term dietary habits affect soy isoflavone metabolism and accumulation in prostatic fluid in Caucasian men. *J. Nutr.* 135: 1400–1406, 2005.

185. Kelly, G.E., Nelson, C., Waring, M.A., Joannou, G.E., and Reeder, A.Y. Metabolites of dietary (soya) isoflavones in human urine. *Clin. Chim. Acta,* 223: 9–22, 1993.

186. Heinonen, S., Wähälä, K., and Adlercreutz, H. Identification of isoflavone metabolites dihydrodaidzein, dihydrogenistein, 6-OH-ODMA, and cis-4-OH-equol in human urine by gas chromatography-mass spectrometry using authentic reference compounds. *Anal. Biochem.* 274: 211–219, 1999.

187. Heinonen, S., Wähälä, K., Liukkonen, K., Aura, A., Poutanen, K., and Adlercreutz, H. Studies of the in vitro intestinal metabolism of isoflavones in the identification of their urinary metabolites. *J. Agric. Food Chem.* 52: 2640–2646, 2004.

188. Simons, A.L., Renouf, M., Hendrich, S., and Murphy, P.A. Metabolism of glycitein (7,4-dihydroxy-6-methoxy-isoflavone) by human gut microflora. *J. Agric. Food Chem.* 53: 8519–8525, 2005.

189. Hendrich, S., Wang, G.-J., Xu, X., Tew, B.-Y., Wang, H.-J., and Murphy, P.A. Human Bioavailability of Soy Bean Isoflavones: Influences of Diet, Dose, Time and Gut Microflora. In *Functional Foods*, ACS Monograph, Ed., Shibamoto, T. ACS Books, Washington, D.C., 1998, pp. 150–156.

190. Wang, G.-J., Human Gut Microfloral Metabolism of Soybean Isoflavones. Iowa State University Master's Thesis, Ames. IA, 1997.

191. Zheng, Y., Hu, J., Murphy, P.A., Alekel, D.L., Franke, W.D., Hendrich, S., Rapid gut transit time and slow fecal isoflavone disappearance phenotype are associated with greater genistein bioavailability in women. *J. Nutr.* 133: 3110–3116, 2003.

192. Winter J., Moore, L.H., Dowell, V.R., Jr., and Bokkenheuser, V.D. C-ring cleavage of flavonoids by human intestinal bacteria. *Appl. Environ. Microbiol.* 55: 1203–1208, 1989.

193. Mitsuoka, T. Recent trends in research on intestinal flora. *Bifidobacteria Microflora* 3, 3–24, 1982.

194. Verdeal, K. and Ryan, D.S. Naturally-occurring estrogens in plant foodstuffs — a review. *J. Food Prot.* 42: 577–583, 1979.

195. Markaverich, B.M., Gregory, R.R., Alejandro, M.A., Clark, J.H., Johnson, G.A., and Middleditch, B.S. Methyl p-hydroxyphenyllactate — an inhibitor of cell growth and proliferation and an endogenous ligand for nuclear type-II binding sites. *J. Biol. Chem.* 263: 7203–7210, 1988.

196. Muyzer, G., De Wall, E.C., and Uitterlinden, A.G. Profiling of complex microbial populations by denaturing gradient gel electrophoresis analysis of polymerase chain reaction-amplified genes coding for 16S rRNA. *Appl. Environ. Microbiol.* 59: 695–700, 1993.

3 Lycopene: Food Sources, Properties, and Health

Richard S. Bruno, Robert E.C. Wildman,
and Steven J. Schwartz

CONTENTS

I. INTRODUCTION

Nearly 200 studies have examined the relationship between fruit and vegetable intake and cancers of the lung, colon, breast, cervix, esophagus, oral cavity, stomach, bladder, pancreas, and ovary.[1] Of these, a protective effect of fruit and vegetable consumption was found in 128 of 156 dietary studies. For most cancer sites, individuals with the lowest fruit and vegetable intake (at least the lower one fourth of the population) had approximately twice the risk of developing cancer compared with those with the highest intakes, even after controlling for potentially confounding factors.

There are innumerous compounds in fruits and vegetables that could individually or synergistically contribute to improvements in human health. Carotenoids are the pigment compounds that contribute to the coloring of fruits and vegetables. For example, lycopene (Figure 3.1) contributes the red pigment found in tomatoes.[2] Lycopene is one of nearly 700 carotenoids that have been

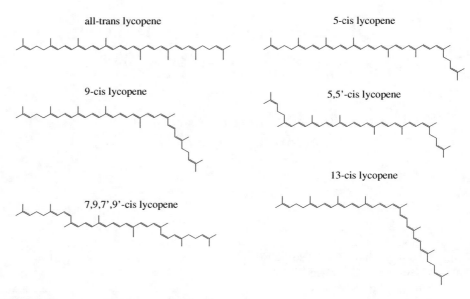

FIGURE 3.1 Structures of lycopene and select isomers.

characterized.[3,4] These compounds share common features including the polyisoprenoid structure and a series of centrally located double bonds.[3,4]

The deep red crystalline pigment produced by lycopene was first isolated from *Tamus communis* berries in 1873 by Hartsen.[5] Subsequently, in 1875, a crude mixture containing lycopene was obtained from tomatoes. However, not until 1903 was *lycopene* coined as it was determined that it had a unique absorption spectrum that differed from carotenes obtained from carrots. In the Western diet, lycopene is the most abundant nonprovitamin A carotenoid in the diet and human plasma.[6] Likewise, it can be readily detected in a variety of biological tissues. Continued studies on lycopene have led to our increased understanding of its potential role in human health.

II. DIETARY SOURCES OF LYCOPENE

In the U.S., it is estimated that lycopene contributes approximately 30% of the total carotenoid intake, which equates to about 3.7 mg/d.[7] For comparison, daily lycopene intake in Great Britain is 1.1 mg/d.[8] Lycopene is unique in that it is primarily represented by a single dietary source: tomatoes and tomato products[6] (Figure 3.2). This is further emphasized by the fact that plasma lycopene concentrations were not correlated with total fruit and vegetable consumption. Despite the numerous cis configurations that can arise with lycopene, lycopene from natural dietary sources is generally found in the all trans configuration (Figure 3.1).[9]

In the U.S., estimates indicated that tomatoes and tomato products contribute more than 80% of the lycopene content to the American diet.[10] Although the lycopene content is dependent on the stage of fruit ripening, fresh tomato contains 31–77 mg/kg.[11,12] Furthermore, tomato variety plays a factor into the lycopene content of the fruit. Redder varieties contain upwards of 50 mg/kg whereas yellower varieties contain 5 mg/kg. Even though tomatoes and tomato products are the predominant source of dietary lycopene (Figure 3.3), other foods including apricots, guava, rose hips, watermelon, papaya, and pink grapefruit also contribute to the dietary lycopene intake.[13]

Changes in carotenoid intake from 1987 to 1992 were evaluated in American adults.[14] Interestingly, during this period, mean lycopene intake increased 5–6% among adults 18–69 years old. Moreover, those with more education (>13 yr), higher incomes (>$20,000), and residing in the West had lycopene intakes that increased by 12.5, 8, and 16%, respectively.

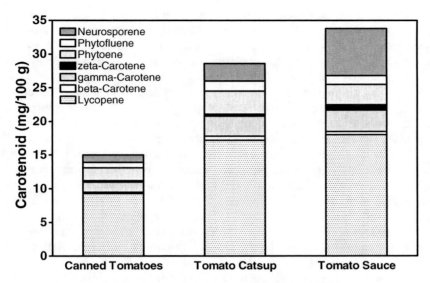

FIGURE 3.2 Carotenoid distribution of tomato products. (Data have been adapted from Johnson, E.J., Human studies on bioavailability and plasma response of lycopene, *Proc Soc Exp Biol Med*, 218(2): 115–20, 1998. With permission.)

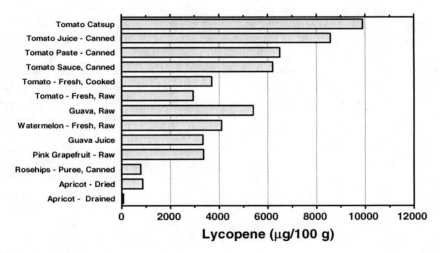

FIGURE 3.3 Lycopene content of select foods.

III. BIOAVAILABILITY, BIOLOGICAL DISTRIBUTION, AND METABOLISM

A. ABSORPTION AND BIOAVAILABILITY

In general, carotenoids found in foods are tightly bound within the food matrix, which may result in absorption difficulties and reduced bioavailability.[15] Because lycopene is lipophilic, its absorption is dependent upon the same processes that enable fat digestion and absorption such as solubilization by bile acids and digestive enzymes, and the incorporation into micelles.[6] The simultaneous presence of dietary fat in the small intestine is recognized as an important factor for the absorption of lycopene.[16] Therefore, any disease, drug, or dietary compound that contributes to lipid malabsorption or that disrupts the micelle-mediated process could potentially reduce the bioavailability of lycopene as well as other carotenoids. Optimal carotenoid absorption occurs if these compounds can be effectively extracted from the food matrix and subsequently incorporated into the lipid phase of the chyme present in the gut. Consequently, patients with cholestatis, who are known to have difficulties with fat absorption, have lower plasma concentrations of lipophilic nutrients including lycopene than healthy control patients.[17]

Dietary fat stimulates bile acid secretion, which assists in the formation of micelles. However, limited data exist regarding the optimal amount of fat required for lycopene absorption, but it has been suggested that only 3–5 g fat were required for optimal α- and β-carotene absorption.[16] Similar to other lipophilic substances, lycopene is likely absorbed through passive diffusion across the small intestines. Subsequently, it is packaged into chylomicrons and secreted into the lymphatic system. Lipoproteins appear to be the only carriers for lycopene because no binding proteins or carriers have been identified for lycopene.[18] The LDL fraction seems to be the predominant carrier for lycopene unlike lutein, zeaxanthin, canthaxanthin, and β-cryptoxanthin, which seem to be more equally distributed between LDL and HDL — which may be explained by the fact that lycopene is a hydrocarbon whereas these other carotenoids are xanthophylls.[19,20] Thus, plasma lycopene seems to peak in chylomicrons in 3–5 h after a meal [21] followed by LDL and HDL peaks occurring by 24–48 h.[20]

Potentially, other carotenoids could compete with lycopene during absorption. An investigation in which 60 mg each of all trans lycopene and β-carotene dispersed in corn oil were coingested with low carotenoid meals demonstrated that the absorption of lycopene was enhanced by β-carotene, but lycopene did not have any significant effect on β-carotene absorption.[22]

Many investigations have examined the bioavailability of lycopene from the food matrix. Fresh tomatoes or tomato paste containing 23 mg lycopene were ingested with 15 g corn oil to healthy participants on a single occasion.[23] The lycopene isomer patterns in both preparations were similar, but ingestion of tomato paste resulted in 2.5-fold higher total and all trans lycopene maximal concentrations and a 3.8-fold higher area under the curve compared to the ingestion of the fresh tomatoes, suggesting that lycopene derived from tomato paste may be more bioavailable.

A trial evaluated carotenoid bioavailability from a salad (containing ~9 mg lycopene) when no-fat (0 g fat), low-fat (6 g fat), or full-fat (28 g fat) salad dressings were also ingested.[21] Following the ingestion of the salad with no-fat dressing, the appearance of lycopene in chylomicrons was negligible. However, maximal plasma chylomicron lycopene concentrations during the low-fat and full-fat dressing trials increased to approximately 1.5 nmol/L and 3.0 nmol/L, respectively, demonstrating that increasing the fat content of a meal enhances the bioavailability of lycopene. Lycopene bioavailability from salsa (containing ~40 mg lycopene) was investigated in healthy participants who also simultaneously ingested avocado as a fat source.[24] When the salsa was consumed alone, a small increase of lycopene in the triglyceride-rich lipoproteins was observed. However, the simultaneous ingestion of avocado (150 g) resulted in a 4.4-fold increase in the area under the curve, which further supported the need of dietary fat for enhanced lycopene absorption.

Serum and tissue lycopene is > 50% cis lycopene whereas tomato and tomato product lycopene is predominately of the trans configuration. This disconnect led to the investigation into the bioavailability of lycopene cis isomers compared to all trans isomers.[25] Cannulated ferrets were used as a model for lycopene absorption. After feeding the ferrets a tomato extract containing 91% all trans lycopene (40 mg), the stomach, intestinal content, and lymph secretions were collected and analyzed for lycopene isomers. In the stomach and intestines, lycopene cis isomers accounted for 6.2–17.5% whereas in the lymph secretion, lycopene was found to be 77.4% cis lycopene. This suggested that cis isomers of lycopene were more bioavailable and the enterocyte may contribute in converting trans lycopene into cis isomers.

Androgen status has also been investigated as a factor that could potentially modulate lycopene bioavailability.[26] Intact and castrated F344 rats were fed lycopene (0–5 g/kg) for 8 weeks, and then tissues were analyzed for lycopene isomers. A plateau in tissue lycopene concentrations was observed at the 0.5 g/kg dose. However, as the lycopene dose increased, the proportion of hepatic cis lycopene also increased. With reduced androgen status (i.e., castration), hepatic lycopene concentrations were doubled compared to controls, but this effect did not extend to serum, adrenal, kidney, adipose, or lung tissue.

Because plasma lycopene is generally found in low quantities, it has been difficult to accurately assess changes in plasma concentrations. To overcome these limitations, stable isotope, deuterium labeled lycopene has been synthesized chemically or by growing hydroponic tomatoes with deuterium labeled water.[27] The advantage here is that participants can safely ingest the deuterated lycopene, and then plasma samples can be extracted for lycopene and analyzed by HPLC with mass spectrometry detection to differentiate between dietary lycopene and the deuterium labeled lycopene on the basis of the difference in molecular weight between the two forms. Utilizing these advances in technology, a pilot study (n = 2 participants or groups) was conducted to evaluate the differences in deuterium labeled lycopene bioavailability between capsules containing 11 μmol $^2H_{10}$ lycopene in 6 g corn oil vs. tomatoes (steamed and pureed) containing ~17 μmol $^2H_{10}$ lycopene. Following the ingestion of a meal containing 25% dietary fat, it appeared that the bioavailability of lycopene was about three times higher from the capsule compared to the tomatoes. Certainly, these novel methodologies will be used in future trials to more accurately evaluate lycopene bioavailability.

B. Effect of Food Processing

With most food-processing techniques, concerns of micronutrient destruction arise due to heating, ultraviolet light exposure, and mechanical processing. Degradation of lycopene during food processing would reduce its purported health benefits.[28] The potential for oxidation to occur during thermal processing (bleaching, retorting, or freezing) is of tremendous concern. Additionally, lycopene from foods predominately exists in the all trans configurations (Figure 3.1), but food processing could increase its isomerization to cis isomers. Furthermore, lycopene from powdered or dehydrated tomato products has poor stability, unless the product is carefully processed and sealed in a package containing inert gas.

In comparison to β-carotene, lycopene was relatively resistant to isomerization during heat-induced food processing of tomato products.[9] Moreover, the percentage of fat, solids, and severity of heat treatment did not contribute to the formation of lycopene isomers. Similar findings were also reported in another investigation when lycopene stability and bioavailability were investigated.[29] In this trial, lycopene from heated tomato juice (boiled with 1% corn oil for 60 min) did not differ from unprocessed juice. However, lycopene bioavailability, as measured by changes in plasma lycopene concentrations, was enhanced two- to threefold by heating of the juice compared to relatively no plasma changes without heat processing, suggesting the possibility that thermal processing promotes tissue cell wall degradation and release of lycopene.

Interestingly, despite concerns of thermal processing on lycopene stability, heating tomatoes at 80°C for 2, 15, and 30 min increased the content of all trans lycopene from 2.01 ± 0.04 mg trans lycopene/g tomato to 3.11 ± 0.04, 5.45 ± 0.02, and 5.32 ± 0.05 mg of trans lycopene/g of tomato, respectively, suggesting that heating increased the bioaccessibility of lycopene.[30] Furthermore, total antioxidant activity significantly increased with heat processing despite the fact that vitamin C was significantly reduced by heat processing.

Tomato peels that are often discarded during food processing are an important source of dietary lycopene. Recognizing this, a trial was designed to evaluate lycopene bioavailability from tomato paste enriched with 6% tomato peel (ETP) compared to classically prepared tomato paste (CTP).[31] It was determined *in vitro*, using Caco-2 cells, that 75% more lycopene from the ETP treatment was absorbed compared to the CTP. In eight healthy male participants who ingested ETP and CTP on separate occasions, the lycopene response assessed in chylomicrons was 34% greater with ETP compared to CTP, but this was not statistically significant (p = 0.09).

C. FACTORS ALTERING ABSORPTION AND PLASMA CONCENTRATIONS

As mentioned previously, lycopene from food is mostly in the all trans configuration. Food processing did not seem to increase lycopene cis-isomerization, but plasma from participants who ingested all trans lycopene had significantly higher concentrations of 9-cis and 13-cis lycopene isomers,[29] suggesting that cis-isomers may be preferentially absorbed. However, since cis-isomers were not formed with heating, it has been speculated that a yet-to-be-determined *in vivo* mechanism must have increased the isomerization to enhance lycopene absorption.[9,29]

Sucrose polyester, or Olestra™, is known to reduce plasma or serum concentrations of lipophilic nutrients, including lycopene. The ingestion of Olestra™, fed at 3 or 12.4 g/d in double-blind, placebo-controlled, crossover studies resulted in reductions of plasma lycopene concentrations by 0.12 μmol/L (38%) and 0.14 μmol/L (52%), respectively.[32] In a 1-year, randomized, double-blind, placebo-controlled investigation, daily ingestion of Olestra™ resulted in a 24% reduction in plasma lycopene.[33] While Olestra™ ingestion seems to have profound effects on lycopene and carotenoid bioavailability, it is likely that these observed effects may be somewhat exaggerated because foods containing Olestra™ are not typically consumed with foods rich in carotenoids.

Dietary fiber is known to reduce the bioavailability of β-carotene.[34] Because lycopene is a hydrocarbon like β-carotene, the potential for these effects were investigated for lycopene.[35] Healthy women ingested a mixture of carotenoids and α-tocopherol with a standard meal containing no fiber or enriched with pectin, guar, alginate, cellulose, or wheat bran. All of these fibers significantly reduced 24-h area under the curves for lycopene by 40–74%.

Aging could potentially effect the efficiency of lycopene absorption. In young (20–35 yr) and older (60–75 yr) adults who consumed three different meals containing 40 g triglycerides and vegetables containing 30 mg lycopene, a 40% reduction in chylomicron or triglyceride adjusted lycopene concentration was observed among the older subjects.[36]

Additional research to define the relations among carotenoid intake, absorption, tissue distribution, and biological effects is clearly necessary to address the potential health benefits of tomato products and lycopene consumption.[37]

D. BIOLOGICAL DISTRIBUTION

The ability of lycopene to reduce the risk of or prevent chronic disease could be limited by its uptake and biological distribution (Figure 3.4). Ferrets and F344 rats were supplemented with 4.6 mg/kg body weight of lycopene from a tomato oleoresin-corn oil mixture for 9 weeks, and tissues were collected for analysis.[38] Ferrets' liver lycopene content was the highest with 933 nmol/kg wet weight followed by intestine, prostate, and stomach with 73, 12.7, and 9.3 nmol/kg wet weight, respectively. Rats had significantly higher lycopene concentrations compared to the ferrets with lycopene concentrations (nmol/kg weight wet) in liver, intestine, stomach, prostate, and testis of 14213, 3125, 78.6, 24, and 3.9, respectively.

Serum lycopene concentrations in men were 0.6–1.9 nmol/L comprised of 27–42% all trans lycopene and 58–73% cis lycopene isomers.[39] In benign prostate tissues, cis lycopene isomers are somewhat higher (79–88%) compared to plasma but importantly, lycopene is present in biological concentrations that could potentially reduce disease risk. In men with clinical stage T1 or T2 prostate adenocarcinoma, prostate biopsies were analyzed for lycopene prior to and after 3-week ingestion of tomato sauce (30 mg lycopene/d).[40] Serum lycopene doubled after dietary intervention whereas total lycopene in prostate tissue tripled. Prior to dietary intervention, prostate tissue all trans lycopene was 12.4% and increased significantly to 22.7% after 3 weeks, but serum all trans lycopene only increased by 2.8%.

Breast milk may also contribute to lycopene status of infants. In lactating women, randomized to low-lycopene or fresh tomatoes and tomato sauce (50 mg lycopene/d) for three days, a significant

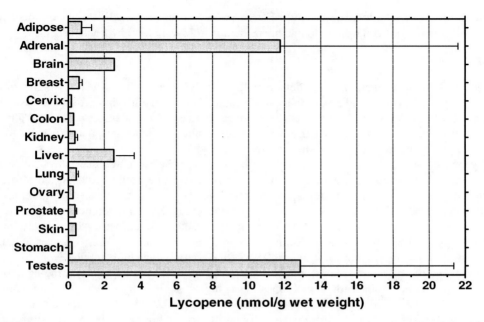

FIGURE 3.4 Lycopene concentrations from select human tissues. Lycopene concentrations from adipose, adrenal, brain, breast, cervix, colon, kidney, liver, lung, ovary, prostate, skin, stomach, and testes. (Adapted from References 10,39,42,83,92–98.)

increase in breast milk lycopene was observed with the 3-d consumption of tomatoes or tomato sauce but not with the low-lycopene diet.[41]

E. METABOLISM

Little is known regarding the metabolism of lycopene. From breast milk, 34-carotenoids, comprised of 13 geometrical isomers and 8 metabolites, were separated and quantified by HPLC with photo-diode array and mass spectrometry detection.[42] Two oxidation products of lycopene were determined as epimeric 2,6-cyclolycopene-1,5-diols and contained a novel five-membered-ring end group. Lycopene metabolism has also been investigated, following the isolation of mitochondria of the rat mucosa.[43] When mitochondria were incubated with lipoxygenase, the increased production of lycopene metabolites occurred. These products were identified as both cleavage and oxidation products. The likely cleavage products were 3-keto-apo-13-lycopene or 6,10, 14-trimethyl-12-one-3,5,7,9,13-pentadecapentaene-2-one and 3,4-dehydro-5,6-dihydro-15,15′-apo-lycopenal, whereas the oxidation products were 2-apo-5,8-lycopenal-furanoxide, lycopene-5, 6, 5′, 6′-diepoxide, lyco-pene-5,8-furanoxide isomer, lycopene-5,8-epoxide isomer, and 3-keto-lycopene-5′,8′-furanoxide. Further investigations are still warranted to determine if these metabolites can be found in humans consuming a lycopene rich diet. Determination of lycopene oxidation products *in vivo* may also require improvements in analytical tools and techniques.

IV. ANTIOXIDANT PROPERTIES

It has been proposed that the antioxidant capability of carotenoids are the basis for their protective effects against cancer.[44] Whereas lycopene has clear antioxidant properties *in vitro*, no clear or specific evidence has indicated similar properties in humans. Some of the best evidence for its protective effect is observed when lycopene is consumed from a diet rich in lycopene such as from tomatoes or tomato products. Most of the antioxidant benefits observed with lycopene are likely attributed to its acyclic structure, its numerous conjugated double bonds, and its relatively high hydrophobicity.[10]

A. IN VITRO

Various *in vitro* investigations have demonstrated that lycopene is an effective singlet oxygen quencher, has an excellent radical-trapping ability, and possesses a high ability to scavenge peroxyl radicals. Singlet oxygen by definition is not a free radical because it does not possess an unpaired electron.[45] However, it is highly reactive, can damage various biomolecules, and is usually formed through light-dependent or photosentization reactions.[10]

Lycopene may quench singlet oxygen through physical or chemical processes. Physical quenching is typically more effective and occurs the majority of the time. In this process, the carotenoid remains undamaged after the transfer of energy from singlet oxygen to the carotenoid, thus enabling itself to undergo additional cycles of singlet oxygen quenching. During this process, singlet oxygen becomes a ground-state oxygen and lycopene in the excited triplet state. Alternatively, during chemical quenching, a bleaching or decomposition of the carotenoid occurs. However, this latter process is believed to account for only < 0.05% of the overall quenching activity.[20]

Compared to other antioxidants, lycopene had the highest singlet oxygen scavenging ability.[46] Its quenching rate constant with singlet oxygen was higher ($k_q = 31 \times 10^9$ M^{-1} s^{-1}) than that of β-carotene ($k_q = 14 \times 10^9$ M^{-1} s^{-1}), albumin-bound bilirubin ($k_q = 3.2 \times 10^9$ M^{-1} s^{-1}), and α-tocopherol ($k_q = 0.3 \times 10^9$ M^{-1} s^{-1}). Similar results were found in another investigation, which demonstrated that lycopene had the highest singlet oxygen quenching rate compared to other compounds: γ-carotene, astaxanthin, canthaxanthin, α-carotene, β-carotene, bixin, zeaxanthin, lutein, bilirubin, biliverdin, tocopherols, and thiols.[47] The higher singlet oxygen quenching rates by lycopene may be explained, in part, by the fact that of all C_{40} carotenoids, lycopene has two additional double bonds, which may improve its chemical reactivity.[20] Interestingly, plasma lycopene occurs in the lowest concentration compared to these other singlet oxygen quenchers but has the highest singlet oxygen quenching capacity. Thus, on the basis of physiological concentrations, lycopene likely has comparable effects to these other compounds.

The imbalance between free radicals and antioxidant defenses, in favor of the former, may result in oxidative stress. Physiologically, innumerous free radicals exist such as superoxide, hydroxyl radical, peroxynitrite, and peroxyl radicals. Concern regarding these free radicals stems from the fact that they may react with biomolecules such as DNA, proteins, and lipids, and contribute to or possibly cause free radical mediated diseases such as cancer, cardiovascular disease, or diabetes. It is believed that lycopene, as well as other carotenoids, may provide protection against these deleterious species, such that chronic disease risk is reduced via the prevention of oxidation of these biomolecules.[48,49]

Cigarette smoke exposure depletes lycopene from plasma, suggesting an antioxidant role in the protection against free radicals found in cigarette smoke.[50] The role of lycopene has also been investigated in experimental models of cataract formation.[51] Supplementation with lycopene *in vitro* improved glutathione and reduced malondialdehyde concentrations, and also improved enzymatic activities of superoxide dismutase, catalase, and glutathione-S-transferase. Further efforts will be necessary to determine the role of lycopene in human eye health. In addition to reacting with reactive oxygen species, lycopene may react with reactive nitrogen species such as peroxynitrite, the product of the reaction between nitric oxide and superoxide.[52] A variety of carotenoids in LDL were treated with peroxynitrite and prevented the formation of rhodamine 123 from dihydro-rhodamine 123 (caused by peroxynitrite).[53] Lycopene, α-carotene, and β-carotene were more effective than oxocarotenoids and may indicate a role for scavenging peroxynitrite *in vivo*.

B. IN VIVO

Modulation of the magnitude of oxidative stress in humans is an area of growing interest since it is speculated that reductions in it would promote optimal health. Resistance to LDL oxidation was determined in healthy individuals who were instructed to follow a lycopene-free diet for 1 week and then randomized to various tomato products (35 ± 1, 23 ± 1, or 25 ±1 mg lycopene/d) for 15 d.[54] During the wash-out periods, plasma lycopene concentrations decreased by 35%. After 15 d consumption of tomato products, total lycopene concentrations increased significantly in all groups compared to their concentrations after the wash-out period, and the *ex vivo* lipoprotein oxidation lag period increased significantly, suggesting a protective role of lycopene from tomato products.

Healthy male and female participants (n = 17) underwent a two-week washout period by following a low lycopene containing diet.[55] Subsequently, they were instructed to follow a high lycopene-containing diet (30 mg/d) for 4 weeks. Serum lycopene significantly increased from 181.8 ± 31 to 684.7 ± 113.9 nmol/L, which paralleled significant increases in plasma total antioxidant potential and significant reductions in lipid and protein oxidation. Thus, it was suggested that diets high in lycopene from tomato products can improve plasma lycopene status while reducing oxidative stress.

In an intervention trial, 19 healthy participants ingested lycopene daily from tomato juice, tomato sauce, and tomato oleoresin for 1 week each, and blood samples were collected at the end of each treatment.[56] Plasma lycopene increased greater than twofold and lipid peroxidation markers were significantly reduced, suggesting a protective effect by the high lycopene diet.

Inflammation measured by C-reactive protein concentrations, were inversely associated with lycopene and other plasma antioxidants after adjustments for age, sex, race or ethnicity, education, cotinine concentration, body mass index, leisure-time physical activity, and aspirin use, suggesting that lycopene and other antioxidants may be depleted with chronic oxidative stress or inflammation.[57] In lymphocytes harvested after participants ingested a lycopene-rich diet, it was demonstrated that lymphocytes were more protective against nitrogen dioxide radical and singlet oxygen treatments.[58]

V. LYCOPENE AND CHRONIC DISEASE

A. Epidemiological Studies

A growing body of literature suggests a protective effect of lycopene, often provided from a high tomato or tomato product diet, in the risk reduction of chronic diseases. Extensive efforts have been taken to evaluate the association between plasma antioxidants and mortality.[59] In statistical models adjusted for age, plasma cholesterol, time-dependent smoking, treatment arm, study site and gender, only plasma lycopene emerged as significantly inversely associated with total mortality (hazard ratio = 0.53).

A review of epidemiological data from 72 studies indicated an inverse relationship between tomato and tomato product consumption and a reduced cancer risk for 57 of these studies.[60] Of these 57 studies, 35 were found to be statistically significant for the inverse relationship between lycopene or tomato consumption and cancer at a defined anatomical site. Interestingly, the strongest relationships were found for cancers of the prostate, lung, and stomach, whereas lesser relationships were determined for cancers of the cervix, colon, pancreas, esophagus, digestive tract, and breast. Because these are observational studies, no cause–effect relationship can be established, but they have paved the way for subsequent animal and human trials to evaluate the efficacy of lycopene and tomato product in the prevention of chronic disease.

Further illustrating the role of lycopene and tomatoes in human health, epidemiological data indicated that the increased consumption of lycopene from tomato products was significantly associated with a lower risk of prostate cancer.[61] Analysis of data from the Health Professionals Follow-Up Study suggested that lycopene intake was associated with a relative risk of 0.84 when high vs. low quintiles of dietary intake were compared, but the consumption of tomato sauce had greater protective effects. Interestingly, foods that accounted for 82% of lycopene intake (tomatoes, tomato sauce, tomato juice, and pizza) were inversely associated with prostate cancer risk (relative risk = 0.65) when >10 servings/week were consumed compared to 1.5 servings/week.[62] These protective effects also persisted for advanced prostate cancer (relative risk = 0.47). In the analysis of lifestyle questionnaires from Seventh-Day Adventist men, it was determined that higher consumption of tomatoes as well as beans, lentils, peas, raisin, dates, and other dried fruits were significantly associated with reduced prostate cancer risk.[63] A recent review summarized the epidemiological literature on tomato products, lycopene, and prostate cancer.[64]

Carotenoids may also modulate the risk of developing lung cancer.[65] In a prospective investigation, carotenoid intakes (α-carotene, β-carotene, lutein, lycopene, and β-cryptoxanthin) were assessed by food frequency questionnaire to determine if their consumption was associated with the reduction of lung cancer. In the pooled analysis of more than 124,000 participants, lycopene and α-carotene intakes were significantly associated with a lower risk of cancer. However, the lowest risk was observed among individuals who consumed the greatest variety of carotenoids.

The relationship between breast cancer risk and dietary nutrients has also been investigated.[66] Using food frequency questionnaires to evaluate dietary history, it was determined that odds ratios (after adjustment for age, education, parity, menopausal status, BMI, and energy and alcohol intake) between total carotenoid (OR = 0.42) or lycopene (OR = 0.43) intakes were inversely related with breast cancer risk. Interestingly, when all nutrients inversely associated with risk-reductions in breast cancer were included in the statistical model, only lycopene and vitamin C intakes continued to have a significant inverse relationship with breast cancer.

Similar findings have also been reported with regard to pancreatic cancer risk.[67] In a case-controlled study of confirmed pancreatic cancer cases and population based controls, it was determined that lycopene intake, particularly from tomatoes, was significantly associated with a 31% reduction in pancreatic cancer risk when highest and lowest quartiles intake were compared. Similar results were observed for β-carotene and total carotenoids, but these effects were only apparent among individuals who never smoked.

B. Tissue and Cell Culture

Numerous *in vitro* studies have been conducted to determine the mechanisms of action of lycopene in modulating disease risk. Lycopene, compared to α- and β-carotenes, more strongly inhibited cellular proliferation in human endometrial, mammary, and lung cancer cell lines.[68] This effect was observed within 24 h of incubation with lycopene and persisted for 3 d. These investigators also demonstrated that lycopene suppressed insulin-like growth factor-I-stimulated growth, suggesting a possibility for lycopene in the modulation of the autocrine and paracrine systems.

The effect of lycopene on the proliferation of human prostate cells (LnCaP) has also been investigated.[69] Lycopene, administered to the media at final concentrations of 10^{-6} and 10^{-5} M, significantly reduced cell growth after 48, 72, and 96 h by 24.4–42.8%. These effects were subsequently tested at lower lycopene doses (10^{-9} and 10^{-7} M) with similar success. Lycopene, as a chemopreventive agent, may also induce phase II detoxification enzymes.[70] In transiently transfected cancer cells, lycopene (compared to other carotenoids tested in this system) more strongly activated the reported genes fused with the antioxidant response element.

High concentrations of insulin-like growth factor-1 are associated with increased risk for breast and prostate cancers.[71] In mammary cancer cells, lycopene inhibited growth stimulation by insulin-like growth factor-1 without inducing apoptosis or necrosis. However, treatment of cells with lycopene decreased insulin-like growth factor-1 stimulation of tyrosine phosphororylation of insulin receptor substrate 1 as well as the binding capacity of AP-1. Furthermore, lycopene slowed cell cycle progression. Thus, the inhibitory effects of lycopene on mammary cancer cells was not due to its possible toxicity to cells, but rather due to its interference with insulin-like growth factor-1 receptor signaling and cell cycle progression.

Similarly, work has been conducted with the leukemia cell line HL-60.[72] Lycopene dose dependently decreased cell growth, inhibited cell cycle progression in the G0 and G1 phase, as well as induced cell differentiation. Interestingly, a synergistic effect of lycopene and vitamin D

(1,25-dihydroxyvitamin D_3) was found for cell proliferation whereas an additive effect was found on cell cycle progression. Thus, lycopene alone or with vitamin D may have potent cancer chemo-preventive properties.

Because lycopene has repeatedly demonstrated a capacity to inhibit the growth of cancerous cell lines, including prostate cancer cells, an investigation was conducted to determine if lycopene has similar effects in normal prostate cells.[73] Treating cells with up to 5 μM lycopene dose dependently inhibited cell growth and significantly increased cell cycle arrest in the G0 and G1 phase. This suggested that lycopene may have a role in the prevention of early prostate cancer events such as prostate hypertrophy or hyperplasia.

C. ANIMAL TRIALS

In recent years, numerous animal trials have been conducted to determine a biological role of lycopene in disease. Rats pretreated for 5 d with lycopene (10mg/kg body weight) had significant reductions in hepatic oxidative DNA damage and lipid peroxidation.[74] Using a DMBA-induced (7,12-dimethylbenz[a]anthracene) buccal pouch model of carcinogenesis induction, it was determined that lycopene significantly decreased the formation of lipid hydroperoxides while increasing glutathione and the activities of hepatic transformation enzymes such as glutathione S-transferase.[75]

Lung cancer has one of the highest incidence rates in American men and women. Thus, treatment of lycopene was tested in a mouse multiorgan carcinogenesis model.[76] After 32 weeks of treatment, the incidence of lung adenomas plus carcinomas was significantly reduced with lycopene treatment, a finding made only in male mice. Unfortunately, no significant effects attributed to lycopene treatment were found for liver, colon, or kidney. Further studies have investigated lycopene in models of cigarette smoke-induced lung cancer.[77] Ferrets subjected to cigarette smoke exposure along with treatment with lycopene had higher concentrations of plasma insulin-like growth factor-binding protein-3 and a lower ratio of insulin-like growth factor 1:insulin-like growth factor-binding protein-3, compared to ferrets exposed to smoke alone. The smoke-exposed ferrets had lower concentrations of lycopene compared to the lycopene supplemented animals and lycopene treatment inhibited squamous lung cell metaplasia and prevented phosphorylation of BAD (a member of the BH3-only subfamily of Bcl-2). Thus, the anticancer properties of lycopene may not be associated with its antioxidant properties but possible through its ability to regulate factors that could promote apoptosis and inhibit cell proliferation.

The effect of lycopene on prostate cancer has also been assessed in a rat carcinogenesis model.[78] Rats were fed tomato powder, lycopene beadlets, or a control diet while being treated with N-methyl-N-nitrosourea and testosterone to induce prostate cancer. Risk of death from prostate cancer was lower among rats fed the tomato powder compared to the control diet. Interestingly, mortality was similar between the control animals and those supplemented with lycopene. Thus, the authors speculated that perhaps tomato products contained compounds in addition to lycopene that could modify prostate cancer risk. Another rat study investigated the effects of lycopene on prostate cancer risk in which rats were supplemented with 200 ppm lycopene for up to 8 weeks.[79] Significant accumulations of lycopene were found in all four prostate lobes, but the lateral lobe had the highest concentration compared to the other three lobes. Lycopene supplementation significantly reduced gene expression for select androgen-metabolizing enzymes and androgen targets and decreased the lateral lobe expression of insulin-like growth factor-1. Significant reductions in transcript levels of proinflammatory cytokines and immunoglobins were also observed with lycopene supplementation. Thus, direct effects of lycopene supplementation on reducing prostate cancer risk were found.

Some data support the role of lycopene in breast cancer prevention as well.[80] In mice supplemented with lycopene, mammary tumor development was inhibited, which was associated with decreased mammary gland activity of thymidylate synthetase and decreased serum concentrations of free fatty acids and prolactin. These studies highlight the need for additional research to establish the role of tomatoes as part of the diet or lycopene as a supplement in cancer prevention.[81]

D. HUMAN INVESTIGATIONS

1. Cancer

Epidemiological tissue culture and animal trials have indicated some beneficial role of lycopene in health. Naturally, these health benefits can only be extended to humans if they are directly tested in humans. Men with confirmed prostate cancer who were scheduled for prostatectomy were provided lycopene (consumed from tomato sauce) for 3 weeks.[82] Compared to baseline serum concentrations and prostate biopsies, lycopene increased nearly 2- and 3-fold respectively in the serum and prostate tissue following the controlled diet. Furthermore, serum PSA and leukocyte DNA damage significantly decreased by 17.5 and 21.3%. Thus, at least in this short-term trial, administration of lycopene rich foods significantly improved prostate lycopene concentrations and simultaneously improved markers of prostate cancer risk. In 26 men with newly diagnosed prostate cancer, half were randomized to receive lycopene (15 mg, twice daily) three weeks prior to radical prostatectomy in order to assess the beneficial effect of lycopene alone.[83] In the men receiving lycopene, PSA decreased by 18% whereas PSA levels rose 14% in the nonsupplemented group. Thus, in contrast to other studies, lycopene supplementation alone may exhibit important benefits.

The relationship between breast cancer risk and plasma carotenoids was assessed using a nested case-referent design.[84] Plasma samples from 201 cases and 290 referents were obtained at study enrollment, and breast cancer incidence was identified via cancer registries. None of the carotenoids measured were related to the risk of developing breast cancer. However, among premenopausal women only, there was a significant inverse relationship between breast cancer and plasma lycopene. Therefore, it seems possible that lycopene may reduce the risk of breast cancer among young, premenopausal women.

Carotenoids and their relationship to cancers of the digestive tract have been evaluated in recent years. In Uruguay, a case-control study was conducted in which 238 cases and 491 hospitalized controls were matched on the basis of age, sex, residence, and urban or rural status. After adjustments for total energy intake, a significant reduction in risk for cancer of the upper digestive tract was found with tomato intake and tomato sauce. Further analysis revealed that lycopene was also strongly associated with a reduced risk of 0.22. Similarly, lower carotenoid intakes have been associated with an increased risk for colorectal cancer. Thus, carotenoid concentrations were evaluated in colorectal adenomas.[85] Comparing colorectal adenoma biopsies to samples obtained from colons of control patients, it was determined that control patients had the highest colon carotenoid concentrations. Although this was not an intervention study, this suggests the possibility that carotenoid status, including lycopene, may be involved in the pathogenesis of colon cancer. To evaluate the role of dietary nutrients in bladder cancer risk, serum was collected from 25,802 individuals residing in Maryland.[86] In the 12-year follow-up period, 35 bladder cancer cases arose and the serum samples were compared between these cases and two matched controls. Although selenium concentrations were significantly lower among the cases compared to controls, a borderline significant reduction in lycopene was also observed. Clearly, additional work is warranted to further assess lycopene in this pathology.

Limited data exists regarding lycopene and skin cancer risk. In a placebo-controlled study that evaluated the effects of β-carotene ingestion on skin and plasma β-carotene and lycopene concentrations, it was determined that β-carotene ingestion had no effect in reducing plasma or skin lycopene levels.[87] These participants were then subjected to UV-light exposure on the forearm which caused a 31–46% reduction in skin lycopene concentration compared to adjacent nonexposed skin whereas skin β-carotene concentrations did not change. Thus, although this study was too short to assess the role of lycopene on the risk of developing skin cancer, it suggested that lycopene may have a protective benefit against UV-light mediated damage.

A National Cancer Institute workshop during 2005 entitled Promises and Perils of Lycopene/Tomato Supplementation and Cancer Prevention identified research priorities and recommendations for future cancer prevention research.

2. Heart Disease

Heart disease is the leading cause of death in the U.S., accounting for nearly 700,000 deaths annually.[88] The recognition of the involvement of oxidative stress in heart disease has spawned innumerous trials to determine if modulation in oxidative stress can improve heart disease risk. Oxidation of LDL is the leading mechanism involved in the etiology of coronary heart disease and atherosclerosis.[89] Thus, antioxidants may have an effect in reducing LDL oxidation and possibly attenuating the risk of developing heart disease. With regard to the role of lycopene in the pathogenesis of heart disease, healthy participants have been supplemented with lycopene in the form of tomato juice, tomato sauce, or soft gel capsules for one week, and LDL oxidation was compared between them and nonsupplemented controls. However, it should be noted that this is an effect that has not been consistently found. In another trial, β-carotene but not lycopene significantly inhibited LDL oxidation.[90] To evaluate the relationship between antioxidant status and acute myocardial infarction, a case-control study was conducted in which myocardial infarction cases and matched controls were recruited.[91] Following infarction, a biopsy was obtained from adipose tissue and analyzed for carotenoids and tocopherols. By conditional logistic regression modeling, controlling for age, BMI, socioeconomic status, smoking, hypertension, and family history, it was determined that lycopene was highly protective (OR = 0.52).

VI. CONCLUSIONS

Data regarding the specific health benefits of lycopene are still limited. To date, no health agencies have formulated dietary recommendations for lycopene because it has yet to be recognized as an essential nutrient. Continued effects will enable the determination if it, or the tomato products in which it is typically found, are the responsible entity for the reduction of chronic disease. Therefore, it is likely premature to recommend a lycopene supplement to a broad population as a dietary strategy to improve health, but individuals should be advised to improve their fruit and vegetable consumption. Fruits and vegetables are rich with innumerable chemical compounds including vitamins, minerals, and other potentially helpful phytochemicals. Furthermore, their consumption leads to higher intakes of dietary fiber while providing lower amounts of dietary fat. However, recall from this chapter that small amounts of dietary fat are necessary to facilitate lycopene absorption. Continued research into the mechanisms by which lycopene and other carotenoids prevent chronic diseases is warranted in order to formulate dietary recommendations. Lastly, additional data are integral to determine the synergistic effects of phytochemicals present in the diet and how they may protect humans from chronic disease.

REFERENCES

1. Block, G., Patterson, B., and Subar, A., Fruit, vegetables, and cancer prevention: a review of the epidemiological evidence, *Nutr Cancer*, 18(1): 1–29, 1992.
2. Heber, D., Vegetables, fruits and phytoestrogens in the prevention of diseases, *J Postgrad Med*, 50(2): 145–9, 2004.
3. Olson, J.A. and Krinsky, N.I., Introduction: the colorful, fascinating world of the carotenoids: important physiologic modulators, *FASEB J*, 9(15): 1547–50, 1995.
4. Britton, G., Structure and properties of carotenoids in relation to function, *FASEB J*, 9(15): 1551–8, 1995.

5. Nguyen, M.L. and Schwartz, S.J., Lycopene: chemical and biological properties, *Food Technol.*, 53(2): 38–45, 1999.

6. Johnson, E.J., Human studies on bioavailability and plasma response of lycopene, *Proc Soc Exp Biol Med*, 218(2): 115–20, 1998.

7. Forman, M.R., Lanza, E., Yong, L.C., Holden, J.M., Graubard, B.I., Beecher, G.R., Meltiz, M., Brown, E.D., and Smith, J.C., The correlation between two dietary assessments of carotenoid intake and plasma carotenoid concentrations: application of a carotenoid food-composition database, *Am J Clin Nutr*, 58(4): 519–24, 1993.

8. Scott, K.J., Thurnham, D.I., Hart, D.J., Bingham, S.A., and Day, K., The correlation between the intake of lutein, lycopene and beta-carotene from vegetables and fruits, and blood plasma concentrations in a group of women aged 50–65 years in the U.K., *Br J Nutr*, 75(3): 409–18, 1996.

9. Nguyen, M.L. and Schwartz, S.J., Lycopene stability during food processing, *Proc Soc Exp Biol Med*, 218(2): 101–5, 1998.

10. Clinton, S.K., Lycopene: chemistry, biology, and implications for human health and disease, *Nutr Rev*, 56(2 Pt. 1): 35–51, 1998.

11. Bramley, P.M., Regulation of carotenoid formation during tomato fruit ripening and development, *J Exp Bot*, 53(377): 2107–13, 2002.

12. Nguyen, M. and Schwartz, S., Lycopene, in *Natural Food Colorants: Science and Technology*, G. Lauro and F. Francis, Eds., Marcel Dekker: New York. 2000, pp. 153–192.

13. Mangels, A.R., Holden, J.M., Beecher, G.R., Forman, M.R., and Lanza, E., Carotenoid content of fruits and vegetables: an evaluation of analytic data, *J Am Diet Assoc*, 93(3): 284–96, 1993.

14. Nebeling, L.C., Forman, M.R., Graubard, B.I., and Snyder, R.A., Changes in carotenoid intake in the U.S.: the 1987 and 1992 National Health Interview Surveys, *J Am Diet Assoc*, 97(9): 991–6, 1997.

15. Zhou, J.R., Gugger, E.T., and Erdman, J.W., Jr., The crystalline form of carotenes and the food matrix in carrot root decrease the relative bioavailability of beta- and alpha-carotene in the ferret model, *J Am Coll Nutr*, 15(1): 84–91, 1996.

16. Roodenburg, A.J., Leenen, R., van het Hof, K.H., Weststrate, J.A., and Tijburg, L.B., Amount of fat in the diet affects bioavailability of lutein esters but not of alpha-carotene, beta-carotene, and vitamin E in humans, *Am J Clin Nutr*, 71(5): 1187–93, 2000.

17. Floreani, A., Baragiotta, A., Martines, D., Naccarato, R., and D'Odorico, A., Plasma antioxidant levels in chronic cholestatic liver diseases, *Aliment Pharmacol Ther*, 14(3): 353–8, 2000.

18. Parker, R.S., Absorption, metabolism, and transport of carotenoids, *FASEB J*, 10(5): 542–51, 1996.

19. Goulinet, S. and Chapman, M.J., Plasma LDL and HDL subspecies are heterogenous in particle content of tocopherols and oxygenated and hydrocarbon carotenoids. Relevance to oxidative resistance and atherogenesis, *Arterioscler Thromb Vasc Biol*, 17(4): 786–96, 1997.

20. Sies, H. and Stahl, W., Lycopene: antioxidant and biological effects and its bioavailability in the human, *Proc Soc Exp Biol Med*, 218(2): 121–4, 1998.

21. Brown, M.J., Ferruzzi, M.G., Nguyen, M.L., Cooper, D.A., Eldridge, A.L., Schwartz, S.J., and White, W.S., Carotenoid bioavailability is higher from salads ingested with full-fat than with fat-reduced salad dressings as measured with electrochemical detection, *Am J Clin Nutr*, 80(2): 396–403, 2004.

22. Johnson, E.J., Qin, J., Krinsky, N.I., and Russell, R.M., Ingestion by men of a combined dose of beta-carotene and lycopene does not affect the absorption of beta-carotene but improves that of lycopene, *J Nutr*, 127(9): 1833–7, 1997.

23. Gartner, C., Stahl, W., and Sies, H., Lycopene is more bioavailable from tomato paste than from fresh tomatoes, *Am J Clin Nutr*, 66(1): 116–22, 1997.

24. Unlu, N.Z., Bohn, T., Clinton, S.K., and Schwartz, S.J., Carotenoid absorption from salad and salsa by humans is enhanced by the addition of avocado or avocado oil, *J Nutr*, 135(3): 431–6, 2005.

25. Boileau, A.C., Merchen, N.R., Wasson, K., Atkinson, C.A., and Erdman, J.W., Jr., Cis-lycopene is more bioavailable than trans-lycopene in vitro and in vivo in lymph-cannulated ferrets, *J Nutr*, 129(6): 1176–81, 1999.

26. Erdman, J.W., Jr., How do nutritional and hormonal status modify the bioavailability, uptake, and distribution of different isomers of lycopene? *J Nutr*, 135(8): 2046S–7S, 2005.

27. Tang, G., Ferreira, A.L., Grusak, M.A., Qin, J., Dolnikowski, G.G., Russell, R.M., and Krinsky, N.I., Bioavailability of synthetic and biosynthetic deuterated lycopene in humans, *J Nutr Biochem*, 16(4): 229–35, 2005.

28. Shi, J. and Le Maguer, M., Lycopene in tomatoes: chemical and physical properties affected by food processing, *Crit Rev Food Sci Nutr*, 40(1): 1–42, 2000.
29. Stahl, W. and Sies, H., Uptake of lycopene and its geometrical isomers is greater from heat-processed than from unprocessed tomato juice in humans, *J Nutr*, 122(11): 2161–6, 1992.
30. Dewanto, V., Wu, X., Adom, K.K., and Liu, R.H., Thermal processing enhances the nutritional value of tomatoes by increasing total antioxidant activity, *J Agric Food Chem*, 50(10): 3010–4, 2002.
31. Reboul, E., Borel, P., Mikail, C., Abou, L., Charbonnier, M., Caris-Veyrat, C., Goupy, P., Portugal, H., Lairon, D., and Amiot, M.J., Enrichment of tomato paste with 6% tomato peel increases lycopene and beta-carotene bioavailability in men, *J Nutr*, 135(4): 790–4, 2005.
32. Weststrate, J.A. and van het Hof, K.H., Sucrose polyester and plasma carotenoid concentrations in healthy subjects, *Am J Clin Nutr*, 62(3): 591–7, 1995.
33. Broekmans, W.M., Klopping-Ketelaars, I.A., Weststrate, J.A., Tijburg, L.B., van Poppel, G., Vink, A.A., Berendschot, T.T., Bots, M.L., Castenmiller, W.A., and Kardinaal, A.F., Decreased carotenoid concentrations due to dietary sucrose polyesters do not affect possible markers of disease risk in humans, *J Nutr*, 133(3): 720–6, 2003.
34. Rock, C.L. and Swendseid, M.E., Plasma beta-carotene response in humans after meals supplemented with dietary pectin, *Am J Clin Nutr*, 55(1): 96–9, 1992.
35. Riedl, J., Linseisen, J., Hoffmann, J., and Wolfram, G., Some dietary fibers reduce the absorption of carotenoids in women, *J Nutr*, 129(12): 2170–6, 1999.
36. Cardinault, N., Tyssandier, V., Grolier, P., Winklhofer-Roob, B.M., Ribalta, J., Bouteloup-Demange, C., Rock, E., and Borel, P., Comparison of the postprandial chylomicron carotenoid responses in young and older subjects, *Eur J Nutr*, 42(6): 315–23, 2003.
37. Schwartz, S.J., How can the metabolomic response to lycopene (exposures, durations, intracellular concentrations) in humans be adequately evaluated? *J Nutr*, 135(8): 2040S–1S, 2005.
38. Ferreira, A.L., Yeum, K.J., Liu, C., Smith, D., Krinsky, N.I., Wang, X.D., and Russell, R.M., Tissue distribution of lycopene in ferrets and rats after lycopene supplementation, *J Nutr*, 130(5): 1256–60, 2000.
39. Clinton, S.K., Emenhiser, C., Schwartz, S.J., Bostwick, D.G., Williams, A.W., Moore, B.J., and Erdman, J.W., Jr., cis-trans lycopene isomers, carotenoids, and retinol in the human prostate, *Cancer Epidemiol Biomarkers Prev*, 5(10): 823–33, 1996.
40. van Breemen, R.B., Xu, X., Viana, M.A., Chen, L., Stacewicz-Sapuntzakis, M., Duncan, C., Bowen, P.E., and Sharifi, R., Liquid chromatography-mass spectrometry of cis- and all-trans-lycopene in human serum and prostate tissue after dietary supplementation with tomato sauce, *J Agric Food Chem*, 50(8): 2214–9, 2002.
41. Alien, C.M., Smith, A.M., Clinton, S.K., and Schwartz, S.J., Tomato consumption increases lycopene isomer concentrations in breast milk and plasma of lactating women, *J Am Diet Assoc*, 102(9): 1257–62, 2002.
42. Khachik, F., Spangler, C.J., Smith, J.C., Jr., Canfield, L.M., Steck, A., and Pfander, H., Identification, quantification, and relative concentrations of carotenoids and their metabolites in human milk and serum, *Anal Chem*, 69(10): 1873–81, 1997.
43. Ferreira, A.L., Yeum, K.J., Russell, R.M., Krinsky, N.I., and Tang, G., Enzymatic and oxidative metabolites of lycopene, *J Nutr Biochem*, 14(9): 531–40, 2003.
44. Khachik, F., Beecher, G.R., and Smith, J.C., Jr., Lutein, lycopene, and their oxidative metabolites in chemoprevention of cancer, *J Cell Biochem*, Suppl. 22: 236–46, 1995.
45. Halliwell, B. and Gutteridge, J.M.C., Free radicals in biology and medicine, 3rd ed., Oxford Science Publications, Oxford New York: Clarendon Press; Oxford University Press, 1999, xxxi, 936.
46. Di Mascio, P., Kaiser, S., and Sies, H., Lycopene as the most efficient biological carotenoid singlet oxygen quencher, *Arch Biochem Biophys*, 274(2): 532–8, 1989.
47. Di Mascio, P., Devasagayam, T.P., Kaiser, S., and Sies, H., Carotenoids, tocopherols and thiols as biological singlet molecular oxygen quenchers, *Biochem Soc Trans*, 18(6): 1054–6, 1990.
48. Gerster, H., The potential role of lycopene for human health, *J Am Coll Nutr*, 16(2): 109–26, 1997.
49. Gerster, H., Anticarcinogenic effect of common carotenoids, *Int J Vitam Nutr Res*, 63(2): 93–121, 1993.
50. Handelman, G.J., Packer, L., and Cross, C.E., Destruction of tocopherols, carotenoids, and retinol in human plasma by cigarette smoke, *Am J Clin Nutr*, 63(4): 559–65, 1996.

51. Gupta, S.K., Trivedi, D., Srivastava, S., Joshi, S., Halder, N., and Verma, S.D., Lycopene attenuates oxidative stress induced experimental cataract development: an in vitro and in vivo study, *Nutrition*, 19(9): 794–9, 2003.

52. Beckman, J.S., Beckman, T.W., Chen, J., Marshall, P.A., and Freeman, B.A., Apparent hydroxyl radical production by peroxynitrite: implications for endothelial injury from nitric oxide and superoxide, *Proc Natl Acad Sci U S A*, 87(4): 1620–4, 1990.

53. Panasenko, O.M., Sharov, V.S., Briviba, K., and Sies, H., Interaction of peroxynitrite with carotenoids in human low density lipoproteins, *Arch Biochem Biophys*, 373(1): 302–5, 2000.

54. Hadley, C.W., Clinton, S.K., and Schwartz, S.J., The consumption of processed tomato products enhances plasma lycopene concentrations in association with a reduced lipoprotein sensitivity to oxidative damage, *J Nutr*, 133(3): 727–32, 2003.

55. Rao, A.V., Processed tomato products as a source of dietary lycopene: bioavailability and antioxidant properties, *Can J Diet Pract Res*, 65(4): 161–5, 2004.

56. Agarwal, S. and Rao, A.V., Tomato lycopene and low density lipoprotein oxidation: a human dietary intervention study, *Lipids*, 33(10): 981–4, 1998.

57. Ford, E.S., Liu, S., Mannino, D.M., Giles, W.H., and Smith, S.J., C-reactive protein concentration and concentrations of blood vitamins, carotenoids, and selenium among U.S. adults, *Eur J Clin Nutr*, 57(9): 1157–63, 2003.

58. Bohm, F., Edge, R., Burke, M., and Truscott, T.G., Dietary uptake of lycopene protects human cells from singlet oxygen and nitrogen dioxide-ROS components from cigarette smoke, *J Photochem Photobiol B*, 64(2–3): 176–8, 2001.

59. Mayne, S.T., Cartmel, B., Lin, H., Zheng, T., and Goodwin, W.J., Jr., Low plasma lycopene concentration is associated with increased mortality in a cohort of patients with prior oral, pharynx or larynx cancers, *J Am Coll Nutr*, 23(1): 34–42, 2004.

60. Giovannucci, E., Tomatoes, tomato-based products, lycopene, and cancer: review of the epidemiologic literature, *J Natl Cancer Inst*, 91(4): 317–31, 1999.

61. Giovannucci, E., Rimm, E.B., Liu, Y., Stampfer, M.J., and Willett, W.C., A prospective study of tomato products, lycopene, and prostate cancer risk, *J Natl Cancer Inst*, 94(5): 391–8, 2002.

62. Giovannucci, E., Ascherio, A., Rimm, E.B., Stampfer, M.J., Colditz, G.A., and Willett, W.C., Intake of carotenoids and retinol in relation to risk of prostate cancer, *J Natl Cancer Inst*, 87(23): 1767–76, 1995.

63. Mills, P.K., Beeson, W.L., Phillips, R.L., and Fraser, G.E., Cohort study of diet, lifestyle, and prostate cancer in Adventist men, *Cancer*, 64(3): 598–604, 1989.

64. Giovannucci, E., Tomato products, lycopene, and prostate cancer: a review of the epidemiological literature, *J Nutr*, 135(8): 2030S–1S, 2005.

65. Michaud, D.S., Feskanich, D., Rimm, E.B., Colditz, G.A., Speizer, F.E., Willett, W.C., and Giovannucci, E., Intake of specific carotenoids and risk of lung cancer in 2 prospective U.S. cohorts, *Am J Clin Nutr*, 72(4): 990–7, 2000.

66. Levi, F., Pasche, C., Lucchini, F., and La Vecchia, C., Dietary intake of selected micronutrients and breast-cancer risk, *Int J Cancer*, 91(2): 260–3, 2001.

67. Nkondjock, A., Ghadirian, P., Johnson, K.C., and Krewski, D., Dietary intake of lycopene is associated with reduced pancreatic cancer risk, *J Nutr*, 135(3): 592–7, 2005.

68. Levy, J., Bosin, E., Feldman, B., Giat, Y., Miinster, A., Danilenko, M., and Sharoni, Y., Lycopene is a more potent inhibitor of human cancer cell proliferation than either alpha-carotene or beta-carotene, *Nutr Cancer*, 24(3): 257–66, 1995.

69. Kim, L., Rao, A.V., and Rao, L.G., Effect of lycopene on prostate LNCaP cancer cells in culture, *J Med Food*, 5(4): 181–7, 2002.

70. Ben-Dor, A., Steiner, M., Gheber, L., Danilenko, M., Dubi, N., Linnewiel, K., Zick, A., Sharoni, Y., and Levy, J., Carotenoids activate the antioxidant response element transcription system, *Mol Cancer Ther*, 4(1): 177–86, 2005.

71. Karas, M., Amir, H., Fishman, D., Danilenko, M., Segal, S., Nahum, A., Koifmann, A., Giat, Y., Levy, J., and Sharoni, Y., Lycopene interferes with cell cycle progression and insulin-like growth factor I signaling in mammary cancer cells, *Nutr Cancer*, 36(1): 101–11, 2000.

72. Amir, H., Karas, M., Giat, J., Danilenko, M., Levy, R., Yermiahu, T., Levy, J., and Sharoni, Y., Lycopene and 1,25-dihydroxyvitamin D3 cooperate in the inhibition of cell cycle progression and induction of differentiation in HL-60 leukemic cells, *Nutr Cancer*, 33(1): 105–12, 1999.

73. Obermuller-Jevic, U.C., Olano-Martin, E., Corbacho, A.M., Eiserich, J.P., van der Vliet, A., Valacchi, G., Cross, C.E., and Packer, L., Lycopene inhibits the growth of normal human prostate epithelial cells in vitro, *J Nutr*, 133(11): 3356–60, 2003.

74. Matos, H.R., Capelozzi, V.L., Gomes, O.F., Mascio, P.D., and Medeiros, M.H., Lycopene inhibits DNA damage and liver necrosis in rats treated with ferric nitrilotriacetate, *Arch Biochem Biophys*, 396(2): 171–7, 2001.

75. Bhuvaneswari, V., Velmurugan, B., and Nagini, S., Induction of glutathione-dependent hepatic biotransformation enzymes by lycopene in the hamster cheek pouch carcinogenesis model, *J Biochem Mol Biol Biophys*, 6(4): 257–60, 2002.

76. Kim, D.J., Takasuka, N., Kim, J.M., Sekine, K., Ota, T., Asamoto, M., Murakoshi, M., Nishino, H., Nir, Z., and Tsuda, H., Chemoprevention by lycopene of mouse lung neoplasia after combined initiation treatment with DEN, MNU and DMH, *Cancer Lett*, 120(1): 15–22, 1997.

77. Liu, C., Lian, F., Smith, D.E., Russell, R.M., and Wang, X.D., Lycopene supplementation inhibits lung squamous metaplasia and induces apoptosis via up-regulating insulin-like growth factor-binding protein 3 in cigarette smoke-exposed ferrets, *Cancer Res*, 63(12): 3138–44, 2003.

78. Boileau, T.W., Liao, Z., Kim, S., Lemeshow, S., Erdman, J.W., Jr., and Clinton, S.K., Prostate carcinogenesis in N-methyl-N-nitrosourea (NMU)-testosterone-treated rats fed tomato powder, lycopene, or energy-restricted diets, *J Natl Cancer Inst*, 95(21): 1578–86, 2003.

79. Herzog, A., Siler, U., Spitzer, V., Seifert, N., Denelavas, A., Hunziker, P.B., Hunziker, W., Goralczyk, R., and Wertz, K., Lycopene reduced gene expression of steroid targets and inflammatory markers in normal rat prostate, *FASEB J*, 19(2): 272–4, 2005.

80. Nagasawa, H., Mitamura, T., Sakamoto, S., and Yamamoto, K., Effects of lycopene on spontaneous mammary tumour development in SHN virgin mice, *Anticancer Res*, 15(4): 1173–8, 1995.

81. Clinton, S.K., Tomatoes or lycopene: a role in prostate carcinogenesis? *J Nutr*, 135(8): 2057S–9S, 2005.

82. Bowen, P., Chen, L., Stacewicz-Sapuntzakis, M., Duncan, C., Sharifi, R., Ghosh, L., Kim, H.S., Christov-Tzelkov, K., and van Breemen, R., Tomato sauce supplementation and prostate cancer: lycopene accumulation and modulation of biomarkers of carcinogenesis, *Exp Biol Med (Maywood)*, 227(10): 886–93, 2002.

83. Kucuk, O., Sarkar, F.H., Sakr, W., Djuric, Z., Pollak, M.N., Khachik, F., Li, Y.W., Banerjee, M., Grignon, D., Bertram, J.S., Crissman, J.D., Pontes, E.J., and Wood, D.P., Jr., Phase II randomized clinical trial of lycopene supplementation before radical prostatectomy, *Cancer Epidemiol Biomarkers Prev*, 10(8): 861–8, 2001.

84. Hulten, K., Van Kappel, A.L., Winkvist, A., Kaaks, R., Hallmans, G., Lenner, P., and Riboli, E., Carotenoids, alpha-tocopherols, and retinol in plasma and breast cancer risk in northern Sweden, *Cancer Causes Control*, 12(6): 529–37, 2001.

85. Muhlhofer, A., Buhler-Ritter, B., Frank, J., Zoller, W.G., Merkle, P., Bosse, A., Heinrich, F., and Biesalski, H.K., Carotenoids are decreased in biopsies from colorectal adenomas, *Clin Nutr*, 22(1): 65–70, 2003.

86. Helzlsouer, K.J., Comstock, G.W., and Morris, J.S., Selenium, lycopene, alpha-tocopherol, beta-carotene, retinol, and subsequent bladder cancer, *Cancer Res*, 49(21): 6144–8, 1989.

87. Ribaya-Mercado, J.D., Garmyn, M., Gilchrest, B.A., and Russell, R.M., Skin lycopene is destroyed preferentially over beta-carotene during ultraviolet irradiation in humans, *J Nutr*, 125(7): 1854–9, 1995.

88. Kochanek, K.D., Murphy, S.L., Anderson, R.N., and Scott, C., Deaths: final data for 2002, *Natl Vital Stat Rep*, 53(5): 1–115, 2004.

89. Rao, A.V., Lycopene, tomatoes, and the prevention of coronary heart disease, *Exp Biol Med (Maywood)*, 227(10): 908–13, 2002.

90. Dugas, T.R., Morel, D.W., and Harrison, E.H., Dietary supplementation with beta-carotene, but not with lycopene, inhibits endothelial cell-mediated oxidation of low-density lipoprotein, *Free Radic Biol Med*, 26(9–10): 1238–44, 1999.

91. Kohlmeier, L., Kark, J.D., Gomez-Gracia, E., Martin, B.C., Steck, S.E., Kardinaal, A.F., Ringstad, J., Thamm, M., Masaev, V., Riemersma, R., Martin-Moreno, J.M., Huttunen, J.K., and Kok, F.J., Lycopene and myocardial infarction risk in the EURAMIC Study, *Am J Epidemiol*, 146(8): 618–26, 1997.

92. Craft, N.E., Haitema, T.B., Garnett, K.M., Fitch, K.A., and Dorey, C.K., Carotenoid, tocopherol, and retinol concentrations in elderly human brain, *J Nutr Health Aging*, 8(3): 156–62, 2004.
93. Rao, A.V., Fleshner, N., and Agarwal, S., Serum and tissue lycopene and biomarkers of oxidation in prostate cancer patients: a case-control study, *Nutr Cancer*, 33(2): 159–64, 1999.
94. Freeman, V.L., Meydani, M., Yong, S., Pyle, J., Wan, Y., Arvizu-Durazo, R., and Liao, Y., Prostatic levels of tocopherols, carotenoids, and retinol in relation to plasma levels and self-reported usual dietary intake, *Am J Epidemiol*, 151(2): 109–18, 2000.
95. Kaplan, L.A., Lau, J.M., and Stein, E.A., Carotenoid composition, concentrations, and relationships in various human organs, *Clin Physiol Biochem*, 8(1): 1–10, 1990.
96. Schmitz, H.H., Poor, C.L., Wellman, R.B., and Erdman, J.W., Jr., Concentrations of selected carotenoids and vitamin A in human liver, kidney and lung tissue, *J Nutr*, 121(10): 1613–21, 1991.
97. Nierenberg, D.W. and Nann, S.L., A method for determining concentrations of retinol, tocopherol, and five carotenoids in human plasma and tissue samples, *Am J Clin Nutr*, 56(2): 417–26, 1992.
98. Stahl, W., Schwarz, W., Sundquist, A.R., and Sies, H., cis-trans isomers of lycopene and beta-carotene in human serum and tissues, *Arch Biochem Biophys*, 294(1): 173–7, 1992.

4 Garlic: The Mystical Food in Health Promotion

Sharon A. Ross and John A. Milner

CONTENTS

I. INTRODUCTION

Garlic (*Allium sativum*) has been valued for its medicinal properties for centuries. This interest has been accelerated in recent years by several publications, which reveal that it may also reduce the risk of heart disease and cancer.[1–5] The ability of garlic and related components to serve as antioxidants,[6] influence immunocompetence,[7] and possibly mental function[8] suggests its health implications may be extremely widespread.

A member of the Alliaceae family, garlic is one of the more economically important cultivated spices. Large amounts of garlic are produced annually in China and India. In 2002, 5.65 million cwt. of garlic was harvested from 32,800 acres in the U.S.[9] About 80% of this amount is produced in California. Although considerable consumption occurs as fresh garlic, it is also found as dehydrates, flakes, and salts in a variety of food preparations. Dozens of garlic supplements are also commercially available as essential oils, garlic-oil macerate, garlic powder, or garlic extract. Garlic has continued to be one of the top selling herbs in the U.S.

Garlic is classified as a spice, herb, or vegetable. Along with onions, leeks, shallots, and chives it is one of the major Allium foods consumed by humans. The garlic bulb consists of several individual pieces, also known as bulblets or cloves, each weighing about 3 g. Actual garlic intakes are not known with certainty, especially as it is not typically considered in dietary assessment surveys. Nevertheless, intakes are thought to vary from region to region and from individual to individual. In 1981, annual per capita retail consumption of fresh garlic was 0.5 of a pound. By 1991, annual consumption had risen to 1.2 lb per person. After peaking at 3.1 lb in 1999, retail consumption dropped to 2 lb per person in 2001.[9] Steinmetz et al.[10] provided evidence that average intakes in parts of the Midwestern U.S. are around 0.6 g per week or less, while intakes in some parts of China may reach 20 g per day. Data used in a meta analysis of colorectal and stomach cancer suggested the mean intake (±SD) of raw and cooked garlic intake across all published reports was 18.3 ± 14.2 g per week, or about 6 cloves garlic per week.[11] Consumption ranged from none to 3.5 g per week (about 1 clove), whereas the highest intake exceeded 28.8 g per week (about 9 to 10 cloves).[11]

Negative consequences are not always an outcome of exaggerated garlic intake, but some individuals may be more susceptible to side effects than others. Although their incidence is low, a spectrum of adverse allergic reactions can occur following contact with garlic.[12] Even though garlic is recognized as a powerful irritant, relatively few reports of allergic contact dermatitis appear in the literature.[13] Avoidance of direct contact seems the most logical approach for food handlers who are sensitive, but this may be more difficult than anticipated as diallyl disulfide (DADS), an active irritant, penetrates most commercially available gloves.[14]

Excess garlic intake has also been reported to lead to hemolytic anemia. The severity of the anemia correlates with a reduction in erythrocyte-reduced glutathione (GSH) and plasma ascorbic acid.[15] Incubations of canine erythrocytes with sodium 2-propanyl thiosulfate from garlic were found to increase methemoglobin concentration and Heinz body occurrences, indicating that this compound may be the cause of oxidative damage in canine erythrocytes.[16] Umar et al.[15] found that ascorbic acid or vitamin E supplements prevented the garlic-precipitated reduction in GSH and plasma ascorbic acid, thereby providing greater protection to the erythrocyte membrane.

II. GARLIC COMPOSITION AND CHEMISTRY

The use of garlic typically centers on its unique flavor and odor characteristics. Unlike other foods, garlic is distinctive in that about 1% of its dry weight is sulfur.[17] Garlic is of somewhat limited nutritional value because its total intake is typically low, although it is more nutritious than onions on a fresh-weight basis. A 3 g serving of garlic provides about 4.5 mg of potassium, 0.6 g of carbohydrate, and trace amounts of calcium, fiber, iron, and vitamin C. Table 4.1 provides some compositional information about garlic. Carbohydrates provide about 33% of garlic's weight, whereas protein accounts for another 6.4%. Whereas much of garlic's health benefits have been attributed to its sulfur components, its other constituents, including arginine, selenium, oligosaccharides and flavonoids, may influence the overall response.[18]

The chemistry of sulfur compounds found in garlic is exceedingly complex and not completely understood.[19–21] Regardless, it is known that the primary sulfur-containing constituents in garlic bulbs are γ-glutamyl-S-alk(en)yl-L-cysteines and S-alk(en)yl-L-cysteine sulfoxides. The content of S-alk(en)ylcysteine sulfoxide in garlic typically ranges between 0.53 to 1.3% of the fresh weight, with alliin (S-allylcysteine sulfoxide) the largest contributor.[22] This variation likely reflects environmental factors including climate or cropping conditions.[23,24] Similarly, the processing method used can markedly influence the amounts and types of individual sulfur compounds.[25] Alliin concentrations can increase during storage as a result of the transformation of γ-glutamylcysteines. In addition to alliin, garlic bulbs contain small amounts of (+)-S-metyl-L-cysteine sulfoxide (methiin) and (+)-S-(trans-1-propenyl)-L-cysteine sulfoxide, S-(2-carboxypropyl)glutathione, γ-

TABLE 4.1
Content of Selected Components in Edible Garlic[a]

Component	Amount/100 g
Water, g	58.6
Energy, kcal	149.0
Protein, g	6.4
Total lipid (fat), g	0.5
Carbohydrate, g	33.1
Fiber, total dietary, g	**2.1**
Calcium, mg	181.0
Magnesium, mg	25.0
Phosphorus, mg	153.0
Potassium, mg	401.0
Selenium, mcg	14.2
Vitamin C, mg	31.2
Folate, µg	3.1

[a] USDA Nutrient Database for Standard Reference, Release 13 (November 1999).

glutamyl-*S*-allyl-L-cysteine, γ-glutamyl-*S*-(*trans*-1-propenyl)-L-cysteine, and γ-glutamyl-*S*-allyl-mercapto-L-cysteine.[17,26]

The characteristic odor of garlic arises from allicin (thio-2-propene-1-sulfinic acid S-allyl ester) and oil-soluble sulfur compounds formed when the bulb is crushed or damaged. This membrane destruction yields a host of organosulfur degradation products as a result of the release of the enzyme alliinase. This enzyme rapidly converts alliin to form the odiferous alkyl alkane-thiosulfinates, including allicin. Because allicin is unstable it further decomposes to sulfides, ajoene, and dithiins.[27–29] Tamaki and Sonoki[29] reported that strong garlic flavor and scent were linked to a higher content of volatile sulfur. Not surprisingly, heating garlic reduced allyl mercaptan (AM), methyl mercaptan, and allyl methyl sulfide (AMS) concentrations and reduced its odor possibly because of an inactivation of alliinase activity.[29]

Studies by Arnault et al.[20] provide evidence that the quality and stability of some preparations currently available in the marketplace is troubling, as the various types of preparations cannot be considered equivalent. Nevertheless, the stability of some of them appears acceptable, according to Lawson and Gardner.[30] They reported that the allyl thiosulfinates of blended fresh garlic were stable for at least 2 years when stored at −80°C. Likewise, they found the dissolution release of thiosulfinates from the enteric-coated garlic tablets was near 95% and the bioavailability, as determined by breath allyl methyl sulfide, was virtually complete and equivalent to that occurring with crushed fresh garlic. The S-allylcysteine (SAC) occurring in deodorized garlic preparations was found to be stable for 12 months when stored at ambient temperature.[30] Undeniably more compositional information should be provided about each garlic preparation available in the marketplace, especially when claims are being made about a specific preparation.[31] Greater attention to the types and amounts of active compounds in the various products will likely resolve some of the inconsistencies in the literature about the potential health benefits of garlic and commercially prepared extracts, solutions, or tablets. Arnault et al.[20] proposed that a high-pressure liquid chromatographic profile may be a useful tool for not only understanding the composition of various garlic preparations, but also in identifying the relative efficacy of these preparations to retard diseases. However, standardization of the various garlic preparations with respect to one constituent is not a possibility as the various preparations available in the marketplace likely have entirely different active components. The development of reference assays that can evaluate the relative bioactivity/potency across preparations may be one of the only solutions for comparing the various preparations available in the marketplace.

Few studies have examined the *in vivo* pharmacokinetics of allyl sulfur compounds. However, Lachmann, et al.[32] have reported the distribution of allicin and vinyldithiines in the form of an oil macerate of the ^{35}S-labeled substance in the rat. Overall, the absorption and the elimination of ^{35}S-alliin was faster than for the other garlic constituents, with maximum blood levels reached within the first 10 min after exposure. Alliin elimination from the blood was almost complete after 6 h. Maximum blood concentrations of ^{35}S-allicin were not reached until 30 to 60 min after treatment, and for vinyldithiines the maximum was not achieved until 120 min. Both allicin and vinyldithiines were present in blood at the end of their 72 -h study. Urinary excretions suggested an absorption rate approximating 65% for allicin and 73% for vinyldithiines.

Lawson and Wang[19] suggest that allicin absorption in humans is about 95%, although precision was limited because of the rapid metabolism and absence in the blood after consumption. Allicin is known to be rapidly transformed in the liver to DADS and allyl mercaptan (AM).[33] DADS can also be further transformed into AM, allyl methyl sulfide, allyl methyl sulfoxide, and allyl methyl sulphone.[34]

Teyssier et al.[35] provided evidence that DADS can be reconverted to diallyl thiosulfinate (allicin) in tissues principally by oxidation arising from cytochrome P450 monooxygenases, and to a limited extent by flavin-containing monooxygenases. Interestingly, their data suggest DADS is preferentially metabolized in human liver to allicin by cytochrome P450 2E1 (CYP2E1). As DADS can also cause the autocatalytic CYP2E1 destruction, it is unclear how much allicin might be formed under physiological conditions. Flavin-containing monooxygenases in liver probably are responsible for the oxidization of S-allyl cysteine (SAC), among many other sulfur compounds.[36] P450 monooxygenases do not appear to be involved in SAC metabolism.

Rarely have comparisons of water- and oil-soluble compounds from garlic been examined in the same study. Nevertheless, available evidence suggests that major differences in efficacy among extracts are not of paramount importance.[37–42] Whereas subtle differences among garlic preparations are likely to occur, quantity rather than source appears to be a key factor influencing the response.[37] Differences that do occur between preparations very likely relate to the content and effectiveness of individual sulfur constituents. The number of sulfur atoms present in the molecule seems to influence the response with diallyl trisulfide (DATS), generally found to be more effective than DADS, which is better than diallyl sulfide (DAS).[43–45] Likewise, the presence of the allyl group generally enhances the response over that provided by the propyl moiety.[44,46]

III. IMPLICATION IN HEALTH

Garlic and a host of its allyl sulfur compounds have been reported to possess a variety of health benefits. Notable among these are the antimicrobial, anticarcinogenic, and protective benefits against cardiovascular disease. Table 4.2 contains a list of some of the most common compounds that have been found to have benefits on a variety of biomarkers that reflect a reduction in risk. While long-term intervention studies are lacking, a variety of laboratory-based and epidemiological studies suggest that key molecular targets involved in the risk of several diseases can be influenced by these organosulfur compounds arising from garlic.

IV. ANTIMICROBIAL EFFECTS

A host of plants are reported to act as antimicrobial agents. Those rich in tannins, terpenoids, alkaloids, flavonoids, and sulfur compounds have been found to be particularly effective. Histori-

TABLE 4.2

Names and Structures of Organosulfur Compounds from Garlic

Scientific Name	Abbreviation	Chemical Structure
Disulfide, 2-propenyl 3-(2-propenylsulfinyl)-1-propenyl	Ajoene	
Diallyl thiosulfinate	Allicin	
S-Allyl-l-cysteine sulfoxide	Alliin	
Allyl mercaptan	AM	
Ddiallyl disulfide	DADS	
Diallyl sulfide (DAS)	DAS	
Diallyl trisulfide	DATS	
γ-Glutamyl-S-allyl-l-cysteine	GLUAICS	
γ-Glutamyl-S-(trans-1-propenyl)-l-cysteine	IsoGLUAICS	
S-Methylcysteine sulfoxide	Methiin	

Continued.

TABLE 4.2 *(Continued)*
Names and Structures of Organosulfur Compounds from Garlic

Scientific Name	Abbreviation	Chemical Structure
S-Allyl-l-cysteine, deoxyalliin,	SAC	
3-Vinyl-[4*H*]-1,2-dithiin	Vinyldithiin I	
2-Vinyl-[4*H*]-1,3-dithiin	Vinyldithiin II	

cally garlic extracts have been labeled as universal antibiotics.[47] Considerable evidence indicates that garlic extracts can inhibit a range of Gram-negative and Gram-positive bacteria and serve as an antifungal agent.[48–50] In addition to allicin, various other sulfur compounds including DAS, DADS, E-ajoene, Z-ajoene, E-4,5,9-trithiadeca-1,6-diene-9-oxide (E-10-devinylajoene, E-10-DA), and E-4,5,9-trithiadeca-1,7-diene-9-oxide (iso-E-10-devinylajoene, iso-E-10-DA) may contribute to garlic's antimicrobial properties.[51–53] For example, *in vivo* protection against methicillin-resistant *Staphylococcus aureus* infection in BALB/cA mice has been shown for orally administered DAS and DADS.[53] Although differences in efficacy among these compounds exist, relatively small amounts are effective microbial-growth deterrents. However, not all microorganisms are equally susceptible to the toxic effects of individual sulfur compounds.[54,55] Ruddock et al.[56] recently examined the microbial activity of several garlic products found in the Canadian marketplace and observed a general trend towards increased *in vitro* antibacterial activity among those products containing higher amounts of allicin. Those products with marginal antibacterial activity often contained lower concentrations of active constituents than their product labels indicated, which suggests the need to standardize garlic preparations used in research.

Recently, a novel protein in garlic, designated alliumin, has been identified that possesses both antimicrobial and antifungal activity.[57] It is noteworthy that the antifungal action of alliumin was preserved after exposure to 100°C for 1 h, suggesting a marked thermostability. Like certain antifungal proteins that inhibit proliferation of tumor cells, alliumin was found to be inhibitory to L1210 cells; but, interestingly, it was shown to be devoid of such activity toward Hep G2 cells. Additional characterization of alliumin will likely shed insight about its antifungal properties and may also provide further evidence for garlic's health-promoting activity.

Helicobacter pylori colonization of the gastric mucosa is increasingly linked with gastritis. Likewise, emerging evidence connects gastritis with a greater propensity to develop gastric cancer. Studies by Cellini et al.[58] provide rather convincing evidence that aqueous garlic extracts (2 to 5 mg/ml) inhibit *Helicobacter pylori* proliferation. Reduced effectiveness occurred when the garlic was heated prior to extraction.[58] This depression in activity suggests the need for breakdown products from alliin to achieve a maximum response. As both DAS and DADS are recognized to elicit a dose-dependent depression in *Helicobacter pylori* proliferation in culture,[59] a reduction in their formation may account for the loss of effectiveness caused by heating. Raw garlic extracts and three commercially available garlic tablets were found to vary in their efficacy, as indicated by a minimum inhibitory concentration in the range between 10 to 17.5 μg dry weight/ml.[60]

An *in vivo* effect of garlic on *H. pylori*-induced gastritis in Mongolian gerbils has also been reported.[61] Although the number of viable *H. pylori* was not changed by the garlic extract treatment, garlic reduced the number of hemorrhagic spots in the glandular stomach and the microscopic score for gastritis, compared to control-fed gerbils. These findings suggest that garlic and its active constituents may display secondary or indirect effects, such as an influence on the inflammatory or immunocompetence pathways, in addition to a direct effect on viability of certain bacterial cells.

The ability of garlic to reduce *H. pylori* infection in humans is inconclusive. Although an epidemiological study suggests an association between increased garlic consumption and reduced *H. pylori* infection,[62] two clinical studies testing different garlic preparations in *H. pylori*-infected subjects did not show efficacy.[63,64] Neither of these interventions resulted in the elimination of the organism, change in the severity of gastritis, or a significant change in symptom scores. Both studies were not randomized and had a small sample size, suggesting that a well-designed clinical trial is still needed to determine the efficacy of garlic consumption in reducing *H. pylori* infection and its symptoms.

Allium foods, including garlic, are also effective in suppressing fungal growth.[50] Allicin has been reported to be protective against *Candida albicans* and a host of other strains. These organisms were extremely sensitive to garlic extracts, some to a greater degree than to nystatin, a known effective antibiotic.[65] Ajoene is also noted for its antimycotic activity both *in vitro* and *in vivo*. A fungal infection of the skin known commonly as ringworm and medically as tinea corporis, can also be influenced by sulfur compounds found in garlic. Ledezma et al.[66] found that treatment with ajoene (0.6% ajoene or 1% ajoene gel) was as effective as terbinafine (1% cream) in healing tinea corporis and tinea cruris in 70 soldiers with dermatophytosis. As ajoene can be prepared easily from garlic it may be particularly useful as a public health strategy, particularly in developing countries.

The primary antimicrobial effect of garlic may reflect chemical reactions that take place with selected thiol groups of various enzymes and/or a change in the overall redox state of the organism. Specifically, the antimicrobial action of allicin and its breakdown products has been suggested to result from its rapid interaction with SH-containing molecules, including amino acids and cellular proteins within microbial organisms.[50] An example of such a putative *in vivo* reaction is that between allicin and glutathione (GSH), which is thought to be the major intracellular mammalian thiol, and investigators have isolated the product of the reaction, established its structure, and examined its interaction with thiol-containing proteins.[67] GSH was observed to react with allicin in the following fashion: $2GSH + CH_2\text{-}CH\text{-}CH_2(SO)\text{-}S\text{-}CH_2\text{-}CH=CH_2(allicin) \rightarrow 2GS\text{-}S\text{-}CH_2\text{-}CH=CH_2(S\text{-}allylmercaptoglutathione) (GSSA) + H_2O$. As proof of principle, in an *in vitro* setting, GSSA was found to react with the thiol-containing proteins papain and alcohol dehydrogenase from *Thermoanaerobium brockii* and inhibit their activity, whereas both proteins were reactivated using either reducing agent dithiothreitol or 2-mercaptoethanol. The concomitant release of allylmercaptan in both of these reactions indicated that the thioallyl moiety binds to inactivated proteins just as allicin has been shown to do. It is interesting to note that one enzyme that may be similarly affected by allicin breakdown products (i.e., DATS, SAC) is squalene monooxygenase.[68] Such activity may explain the antifungal properties of allicin as squalene monooxygenase is an important enzyme for the formation of the fungal-cell wall.[69] Changes in thiol status have been suggested as one possible mechanism by which garlic and related sulfur compounds might also suppress tumor proliferation.

V. CANCER

Scientists, legislators, and consumers are becoming increasingly aware that several foods may contribute to health, including a reduction in cancer risk.[70,71] Although limitations exist in defining the precise role that garlic has in the cancer process, the likelihood of its significance is underscored by both epidemiological and laboratory investigations. Although there is epidemiological support for the association between increased intake of garlic, and/or its active constituents, with certain cancers, the data are very limited.[10,72,73] Results from the Iowa Women's Health Study, a prospective cohort study, found that the strongest association among fruits and vegetables for colon cancer risk reduction was for garlic consumption, with a reduced risk of approximately 50% in distal colon cancer associated with high garlic consumption.[10] Additionally, a meta-analysis of data from seven epidemiological studies found an inverse association between raw and cooked garlic consumption and both stomach and colorectal cancer risk.[72] Furthermore, Hsing et al.[73] reported that the reduced risk of prostate cancer in those consuming increasing quantities of allium vegetables was independent of body size, intake of other foods, and total calorie intake, as well.

Few intervention studies have been performed to examine the efficacy of garlic in preventing or treating cancer. In a double-blind, randomized study of Japanese patients with colorectal adenomas, a higher-dose aged garlic extract was shown to reduce the risk of new colorectal adenomas compared to a lower-dose garlic extract.[74] Due to observations of a case-control study of gastric cancer in Shandong, China, which indicated that persons in the highest quartile of intake of allium-containing vegetables (including garlic, garlic stalks, scallions, chives, and onions) had only 40% of the risk of those in the lowest quartile of intake,[75] investigators included a garlic-supplementation arm (800 mg of garlic extract plus 4 mg steam-distilled garlic oil daily) in a randomized multi-intervention trial to inhibit the progression of precancerous gastric lesion in this same region of China.[76] Compliance rates following 39 months of treatment with the garlic preparation were 92.9% as measured by pill count;[77] the results of the study are not yet available.

Preclinical models (Table 4.3) provide some of the most compelling evidence that garlic and its related sulfur components suppress cancer risk and alter the biological behavior of tumors. Overall, garlic and its associated sulfur components have been found to suppress the incidence of mammary, colon, skin, uterine, esophageal, lung, renal, forestomach and liver cancers.[38,78–85] Aberrant crypt foci (ACF) are a proposed early preneoplastic lesion of adenoma-carcinoma in humans and chemically induced colon cancer in rodents. In many preclinical studies, both water- and lipid-soluble allyl sulfur compounds administered to animals through their diet have been reported to inhibit ACF.[86–88]

Cancer protection may arise from several mechanisms including blockage of carcinogen formation, suppressed bioactivation of carcinogens, enhanced DNA repair, reduced cell proliferation, and/or induction of apoptosis. It is possible, and quite probable, that several of these cellular events are modified simultaneously.

A. Nitrosamine and Heterocyclic Amine Formation

Human beings are exposed to a complex array of substances that may be involved in cancer causation through food sources. Nitrosamines, heterocyclic amines, and polycyclic aromatic hydrocarbons are potential dietary carcinogens that are not normally present in foods but may arise during preservation or cooking.[89] Human exposure to these suspect carcinogens occurs through the ingestion or inhalation of preformed NOCs or by the ingestion of precursors that are combined endogenously.[90] Considerable evidence points to the ability of garlic to suppress the formation of several N-nitroso compounds (NOCs).[91,92] The ability of garlic to reduce NOCs may actually be secondary to an increase in the formation of nitrosothiols. Williams[93] proposed that several sulfur compounds could foster the formation of nitrosothiols, thereby reducing the quantity of nitrite available for NOC formation. Studies by Dion et al.[51] revealed that not all allyl sulfur compounds are equally effective in stopping the formation of NOCs. The ability of SAC and its nonallyl analog S-propyl cysteine to retard NOC formation — but not DADS, dipropyl disulfide, and DAS — reveal the critical role that the cysteine residue has in this inhibition.[51] As the content of allyl sulfur can vary among preparations, it is likely that not all garlic sources are equal in the protection they provide

TABLE 4.3
Anticarcinogenic Effects of Garlic and/or Associated Allyl Sulfur Compounds[a]

Site	Host
Bone marrow	
Benzo[a]pyrene	Mouse[189]
Buccal Pouch	
7,12-dimethylbenz[a]anthracene	Hamster[39]
Colon	
1,2-dimethylhydrazine	Rat[190]
	Mouse[79]
Azoxymethane	Rat[191]
N-nitrosodiethylamine	Rat[192]
Cervix	
3-methylcholanthrene	Mouse[80]
Esophagus	
N-nitrosomethylbenzylamine	Rat[81]
Forestomach	
7,12-dimethylbenz[a]anthracene	Hamster[84]
Benzo(a)pyrene	Mouse[193]
N-nitrosodiethylamine	Mice[192]
Gastric	
Methylnitronitrosoguanidine	Rat[194]
Liver	
Aflatoxin B1	Toad[195]
	Rat[196]
N-nitrosodimethylamine	Rat[197]
Lung	
Benzo(a)pyrene	Mouse[193]
Mammary	
7,12 Dimethylbenz(a)anthracene	Rat[78,154]
N-methyl-N-nitrosourea	Rat[41]
2-amino-1-methyl-6-phenylimidazo[4,5-b]pyridine (PhIP)	Rat[198]
Nasal	
4-(methylnitrosamino)-1-(3-pyridyl)-1-butanone	Rat[199]
	Mouse[82]
N-nitrosodiethylamine	Rat[199]
N-nitrosodimethylamine	Rat[199]
Renal	
N-diethylnitrosamine	Rat[83]
Skin	
7,12 Dimethylbenz(a)anthracene	Mouse[200]
Benzo(a)pyrene	Mouse[201]
Vinyl carbamate	Mouse[202]

[a] The overall response to garlic and/or specific allyl sulfur components depends on the quantity provided and the amount of carcinogen administered.

against NOC formation. Some of the protection against NOC exposure may also relate to antimicrobial properties associated with garlic and some of its components as discussed above.

Some of the most compelling evidence that garlic depresses nitrosamine formation in humans comes from studies by Mei et al.[94] In their studies, providing 5 g garlic per day completely blocked the enhanced urinary excretion of nitrosoproline that occurred as a result of ingesting supplemental nitrate and proline. The significance of this observation comes from the predictive value that nitrosoproline has for the synthesis of potential carcinogenic nitrosamines.[95] Evidence that the effect of garlic occurs with nitrosamines other than those excreted in urine comes from data from Lin et al.[96] Their studies provided evidence that garlic was effective in blocking liver-DNA adducts resulting from the feeding of NOC precursors.

The anticancer benefits attributed to garlic are also associated with the ability of its allyl sulfur compounds to suppress carcinogen bioactivation. Evidence from a variety of sources reveals that garlic is effective in blocking DNA alkylation, a primary step in nitrosamine carcinogenesis.[82,97] Consistent with this reduction in bioactivation, Dion et al.[51] found that both water-soluble SAC and lipid-soluble DADS were effective in retarding the mutagenicity of N-nitrosomorpholine in *Salmonella typhimurium* TA100. A block in mutagenicity following aqueous garlic-extract exposure has also been noted following treatment with ionizing radiation, peroxides, adriamycin, and N-methyl-N-nitro-nitrosoguanidine.[98]

A block in nitrosamine bioactivation may reflect changes in several enzymes. However, substantial evidence points to the involvement of CYP2E1.[99,100] An autocatalytic destruction of CYP2E1 may account for some of the chemoprotective effects of DAS, and possibly other allyl sulfur compounds.[101] Variation in the content and overall activity of P4502E1 may be an important variable in the degree of protection provided by garlic and associated allyl sulfur components.

The *in vivo* bioactivation of heterocyclic amines to carcinogenic species is known to be initiated by N-oxidation. This reaction occurs primarily in the liver, and in humans is catalyzed by cytochrome P4501A2 (CYP1A2). Davenport and Wargovich[102] reported that in rats the administration of a single bolus of 200 mg/kg DAS and AMS increased hepatic CYP1A2 protein (but not mRNA) by 282 and 70%, respectively. Acetylation or sulfation of the N-hydroxy-HCA can also occur through the action of acetyltransferases (NAT) and sulfotransferases, which generate N-acetoxy and N-sulfonyloxy esters, electrophiles that are much more reactive with DNA. Several studies provide evidence that organosulfur compounds arising from garlic can effectively reduce NAT activity. Recent studies by Yu et al.[103] demonstrated that a suppression in NAT mRNA expression accounts for the majority of the reduction in activity.

B. Carcinogen Activity Modulation

Garlic and several of its allyl sulfur compounds can also effectively block the bioactivation and carcinogenicity of non NOCs (Table 4.3). This protection, which involves a diverse array of compounds and several target-tissue sites, suggests either multiple mechanisms of action, or a widespread biological effect.

Garlic has also been found to reduce the incidence of tumors resulting from treatment with methylnitrosurea (MNU), a known direct-acting carcinogen.[96] Providing water-soluble S-allyl cysteine and lipid-soluble DADS at 57 μmol/kg diet has been reported to cause a comparable reduction in MNU-induced O6-methylguanine adducts bound to mammary cell DNA.[41] Studies by Ludeke et al.[104] revealed that DAS diminished the DNA hypermethylation of esophagus, liver, and nasal mucosa that arose from treatment with N-nitrosomethylbenzylamine. This finding suggests that the bioactivation of several carcinogens known to influence DNA methylation patterns[105] may also be influenced by garlic and many of its sulfur constituents.[92] However, not all evidence supports SAC as protection against MNU-induced mammary tumors.[106] The reason for this discrepancy is unknown but may relate to the quantity of lipid in the diet or the quantity of carcinogen provided. If DADS and/or SAC are effective blockers of MNU carcinogenesis, the mechanism(s) remain unresolved.

As metabolic activation is required for many of these carcinogens used in studies aimed at examining the anticarcinogenic properties of garlic, it is likely that phase I and II enzymes are involved. Recent observations show that the activity of several phase I enzymes, in addition to P450-1A2 and -2E1, are modified following treatment with garlic or related sulfur compounds.[102,107–109]

The influence of organosulfur compounds (OSCs) on phase I metabolizing enzymes is reportedly quite diverse. For example, previous studies demonstrated that DAS competitively inhibited CYP2E1 activity, but robustly increased the transcriptional levels of CYP1A1, CYP2B1, and CYP3A1 in rat liver.[108,110] Therefore, the role of garlic OSCs in carcinogenic biotransformation may be substrate-specific.

The significance of any slight induction of certain P450 activities is not clear, but some reports suggest the induction of P450 metabolic enzymes may increase the rate of clearance of toxic metabolites.[111] Other enzymes and pathways are involved in the bioactivation or removal of carcinogenic metabolites in the observed protection from garlic supplements. Singh et al.[112] provided evidence that the efficacy of various organosulfides to suppress benzo(a)pyrene tumorigenesis was correlated with their ability to induce NAD(P)H:quinone oxidoreductase (NQO), an enzyme involved with the removal of quinones associated with this carcinogen. Investigators have recently discovered that this inductive effect of organosulfur compounds appears to be mediated by the resident antioxidant response element (ARE) enhancer sequence bound by the nuclear factor E2-related factor 2 (Nrf2) in the NQO1 and the heme oxygenase 1(HO1) gene promoters.[113] In fact, it was found that the organosulfur compounds — DAS, DADS, or DATS — differentially mediated the transcriptional levels of NQO1 and HO1. The third sulfur in the structure of OSCs appeared to have a major contribution to this bioactivity, and the allyl-containing OSCs were more potent than the propyl-containing OSCs. The data also suggested that the up regulation of detoxifying enzymes by garlic OSCs through Nrf2 protein accumulation and ARE activation might be partly due to the stress signals originating from the oxidative stress and/or calcium-dependent signaling pathways.[113]

Changes in glutathione concentration and the activity of specific glutathione-S-transferase, both factors involved in phase II detoxification, may be important in the protection provided by garlic. Both DADS and DATS have been shown to increase the activity of the GST in a variety of rat tissues.[114] The preventive effects of garlic powders, containing variable levels of sulfur compounds, on the development of preneoplastic foci initiated by aflatoxin B1 (AFB1) in rats was recently characterized.[24] The ultimate metabolite of AFB1, AFBO, is conjugated with glutathione by GST and more specifically by GST A5; thus, GST was explored as a mechanism responsible for any chemoprotective properties of garlic against AFB1-induced carcinogenesis. Consumption of garlic was efficient in protecting against AFB1 carcinogenesis, and DADS treatment induced GST protein levels and activity, particularly GST A5. Thus, not all GST isozymes may be influenced equally. Earlier evidence from Hu et al.[46] provided support that the induction of glutathione (GSH) S-transferase pi (mGSTP1-1) may be particularly important in the anticarcinogenic properties associated with garlic and allyl sulfur components.

C. CELL CYCLE ARREST/APOPTOSIS

Recent evidence indicates that garlic constituents (i.e., DADS, DATS, SAMC, ajoene) have the ability to suppress proliferation of several different cancer cells by blocking cell-cycle progression and/or causing apoptosis (also known as programmed cell death).[115–117] Current knowledge of the mechanisms by which these compounds cause apoptosis indicates that the garlic constituents target various apoptosis-signaling molecules from initiation to execution, including MAPKs (JNK, ERK1/2, and p38), P53, NF–kB, bcl-2 family, and caspases,[116] but not all of the signaling molecules were affected by each of the garlic constituents. In many studies, however, the apoptotic effects of garlic constituents were triggered by increased intracellular production of reactive oxygen species (ROS), suggesting the importance of the intracellular redox environment for apoptosis induction. An example is shown by the ability of DADS to induce apoptosis, as well as cell-cycle arrest at the G2/M phase, in human A549 lung cancer cells in a time- and dose-dependent manner.[117] In this study, DADS caused not only a dose-dependent increase, but also a time-dependent change of ROS production and an oxidative burst was found to be an early event, occurring less than 0.5 h after DADS treatment. These investigators hypothesized that the increased ROS may also act on the important signaling molecule in the observed DADS-induced cell cycle arrest.

Several mechanisms have been cited for the effect of garlic constituents on cell cycle arrest, including reduced Cdk1/cyclin B kinase activity, or activation of extracellular signal-regulated kinases (ERK1/2).[115,118] Knowles and Milner[119] showed that the DADS-mediated suppression of Cdk1 kinase activity during cell-cycle arrest in G2/M was not due to direct interaction with the protein, but was associated with (a) a temporal and dose-dependent increase in cyclin B1 protein level, (b) a reduction in the level of Cdk1–cyclin B1 complex formation, (c) inactivating hyper-phosphorylation of Cdk1, and (d) a decrease in Cdc25C protein level. The evidence suggests a complex and coordinated interaction of many factors for the observed DADS-induced cell-cycle arrest. Furthermore, gene expression analysis suggested that alterations in DNA repair and cellular adhesion factors may also be involved in the G2/M block following DADS exposure.[120]

D. DNA Repair

Exposing cells to mutagens including intracellular by-products of cellular metabolism (ROS, endog-enous alkylating agents) or extracellular influences (carcinogens, UV, or ionizing radiation) can cause DNA damage that is manifested as genomic instability, cellular senescence, and/or cell death. Initially the cell attempts to repair the damage, but if too extensive, a cascade of alternative cellular responses including cell-cycle arrest or the induction of apoptosis may occur.

There are three major DNA repairing mechanisms: base excision, nucleotide excision, and mismatch repair. Very little information exists about garlic or its organosulfur constituents as a modifier of DNA repair, although evidence exists that pretreatment with garlic extracts have been reported to stimulate DNA repair in human fibroblasts following cadmium chloride, gamma-radiation, and 4-nitroquinoline-1-oxide treatment.[121] Regardless, several studies have demonstrated that histone/chromatin modifications such as acetylation, methylation, and phosphorylation have a crucial role in DNA-repair processes and some evidence suggests that garlic could influence one or more of these determinants of repair.

E. Epigenetic Modulation

Cancer progression is probably also highly dependent on epigenetic changes. Several regulatory proteins including DNA methyltransferases, methyl-cytosine guanine dinucleotide binding proteins, histone-modifying enzymes, chromatin-remodeling factors, and their multimolecular complexes are involved in controlling the epigenetic process.[122] Because epigenetic events can be influenced by several dietary components, they represent another plausible site for intervention with bioactive food components.[122]

As previously mentioned, there is evidence that some garlic constituents can influence another aspect of epigenomics, namely histone homeostasis. Lea et al.[123] reported that at least part of the ability of DADS to induce differentiation in DS19 mouse erythroleukemic cells might relate to its ability to increase histone acetylation. DADS caused a marked increase in the acetylation of H4 and H3 histones in DS19 and K562 human leukemic cells. Consistent with other studies the disulfide was found more effective than the monosulfide. In a more recent paper, these investigators found that the inhibition of cell proliferation by SAC and SAMC of DS19, Caco-2 human colon cancer, and T47D human breast cancer cells was associated with increased histone acetylation.[124] More recently, Druesne et al.[125] reported DADS and AM effectively increased histone H3 acetylation in cultured Caco-2 and HT-29 cells. The histone H4 hyperacetylation was found to occur preferentially at the lysine residues 12 and 16. The reason for this hyperacetylation may relate to the observed reduction in histone deacetylase activity.[125] This change in hyperacetylation was also accompanied by an increase in p21(waf1/cip1) expression, at mRNA and protein levels, again demonstrating that epigenomic events can influence subsequent gene-expression patterns and lead to the accumulation of cells in the G2 phase of the cell cycle.[125] DADS and AM are rather unique in that they join a relatively few food components, butyrate and sulfloraphane, as modifiers of histone homeostasis.[126]

F. REDOX AND ANTIOXIDANT CAPACITY

It is well documented that ROS are involved in the etiology of a variety of diseases. As a result special attention has been given to the identification of antioxidants in human foods. A variety of methods have been used to evaluate the total antioxidant activity of garlic preparations available in the marketplace. Undeniably, any single method is insufficient as the response depends not only on its ability to reduce oxidation radicals, but on its metal-chelating capabilities. Regardless, both alliin and allicin are recognized to possess antioxidant properties in a Fenton oxygen-radical generating system [H_2O_2-Fe(II)].[67,127] Additionally, the antioxidant actions of garlic and its constituents have been documented through their ability to scavenge ROS, inhibit lipid peroxide formation, retard LDL oxidation, and by enhancing endogenous antioxidant systems.[6,128]

A variety of organosulfur compounds, although not all, have been reported to exhibit antioxidant properties. DADS, but not DAS, dipropyl sulfide or dipropyl disulfide, has been found to inhibit liver microsomal-lipid peroxidation induced by NADPH, ascorbate, and doxorubicin.[129] The presence of both the allyl and sulfur groups appears to magnify the antioxidant capabilities of the molecule. Both the number of sulfur atoms and the oxidation state of sulfur atoms can influence the overall antioxidant potential.[130] Whereas allicin is effective in retarding methyl linoleate oxidation, it is less than that caused by α-tocopherol.[131] Organosulfur compounds such as SAC are recognized to be powerful antioxidants and radical scavengers with the strong capacity to minimize oxidization.[128] Garlic oil is also an effective antioxidant against the oxidative damage caused by various agents indicating that both water- and lipid-soluble organosulfur compounds can be effective antioxidants. Although some ether-extracted garlic oil preparations in the marketplace may contain about nine times as much vinyl-dithiins and four times as much ajoene, these preparations had no free-radical scavenging properties, again indicating not all organosulfur constituents have antioxidant properties.[132] It is also clear that the heating of garlic can not only denature proteins, but also its antioxidant properties.[133]

G. IMMUNOCOMPETENCE/IMMUNONUTRITION

Diet is increasingly recognized to play an important role in the development and functionality of immunocompetent cells. Several dietary components, including garlic extracts and allyl sulfur compounds, may have physiologically important immunomodulatory effects.[7,134,135] Both an aqueous and an ethanolic extract prepared from a garlic powder sample significantly stimulated proliferation of rat spleen lymphocytes in culture, which was correlated with the up regulation of the Interleukin 2-receptor alpha expression and an increase in IL-2 production.[135] These data also suggested that the potentiating effect of the garlic extract on lymphocyte proliferation *in vitro* differed, depending on specific stimulators of cell proliferation; speculating that the *in vivo* response would depend on the type of responding cells. These investigators also demonstrated that aqueous and ethanolic extracts from two garlic powders significantly modulated proliferation of rat thymocytes and splenocytes *in vitro* to concanavalin A.[136] Both garlic extracts significantly modulated lymphocyte proliferation, triggered by this potent T-cell mitogen, but the response was dependent on the type and dilutions of extracts, and concentrations of concanavalin A. Interestingly, at higher concentrations of the extracts an inhibitory effect on T-cell proliferation was observed, whereas at lower concentrations a significant increase in T-cell proliferation occurred. Ghazanfari et al.[137] found that a garlic extract given i.p. to BALB/c mice was effective in reducing *Leishmania major* infection, and this response was associated with increased TH1 immune response manifested by higher IFNg and IL-2 production. These results support the concept that garlic may be a potent modulator of T cell-mediated immune functions *in vivo*. In another *in vivo* study, DAS treatment of BALB/c mice has been reported to block the suppression of the antibody response caused by N-nitrosodimethylamine to T-cell-dependent antigens, and the lymphoproliferative response to T-cell and the B-cell mitogens.[100] However, the effects are not limited to sulfur compounds as a protein fraction isolated from aged-garlic extract was found to enhance cytotoxicity of human peripheral blood lymphocytes (PBL) against both natural killer-sensitive K562 and NK-resistant M14 cell lines.[138] More recently, a 14-kDa glycoprotein isolated from garlic was found to augment a delayed type hypersensitivity response,[139] as well as increase natural killer-cell activity in BALB/c mice when administered i.p.[140] The mechanism(s) by which sulfur or non sulfur components of garlic influence immunocompetence remains to be determined.

Garlic compounds may also be modulators of inflammatory molecules, including cytokines that exhibit a vast array of regulatory functions in both adaptive and innate immunity. DADS and AMS, in addition to DAS,[141] demonstrated different effects on the production of cytokines in LPS-activated macrophages. DAS inhibited both pro- and anti-inflammatory cytokines, including TNF-α, IL-β, IL-6, and IL-10, in stimulated macrophages. DADS enhanced proinflammatory cytokines IL-β and IL-6, but suppressed anti-inflammatory cytokine IL-10, indicating the effect of DADS may be more toward proinflammation. On the other hand, AMS, to a lesser extent, decreased production of NO and TNF-α in activated macrophages, but significantly enhanced IL-10 production, suggesting that AMS may be a potential anti-inflammation compound.

Allicin and ajoene have been reported to cause a dose-dependent inhibition of the inducible nitric oxide synthase (iNOS) system in lipopolysaccharide (LPS)-stimulated RAW 264.7 macrophages.[142] Such inhibition has been correlated with a reduction in iNOS protein, as well as in its mRNA. Thus, changes in the amount or ratio of NO and peroxynitrite concentrations may be significant in the observed lowering of inflammation by garlic and associated sulfur components. More recently DAS, DADS, and AMS had unique regulatory properties in suppressing NO in stimulated macrophages.[143] DAS was found to decrease stimulated NO and PGE2 production by inhibiting inducible NO synthase and cyclooxygenase-2 expressions, and to indirectly enhance NO clearance. DADS inhibited activated NO production by decreasing inducible NO synthase expression and by directly clearing NO, whereas AMS suppressed NO mainly through its direct NO clearance activity. These findings suggest that the antitumor effect of allyl sulfurs may be related to their antiinflammatory as well as immune-stimulatory properties.

H. COX/LOX PATHWAYS

Smith et al.[144] reported that prostaglandin H synthase could metabolize the bay region diol of benzo(a)pyrene to electrophilic diol epoxides that were capable of binding to DNA. More recently Li et al.[145] have reported that both cyclooxygenase and lipoxygenase are involved with DMBA bioactivation. Ali[146] provided evidence that garlic could block cyclooxygenase activity. McGrath and Milner[147] reported that lipoxygenase bioactivated DMBA at a rate that was about 10 times greater than that caused by cyclooxygenase. While limited, there is evidence that garlic and associated sulfur components can inhibit lipoxygenase activity.[148] Finally, evidence for the involvement of lipoxygenase in the bioactivation of DMBA comes from Song and Milner[149] who found that feeding a known lipoxygenase inhibitor, Nordihydroguaiaretic acid (NDGA), markedly reduced DMBA-induced DNA adducts in rat mammary tissue.

With regard to the influence of allyl sulfur compounds on the lipoxygenase and cyclooxygenase signaling pathways, DAS, DADS, and to a lesser extent, AMS, were found to differentially regulate NO and PGE2 production in mouse RAW 264.7 macrophages stimulated by LPS.[143] In another recent study, ajoene was found to act similarly to several non steroidal anti-inflammatory drugs in that this garlic compound inhibited, in a dose-dependent fashion, the release of PGE2 from LPS-activated RAW 264.7 cells, which was associated with a dose-dependent inhibition of COX-2 enzyme activity.[150] Collectively, these studies pose interesting questions about the role of both cyclooxygenase and lipoxygenase in not only forming prostaglandins, and therefore modulating tumor cell proliferation and immunocompetence, but also their involvement in the bioactivation of carcinogens. Clearly additional attention is needed to clarify what role, if any, these enzymes have in determining the biological response to dietary garlic or its allyl sulfur components.

I. DIET AS A MODIFIER

Garlic's influence on cancer processes cannot be considered in isolation as several dietary components can influence the overall response. Recently, the effects of combining tomato and garlic were examined using several carcinogenesis models.[151–153] The combination suppressed the incidence and mean tumor burden of hamster buccal-pouch carcinomas more than either alone, and appeared to relate to a decrease in phase I enzymes and to an increase in phase II enzyme activities.

A variety of individual food components may also influence the response to garlic. Notable are the modifications made by the quantity of fat, selenium, methionine, and vitamin A in the diet.[42,154,155] Amagase et al.[154] and Ip et al.[155] reported that selenium supplied either as a component of the diet or as a constituent of the garlic supplement enhanced the protection against 7,12 dimethylbenz(a)anthracene (DMBA) mammary carcinogenesis beyond that provided by garlic alone. Suppression in carcinogen bioactivation, as indicated by a reduction in DNA adducts, may partially account for this combined benefit of garlic and selenium.[42] Because both selenium and allyl sulfur compounds are recognized to suppress tumor-cell proliferation and to induce apoptosis,[156–158] the synergistic response to allyl sulfur and selenium may relate to changes in cancer-related processes other than those associated with carcinogen metabolism.

Dietary fatty acid supply can influence the bioactivation of DMBA and ultimately the metabolites of this carcinogen, which binds to rat mammary cell DNA. A significant portion of the enhancement in mammary DNA adducts caused by increasing dietary corn oil consumption can be attributed to linoleic acid intake.[159] Whereas exaggerated oleic acid consumption also increases DMBA-induced DNA adducts, it was found to be far less effective in promoting adduct formation than was linoleic acid.

The diversity of molecular targets that can be influenced by various food components demonstrates the complexity in dealing with nutrient–nutrient interactions. Although the effect of combining bioactive food components on garlic's ability to influence cellular proliferation has not been adequately examined, there are potentially several combinations that would produce more dramatic effects. For example, and similar to information with chemical carcinogenesis, there is evidence of a greater effect of allyl sulfur when combined with selenium than when provided alone.[160] Likewise, a combination of garlic and onion oils was more effective in blocking the proliferation of HL60 cells in culture than when used singly.[161] Although the molecular basis for these enhanced effects needs to be investigated in more detail, they serve as proof-of-principal that interactions among food components must be considered when developing strategies for using diet for cancer prevention.

VI. HEART DISEASE

Garlic may have a role in the genesis and progression of cardiovascular disease. These effects may be mediated through a variety of biological responses including a decrease in total and LDL-cholesterol, increase in HDL-cholesterol, reduction of serum triglyceride and fibrinogen concentrations, lowering of arterial blood pressure, and/or an inhibition of platelet aggregation.

A. CHOLESTEROL AND LIPOPROTEINS

Several studies have attempted to clarify the exact role that garlic has on serum cholesterol, LDL, HDL, and triglycerides as these might be the signal of protection.[162,163] While some studies have reported that garlic reduces LDL concentrations,[164,165] others have not.[166,167] Eliciting the true response is made complicated by the use of various quantities of garlic, different preparations and standardizations, and variation in the duration of treatment. Nevertheless, many do provide evidence that garlic can decrease cholesterol and triglyceride concentrations in some, but probably not all, patients. A recent systematic review undertaken by Adler et al.[163] indicated that several studies provided evidence that garlic was effective in lowering cholesterol. The average decrease in total cholesterol was 24.8 mg/dl (9.9%), LDL 15.3 mg/dl (11.4%), and triglycerides 38 mg/dl (9.9%). The overall average Boyack and Lookinland Methodological Quality Index (MQI) score was 39.6% (18 to 70%). While a reduction in cholesterol in the range of 7 to 15% was relatively common this in itself is a rather large variation in response. As demonstrated for cancer models, it appears that the response to cholesterol is dependent on the formation of bioactive sulfur compounds. Jabbari et al.[168] found that swallowing undamaged garlic had little or no lowering effect on serum lipids but consuming crushed garlic reduced cholesterol, triglyceride, malondialdehyde, and blood pressure. Thus, similar to other processes, the active compound arising from garlic requires time for formation and if not formed there is no biological response.[149]

LDL oxidation is increasingly being recognized as a contributor to the initiation and progression of atherosclerosis.[169] Munday et al.[170] found a modest reduced susceptibility of LDL particles to Cu^{+2}-mediated oxidation from subjects given daily 2.4 g aged garlic extract (AGE) for 7 d. Interestingly, a similar response was not observed when subjects were given 6 g raw garlic as a daily supplement for 7 d. Byrne et al.[166] did not find that 900mg Kwai garlic powder (Lichtwer Pharma, Berlin) for 6 months had an impact on LDL susceptibility to oxidation. It is unclear if the discrepancies in the literature about garlic and LDL oxidation relate to the subjects examined or the preparations used. DADS has been reported to protect human LDL, erythrocyte membranes, and platelets from oxidation and/or glycation.[171] Recently the protective effects of six organosulfur compounds (DAS, DADS, SAC, S-ethylcysteine, S-methylcysteine, and S-propylcysteine) were tested for their ability to reduce further oxidation and glycation in already partially oxidized and glycated samples from patients with non-insulin-dependent diabetes.[172] Their studies revealed that DAS and DADS were superior in delaying LDL oxidation compared to the four cysteine-containing compounds tested. However, the cysteine-containing agents were superior to DAS and DADS in delaying glycative deterioration in already partially glycated LDL. Both responses were highly concentration-dependent. Thus, the content or potential for forming active intermediates likely explains much of the variability that has been observed in the published literature.

B. BLOOD PRESSURE

Aortic stiffening is also an important risk factor in cardiovascular morbidity and mortality. This stiffness coincides with a high systolic blood pressure and augmented pulse pressure. Diet in addition to age, gender, hormonal state, and genetic factors probably influences aortic stiffening. Increasing evidence suggests garlic may be a dietary component with the ability to reduce blood pressure and cause relaxation in arterial walls. Garlic treatment has also been found to lead to a dose-dependent vaso-relaxation in both endothelium-intact and mechanically endothelium-disrupted pulmonary arterial rings.[173] This vaso-relaxation was diminished by the administration of NG-nitro-L-arginine methyl ester, a nitric oxide synthase inhibitor. The inducible nitric oxide synthase is recognized to occur in human atherosclerotic lesions. Recent studies have demonstrated that garlic exerts its therapeutic effect by increasing NO production.[174] The relaxant effect on vascular smooth muscle appears to be mediated through a decrease in cGMP and the subsequent release in endothelium-derived relaxing factors, as well as a depression in prostaglandins via a suppression in cyclooxygenase activity.[175,176] It is known that ROS counteract the vaso-dilating and antiproliferative actions of nitric oxide by rapidly degrading it to peroxynitrites. It is possible that part of the blood pressure changes caused by garlic may relate to its ability to reduce radical formation.

Recently, garlic was found in the Goldblatt model for hypertension to exert a sustained depression in arterial blood pressure.[177] An extract of garlic has been reported to serve as an antihypertensive in this two-kidney, one-clip (2K-1C) renovascular rat model for hypertension. At least part of the protection appears to be mediated through a normalization of prostaglandin E2 and thromboxane B2.[178] A change in the activity of the Na/H exchanger (NHE) may also be involved.[179]

C. Plaque and Platelet Aggregation

Acute coronary syndromes can occur when an unstable atherosclerotic plaque erodes or ruptures, thereby exposing the highly thrombogenic material inside the plaque to the circulating blood.[180] This exposure triggers a rapid formation of a thrombus that occludes the artery. Efendy et al.[181] found that feeding a deodorized garlic preparation (Kyolic) reduced the fatty streak development and vessel-wall cholesterol accumulation in cholesterol-fed rabbits. More recently Budoff et al.[182] found in a pilot study that providing an AGE extract for a year inhibited the rate of progression of coronary calcification compared to a placebo. Regular odor garlic preparations have also been reported to inhibit plaque formation in humans. Providing garlic powder (Lichtwer Pharma AG, Berlin, Germany) for 48 weeks in a randomized trial reduced arteriosclerotic plaque volumes in both the carotid and femoral arteries by 5 to 18%.[183] Zahid et al.[184] suggest that garlic may exert its beneficial effect on plaque formation by reducing cholesterol and maintaining the NO-mediated endothelial function, possibly secondary to an inhibition of LDL oxidation and an increase in HDL.

Aggregates of activated platelets also likely have a pivotal role in coronary syndromes. Garlic and some of its organosulfur components have been found to be potent inhibitors of platelet aggregation in vitro.[175,185–187] Some of the platelet-inhibitory compounds arising from allium plants include ajoene, allicin, SAC, methylallyl trisulfide, and alk(en)nyl thiosulfates such as sodium 2-propenyl thiosulfate and sodium n-propyl thiosulfate. Heating garlic by boiling retards its ability to inhibit platelet aggregation.[185] Unfortunately, few studies have documented that garlic can inhibit platelet aggregation in vivo. Regardless, Steiner and Lin[188] provided evidence that consumption of aged garlic extract reduced epinephrine and collagen-induced platelet aggregation, although it failed to influence adenosine diphosphate-induced aggregation. Their studies also provided evidence that platelet adhesion to fibrinogen could be suppressed by consumption of this garlic supplement.

Overall, garlic's ability to reduce hyperlipidemia, hypertension, sterol synthesis, and thrombus formation make it a strong candidate for lowering the risk of heart disease and stroke. Nevertheless, the literature provides evidence for considerable variability in response. Additional studies are needed to help clarify who might benefit most from added garlic.

VII. SUMMARY AND CONCLUSIONS

Garlic does have significant physiological attributes for promoting health. Although it is possible that other allium foods possess similar health attributes, few comparative studies have been undertaken. As garlic causes relatively few side-effects, except for possibly its lingering odor, there is little reason to avoid its use. Nevertheless, odor does not appear to be a necessary prerequisite for many of the benefits as water-soluble SAC generally gives comparable benefits to those compounds associated with smell. Although garlic and its bioactive components may influence a number of key molecular events that are involved with health, to do so it must achieve an effective concentration within the target site, be in the correct metabolic form, and lead to changes in small molecular-weight signals in the cellular milieu (metabolomic effects). Whereas most can savor the culinary experiences identified with garlic, some individuals, because of their gene profile and/or environmental exposure, may be particularly responsive to more exaggerated intakes.

REFERENCES

1. Tattelman, E., Health effects of garlic, *Am. Fam. Physician*, 72(1): 103–106, 2005.

2. Khanum, F., Anilakumar, K.R., and Viswanathan, K.R., Anticarcinogenic properties of garlic: a review, *Crit. Rev. Food Sci. Nutr.*, 44(6): 479–488, 2004.
3. Williams, M.J., Sutherland, W.H., McCormick, M.P., Yeoman, D.J., and de Jong, S.A., Aged garlic extract improves endothelial function in men with coronary artery disease, *Phytother. Res.*, 19(4): 314–319, 2005.
4. Sengupta, A., Ghosh, S., and Bhattacharjee, S., Allium vegetables in cancer prevention: an overview, *Asian Pac. J. Cancer Prev.*, 5(3): 237–245, 2004.
5. Blomhoff, R., Dietary antioxidants and cardiovascular disease, *Curr. Opin. Lipidol.*, 16(1): 47–54, 2005.
6. Banerjee, S.K., Mukherjee, P.K., and Maulik, S.K., Garlic as an antioxidant: the good, the bad and the ugly, *Phytother. Res.*, 17(2): 97–106, 2003.
7. Kyo, E., Uda, N., Kasuga, S., and Itakura, Y., Immunomodulatory effect of aged garlic extract, *J. Nutr.*, 131(3S): 1075S–1079S, 2001.
8. Yamada, N., Hattori, A., Hayashi, T., Nishikawa, T., Fukuda, H., and Fujino, T., Improvement of scopolamine-induced memory impairment by Z-ajoene in the water maze in mice, *Pharmacol. Biochem. Behav.*, 78(4): 787–791, 2004.
9. Hartsook, C., Herb Profile, United States Department of Agriculture, Economic Research Service, AgMRC, Iowa State University, Agricultural Outlook, 2003.
10. Steinmetz, K.A., Kushi, L.H., Bostick, R.M., Folsom, A.R., and Potter, J.D., Vegetables, fruit, and colon cancer in the Iowa Women's Health Study, *Am. J. Epidemiol.*, 139(1): 1–15, 1994.
11. Fleischauer, A.T., Poole, C., and Arab, L., Garlic consumption and cancer prevention: meta-analyses of colorectal and stomach cancers, *Am. J. Clin. Nutr.*, 72(4): 1047–1052, 2000.
12. Jappe, U., Bonnekoh, B., Hausen, B.M., and Gollnick, H., Garlic-related dermatoses: case report and review of the literature, *Am. J. Contact. Dermatitis*, 10(1): 37–39, 1999.
13. Burden, A.D., Wilkinson, S.M., Beck, M.H., and Chalmers, R.J., Garlic induced systemic contact dermatitis, *Contact Dermatitis*, 30(5): 299–300, 1994.
14. Moyle, M., Frowen, K., and Nixon, R., Use of gloves in protection from diallyl disulphide allergy, *Australas. J. Dermatol.*, 45(4): 223–225, 2004.
15. Umar, I.A., Arjinoma, Z.G., Gidado, A., and Hamza, H.H., Prevention of garlic (Allium sativum Linn)-induced anaemia in rats by supplementation with ascorbic acid and vitamin E, *Nig. J. Biochem. Mol. Biol.*, 13: 31–40, 1998.
16. Yamato, O., Sugiyama, Y., Matsuura, H., Lee, K.W., Goto, K., Hossain, M.A., Maede, Y., and Yoshihara, T., Isolation and identification of sodium 2-propenyl thiosulfate from boiled garlic (Allium sativum) that oxidizes canine erythrocytes, *Biosci. Biotechnol. Biochem.*, 67(7): 1594–1596, 2003.
17. Fenwick, G.R. and Hanley, A.B., The genus Allium, Part 2, *Crit. Rev. Food Sci. Nutr.*, 22(4): 273–277, 1985.
18. Milner, J.A., Garlic: its anticarcinogenic and antitumorigenic properties, *Nutr. Rev.*, 54(11 Pt. 2): S82–S86, 1996.
19. Lawson, L.D. and Wang, Z.J., Allicin and allicin-derived garlic compounds increase breath acetone through allyl methyl sulfide: use in measuring allicin bioavailability, *J. Agric. Food Chem.*, 53(6): 1974–1983, 2005.
20. Arnault, I., Haffner, T., Siess, M.H., Vollmar, A., Kahane, R., and Auger, J., Analytical method for appreciation of garlic therapeutic potential and for validation of a new formulation, *J. Pharm. Biomed. Anal.*, 37(5): 963–970, 2005.
21. Rose, P., Whiteman, M., Moore, P.K., and Zhu, Y.Z., Bioactive S-alk(en)yl cysteine sulfoxide metabolites in the genus Allium: the chemistry of potential therapeutic agents, *Nat. Prod. Rep.*, 22(3): 351–368, 2005.
22. Kubec, R., Svobodova, M., and Velisek, J., Gas chromatographic determination of S-alk(en)ylcysteine sulfoxides, *J. Chromatogr. A.*, 862(1): 85–94, 1999.
23. Freeman, G.G. and Mossadeghi, N., Influence of sulphate nutrition on the flavour components of garlic (Allium sativum) and wild onions (Allium vineale), *J. Sci. Food Agric.*, 22: 330–334, 1971.
24. Berges, R., Siess, M.H., Arnault, I., Auger, J., Kahane, R., Pinnert, M.F., Vernevaut, M.F., and le Bon, A.M., Comparison of the chemopreventive efficacies of garlic powders with different alliin contents against aflatoxin B1 carcinogenicity in rats, *Carcinogenesis*, 25(10): 1953–1959, 2004.

25. Lawson, L.D., Garlic: a review of its medicinal effects and indicated active compounds, in *Phytomedicines of Europe: Chemistry and Biological Activity*, Lawson, L.D., and Bauer, R., Eds., American Chemical Society, Washington, D.C., 1998.

26. Sugii, M., Suzuki, T., Nagasawa, S., and Kawashima, K., Isolation of Gamma-1-Glutamyl-S-allylmercapto-L-cysteine and S-allylmercapto-L-cysteine from garlic, *Chem. Pharm. Bull. (Tokyo)*, 12: 1114–1115, 1964.

27. Block, E., The chemistry of garlic and onion, *Sci. Am.*, 252(3): 114–119, 1985.

28. Lawson, L.D., Wang, Z.J., and Hughes, B.G., Identification and HPLC quantitation of the sulfides and dialk(en)yl thiosulfinates in commercial garlic products, *Planta Med.*, 57(4): 363–370, 1991.

29. Tamaki, T. and Sonoki, S., Volatile sulfur compounds in human expiration after eating raw or heat-treated garlic, *J. Nutr. Sci. Vitaminol. (Tokyo)*, 45(2): 213–222, 1999.

30. Lawson, L.D. and Gardner, C.D., Composition, stability, and bioavailability of garlic products used in a clinical trial, *J. Agric. Food Chem.*, 53(16): 6254–6261, 2005.

31. Staba, E.J., Lash, L., and Staba, J.E., A commentary on the effects of garlic extraction and formulation on product composition, *J. Nutr.*, 131(3S): 1118S–1119S, 2001.

32. Lachmann, G., Lorenz, D., Radeck, W., and Steiper, M., The pharmacokinetics of the S35 labeled garlic constituents alliin, allicin, and vinyldithiine, *Arzneimittelforschung*, 44(6): 734–743, 1994.

33. Egen-Schwind, C., Eckard, R., and Kemper, F.H., Metabolism of garlic constituents in the isolated perfused rat liver, *Planta Med.*, 58(4): 301–305, 1992.

34. Germain, E., Auger, J., Ginies, C., Siess, M.H., and Teyssier, C., In vivo metabolism of diallyl disulphide in the rat: identification of two new metabolites, *Xenobiotica*, 32(12): 1127–1138, 2002.

35. Teyssier, C., Guenot, L., Suschetet, M., and Siess, M.H., Metabolism of diallyl disulfide by human liver microsomal cytochromes P-450 and flavin-containing monooxygenases, *Drug Metab. Dispos.*, 27(7): 835–841, 1999.

36. Ripp, S.L., Overby, L.H., Philpot, R.M., and Elfarra, A.A., Oxidation of cysteine S-conjugates by rabbit liver microsomes and cDNA-expressed flavin-containing mono-oxygenases: studies with S-(1,2-dichlorovinyl)-L-cysteine, S-(1,2,2 trichlorovinyl)-L-cysteine, S-allyl-L-cysteine, and S-benzyl-L-cysteine, *Mol. Pharmacol.*, 51(3): 507–515, 1997.

37. Liu, J.Z., Lin, R.I., and Milner, J.A., Inhibition of 7,12-dimethylbenz(a)-anthracene induced mammary tumors and DNA adducts by garlic powder, *Carcinogenesis*, 13(10): 1847–1851, 1992.

38. Singh, A. and Shukla, Y., Antitumour activity of diallyl sulfide on polycyclic aromatic hydrocarbon-induced mouse skin carcinogenesis, *Cancer Lett.*, 131(2): 209–214, 1998.

39. Balasenthil, S., Arivazhagan, S., Ramachandran, C.R., and Nagini, S., Effects of garlic on 7,12-dimethylbenz[a]anthracene-induced hamster buccal pouch carcinogenesis, *Cancer Detect. Prev.*, 23(6): 534–538, 1999.

40. Amagase, H. and Milner, J.A., Impact of various sources of garlic and their constituents on 7,12-dimethylbenz(a)anthracene binding to mammary cell DNA, *Carcinogenesis*, 14(8): 1627–1631, 1993.

41. Schaffer, E.M., Liu, J.Z., Green, J., Dangler, C.A., and Milner, J.A., Garlic and associated allyl sulfur components inhibit N-methyl-N-nitrosourea induced rat mammary carcinogenesis, *Cancer Lett.*, 102(1–2): 199–204, 1996.

42. Schaffer, E.M., Liu, J.Z., and Milner, J.A., Garlic powder and allyl sulfur compounds enhance the ability of dietary selenite to inhibit 7,12-dimethylbenz[a]anthracene-induced mammary DNA adducts, *Nutr. Cancer*, 27(2): 162–168, 1997.

43. Sakamoto, K., Lawson, L.D., and Milner, J., Allyl sulfides from garlic suppress the in vitro proliferation of human A549 lung tumor cells, *Nutr. Cancer*, 29(2): 152–156, 1997.

44. Sundaram, S.G. and Milner, J.A., Diallyl disulfide induces apoptosis of human colon tumor cells, *Carcinogenesis*, 17(4): 669–673, 1996.

45. Tsai, S.J., Jenq, S.N., and Lee, H., Naturally occurring diallyl disulfide inhibits the formation of carcinogenic heterocyclic aromatic amines in boiled pork juice, *Mutagenesis*, 11(3): 235–240, 1996.

46. Hu, X., Benson, P.J., Srivastava, S.K., Xia, H., Bleicher, R.J., Zaren, H.A., Awasthi, S., Awasthi, Y.C., and Singh, S.V., Induction of glutathione S-transferase pi as a bioassay for the evaluation of potency of inhibitors of benzo(a)pyrene-induced cancer in a murine model, *Int. J. Cancer*, 73(6): 897–902, 1997.

47. Adetumbi, M.A. and Lau, B.H., Allium sativum (garlic) — a natural antibiotic, *Med. Hypotheses*, 12(3): 227–237, 1983.

48. Lee, Y.L., Cesario, T., Wang, Y., Shanbrom, E., and Thrupp, L., Antibacterial activity of vegetables and juices, *Nutrition*, 19(11–12): 994–996, 2003.

49. Lai, P.K. and Roy, J., Antimicrobial and chemopreventive properties of herbs and spices, *Curr. Med. Chem.*, 11(11):.1451–1460, 2004.

50. Davis, S.R., An overview of the antifungal properties of allicin and its breakdown products — the possibility of a safe and effective antifungal prophylactic, *Mycoses*, 48(2): 95–100, 2005.

51. Dion, M.E., Agler, M., and Milner, J.A., S-allyl cysteine inhibits nitrosomorpholine formation and bioactivation, *Nutr. Cancer*, 28(1): 1–6, 1997.

52. Yoshida, H., Katsuzaki, H., Ohta, R., Ishikawa, K., Fukuda, H., Fujino, T., and Suzuki, A., An organosulfur compound isolated from oil-macerated garlic extract, and its antimicrobial effect, *Biosci. Biotechnol. Biochem.*, 63(3): 588–590, 1999.

53. Tsao, S.M., Hsu, C.C., and Yin, M.C., Garlic extract and two diallyl sulphides inhibit methicillin-resistant Staphylococcus aureus infection in BALB/cA mice, *J. Antimicrob. Chemother.*, 52(6): 974–980, 2003.

54. Avato, P., Tursil, E., Vitali, C., Miccolis, V., and Candido, V., Allylsulfide constituents of garlic volatile oil as antimicrobial agents, *Phytomedicine*, 7(3): 239–243, 2000.

55. Kim, J.W., Kim, Y.S., and Kyung, K.H., Inhibitory activity of essential oils of garlic and onion against bacteria and yeasts, *J. Food Prot.*, 67(3): 499–504, 2004.

56. Ruddock, P.S., Liao, M., Foster, B.C., Lawson, L., Arnason, J.T., and Dillon, J.A., Garlic natural health products exhibit variable constituent levels and antimicrobial activity against *Neisseria gonorrhoeae*, *Staphylococcus aureus* and *Enterococcus faecalis*, *Phytother. Res.*, 19(4): 327–334, 2005.

57. Xia, L. and Ng, T.B., Isolation of alliumin, a novel protein with antimicrobial and antiproliferative activities from multiple-cloved garlic bulbs, *Peptides*, 26(2): 177–183, 2005.

58. Cellini, L., Di Campli, E., Masulli, M., Di Bartolomeo, S., and Allocati, N., Inhibition of Helicobacter pylori by garlic extract (Allium sativum), *FEMS Immunol. Med. Microbiol.*, 13(4): 273–277, 1996.

59. Chung, J.G., Chen, G.W., Wu, L.T., Chang, H.L., Lin, J.G., Yeh, C.C., and Wang, T.F., Effects of garlic compounds diallyl sulfide and diallyl disulfide on arylamine N-acetyltransferase activity in strains of Helicobacter pylori from peptic ulcer patients, *Am. J. Chin. Med.*, 26(3–4): 353–364, 1998.

60. Jonkers, D., van den Broek, E., van Dooren, I., Thijs, C., Dorant, E., Hageman, G., and Stobberingh, E., Antibacterial effect of garlic and omeprazole on Helicobacter pylori, *J. Antimicrob. Chemother.*, 43(6): 837–839, 1999.

61. Iimuro, M., Shibata, H., Kawamori, T., Matsumoto, T., Arakawa, T., Sugimura, T., and Wakabayashi, K., Suppressive effects of garlic extract on Helicobacter pylori-induced gastritis in Mongolian gerbils, *Cancer Lett.*, 187(1–2): 61–68, 2002.

62. You, W.C., Zhang, L., Gail, M.H., Ma, J.L., Chang, Y.S., Blot, W.J., Li, J.Y., Zhao, C.L., Liu, W.D., Li, H.Q., Hu, Y.R., Bravo, J.C., Correa, P., Xu, G.W., and Fraumeni, J.F., Jr., Helicobacter pylori infection, garlic intake and precancerous lesions in a Chinese population at low risk of gastric cancer, *Int. J. Epidemiol.*, 27(6): 941–944, 1998.

63. Aydin, A., Ersoz, G., Tekesin, O., Akcicek, E., and Tuncyurek, M., Garlic oil and Helicobacter pylori infection, *Am. J. Gastroenterol.*, 95(2): 563–564, 2000.

64. Graham, D.Y., Anderson, S.Y., and Lang, T., Garlic or jalapeno peppers for treatment of Helicobacter pylori infection, *Am. J. Gastroenterol.*, 94(5): 1200–1202, 1999.

65. Arora, D.S. and Kaur, J., Antimicrobial activity of spices, *Int. J. Antimicrob. Agents*, 12(3): 257–262, 1999.

66. Ledezma, E., Marcano, K., Jorquera, A., De Sousa, L., Padilla, M., Pulgar, M., and Apitz-Castro, R., Efficacy of ajoene in the treatment of tinea pedis: a double-blind and comparative study with terbinafine, *J. Am. Acad. Dermatol.*, 43(5 Pt. 1): 829–832, 2000.

67. Rabinkov, A., Miron, T., Mirelman, D., Wilchek, M., Glozman, S., Yavin, E., and Weiner, L., S-Allylmercaptoglutathione: the reaction product of allicin with glutathione possesses SH-modifying and antioxidant properties, *Biochim. Biophys. Acta*, 1499(1–2):.144–153, 2000.

68. Gupta, N. and Porter, T.D., Garlic and garlic-derived compounds inhibit human squalene monooxygenase, *J. Nutr.*, 131(6): 1662–1667, 2001.

69. Balkis, M.M., Leidich, S.D., Mukherjee, P.K., and Ghannoum, M.A., Mechanisms of fungal resistance: an overview, *Drugs*, 62(7): 1025–1040, 2002.

70. Castro, I.A., Barroso, L.P., and Sinnecker, P., Functional foods for coronary heart disease risk reduction: a meta-analysis using a multivariate approach, *Am. J. Clin. Nutr.*, 82(1): 32–40, 2005.
71. Milner, J.A., Molecular targets for bioactive food components, *J. Nutr.*, 134(9): 2492S–2498S, 2004.
72. Fleischauer, A.T. and Arab, L., Garlic and cancer: a critical review of the epidemiologic literature, *J. Nutr.*, 131(3S): 1032S–1040S, 2001.
73. Hsing, A.W., Chokkalingam, A.P., Gao, Y.T., Madigan, M.P., Deng, J., Gridley, G., and Fraumeni, J.F. Jr., Allium vegetables and risk of prostate cancer: a population-based study, *J. Natl. Cancer Inst.*, 94(21): 1648–1651, 2002.
74. Tanaka, S., Haruma, K., Kunihiro, M., Nagata, S., Kitadai, Y., Manabe, N., Sumii, M., Yoshihara, M., Kajiyama, G., and Chayama, K., Effects of aged garlic extract (AGE) on colorectal adenomas: a double-blinded study, *Hiroshima J. Med. Sci.*, 53(3–4): 39–45, 2004.
75. You, W.C., Blot, W.J., Chang, Y.S., Ershow, A., Yang, Z.T., An, Q., Henderson, B.E., Fraumeni, J.F., Jr., and Wang, T.G., Allium vegetables and reduced risk of stomach cancer, *J. Natl. Cancer Inst.*, 81(2): 162–164, 1989.
76. Gail, M.H., You, W.C., Chang, Y.S., Zhang, L., Blot, W.J., Brown, L.M., Groves, F.D., Heinrich, J.P., Hu, J., Jin, M.L., Li, J.Y., Liu, W.D., Ma, J.L., Mark, S.D., Rabkin, C.S., Fraumeni, J.F., Jr., and Xu, G.W., Factorial trial of three interventions to reduce the progression of precancerous gastric lesions in Shandong, China: design issues and initial data, *Control Clin. Trials*, 19(4): 352–369, 1998.
77. You, W.C., Chang, Y.S., Heinrich, J., Ma, J.L., Liu, W.D., Zhang, L., Brown, L.M., Yang, C.S., Gail, M.H., Fraumeni, J.F., Jr., and Xu, G.W., An intervention trial to inhibit the progression of precancerous gastric lesions: compliance, serum micronutrients and S-allyl cysteine levels, and toxicity, *Eur. J. Cancer Prev.*, 10(3): 257–263, 2001.
78. Ip, C., Lisk, D.J., and Stoewsand, G.S., Mammary cancer prevention by regular garlic and selenium-enriched garlic, *Nutr. Cancer*, 17(3): 279–286, 1992.
79. Wargovich, M.J., Diallyl sulfide, a flavor component of garlic (Allium sativum), inhibits dimethylhydrazine-induced colon cancer, *Carcinogenesis*, 8(3): 487–489, 1987.
80. Hussain, S.P., Jannu, L.N., and Rao, A.R., Chemopreventive action of garlic on methylcholanthrene-induced carcinogenesis in the uterine cervix of mice, *Cancer Lett.*, 49(2): 175–180, 1990.
81. Wargovich, M.J., Woods, C., Eng, V.W., Stephens, L.C., and Gray, K., Chemoprevention of N-nitrosomethylbenzylamine-induced esophageal cancer in rats by the naturally occurring thioether, diallyl sulfide, *Cancer Res.*, 48(23): 6872–6875, 1988.
82. Hong, J.Y., Wang, Z.Y., Smith, T.J., Zhou, S., Shi, S., Pan, J., and Yang, C.S., Inhibitory effects of diallyl sulfide on the metabolism and tumorigenicity of the tobacco-specific carcinogen 4-(methylnitrosamino)-1-(3-pyridyl)-1-butanone (NNK) in A/J mouse lung, *Carcinogenesis*, 13(5): 901–904, 1992.
83. Takahashi, S., Hakoi, K., Yada, H., Hirose, M., Ito, N., and Fukushima, S., Enhancing effects of diallyl sulfide on hepatocarcinogenesis and inhibitory actions of the related diallyl disulfide on colon and renal carcinogenesis in rats, *Carcinogenesis*, 13(9): 1513–1518, 1992.
84. Nagabhushan, M., Line, D., Polverini, P.J., and Solt, D.B., Anticarcinogenic action of diallyl sulfide in hamster buccal pouch and forestomach, *Cancer Lett.*, 66(3): 207–216, 1992.
85. Park, K.A., Kweon, S., and Choi, H., Anticarcinogenic effect and modification of cytochrome P450 2E1 by dietary garlic powder in diethylnitrosamine-initiated rat hepatocarcinogenesis, *J. Biochem. Mol. Biol.*, 35(6): 615–622, 2002.
86. Wargovich, M.J., Chen, C.D., Jimenez, A., Steele, V.E., Velasco, M., Stephens, L.C., Price, R., Gray, K., and Kelloff, G.J., Aberrant crypts as a biomarker for colon cancer: evaluation of potential chemopreventive agents in the rat, *Cancer Epidemiol. Biomarkers Prev.*, 5(5): 355–360, 1996.
87. Wargovich, M.J., Jimenez, A., McKee, K., Steele, V.E., Velasco, M., Woods, J., Price, R., Gray, K., and Kelloff, G.J., Efficacy of potential chemopreventive agents on rat colon aberrant crypt formation and progression, *Carcinogenesis*, 21(6): 1149–1155, 2000.
88. Ross, S.A., Finley, J.W., Leary, P., Gregoire, B., and Milner, J., Speciation effects of allyl sulfur compounds on aberrant crypt formation [abstract], *FASEB J.*, 19(4): A72.13, 2005.
89. Jakszyn, P., Agudo, A., Ibanez, R., Garcia-Closas, R., Pera, G., Amiano, P., and Gonzalez, C.A., Development of a food database of nitrosamines, heterocyclic amines, and polycyclic aromatic hydrocarbons, *J. Nutr.*, 134(8): 2011–2014, 2004.
90. Lijinsky, W., N-Nitroso compounds in the diet, *Mutat. Res.*, 443(1–2): 129–138, 1999.

91. Shenoy, N.R. and Choughuley, A.S., Inhibitory effect of diet related sulphydryl compounds on the formation of carcinogenic nitrosamines, *Cancer Lett.*, 65(3): 227–232, 1992.

92. Milner, J.A., Mechanisms by which garlic and allyl sulfur compounds suppress carcinogen bioactivation. Garlic and carcinogenesis, *Adv. Exp. Med. Biol.*, 492: 69–81, 2001.

93. Williams, D.H,. S-Nitrosation and the reactions of S-Nitroso compounds, *Chem. Soc. Rev.*, 15: 171–196, 1983.

94. Mei, X., Lin, X., Liu, J., Lin, X.Y., Song, P.J., Hu, J.F., and Liang, X.J., The blocking effect of garlic on the formation of N-nitrosoproline in humans, *Acta Nutrimenta Sinica*, 11: 141–145, 1989.

95. Ohshima, H. and Bartsch, H., Quantitative estimation of endogenous N-nitrosation in humans by monitoring N-nitrosoproline in urine, *Methods Enzymol.*, 301: 40–49, 1999.

96. Lin, X-Y., Liu, J.Z., Milner, J.A., Dietary garlic suppresses DNA adducts caused by N-nitroso compounds, *Carcinogenesis*, 15(2): 349–352, 1994.

97. Haber-Mignard, D., Suschetet, M., Berges, R., Astorg, P., and Siess, M.H., Inhibition of aflatoxin B1- and N-nitrosodiethylamine-induced liver preneoplastic foci in rats fed naturally occurring allyl sulfides, *Nutr. Cancer*, 25(1): 61–70, 1996.

98. Knasmuller, S., de Martin, R., Domjan, G., and Szakmary, A., Studies on the antimutagenic activities of garlic extract, *Environ. Mol. Mutagen.*, 13(4): 357–365, 1989.

99. Chen, L., Lee, M., Hong, J.Y., Huang, W., Wang, E., and Yang, C.S., Relationship between cytochrome P450 2E1 and acetone catabolism in rats as studied with diallyl sulfide as an inhibitor, *Biochem. Pharmacol.*, 48(12): 2199–2205, 1994.

100. Jeong, H.G. and Lee, Y.W., Protective effects of diallyl sulfide on N-nitrosodimethylamine-induced immunosuppression in mice, *Cancer Lett.*, 134(1): 73–79, 1998.

101. Jin, L. and Baillie, T.A., Metabolism of the chemoprotective agent diallyl sulfide to glutathione conjugates in rats, *Chem. Res. Toxicol.*, 10(3): 318–327, 1997.

102. Davenport, D.M. and Wargovich, M.J., Modulation of cytochrome P450 enzymes by organosulfur compounds from garlic, *Food Chem. Toxicol.*, July 4 [Epub ahead of print] 2005.

103. Yu, F.S., Yu, C.S., Lin, J.P., Chen, S.C., Lai, W.W., and Chung, J.G., Diallyl disulfide inhibits N-acetyltransferase activity and gene expression in human esophagus epidermoid carcinoma CE 81T/VGH cells, *Food Chem. Toxicol.*, 43(7): 1029–1036, 2005.

104. Ludeke, B.I., Domine, F., Ohgaki, H., and Kleihues, P., Modulation of N-nitrosomethylbenzylamine bioactivation by diallyl sulfide in vivo, *Carcinogenesis*, 13(12): 2467–2470, 1992.

105. Zhang, Y.J., Chen, Y., Ahsan, H., Lunn, R.M., Chen, S.Y., Lee, P.H., Chen, C.J., and Santella, R.M., Silencing of glutathione S-transferase P1 by promoter hypermethylation and its relationship to environmental chemical carcinogens in hepatocellular carcinoma, *Cancer Lett.*, 221(2): 135–143, 2005.

106. Cohen, L.A., Zhao, Z., Pittman, B., and Lubet, R., S-allylcysteine, a garlic constituent, fails to inhibit N-methylnitrosourea-induced rat mammary tumorigenesis, *Nutr. Cancer*, 35(1): 58–63, 1999.

107. Le Bon, A.M., Vernevaut, M.F., Guenot, L., Kahane, R., Auger, J., Arnault, I., Haffner, T., and Siess, M.H., Effects of garlic powders with varying alliin contents on hepatic drug metabolizing enzymes in rats, *J. Agric. Food Chem.*, 51(26): 7617–7623, 2003.

108. Wu, C.C., Sheen, L.Y., Chen, H.W., Kuo, W.W., Tsai, S.J., and Lii, C.K., Differential effects of garlic oil and its three major organosulfur components on the hepatic detoxification system in rats, *J. Agric. Food Chem.*, 50(2): 378–383, 2002.

109. Foster, B.C., Foster, M.S., Vandenhoek, S., Krantis, A., Budzinski, J.W., Arnason, J.T., Gallicano, K.D., and Choudri, S., An in vitro evaluation of human cytochrome P450 3A4 and P-glycoprotein inhibition by garlic, *J. Pharm. Pharm. Sci.*, 4(2): 176–184, 2001.

110. Brady, J.F., Ishizaki, H., Fukuto, J.M., Lin, M.C., Fadel, A., Gapac, J.M., and Yang, C.S., Inhibition of cytochrome P-450 2E1 by diallyl sulfide and its metabolites, *Chem. Res. Toxicol.*, **4(6):** 642–647, 1991.

111. Uno, S., Dalton, T.P., Derkenne, S., Curran, C.P., Miller, M.L., Shertzer, H.G., and Nebert, D.W., Oral exposure to benzo[a]pyrene in the mouse: detoxication by inducible cytochrome P450 is more important than metabolic activation, *Mol. Pharmacol.*, 65(5): 1225–1237, 2004.

112. Singh, S.V., Pan, S.S., Srivastava, S.K., Xia, H., Hu, X., Zaren, H.A., and Orchard, J.L., Differential induction of NAD(P)H: quinone oxidoreductase by anti-carcinogenic organosulfides from garlic, *Biochem. Biophys. Res. Commun.*, 244(3): 917–920, 1998.

113. Chen, C., Pung, D., Leong, V., Hebbar, V., Shen, G., Nair, S., Li, W., and Kong, A.N., Induction of detoxifying enzymes by garlic organosulfur compounds through transcription factor Nrf2: effect of chemical structure and stress signals, *Free Radic. Biol. Med.*, 37(10): 1578–1590, 2004.

114. Munday, R. and Munday, C.M., Relative activities of organosulfur compounds derived from onions and garlic in increasing tissue activities of quinone reductase and glutathione transferase in rat tissues, *Nutr. Cancer*, 40(2): 205–210, 2001.

115. Herman-Antosiewicz, A. and Singh, S.V., Signal transduction pathways leading to cell cycle arrest and apoptosis induction in cancer cells by Allium vegetable-derived organosulfur compounds: a review, *Mutat. Res.*, 555(1–2): 121–131, 2004.

116. Wu, X., Kassie, F., and Mersch-Sundermann, V., Induction of apoptosis in tumor cells by naturally occurring sulfur-containing compounds, *Mutat. Res.*, 589(2): 81–102, 2005.

117. Wu, X.J., Kassie, F., and Mersch-Sundermann, V., The role of reactive oxygen species (ROS) production on diallyl disulfide (DADS) induced apoptosis and cell cycle arrest in human A549 lung carcinoma cells, *Mutat. Res.*, July 14 [Epub ahead of print] 2005.

118. Knowles, L.M. and Milner, J.A., Possible mechanism by which allyl sulfides suppress neoplastic cell proliferation, *J. Nutr.*, 131(3S): 1061S–1066S, 2001.

119. Knowles, L.M. and Milner, J.A., Diallyl disulfide inhibits p34(cdc2) kinase activity through changes in complex formation and phosphorylation, *Carcinogenesis* **21(6):** 1129–1134, 2000.

120. Knowles, L.M. and Milner, J.A., Diallyl disulfide induces ERK phosphorylation and alters gene expression profiles in human colon tumor cells, *J. Nutr.*, 133(9): 2901–2906, 2003.

121. L'vova, G.N. and Zasukhina, G.D., Modification of repair DNA synthesis in mutagen-treated human fibroblasts during adaptive response and the antimutagenic effect of garlic extract, *Genetika*, 38(3): 306–309, 2002.

122. Ross, S.A., Diet and DNA methylation interactions in cancer prevention, *Ann. N.Y. Acad. Sci.*, 983: 197–207, 2003.

123. Lea, M.A., Randolph, V.M., and Patel, M., Increased acetylation of histones induced by diallyl disulfide and structurally related molecules, *Int. J. Oncol.*, 15(2): 347–352, 1999.

124. Lea, M.A., Rasheed, M., Randolph, V.M., Khan, F., Shareef, A., and desBordes, C., Induction of histone acetylation and inhibition of growth of mouse erythroleukemia cells by S-allylmercaptocysteine, *Nutr. Cancer*, **43(1):** 90–102, 2002.

125. Druesne, N., Pagniez, A., Mayeur, C., Thomas, M., Cherbuy, C., Duee, P.H., Martel, P., and Chaumontet, C., Diallyl disulfide (DADS) increases histone acetylation and p21(waf1/cip1) expression in human colon tumor cell lines, *Carcinogenesis*, 25(7): 1227–1236, 2004.

126. Myzak, M.C., Karplus, P.A., Chung, F.L., and Dashwood, R.H., A novel mechanism of chemoprotection by sulforaphane: inhibition of histone deacetylase, *Cancer Res.*, 64(16): 5767–5774, 2004.

127. Rabinkov, A., Miron, T., Konstantinovski, L., Wilchek, M., Mirelman, D., and Weiner, L., The mode of action of allicin: trapping of radicals and interaction with thiol containing proteins, *Biochim. Biophys. Acta*, 1379(2): 233–244, 1998.

128. Rahman, K., Garlic and aging: new insights into an old remedy, *Ageing Res. Rev.*, 2(1): 39–56, 2003.

129. Dwivedi, C., John, L.M., Schmidt, D.S., and Engineer, F.N., Effects of oil-soluble organosulfur compounds from garlic on doxorubicin-induced lipid peroxidation, *Anticancer Drugs*, 9(3): 291–294, 1998.

130. Atmaca, G., Antioxidant effects of sulfur-containing amino acids, *Yonsei Med. J.*, 45(5): 776–788, 2004.

131. Okada, Y., Tanaka, K., Fujita, I., Sato, E., and Okajima, H., Antioxidant activity of thiosulfinates derived from garlic, *Redox Rep.*, 10(2): 96–102, 2005.

132. Lawson, L.D., Bioactive organosulfur compounds of garlic and garlic products, in *Human Medicinal Agents from Plants*, Kinghorn, A.D. and Balandrin, M.F., Eds., American Chemical Society, Washington D.C., 1994.

133. Gorinstein, S., Drzewiecki, J., Leontowicz, H., Leontowicz, M., Najman, K., Jastrzebski, Z., Zachwieja, Z., Barton, H., Shtabsky, B., Katrich, E., and Trakhtenberg, S., Comparison of the bioactive compounds and antioxidant potentials of fresh and cooked Polish, Ukrainian, and Israeli garlic, *Agric. Food Chem.*, 53(7): 2726–2732, 2005.

134. Lamm, D.L. and Riggs, D.R., Enhanced immuno competence by garlic: role in bladder cancer and other malignancies, *J. Nutr.*, 131(3S): 1067S–1070S, 2001.

135. Colic, M. and Savic, M., Garlic extracts stimulate proliferation of rat lymphocyte in vitro increasing IL-2 and IL-4 production, *Immunopharmacol. Immunotoxicol.*, 22(1): 163–181, 2000.
136. Colic, M., Vucevic, D., Kilibarda, V., Radicevic, N., and Savic, M., Modulatory effects of garlic extracts on proliferation of T-lymphocytes in vitro stimulated with concanavalin A, *Phytomedicine*, 9(2): 117–124, 2002.
137. Ghazanfari, T., Hassan, Z.M., Ebtekar, M., Ahmadiani, A., Naderi, G., and Azar, A., Garlic induces a shift in cytokine pattern in *Leishmania major*-infected BALB/c mice, *Scand. J. Immunol.*, 52(5): 491–495, 2000.
138. Morioka, N., Sze, L.L., Morton, D.L., and Irie, R.F., A protein fraction from aged garlic extract enhances cytotoxicity and proliferation of human lymphocytes mediated by interleukin-2 and concanavalin A, *Cancer Immunol. Immunother.*, 37(5): 316–322, 1993.
139. Ghazanfari, T., Hassan, Z.M., and Ebrahimi, M., Immunomodulatory activity of a protein isolated from garlic extract on delayed type hypersensitivity, *Int. Immunopharmacol.*, 2 (11): 1541–1559, 2002.
140. Ghazanfari, T., Hassan, Z.M., and Ebrahimi, M., Immunomodulatory affect of R10 fraction of garlic extract on natural killer activity, *Int. Immunopharmacol.*, 3(10–11): 1483–1489, 2003.
141. Chang, H.P., Huang, S.Y., and Chen, Y.H., Modulation of cytokine secretion by garlic oil derivatives is associated with suppressed nitric oxide production in stimulated macrophages, *J. Agric. Food Chem.*, 53(7): 2530–2534, 2005.
142. Dirsch, V.M., Kiemer, A.K., Wagner, H., and Vollmar, A.M., Effect of allicin and ajoene, two compounds of garlic, on inducible nitric oxide synthase, *Atherosclerosis*, 139(2): 333–339, 1998.
143. Chang, H.P. and Chen, Y.H., Differential effects of organosulfur compounds from garlic oil on nitric oxide and prostaglandin E2 in stimulated macrophages, *Nutrition*, 21(4): 530–536, 2005.
144. Smith, B.J., Curtis, J.F., and Eling, T.E., Bioactivation of xenobiotics by prostaglandin H synthase, *Chem-Biol Interactions*, 79(3): 245–264, 1991.
145. Li, N., Sood, S., Wang, S., Fang, M., Wang, P., Sun, Z., Yang, C.S., and Chen, X., Overexpression of 5-lipoxygenase and cyclooxygenase 2 in hamster and human oral cancer and chemopreventive effects of zileuton and celecoxib, *Clin. Cancer Res.*, 11(5): 2089–2096, 2005.
146. Ali, M., Mechanism by which garlic (Allium sativum) inhibits cyclooxygenase activity: effect of raw versus boiled garlic extract on the synthesis of prostanoids, *Prostaglandins Leukot. Essent. Fatty Acids*, 53(6): 397–400, 1995.
147. McGrath, B.C. and Milner, J.A., Diallyl Disulfide, S-Allyl Sulfide and Conjugated Linoleic Acid Retard 12/15-Lipoxygenase-Mediated Bioactivation of 7,12-Dimethylbenz(a)anthracene (DMBA) In Vitro, *FASEB J.*, 13(4): A540, 1999.
148. Belman, S., Solomon, J., Segal, A., Block, E., and Barany, G., Inhibition of soybean lipoxygenase and mouse skin tumor promotion by onion and garlic components, *J. Biochem. Toxicol.*, 4(3): 151–160, 1989.
149. Song, K. and Milner, J.A., Heating garlic inhibits its ability to suppress 7, 12-dimethylbenz(a)anthracene-induced DNA adduct formation in rat mammary tissue, *J. Nutr.*, 129(3): 657–661, 1999.
150. Dirsch, V.M. and Vollmar, A.M., Ajoene, a natural product with non-steroidal anti-inflammatory drug (NSAID)-like properties, *Biochem. Pharmacol*, 61(5): 587–593, 2001.
151. Velmurugan, B., Bhuvaneswari, V., Abraham, S.K., and Nagini, S., Protective effect of tomato against N-methyl-N-nitro-N-nitrosoguanidine-induced in vivo clastogenicity and oxidative stress, *Nutrition*, 20(9): 812–816, 2004.
152. Bhuvaneswari, V., Abraham, S.K., and Nagini, S., Combinatorial antigenotoxic and anticarcinogenic effects of tomato and garlic through modulation of xenobiotic-metabolizing enzymes during hamster buccal pouch carcinogenesis, *Nutrition*, 21(6): 726–731, 2005.
153. Kumaraguruparan, R., Chandra Mohan, K.V., Abraham, S.K., Nagini, S., Attenuation of N-methyl-N-nitro-N-nitrosoguanidine induced genotoxicity and oxidative stress by tomato and garlic combination. *Life Sci.*, 76(19): 2247–55, 2005.
154. Amagase, H., Schaffer, E.M., and Milner, J.A., Dietary components modify the ability of garlic to suppress 7,12-dimethylbenz(a)anthracene-induced mammary DNA adducts, *J. Nutr.*, 126(4): 817–824, 1996.
155. Ip, C., Lisk, D.J., and Thompson, H.J., Selenium-enriched garlic inhibits the early stage but not the late stage of mammary carcinogenesis, *Carcinogenesis*, 17(9): 1979–1982, 1996.

156. Ganther, H.E., Selenium metabolism, selenoproteins and mechanisms of cancer prevention: complexities with thioredoxin reductase, *Carcinogenesis*, 20(9): 1657–1666, 1999.
157. Sundaram, S.G. and Milner, J.A., Diallyl Disulfide Inhibits the Proliferation of Human Tumor Cells in Culture, *Biochim. Biophys. Acta*, 1315(1): 15–20, 1996.
158. Knowles, L.M. and Milner, J.A., Depressed p34cdc2 kinase activity and G2/M phase arrest induced by diallyl disulfide in HCT-15 cells, *Nutr. Cancer*, 30(3): 169–174, 1998.
159. Schaffer, E.M. and Milner, J.A., Impact of dietary fatty acids on 7,12-dimethylbenz[a]anthracene-induced mammary DNA adducts, *Cancer Lett.*, 106(2): 177–183, 1996.
160. Tang, F., Zhou, J., and Gu, L., In vivo and in vitro effects of selenium-enriched garlic on growth of human gastric carcinoma cells, *Zhonghua Zhong Liu Za Zhi* [Chinese journal of oncology], 23(6): 461–464, 2001.
161. Seki, T., Tsuji, K., Hayato, Y., Moritomo, T., and Ariga, T., Garlic and onion oils inhibit proliferation and induce differentiation of HL-60 cells, *Cancer Lett.*, 160(1): 29–35, 2000.
162. Banerjee, S.K. and Maulik, S.K., Effect of garlic on cardiovascular disorders: a review, *Nutr. J.*, 19(1): 4, 2002.
163. Alder, R., Lookinland, S., Berry, J.A., and Williams, M.A., Systematic review of the effectiveness of garlic as an anti-hyperlipidemic agent, *J. Am. Acad. Nurse Pract.*, 15(3): 120–129, 2003.
164. Adler, A.J. and Holub, B.J., Effect of garlic and fish-oil supplementation on serum lipid, *Am. J. Clin. Nutr.*, 65(2): 445–450, 1997.
165. Steiner, M., Khan, A.H., Holbert, D., and Lin, R.I., A double-blind crossover study in moderately hypercholesterolemic men that compared the effect of aged garlic extract and placebo administration on blood lipids, *Am. J. Clin. Nutr.*, 64(6): 866–870, 1996.
166. Byrne, D.J., Neil, H.A., Vallance, D.T., and Winder, A.F., A pilot study of garlic consumption shows no significant effect on markers of oxidation or sub-fraction composition of low-density lipoprotein including lipoprotein(a) after allowance for non-compliance and the placebo effect, *Clin. Chim. Acta*, 285(1–2): 21–33, 1999.
167. Tanamai, J., Veeramanomai, S., and Indrakosas, N., The efficacy of cholesterol-lowering action and side effects of garlic enteric coated tablets in man, *J. Med. Assoc. Thai.*, 87(10): 1156–1161, 2004.
168. Jabbari, A., Argani, H., Ghorbanihaghjo, A., and Mahdavi, R., Comparison between swallowing and chewing of garlic on levels of serum lipids, cyclosporine, creatinine and lipid peroxidation in Renal Transplant Recipients, *Lipids Health Dis.*, 4: 11, 2005.
169. Holvoet, P., Oxidized LDL and coronary heart disease, *Acta Cardiol.*, 59(5): 479–484, 2004.
170. Munday, J.S., James, K.A., Fray, L.M., Kirkwood, S.W., and Thompson, K.G., Daily supplementation with aged garlic extract, but not raw garlic, protects low density lipoprotein against in vitro, *Atherosclerosis*, 143(2): 399–404, 1999.
171. Ou, C.C., Tsao, S.M., Lin, M.C., and Yin, M.C., Protective action on human LDL against oxidation and glycation by four organosulfur compounds derived from garlic, *Lipids*, 38(3): 219–224, 2003.
172. Huang, C.N., Horng, J.S., and Yin, M.C., Antioxidative and antiglycative effects of six organosulfur compounds in low-density lipoprotein and plasma, *J. Agric. Food Chem.*, 52(11): 3674–3678, 2004.
173. Fallon, M.B., Abrams, G.A., Abdel-Razek, T.T., Dai, J., Chen, S.J., Chen, Y.F., Luo, B., Oparil, S., and Ku, D.D., Garlic prevents hypoxic pulmonary hypertension in rats, *Am. J. Physiol.*, 275(2 Pt. 1): L283–L287, 1998.
174. Maslin, D.J., Brown, C.A., Das, I., and Zhang, X.H., Nitric oxide — a mediator of the effects of garlic?, *Biochem. Soc. Trans.*, 25(3): 408S, 1997.
175. Aqel, M.B., Gharaibah, M.N., and Salhab, A.S., Direct relaxant effects of garlic juice on smooth and cardiac muscles, *J. Ethnopharmacol*, 33(1–2): 13–19, 1991.
176. Ashraf, M.Z., Hussain, M.E., and Fahim, M., Endothelium mediated vasorelaxant response of garlic in isolated rat aorta: role of nitric oxide, *J. Ethnopharmacol*, 90(1): 5–9, 2004.
177. Al-Qattan, K.K., Alnaqeeb, M.A., and Ali, M., The antihypertensive effect of garlic (Allium sativum) in the rat two-kidney — one-clip Goldblatt model, *J. Ethnopharmacol.*, 66(2): 217–222, 1999.
178. Al-Qattan, K.K., Khan, I., Alnaqeeb, M.A, and Ali, M., Thromboxane-B2, prostaglandin-E2 and hypertension in the rat 2-kidney 1-clip model: a possible mechanism of the garlic induced hypotension, *Prostaglandins Leukot. Essent. Fatty Acids*, 64(1): 5–10, 2001.

179. Al-Qattan, K.K., Khan, I., Alnaqeeb, M.A., and Ali, M., Mechanism of garlic (Allium sativum) induced reduction of hypertension in 2K-1C rats: a possible mediation of Na/H exchanger isoform-1, *Prostaglandins Leukot. Essent. Fatty Acids*, 69(4): 217–222, 2003.

180. Patel, V.B. and Topol, E.J., The pathogenesis and spectrum of acute coronary syndromes: from plaque formation to thrombosis, *Cleve. Clin. J. Med.*, 66(9): 561–571, 1999.

181. Efendy, J.L., Simmons, D.L., Campbell, G.R., and Campbell, J.H., The effect of the aged garlic extract, 'Kyolic', on the development of experimental atherosclerosis, *Atherosclerosis*, 132(1): 37–42, 1997.

182. Budoff, M.J., Takasu, J., Flores, F.R., Niihara, Y., Lu, B., Lau, B.H., Rosen, R.T., and Amagase, H., Inhibiting progression of coronary calcification using Aged Garlic Extract in patients receiving statin therapy: a preliminary study, *Prev. Med.*, 39(5): 985–991, 2004.

183. Koscielny, J., Klussendorf, D., Latza, R., Schmitt, R., Radtke, H., Siegel, G., and Kiesewetter, H., The antiatherosclerotic effect of Allium sativum, *Atherosclerosis*, 144(1): 237–249, 1999.

184. Zahid, A.M., Hussain, M.E., and Fahim, M., Antiatherosclerotic effects of dietary supplementations of garlic and turmeric: Restoration of endothelial function in rats, *Life Sci.*, 77(8): 837–857, 2005.

185. Ali, M., Bordia, T., and Mustafa, T., Effect of raw versus boiled aqueous extract of garlic and onion on platelet aggregation, *Prostaglandins Leukot. Essent. Fatty Acids*, 60(1): 43–47, 1999.

186. Rahman, K. and Billington, D., Dietary supplementation with aged garlic extract inhibits ADP-induced platelet aggregation in humans, *J. Nutr.* 130(11): 2662–2665, 2000.

187. Chang, H.S., Yamato, O., Yamasaki, M., and Maede, Y., Modulatory influence of sodium 2-propenyl thiosulfate from garlic on cyclooxygenase activity in canine platelets: possible mechanism for the anti-aggregatory effect, *Prostaglandins Leukot. Essent. Fatty Acids*, 72(5): 351–355, 2005.

188. Steiner, M. and Lin, R.S., Changes in platelet function and susceptibility of lipoproteins to oxidation associated with administration of aged garlic extract, *J. Cardiovasc. Pharmacol.*, 31(6): 904–908, 1998.

189. Marks, H.S., Anderson, J.L., and Stoewsand, G.S., Inhibition of benzo[a]pyrene-induced bone marrow micronuclei formation by diallyl thioethers in mice, *J. Toxicol. Environ. Health.*, 37(1): 1–9, 1992.

190. Hatono, S., Jimenez, A., and Wargovich, M.J., Chemopreventive effect of S-allylcysteine and its relationship to the detoxification enzyme glutathione S-transferase, *Carcinogenesis*, 17(5): 1041–1044, 1996.

191. Sengupta, A., Ghosh, S., and Das, S., Tomato and garlic can modulate azoxymethane-induced colon carcinogenesis in rats, *Eur. J. Cancer Prev.*, 12(3): 195–200, 2003.

192. Wattenberg, L.W., Sparnins, V.L., and Barany, G., Inhibition of N-nitrosodiethylamine carcinogenesis in mice by naturally occurring organosulfur compounds and monoterpenes, *Cancer Res.*, 49(10): 2689–2692, 1989.

193. Sparnins, V.L., Barany, G., and Wattenberg, L.W., Effects of organosulfur compounds from garlic and onions on benzo[a]pyrene-induced neoplasia and glutathione S-transferase activity in the mouse, *Carcinogenesis*, 9(1): 131–134, 1988.

194. Hu, P.J. and Wargovich, M.J., Effect of diallyl sulfide on MNNG-induced nuclear aberrations and ornithine decarboxylase activity in the glandular stomach mucosa of the Wistar rat, *Cancer Lett.*, 47(1–2): 153–158, 1989.

195. el-Mofty, M.M., Sakr, S.A., Essawy, A., and Abdel Gawad, H.S., Preventive action of garlic on aflatoxin B1-induced carcinogenesis in the toad *Bufo regularis*, *Nutr. Cancer.*, 21(1): 95–100, 1994.

196. Guyonnet, D., Belloir, C., Suschetet, M., Siess, M.H., and Le Bon, A.M., Mechanisms of protection against aflatoxin B(1) genotoxicity in rats treated by organosulfur compounds from garlic, *Carcinogenesis*, 23(8): 1335–1341, 2002.

197. Samaranayake, M.D., Wickramasinghe, S.M., Angunawela, P., Jayasekera, S., Iwai, S., and Fukushima, S., Inhibition of chemically induced liver carcinogenesis in Wistar rats by garlic (Allium sativum), *Phytother. Res.*, 14(7): 564–567, 2000.

198. Suzui, N., Sugie, S., Rahman, K.M., Ohnishi, M., Yoshimi, N., Wakabayashi K., and Mori, H., Inhibitory effects of diallyl disulfide or aspirin on 2-amino-1-methyl-6 -phenylimidazo[4,5-b]pyridine-induced mammary carcinogenesis in rats, *Jpn. J. Cancer Res.*, 88(8): 705–711, 1997.

199. Hong, J.Y., Smith, T., Lee, M.J., Li, W.S., Ma, B.L., Ning, S.M., Brady, J.F., Thomas, P.E., and Yang, C.S., Metabolism of carcinogenic nitrosamines by rat nasal mucosa and the effect of diallyl sulfide, *Cancer Res.*, 51(5): 1509–1514, 1991.

200. Dwivedi, C., Rohlfs, S., Jarvis, D., and Engineer, F.N., Chemoprevention of chemically induced skin tumor development by diallyl sulfide and diallyl disulfide, *Pharm. Res.*, 9(12): 1668–1670, 1992.
201. Arora, A. and Shukla, Y., Induction of apoptosis by diallyl sulfide in DMBA-induced mouse skin tumors, *Nutr. Cancer*, 44(1): 89–94, 2002.
202. Surh, Y.J., Lee, R.C., Park, K.K., Mayne, S.T., Liem, A., and Miller, J.A., Chemoprotective effects of capsaicin and diallyl sulfide against mutagenesis or tumorigenesis by vinyl carbamate and N-nitrosodimethylamine, *Carcinogenesis*, 16(10): 2467–2471, 1995.

5 Grape Wine and Tea Polyphenols in the Modulation of Atherosclerosis and Heart Disease

Michael A. Dubick and Stanley T. Omaye

CONTENTS

I. INTRODUCTION

Human cultures have a long history of using wines and teas for the promotion of health and for treatment of disease. Recently, some wineries have requested permission to add resveratrol content to their label, and legislation has been proposed in Oregon and New York to allow the wine's antioxidant content to be added to labels on wine sold within their respective states. What is it about these beverages that has given them recognition over the years as health-promoting foods? This chapter addresses the recent explosion of papers in this field exploring the health-promoting benefits of these beverages.

A number of epidemiologic studies observed that moderate alcohol intake appeared to be inversely related to incidences of myocardial infarctions, angina pectoris, or coronary-related deaths.[1–15] These studies examined subjects ranging in age from 25 to 84 years old and involved hundreds to thousands of people in a number of different countries. Further analyses revealed that this negative association was not truly linear, but followed a U- or J-shaped curve.[11,15–17] That is, at low to moderate ethanol intake, the risk of heart disease or death is lower than in abstainers, but at high intake levels, these risks rise again, consistent with the principles of hormesis.[18] Although the mechanisms for this reduced risk are not well understood, ethanol intake has been reported to raise the plasma levels of high-density lipoproteins (HDL) and/or lower the levels and rate of oxidation of low-density lipoproteins (LDL).[3,19–21] Ethanol intake is also known to prolong the clotting times of blood.[22,23]

This association between moderate alcohol consumption and risk of ischemic heart disease has caught the public's attention in what has been labeled the "French Paradox." Epidemiologic studies have observed that in southern France mortality rates from heart disease were lower than expected despite the consumption of diets high in saturated fats and the tendency to smoke cigarettes.[23,24] These coronary-related deaths in France were reportedly about one third the rate in Great Britain and lower than any country examined except for China and Japan, where diets are generally low in saturated fats.[23] Both dietary and nondietary factors such as lower levels of stress, underreporting of deaths and, recently, a time-lag association similar to that observed between cigarette smoking and incidence of lung cancer in women, have been proposed to explain this so-called "paradox."[8,25–29]

Nevertheless, in addition to their Mediterranean-style diet, most of the attention in explaining the French paradox has focused on the common practice of wine consumption by the French, particularly red wine, with their meals.[4,7,8,26] France has the highest per capita consumption of grape wine than any other developed country.[26,27] Indeed, epidemiologic studies suggested that the consumption of wine at the level of intake in France could explain a 40% reduction in heart disease.[23] However, it should be noted that this relationship does not appear to hold for other regions of France, and overall longevity and mortality rates from all causes in France is similar to that in other industrialized countries.[26]

Epidemiologic studies evaluating the protective effect of drinking tea on the development or incidence of cardiovascular disease are far fewer in comparison to the number of studies examining ethanol or wine intake. Nevertheless, tea consumption is reported to have similar protective effects.[30–33] For example, a study in men and women 30 to 49 years old found that tea consumption was inversely related to serum cholesterol levels and systolic blood pressure, and there was a slightly, but not significantly, lower mortality in those individuals who drank one or more cups of tea/d compared to those who drank less than a cup/d.[33] In addition, a recent study in Japan noted that green tea consumption was directly related to lower serum cholesterol concentrations, higher HDL, and lower LDLs.[34] Tea consumption also contributed to a lower mortality after acute myocardial infarction.[35] In contrast, a British study saw no inverse relation between tea consumption and coronary heart disease, and in healthy adults drinking black tea for 4 weeks, no statistically significant effects on plasma cholesterol, HDL, LDL, or triglycerides were observed except in individuals who had specific atherogenic apoE genotypes.[36,37]

Although the exact mechanisms by which wine or tea consumption could offer protection against atherosclerosis and ischemic heart disease are not fully known, a large body of literature has emerged which suggests that the actions of polyphenolic compounds found in these beverages may account for this protection.[38–41] Table 5.1 lists the various actions suggested through which these compounds could impact on the development of cardiovascular diseases (CVD). This chapter will discuss these polyphenolic substances, the epidemiological evidence that they may protect against CVD, and the evidence for the proposed mechanisms through which these substances may reduce the risk of CVD.

TABLE 5.1
Proposed Properties of Wine and Tea Polyphenols
to Reduce Risk of Atherosclerosis or Heart Disease

I. Effects on Plasma Lipids

Increase HDL levels
Decrease LDL levels
Inhibit lipoprotein synthesis
Decrease lipoprotein (a) levels
Decrease in total lipid

II. General Antioxidant Activity

Chelate transition metals
Inhibit oxidation of LDL
Maintain plasma levels of antioxidant vitamins
Scavenge oxygen free radicals
Modulate activity of antioxidant enzymes.

III. Other Effects

Anticoagulant effects
Inhibit platelet aggregation, including aspirin-like activity
Enhance nitric oxide synthesis to keep blood vessels patent
General antiinflammatory activity
Up-regulation of anti-inflammatory signal transductions pathways.
Reduced body weight (?)

II. POLYPHENOLS

A. CHEMICAL BACKGROUND AND NOMENCLATURE

Wine, grapes, and tea are known to contain a variety of polyphenolic compounds.[42–49] The terms *polyphenols* and *phenolic* are all-encompassing, ranging from simple phenolic acid to polymerized compounds like tannins. Overall in the plant kingdom, polyphenols or phenolic compounds account for more than 800 chemical structures, translating into over 4000 individual compounds.[39,42,45–47] These compounds are the secondary byproducts of plant metabolisms, and their large numbers are indicative of what can arise from various hydroxylation, methoxylation, glycosylation, and acylation reactions during their biosynthesis. Consequently, in addition to teas and wine, they are found in many commonly eaten fruits and vegetables, such as grapes, apples, berries, grapefruit, onion, eggplant, and kale, as well as herbs and spices and dark chocolate.[39,47]

Polyphenols have generally been classified into 3 major groups: (1) simple phenols and phenolic acids, (2) flavonoids, and (3) hydroxycinnamic acid derivatives.[39] Many of the compounds found in tea and wine are low-molecular weight polyphenols such as flavonoids, also loosely referred to as bioflavonoids.[42–49] Many flavonoid compounds occur as sugars (glycosides) and tend to be water-soluble. Flavonoids play significant roles in the plant kingdom. Many flavonoids, especially the flavanols, are astringents, whereas others have evolved to protect plants against microbes, parasites, and oxidative injury.

The flavonoids are based on the flavan nucleus consisting of 15 carbons within three rings recognized as A, B, and C (Figure 5.1A).[42,45–47] The basic structure is a phenyl benzopyrone derivative. The differences between the various subclasses of polyphenolic compounds are due to the presence of 3-hydroxyl and/or 2 oxy groups, the number of hydroxyls in the A and B rings, and the absence/presence of double bonds in the pyrane ring. The chemical substitutions and structures that define the various flavonoids have been reviewed by Bravo.[47] Flavonoids may occur as monomeric, dimeric biflavonoids (not to be confused with bioflavonoids), or oligomeric compounds. Tannins, illustrated in Figure 5.1B, are polymeric derivatives that are classified into two groups: (1) condensed (polymers of flavonoids) or (2) hydrolysable, which often contain gallic acid. An example is epicatechin gallate (ECG), shown in Figure 5.1C, often found in teas.

As might be anticipated, because of the large spectrum of compounds that can be listed as polyphenols or flavonoids, there is a lack of agreement on nomenclature and classification. Using chemical structures, flavonoids can be subdivided into flavonols, flavones, flavanones, flavanols (catechins), anthocyanidins, isoflavones, dihydroflavonols, and chalcones.[47] Another classification system uses the phrase *minor flavonoids* to include flavanones, flavanols, and dihydroflavonols, or those flavonoids with limited natural distribution.[50] With respect to mammalian biological activity, much of the current interest in flavonoids is related to the 4 oxo-flavonoid structures, i.e., flavonols, flavones, flavanones, isoflavones, and dihydroflavonols.[47] Flavonols, flavones, and anthocyanidines are second only to the carotenoids with respect to being compounds of vivid color, and are likely to be a visual signal for insects who provide pollination.[45–47]

Although our infatuation with flavonoids as potential health promoters seems recent, over a dozen flavonoid-containing medicinals have been known and used in traditional medicine.[51] More than 40 species of plants, because of their natural content of flavonoids, have been used throughout the world for various medicinal purposes. They are used as anti-inflammatory, antiseptic, antiarrhythmic, antispasmodic and anxiolytic agents, as sedatives and for wound-healing, to name a few.[52–54] In general, as a group, the polyphenols have been recognized to possess antioxidant activities (Table 5.1).

B. POLYPHENOLS IN WINES AND GRAPES

The polyphenols in wine include phenolic acids, anthocyanins, tannins, and various flavonoids (caffeic acid, rutin, catechin, myricetin, quercetin, epicatechin), among others. Proanthocyanidins, polymers, or oligomers of catechin units are the major polyphenols in red wine and especially in grape seeds.[55,56] Grape skins and juice contain anthrocyanins and flavonoids (quercetin and myricetin).[57] Nonflavonoids are derivatives of cinnamates, tyrosol, volatile phenols, and hydrolyzable tannins. Of the nonflavonoids in wine, resveratrol (3,4′,5-trihydoxystilbene) (Figure 5.1D) has sparked much interest for its potential health-enhancing effects. Besides grapes, only a few other plant species, such as peanuts, contain resveratrol.[57] These stilbenes and stilbene glycosides have antifungal activity, and their health benefits have been attributed to their phytoestrogen properties, to metal-ion chelation, or to general antioxidant activity.[52,54,57–59] Many of the properties of resveratrol have been reviewed recently.[60]

The total polyphenolic content of red wines has been estimated to be about 1200 mg/l, whereas others have reported concentrations as high as 4000 mg/l. [61] In contrast, the polyphenolic content of white wine is about 200 to 300 mg/l.[48] Thus, the total flavonoid content of red wine can be about 20-fold higher than in white wine, whereas grape juice has about one half the flavonoid content of red wine by volume.[61,16] For example, the concentrations of epicatechin and related compounds in wine have been estimated at 150 mg/l and 15 mg/l for red and white wine, respectively.[62] It has also been estimated that quercetin concentrations in wine are about 25 mg/l. Nonflavonoids, such as hydroxybenzoate and hydroxycinnamate, do not differ significantly between red and white wine.[61] Resveratrol, being present in grape skins, is found primarily in red wines, with concentrations around 1 mg/l.[62] The concentrations of select polyphenols in wine are summarized in Table 5.2.

It is also realized that aged wines differ in the nature of their polyphenols compared to young wines or, for the most part, those found in grape juices.[47,55,62] Phenolic concentrations in wine increase during skin fermentation and decrease as phenols interact with proteins and yeast-cell membranes and precipitate. Wine aging results in further modification in the phenolic content. In addition, herbicides and insecticides are known to modulate the concentration of polyphenolic

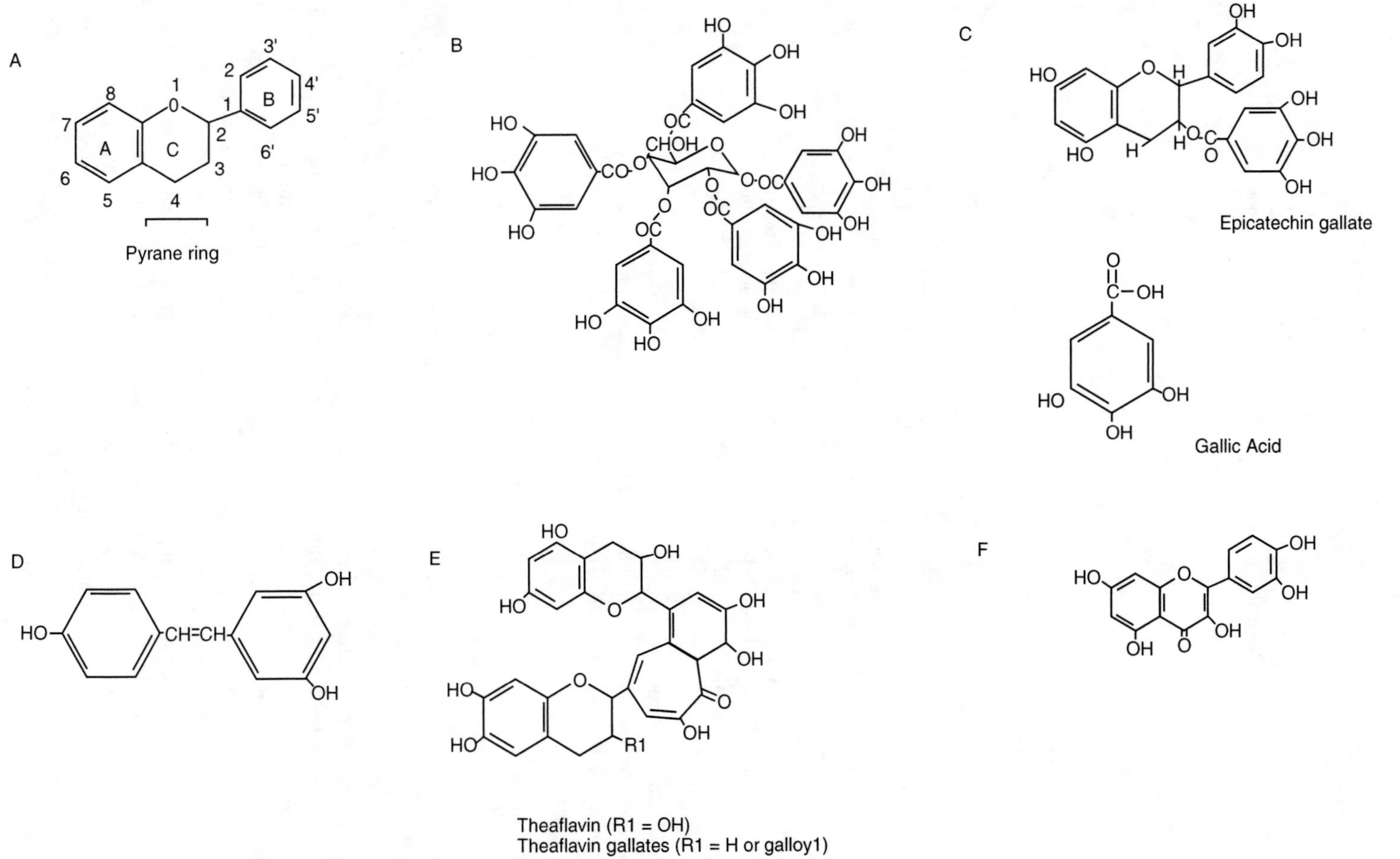

FIGURE 5.1 Select polyphenols from wine and tea. (A) flavonoid base structure with carbon numbering; (B) tannin chemical structure; (C) epicatechin gallate and gallic acid chemical structures; (D) resveratrol (3,5,4'-trihydroxystilbene) structure (resveratrol can exist in the *cis* or *trans* configuration); (E) theaflavin and theaflavin gallate (example of flavonoid oxidation by-product); and (F) structure of quercetin.

TABLE 5.2
Concentrations of Select Flavonoids and Resveratrol in Wine

Subclasses of Flavonoid	Compound	Quantity, mg/l	
		White Wines	Red Wines
Flavonols	Myricetin	0	8.5
	Rutin	0	9
	Quercetin	0	7
Flavanols		56	274
	Catechin	35	191
	Epicatechin	21	82
Anthocyanins	Cyanidin	0	2.8
Resveratrol		0.027	1.5

Source: From Frankel, E., Waterhouse, A., and Teissedre, P., Principal phenolic phytochemicals in selected California wines and their antioxidant activity in inhibiting oxidation of human low-density lipoproteins, *J Agric Food Chem*, 43: 890–894, 1995; Soleas, G., Diamandis, E., and Goldberg, D., Wine as a biological fluid: history, production, and role in disease prevention, *J Clin Lab Anal*, 11(5): 287–313, 1997; Frankel, E.N., Waterhouse, A., and Kinsella, J., Inhibition of human LDL oxidation by resveratrol, *Lancet*, 341(8852): 1103–1104, 1993; Clifford, A.J., Ebeler, S., Ebeler, J., Bills, N., Hinrichs, S., Teissedre, P., and Waterhouse, A., Delayed tumor onset in transgenic mice fed an amino acid-based diet supplemented with red wine solids, *Am J Clin Nutr*, 64(5): 748–756, 1996.

compounds and secondary compounds through reduction of carbon fixation in plants. In summary, the amount of flavonoids in wine can be influenced by several factors, including temperature, sulfite, and ethanol concentrations; the type of fermentation vessel; pH; and yeast strain.[55,58] However, if open wine is protected from light, the polyphenols appear to be stable for about 1 week at room or refrigeration temperatures.[64]

C. COMPOUNDS FOUND IN TEAS

Tea is second only to water as the most consumed beverage in the world.[42] The average consumption of tea is greater than 100 ml per d, and in some locations can be up to 5 l per d, with world-wide per capita consumption being about 0.12 l/d.[44,65] Tea is the beverage originating from the leaf of the plant *Camellia sinensis*, varieties *sinensis* and *assamica*. The tea leaves contain more than 35% of their dry weight as polyphenols. Breeding and selection have resulted in the hybridization and emergence of thousands of types of teas with varying properties and composition.

Green tea is the product produced from fresh leaf. Rapid inactivation of the enzyme, polyphenol oxidase, by steaming or rapid pan firing, rolling, and high temperature air drying, is used to make green tea in Japan and China, and preserves the polyphenol content. Thus, green tea is rich in the flavanols catechin, epicatechin, epicatechin gallate (ECG), gallocatechin, epigallocatechin (EGC), and epigallocatechin gallate (EGCG) — the flavanols that have generated the most interest for human health. It has been estimated that one cup of green tea can contain 100 to 200 mg catechins.[66] In general, green tea contains higher concentrations of the catechins than wine. In addition, green tea contains quercetin, kaempferol, myricetin and their glycosides, apigenin glycosides, and lignans, but at lower concentrations.[67,68] A summary of the most common flavonoids in teas are presented in Table 5.3.

TABLE 5.3
Concentrations of Phenolic Acid, Flavonoids, and Their Oxidation Products in Tea

Subclasses of Flavonoid	Compound	Quantity (mg/g)	
		Green Tea	Black Tea
Flavonols		50–100	60–80
	Quercetin		10–20
	Kaempferol	20–45	14–16
	Myricetin		2–5
Flavanols		300–400	50–100
	Catechin	10–20	5
	Epicatechin (EGC)	10–50	10–20
	Epigallocatechin	30–100	10–20
	Gallocatechin	10–30	
	Epicatechin gallate (EGC)	30–100	30–40
	Epigallocatechin gallate (EGGG)	100–150	300–600
Flavandiols		20–30	
Phenolic acids		30–50	100–120
Theaflavins			30–60
Thearubigens			30–50

Source: From Dreosti, I., Bioactive ingredients: antioxidants and polyphenols in tea, *Nutr Rev*, 54(11 Pt. 2): S51–S58, 1996; Graham, H., Green tea composition, consumption, and polyphenol chemistry, *Prev Med*, 21(3): 334–350, 1992; Hertog, M., Hollman, P., and van de Purtte, B., Content of potentially anticarcinogenic flavonoids of tea infusions, wines, and fruit juices, *J Agric Food Chem*, 41: 1242–1246, 1993; van het Hof, K., Wiseman, S., Yang, C., and Tijburg, L., Plasma and lipoprotein levels of tea catechins following repeated tea consumption, *Proc Soc Exp Biol Med*, 220(4): 203–209, 1999; Price, K., Rhodes, M., and Barnes, K., The chemical pathogenesis of alcohol-induced tissue injury, *J Agric Food Chem*, 46: 2517–2522, 1998.

Black tea is derived from aged tea leaves that have undergone enzymatically catalyzed aerobic oxidation and chemical condensation, particularly of the catechins. Consequently, catechin levels are lower in black than in green tea. Interestingly, in food science, oxidation properties of catechins have been adopted for use as food antioxidants similar to that of BHA.[67–69] The principal products of catechin oxidation are the formation of quinones which in turn form seven-membered ring theaflavin or theaflavin gallate compounds (Figure 5.1.E), as well as thearubigins.[68–70] Theaflavins (1 to 2% by dry weight) are mostly responsible for the reddish color and astringency of black tea. In between green and black tea is Oolong tea, which is partially oxidized but retains much of the original polyphenol content of the leaf.

D. ABSORPTION AND METABOLISM OF POLYPHENOLS

Crucial to any discussion regarding the efficacy of wine and tea polyphenols in the prevention of atherosclerosis and heart disease is how well such compounds are absorbed through the intestinal tract wall, how well they are distributed into various tissues, especially blood plasma, and their metabolism and rate of elimination. Unfortunately, there is limited information in humans, which has led to the uncertainty that these compounds could express *in vivo* antioxidant activity of physiologic significance. Because such compounds occur as complex mixtures in plant materials and have enormous variability, it is difficult to study bioavailability and physiologic effects.

However, not all polyphenols are created equally with respect to bioavailability. The most common polyphenols in our diets are not necessarily the most active within our body. They are not absorbed with equal efficacy, some are extensively metabolized both at the level of the intestine and by the liver, and some may be rapidly eliminated or excreted.[71] Polyphenols only sparingly occur in the free form.

Earlier studies in the U.S. estimated that the daily intake of flavonoids was about 1 g/d when expressed as glycosides, or 650 mg/d when expressed as aglycones.[72] Hollman et al.,[41] however, have raised concern that these values are too high and others have estimated that the average intake of all flavonoids from dietary sources is between 23 and 170 mg/d.[30,40,70] In the Dutch study, daily intake of all flavonoids was estimated at 23 mg/d with quercetin accounting for 16 mg/d.[30,73] This is in keeping with the observation that of the flavonoids, quercetin is generally found in the highest concentration in food. Its concentration in grapes is reportedly 1.4 mg/kg, whereas green tea contains >10,000 mg/kg quercetin glycosides and kaempferol.[74] In addition, Hollman et al. summarized the average daily flavonol intake from 6 studies as 4 to 68 mg/d.[41] Interestingly, on a mg/d basis, flavonoid intake exceeds the average daily intake of vitamin E and β-carotene.

The absorption of polyphenols varies depending on the type of food, the chemical form of the polyphenols, and their interactions with other substances in food, such as protein, ethanol and fiber. As an example, quercetin absorption was $52 \pm 15\%$ from quercetin glucosides in onions, $17 \pm 15\%$ from quercetin rutinoside and $24 \pm 9\%$ from quercetin aglycone.[74] Urinary excretion was about 0.5% of the amount absorbed. Flavonoids, such as quercetin and other flavonoids can be absorbed either as free aglycone and glycoside, as demonstrated by detection in blood and urine following feeding both forms of the substance.[46,75,76] It has also been reported that polyphenols from wine may be absorbed better than the same substances from fruits and vegetables, because the ethanol may enhance the breakdown of the polyphenols into smaller products that are absorbed more readily.[40]

Data suggest that glycosidases from bacteria that colonize the ileum and cecum are involved in the breakdown of flavonoids. For example, it has been shown that flavonoid glycosides ingested by germ-free rats are recovered intact in the feces.[77] Others have found that the administration of 0.5 g/d of catechin or tannic acid to rats over a 3-week period resulted in less than 5% excreted unchanged in the feces.[78] Glycones from onions have been shown to cross the mucosal layer of the intestinal cells, suggesting that humans may have hydrolases to remove sugar components to form aglycones.[79] However, it remains uncertain if the hydrolysis of flavonoid glycosides is necessary for absorption in humans. Also, further research is needed to determine whether deglycosylation of flavonoids occurs independent of gut-microbial action.

Nevertheless, studies in experimental animals and humans indicate that some polyphenols, at least, can be absorbed. Most polyphenols likely do not penetrate the gut wall by passive diffusion because of their hydrophilic nature. Information is scarce, although a unique active-transport mechanism has been described for cinnamic and ferulic acid absorption in the rat jejunum.[80] Absorption is influenced by compound glycosylation and most flavonoids, except flavanols, are found in foods as glycosylated forms. Glycosylated polyphenols are likely to be resistant to acid hydrolysis and are presented to the upper small intestine unchanged.[81] Apparently, only aglycones and perhaps glucosides are absorbed in the small intestine. Proanthocyanidins, because of their polymeric nature, have limited absorption. The majority of the polymeric proanthocyanidins pass unaltered through the small intestine where they are degraded by the colonic microflora.[82] Proanthocyanidins, being one of the more abundant polyphenol constituents in the diet, may exert only local gut effects, such as antioxidant and anti-inflammatory activities, which in turn may be crucial for modulating chronic diseases.[83] Identification and quantification of microbial metabolites of polyphenols is an extremely active field of research, which has the goal of isolating specific bioactive compounds that may modulate atherosclerosis and other chronic diseases.

Accumulation of flavonoids in plasma can be reportedly up to 100 μmol/l.[84,85] Polyphenol metabolites are not free in blood, but bound to plasma proteins. For example, albumin is the primary protein responsible for binding of the metabolites of quercetin.[85] The degree of binding to albumin may affect the rate of clearance of metabolites and their delivery to cells and tissues. The partitioning of polyphenols and their metabolites, between aqueous and lipid phases, favors retention in the aqueous phase because of their hydrophilicity and binding to albumin.

In animal and human studies, between 10 to 20% of an oral dose of quercetin was absorbed.[86] After tea drinking, only 0.5% of the quercetin was excreted unchanged.[87] These authors concluded that plasma concentrations of quercetin and kaempferol reflected short-term intake. In general, peak blood levels of flavonoids occur between 2 and 3 h after consumption and the elimination half-life varied between 5 and 17 h depending on the particular flavonoid or the food source.[88,89] In addition, a recent study reported that in rats fed red wine containing 6.5 mg/l of resveratrol for up to 15 d, some of the intact compound was detected in plasma and tissues, but the concentrations found were considered lower than would be expected to be pharmacologically active.[90] However, it remains to be determined whether repeated intake would increase these tissue levels further.

Clifford et al. detected catechin in plasma from mice fed a diet containing red wine solids.[91] EGCG was detected in plasma 30 min after drinking 300 ml of green tea.[92] Studies with EGCG found that in male adults drinking decaffeinated green tea containing 88 mg EGCG and 82 mg EGC, plasma concentrations 1 h after ingestion ranged from 46 to 268 ng/ml for EGCG and from 82 to 206 ng/ml for EGC.[93] It was also found that addition of milk to black tea did not affect catechin absorption and after a single tea consumption, the half-life of catechins in blood varied from 4.8 h for green tea to 6.9 h for black tea.[94] However, some studies of polyphenol absorption and metabolism may be misleading due to administration of pharmacologic doses in some human studies.[95] Using pharmacologic doses may not reflect the mechanisms of absorption and metabolism of dietary flavonoids at more physiologic levels of intake.

Studies also indicate that the liver is the primary site of polyphenol metabolism, although other sites such as kidney or intestinal mucosa may be involved. In the liver, these compounds can undergo (1) methylation, (2) hydroxylation, (3) reduction of the carbonyl group in the pyrane ring, (4) and conjugation reactions. The most common degradation pathway for flavonoids is through conjugation with glucuronides or sulfate.[96] Polyphenols are known to, directly or indirectly, induce phase II enzyme, such as glutathione transferases (GSTs), NAD(P)H:quinone reductases, epoxide hydrolases, and UDP-glucuronosyltransferases.[97,98] Polyphenols also influence phase I enzymes such as cytochrome P450.[99] In addition, some flavonoid metabolites can be recycled via the enterohepatic biliary route.

III. EPIDEMIOLOGY OF POLYPHENOLS AND ATHEROSCLEROSIS

Evidence that dietary flavonoid intake was inversely related to mortality from coronary heart disease has been supported by numerous epidemiologic studies.[30,32,100–102] In the Zutphen Elderly study, Hertog et al. showed that after adjustment for age, weight, certain risk factors of coronary artery disease, and intake of antioxidant vitamins, the highest tertile of flavonoid intake, primarily from tea, onions, and apples, had a relative risk of heart disease of 0.32 compared with the lowest tertile.[30,101] Although the magnitude of relative risk was less in a Finnish study, the data were similar to that observed in the Dutch study.[32] It should be noted that tea and grape-wine consumption is rather low in Finland. A recent study found a negative relation between high-dose flavonoid intake and risks of heart disease in healthy French women but not men.[103] Also, it was reported that flavonoids found in wine and tea were associated negatively with risk of CVD.[104] Catechin intake has been suggested to explain this negative association,[105] but further confirmation is required.

However, not all studies have seen protective effects. A U.S. study of a large cohort of male health professionals, and of French men or women, did not observe such a negative correlation between flavonoid intake and incidence of coronary heart disease, although there was a trend of protection in men with established heart disease.[102,103,106] In a large U.S. study of college alumni or women, flavonoid or tea intake was not associated with a reduction in CVD risk.[106,107] In addition, a Welsh study observed higher mortality from heart disease associated with high flavonol intake, primarily from tea consumed with milk.[108] In this study, however, it was noted that tea consumption was associated with a lower social class and a less healthy lifestyle, which included cigarette smoking and a higher fat consumption. In contrast, tea consumption in the above Dutch studies was associated with a higher social class and healthier lifestyle. Thus, the evidence supporting a protective effect of polyphenol intake against ischemic heart disease is suggestive but still inconclusive.

IV. ETIOLOGY OF ATHEROSCLEROSIS

Although the etiology of atherosclerosis and the development of heart disease is complex, it is generally agreed that the process of atherosclerosis begins with the accretion of soft fatty streaks along the inner arterial walls.[109,110] It is now hypothesized that blood cholesterol is linked to atherosclerosis and the risk of ischemic heart disease by its presence in low-density lipoprotein (LDL) cholesterol.[109] Although the mechanisms through which high plasma LDL concentrations increase the risk of CVD are not completely understood, evidence is emerging to implicate the oxidation of LDL by free radical byproducts or via an inflammatory process resulting in oxidative injury as an important factor.[110]

V. ACTIONS OF POLYPHENOLS ON RISK FACTORS ASSOCIATED WITH CVD

A. EFFECTS ON CHOLESTEROL AND LIPIDS

As noted in earlier text, several studies in experimental animals and humans have suggested that the consumption of wine or grape polyphenols was associated with lower serum cholesterol, LDLs, and higher HDLs.[9,10,111] Also, wine was observed to be more effective than ethanol in preventing the development of atherosclerotic lesions in cholesterol-fed rabbits.[112]

Likewise, consumption of green tea has been associated with decreased serum triacylglycerols and cholesterol.[42,113] Recently, Unno et al. observed that consumption of 224 mg or 674 mg of tea catechins attenuated the postprandial rise in plasma triacylglycerol levels after a fat load, but did not affect plasma cholesterol.[114] In rabbits fed a high-fat diet, green, but not black tea consumption, reduced aortic lesion formation by 31% compared with controls. Green tea given to hypercholesterolemic rats and spontaneously hypertensive animals lowered blood cholesterol and blood pressure, respectively.[42] In mice fed an atherogenic diet, green tea extract prevented the increase in serum and liver cholesterol levels observed in controls.[116] These protective effects of tea, such as decreasing LDLs and increasing HDLs, seem to be correlated best with green tea rather than black tea.[34,117] Thus, the potential health benefit of drinking tea may be a function of the intake of tea catechins. For example, Xu et al. reported that in hamsters fed a hypercholesterolemic diet for 16 weeks, catechin supplementation was as effective as vitamin E in inhibiting plaque formation.[118] Recent work suggests that the hypolipidemic activity of dietary tea catechins may also reflect inhibition of the absorption of dietary fat and cholesterol.[119]

It was also observed that red wine consumption decreased plasma concentrations of lipoprotein (a), identified as an independent risk factor for atherosclerosis.[120,121] In contrast, another clinical study failed to observe such an effect.[122] In addition, grape seed extract has been observed to inhibit the activity of different lipids *in vitro,* which has led to the suggestion that it may be effective for weight control,[123] but this area is beyond the scope of this review.

B. GENERAL ANTIOXIDANT EFFECTS

It is likely that various polyphenols, including flavonoids, act similarly to dietary antioxidants and that collectively they may bestow protection from the development of heart disease. Physical and chemical properties of individual polyphenolic compounds impact strongly on their abilities to be potent antioxidants and these properties have been well described.[52,124] The antioxidant activity of polyphenols has been related to their ability to: (1) delay or prevent autoxidation at low concentrations compared to the oxidizable substrate, (2) form free radicals that are relatively stable against further oxidation, and (3) induce other antioxidants at both the transcriptional and translational levels. In addition, an antioxidant effect may be induction of antioxidant enzymes. For example, *in vitro*, <20 μM resveratrol induced HO-1 that appeared to be via an NFκB mechanism.[125] Quercetin also induced HO-1 gene expression in a macrophage cell line.[126] Therefore, flavonoids that have the physical and chemical properties of antioxidants are capable of reacting with a variety of disease-promoting free radicals including superoxide, hydroxyl, peroxyl, alkoxyl, and nonradical species, e.g., singlet oxygen, peroxynitrite, and hydrogen peroxide.[52, 124,127] It has been proposed that quercetin possesses many of the properties considered essential for the ideal antioxidant (Figure 5.1F).

In vitro studies have supported the idea that wines possess intrinsic antioxidant activity. Maxwell et al. observed that red wines had about 30-fold greater antioxidant activity than normal human serum.[128] It was also observed that the total reactive antioxidant potential of red wines was 6 to 10 times higher than white wine.[129] Both green and black tea also exhibit significant antioxidant potential. For example, Halder and Bhaduri reported that black tea extracts could prevent lipid peroxidation of red blood cell (RBC) membranes and whole RBCs better than pure catechins in these systems.[130] It also appears that adding milk to tea resulted in significant loss of tea antioxidant activity, likely due to complex formation of tea polyphenols with milk proteins.[99] The antioxidant activity of tea relative to other fruits and vegetables has been summarized by Prior and Cao.[131] Interestingly, Vinson and Debbagh reported that green and black tea have a greater antioxidant index than grape juice or wine.[132] However, Serafini et al reported that the *in vitro* antioxidant activity of black tea was 3 to 4 mM, or about 1/3 the activity reported for red wine, but the contribution of alcohol to these values is not fully known.[128,133] It should be noted that although all fractions of wine polyphenols may display antioxidant activity, not all have cytoprotective properties.[134]

Antioxidant properties of wine have also been observed *in vivo*. Whitehead, et al. fed 9 healthy subjects 300 ml of red wine and observed 18% and 11% increases in serum antioxidant capacity after 1h and 2 h, respectively, compared with 22% and 29% increases at these times in subjects who took 1000 mg ascorbic acid.[135] Lower increases in serum antioxidant capacity were observed if the subjects drank white wine, or apple, grape, or orange juice. However, Durak et al. observed that plasma antioxidant potential was about 20% higher than baseline 4 h after normal subjects ate 1g/kg (body weight) of black grapes.[136] Maxwell et al. observed that 4 h after 10 healthy students consumed red wine with their meal, serum antioxidant status was about 13% higher than baseline values.[128] Others have reported that consumption of red wine polyphenols (1 or 2 g/d) increased total plasma antioxidants by 11 and 15%, respectively, in comparison to a 7% increase by vitamin E.[137,138] Struck et al. observed an antioxidant effect of wine, defined as a reduction in thiobarbituric acid reactive substances, in 20 hypercholesterolemic subjects who drank 180 ml/d of red or white wine for 28 d.[139] In contrast to other studies, Serafini et al. observed a greater effect when the subjects drank white wine compared to the red wine.[133] In addition, they observed no changes in plasma vitamin E, vitamin C, or β-carotene, but consumption of either wine resulted in a 23% reduction from baseline in plasma retinol levels. Although these results suggest that the enhanced antioxidant potential observed after drinking wine can be independent of plasma antioxidant vitamins or antioxidant enzymes, a study by Day and Stansbie reported that 73% of the increase in serum antioxidant capacity following consumption of port wine in 6 individuals could be attributed to an increase in serum uric acid levels, a well-recognized antioxidant.[140-142] However, Cao et al. observed an 8% increase in serum antioxidant capacity in elderly women who drank 300 ml of red wine, that could not be ascribed to an increase in uric acid or vitamin C.[143] Others have demonstrated that both red and white wine could inhibit hydrogen peroxide-induced DNA damage in human lymphocytes or decrease the amount of unstable acetaldehyde-albumin complexes in individuals drinking excessive amounts of wine.[144,145]

As tea contains polyphenols also present in wine, it would be expected that this beverage would also possess antioxidant properties. For example, Rah et al. reported that green tea polyphenols could inhibit oxidant generation *in vitro* in human endothelial cells.[146] Green tea consumption also reduced DNA markers of oxidative stress in smokers more than in nonsmokers.[147] In addition, green tea polyphenols have been observed to scavenge peroxynitrite by preventing tyrosine nitration.[148,149]

It should be noted that studies that did not observe an effect of red wine on plasma antioxidant status may reflect too low a consumption or, as in a rat study, may reflect the limited effects polyphenols may exert when a well-balanced diet with more than adequate intake of micronutrients is consumed.[120,150] Thus, from the above studies it would appear that polyphenols in wine and tea demonstrate antioxidant activity, but the expression of this activity depends on a variety of dietary and other health-related factors. As an example, although dry tea showed high antioxidant activity when expressed as Trolox equivalents, brewing conditions can influence the final values obtained.[131]

C. LDL OXIDATION

Most flavonoids found in teas and wines have a lower oxidation potential than the vitamin E radical. Therefore, analogous to ascorbic acid, flavonoids have the ability to reduce vitamin E radical or to recycle vitamin E as an antioxidant. This is significant in LDL oxidation, because vitamin E represents the first line of defense against LDL oxidation.[151] Once vitamin E is exhausted, the LDL is no longer protected, unless vitamin E can be recycled by appropriate reducing agents, e.g., flavonoids. Evidence that the flavonoid caffeic acid can increase plasma and lipoprotein vitamin E levels has been observed in rats.[152] Finally, flavonoids may protect vitamin E in lipid oxidation by being oxidized themselves in preference to vitamin E or by delaying the initiation of lipid peroxidation. For example, healthy volunteers who drank green tea (100 mg total catechins/d) for 4 weeks showed sparing of their plasma vitamin E and β-carotene levels.[153] Also, flavonoids may inhibit LDL oxidation by scavenging superoxide anions, hydroxyl radicals, or lipid peroxyl radicals. Alternatively, flavonoids may chemically modify LDL and such modification results in LDL being less susceptible to oxidation.

As most polyphenols are water-soluble, it is speculated that they should work in the aqueous phase of plasma and at the surface of lipoproteins. Binding to lipoprotein is not significant and likely less than 0.5%.[85] Vinson and Debbagh showed that catechins or green and black tea exhibited potent lipoprotein-bound antioxidant activity.[132] However, van het Hof observed that catechins were associated with HDLs, but the concentrations found in LDLs did not appear sufficient to enhance the resistance of LDLs to oxidation.[94] In addition, it was proposed that resveratrol was associated with lipoproteins where it could scavenge oxygen free radicals.[154]

However, a number of *in vitro* studies have reported that wine, tea, or select polyphenols could inhibit LDL oxidation. Ishikawa et al. observed that catechins could inhibit LDL oxidation in a dose-dependent manner *in vitro*, and EGCG appeared to be more potent than vitamin E.[155] Interestingly, black tea theaflavins were more effective than catechins. A number of studies have also shown that wine and select individual polyphenols from wine can inhibit oxidative changes of LDL, and red wine appeared more potent than white wine.[156,157] For example, the addition of 3.8 µM and 10 µM polyphenols extracted from red wine to LDLs *in vitro* inhibited its oxidation by 60% and 98%, respectively.[158] Red wine also inhibited cell-mediated LDL oxidation, whereas white wine and ethanol were not effective.[157] Red wine, catechin, or quercetin also inhibited development of aortic atherosclerotic lesions, and reduced the susceptibility of LDL to aggregation and subsequent atherogenic modification of LDL, in atherosclerotic vitamin E deficient mice.[159,160] Polyphenols from grape extract also have the ability to inhibit oxidative changes of LDL.[161] However, although red wine and grape juice could inhibit LDL oxidation *in vitro*, LDL oxidation was only inhibited *in vivo* in those who drank wine.[162] Incubation of LDL with cupric chloride produced a lag phase of 130 min before the onset of a propagation phase. In the presence of grape extract the lag phase was extended 185, 250, and 465 min, respectively, when an 8000-fold, 4000-fold, and

2000-fold diluted grape extract was added to the LDL suspension. Frankel et al. further observed that the inhibition of copper-catalyzed LDL oxidation by dilutions of wine could be mimicked by equal concentrations of quercetin.[158] Resveratrol also was observed to inhibit LDL oxidation *in vitro*, but its potency was only about one-half that of quercetin or epicatechin.[62]

White wines have the ability to inhibit oxidation of LDL *in vitro*, but generally are not as effective as red wines.[156,157] About eight times more white wine was required to produce the equivalent effect of red wines on LDL oxidation and HDL concentration increases. However, if equal concentrations of wine polyphenols extracted from red or white wine were compared, inhibition of LDL oxidation was similar. Comparing dilutions of red or white wine, red grape juice or beer, LDL oxidation was inhibited in a dose-dependent manner depending on the polyphenol concentration.[163] Concentrations of ethanol ranging from 0.1 to 0.5% showed no inhibition, suggesting that it was the polyphenols in these beverages that were responsible for inhibiting LDL oxidation. Taken together, these studies suggest that the reported advantage of red wine over white wine in inhibiting LDL oxidation reflects the higher concentrations of polyphenols in red rather than white wine, red wine polyphenols being more potent on a mole-per-mole basis than white wine polyphenols. However, the potencies of the various polyphenols, acting alone vs. potential additive or synergistic effects of the combinations found in wines and tea, have been little studied in the assay systems examined.

The relative potency of polyphenols compared to traditional antioxidants have been estimated in several studies. The model often used is the *in vitro* oxidation of LDL suspension with cupric iron in the presence of different concentrations of polyphenols or antioxidants. The quality of the antioxidant is expressed as the concentration of the substance needed to produce 50% inhibition of oxidation (IC50). As listed in Table 5.4, individual polyphenols and the beverages containing mixtures of polyphenols have enormous potential to deter oxidative damage. Vitamin C, vitamin E, and β-carotenes are relatively weak antioxidants when compared to pure polyphenols or beverages containing polyphenols. Particularly strong antioxidant quality is expressed by the individual flavonoids, quercetin and EGC, wine, tea, and grapes. It should be noted, however, that the greater ability of wine polyphenols to inhibit LDL oxidation *in vitro* than equal concentrations of vitamin E may simply reflect the limited availability of vitamin E to LDL when incubated *in vitro*.[164] Therefore, although the interpretation of the data presented in Table 5.4 may be difficult relative to vitamin E, the overall picture illustrates the potency of flavonoids. The data, however, also indicate that care must be taken in reaching conclusions based solely on a single *in vitro* assay.

Despite the positive results suggesting that wine polyphenols can inhibit LDL oxidation *in vitro*, few studies have examined these effects *in vivo*. Hayek et al. fed atherosclerotic apolipoprotein-E-deficient mice red wine, quercetin, or catechin in their drinking water for 42 d.[160] They observed that LDLs isolated from these mice were more resistant to oxidation than LDLs isolated from ethanol-fed control mice, and quercetin appeared to inhibit LDL oxidation more than catechin, whereas catechin appeared more effective in inhibiting LDL aggregation. When red or white wine polyphenols were fed to healthy men (1 g/d equivalent to 375 ml of wine for 2 weeks), the red wine group showed a greater increase in the LDL oxidation lag time than the white wine group.[137] Others have demonstrated that red wine consumption by healthy volunteers reduced the susceptibility of their LDL to oxidative damage.[111,165] To date, the study by Fuhrman et al. shows the most significant *in vivo* effects of red wine consumption on inhibiting LDL oxidation.[166] They fed 17 healthy men 400 ml of red or white wine for 14 d. Plasma collected from red wine drinkers at the end of the study was about 20% less likely to peroxidize than plasma collected at baseline, and LDLs isolated from these subjects were more resistant to oxidation; effects independent of plasma vitamin E or β-carotene concentrations. Interestingly, they reported that plasma taken from white wine drinkers showed a 34% increase in lipid peroxidation compared with baseline, and LDLs isolated from these subjects were more prone to oxidation. However, the study has come under question because the results obtained far exceeded the clinical benefit obtained previously by dietary or pharmacologic interventions to prevent LDL oxidation.[167] In contrast, in 24 healthy subjects who

TABLE 5.4
Antioxidant Quality of Selected Polyphenols and Antioxidants

Antioxidant/Polyphenol	Antioxidant Quality, IC_{50} (µM)
Vitamin C	1.45
Vitamin E	2.40
β-Carotene	4.30
Quercetin	0.22
Rutin	0.51
Myrcetin	0.48
Kaempferol	1.82
Epigallocatechin	0.075
Resveratrol	0.33
Red wines[a]	0.72
White wines[a]	0.71
Grapes[a]	0.2–0.65
Black teas[a]	0.86
Oolong teas[a]	0.60
Green teas[a]	0.52

Note: Units of µm/l for beverages.

[a] Inhibit oxidation by 50% (IC50).

Source: Modified From Salah, N., Miller, N., Paganga, G., Tijburg, L., Bolwell, G., and Rice-Evans, C., Polyphenolic flavanols as scavengers of aqueous phase radicals and as chain-breaking antioxidants, *Arch Biochem Biophys*, 322(2): 339–346, 1995; Vinson, J., Flavonoids in foods as in vitro and in vivo antioxidants, *Adv Exp Med Biol*, 439: 151–164, 1998; Fenech, M., Stockley, C., and Aitken, C., Moderate wine consumption protects against hydrogen peroxide-induced DNA damage, *Mutagenesis*, 12(4): 289–296, 1997.

drank 550 ml of red or white wine containing 3.5% ethanol for 28 d, no significant inhibition of copper-catalyzed LDL oxidation was observed.[167] Similar negative results were seen in 20 volunteers who drank 200 ml of red or white wine for 10 d.[120]

Consumption of teas or their polyphenols have also been reported to inhibit LDL oxidation. Green and black tea were observed to inhibit LDL oxidation in rabbits by 13% and 15%, respectively, and LDL oxidation was inhibited when compared with controls, in LDL-receptor deficient mice fed black tea for 8 weeks.[115,168] In 14 healthy volunteers, consumption of 750 ml of black tea for 4 weeks prolonged the lag phase for LDL oxidation from 54 to 62 min whereas no change was seen in control subjects.[155] LDL oxidation and body fat were both reduced in healthy men consuming 690 mg/d catechins in a green tea extract for 12 weeks.[169] In contrast, in 32 healthy volunteers consuming about 9 mg/d quercetin from onion and black tea for 14 d, no significant difference in plasma oxidized LDL or markers of lipid peroxidation were observed compared to those fed a low flavonoid diet.[170] Whether these contrasting results reflect a difference in dose, formulation of polyphenols, or a combination of these or other factors requires further investigation.

However, it was also reported that flavonoids could accelerate LDL oxidation if they were added to minimally oxidized LDL.[171] As atherosclerotic plaque contains high concentrations of copper and iron, the net *in vivo* effect of polyphenols on LDL oxidation cannot be predicted easily.[172]

Therefore, despite the *in vitro* inhibition of LDL oxidation and the acute rise in serum antioxidant potential following consumption of red wine, or tea in particular, the limited human data do not provide strong evidence that a major *in vivo* effect of wine or tea polyphenols is inhibition of LDL oxidation. Further work is needed to define whether these results simply reflect insufficient absorption or deposition of the necessary polyphenols into the target tissues.

D. Vasodilatory and Nitric Oxide-Related Effects

Nitric oxide (NO) synthesized from arginine is a major promoter of vascular relaxation that also inhibits platelet adherence to endothelium. Over the past few years, a large number of *in vitro* studies have explored the vasodilatory and NO effects of wine and tea and their polyphenols. Evidence suggests that wine polyphenols may modulate the production of nitric oxide.[173] This is illustrated by the observation that wines, grape juices, and extracts from grape skins can inhibit the contraction of rat aortic rings or induce dilation of mesenteric vascular blood vessels.[173,174] In addition, quercetin and tannic acid reproduced the effects of wine and grape fractions through enhanced NO synthesis.[175-179] Resveratrol has also been shown to improve vasodilation and cardiac function via an NO-dependent mechanism after ischemia/reperfusion in rats.[180] Anthocyanidins and catechin in pure forms exhibited NO-scavenging properties, which may account for the observation that catechin did not induce vasorelaxation.[181,182]

The effects of tea on NO-related vasodilation have received little attention to date. In one study of 20 volunteers with coronary artery disease, consumption of 3 cups of black tea had no significant effect on dilation of the brachial artery.[183]

It was also noted that both red and white wine are excellent sources of salicylic acid and its dihydroxybenzoic acid metabolites, which have vasodilator and anti-inflammatory activities.[184] It was determined further that the concentrations of these compounds in wine range from 11 to 28.5 mg/l, with the concentrations being higher in red than white wine. Again, the *in vitro* effects are suggestive, but additional studies are needed to determine whether these pharmacologic effects observed *in vitro* occur after *in vivo* consumption of wine and tea.

E. Effects on Hemostasis

Wine and tea may also have a positive effect on reducing risk factors of CVD by inhibition of platelet aggregation and prolongation of clotting times. Ethanol has long been known to exert an aspirin-like effect on clotting mechanisms; however, the concentrations required to inhibit platelet aggregation have generally been high.[23,24,185] In patients with coronary artery disease, those who drank 330 ml of beer per d for 30 d showed evidence of reduced thrombogenic activity compared with patients who did not consume an alcoholic beverage.[186]

Wine or its polyphenols have been shown to have effects on platelet function. For example, de Lange et al. showed that red wine or grape extract inhibited platelet adhesion to fibrinogen but not collagen *in vitro*.[187] Both intravenous or intragastric administration of red wine or grape juice inhibited platelet-mediated thrombus formation acutely in stenosed coronary arteries in dogs.[185] White wine had no effect in this model. In addition, low concentrations (n*M*) of quercetin dispersed platelet thrombi that adhered to rabbit aortic endothelium *in vitro*.[188] It was also shown that platelet aggregation was inhibited by about 70%, compared with controls, in rats fed ethanol, white wine, or red wine in their drinking water for 2 or 4 months.[189] However, if the ethanol or wine was withheld for 18 h, platelet aggregation returned to greater than control levels in the ethanol or white wine-fed groups, whereas aggregation was still inhibited in the red wine group. In this study, the authors focused on the role of tannins in red wine on inhibition of platelet aggregation. In an interesting study in pigs fed 30 g red wine-ethanol/d for 100 d, platelet aggregation at damaged vessel wall sites was significantly reduced.[190]

A number of investigations have examined the effects of wine on hemostasis in humans. Blann et al. actually observed platelet aggregation in 90 volunteers, suggesting a potential deleterious effect after bolus consumption of 375 ml of red but not white wine.[191] In another study, Lavy et al. observed that in 20 healthy males who consumed 400 ml of red or white wine for 14 d, prothrombin time increased significantly, but partial thromboplastin time decreased in both groups.[111] When collagen was employed as an agonist, no significant change in platelet aggregation was observed following consumption of either red or white wine. Also, no significant effects on platelet aggregation were observed in 20 hypercholesterolemic subjects who drank red or white wine for 28 d.[139] In contrast, collagen-induced platelet aggregation was lower in male volunteers who consumed 30 g of ethanol/d (about 2 to 3 drinks) in the form of red wine or ethanol-spiked clear fruit juice for 28 d when compared to subjects who drank dealcoholized red wine.[192] However, no difference in platelet aggregation was observed if ADP was employed as agonist. These data prompted the authors to conclude that their observations were due to ethanol and not to components in red wine. On the other hand, Seigneur et al. reported that ADP-induced platelet aggregation was inhibited in 16 subjects who drank red wine for 15 d.[165] Epinephrine or arachidonic acid-induced platelet aggregation were not affected in these subjects nor was aggregation affected in subjects who drank white wine or an ethanol solution.

A comprehensive study by Pace-Asciak et al. had 24 healthy males consume 375 ml/d of red or white wine or grape juice without or with added trans-resveratrol (4 mg/l) with meals for 28 d.[193] Only white wine inhibited ADP-induced platelet aggregation, whereas red and white wine and resveratrol-supplemented grape juice inhibited thrombin-induced platelet aggregation. *In vitro*, these authors observed that ADP- and thrombin-induced platelet aggregation was inhibited by about 50% by grape juice, without or with resveratrol, whereas red wine nearly abolished platelet aggregation and white wine had no appreciable effect.[193] In a previous *in vitro* study these authors reported that platelet aggregation could be inhibited by dealcoholized red wine, quercetin, and resveratrol in a dose-dependent manner.[194] Also, additional studies on the effects of combinations of polyphenols seem warranted. Again, these data suggest that the *in vitro* effects of wine and its polyphenols on platelet aggregation are more pronounced than the *in vivo* effects. It should also be noted that a recent study showed that combination of grape seed and grape skin polyphenols had a greater antiplatelet effect than either alone in both dogs and humans.[195] Nevertheless, it remains to be determined whether these effects on platelet aggregation are of clinical importance and can translate into reduced risk from thrombi formation that could lead to serious stenosis or a coronary event.

Only a few studies have investigated tea or its polyphenols or platelet function. *In vitro* theaflavin and EGCG inhibited platelet aggregation and platelet activation factor synthesis; however, other catechins were found to actually stimulate platelet aggregation.[196,197] Tea consumption was reported to reduce blood coagulation, but in another study, Vorster et al. did not observe any significant effect of black tea on fibrinogen or other coagulation variables.[198,199] Certainly, more studies are needed to resolve the effects of tea consumption on platelet aggregation.

F. ATHEROSCLEROSIS AND INFLAMMATION

Few studies have directly examined the effects of wine or tea polyphenols on inhibiting inflammation or the atherosclerosis process itself.[159,160] Recently, Fuhrman et al. fed atherosclerotic apo-E-deficient mice a diet containing 150 mg/d total polyphenols or grape powder for 10 weeks.[201] They observed 41% decrease in the atherosclerotic lesion area compared to controls, which was associated with a significant increase in antioxidant capacity. In a hamster atherosclerosis model, green and black tea inhibited disease formation up to 63% and inhibited LDL oxidation compared to conrols.[202] In addition, green tea polyphenols have recently been shown to downregulate genes that may be proatherogenic.[200]

Studies of anti-inflammatory activity of wine and tea have focused on ischemia/reperfusion models in experimental animals. For example, wine and tea polyphenols were reported to reduce ischemia/reperfusion injury in the heart. In rats, oral treatment with 20 mg/kg/d red wine polyphenols for 7 d reduced infarct size compared with controls via a mechanism that appeared to be NO-dependent.[203] Brookes et al. showed similar protective effects in an *ex vivo* rat myocardial ischemia/reperfusion model using doses of quercetin that may be found in 1 to 2 glasses of red wine (0.033 mg/kg/d for 4 d).[204] In addition, EGCG (10mg/kg iv) was shown recently to reduce myocardial damage compared to controls. [205]

A new area of research in this field relates to the effects of polyphenols on gene expression and signal transduction pathways. Utilizing tools of global mRNA profiling, we are becoming more aware of genome-wide responses to nutrients and micronutrients.[206] For example, the Sir2 (silencing information regulator 2) gene in yeast (*S. cerevisiae*) and SIRT1, the mammalian counterpart, are reported to be the gene link between caloric restriction and longevity.[207,208] In response to cellular damage or stresses, SIRT deacetylates the DNA repair factor Ku70, causing it to sequester the proapoptotic factor Bax away from the mitochondria, thereby inhibiting stress-induced apoptotic cell death. Several plant polyphenols have been found to increase SIRT1 activity and preserve cell survival. Resveratrol reduces the K_m of SIRT1 up to 35-fold, to stimulate p53 deacetylation. Thus, polyphenols, similar to caloric restriction, upregulate stress-response pathways involving sirtuins, to suppress p53 and delay apoptosis, likely preventing cell death.[205,209]

In addition, resveratrol has been shown to act on the mitogen-activated protein kinase (MAPK) cascade by inhibiting protein kinase C (PKC)-catalyzed phosphorylation of arginine-rich protein substrates.[210] Inhibition of phosphorylation and other effects in the nucleus reduce expression of various genes implicated in vasoconstriction, angiogenesis, proliferation, and differentiation.[211] Polyphenols are also reported to affect NFkB, which activates the transcription of several target genes implicated in initiation and progression of atherosclerosis, inflammation, and cancer.[212] Notably, many stimuli, such as oxidized LDL, oxidants, and PKC, have the potential to activate the NFkB pathway, which can modulate the transcription of target genes, such as cyclooxygenase (COX), inducible nitric oxide synthase, cytokines, etc.

Further studies in these areas seem warranted to determine how these observations fit into the overall scheme of wine and tea and their polyphenols in the protection from CVD and whether the doses of these compounds needed to produce these effects are relevant to normal consumption and use.

VI. POTENTIAL ADVERSE EFFECTS OF POLYPHENOLS

Consumption of polyphenols through a variety of foods is not likely to produce adverse effects because of the diversity and varying quantities of polyphenols in plant sources. However, chronic intake of pharmacologic doses have been reported to produce adverse effects.[213] For example, doses of 1 to 1.5 g/d of cianidanol, a flavonoid drug, produced renal failure, hepatitis, fever, hemolytic anemia, thrombocytopenia, and skin disorders. In addition, hydrolyzable tannins in black teas are well-known to inhibit iron absorption.[47,214] Green tea consumption has also been reported to reduce iron status, but neither black nor green tea significantly affected calcium, copper, zinc, or magnesium status.[215] However, the nutritional significance of these observations may be minimal but is not fully known.

Daily high doses of green tea extract (5% of diet) was goitrogenic in rats, but dietary levels of 0.625% appeared to be safe.[216] In subjects consuming about 1 g/d EGCG supplements, approximately the dose found in people who drink >10 cups of green tea/day, some stomach discomfort was noted that resolved if the tablets were taken after a meal. Some transient sleeplessness was also reported but could be due to caffeine contamination of the extract. The LD50 in rats is reported to be 5g/kg in males and 3.1 g/kg in females, suggesting that EGCG has relatively low acute toxicity, but may have teratogenicity at concentrations potentially achievable with daily consumption. It should be noted that sensitivity to EGCG reportedly induced asthma in workers at a green tea factory.[93]

Grape seed was found to have a LD50 in rats that exceeded 5000mg/kg, suggesting very low toxicity.[217,218] In addition daily consumption of up to 2% proanthocyanidin-rich grape seed extract appeared to be safe in rats.[218]

Quercetin also appears to be relatively nontoxic with an LD50 in mice over 100 mg/kg. In a phase I clinical study, toxicity, expressed as nephrotoxicity, was not observed until a cumulative dose of 1700 mg/m[2] was achieved.[93] No evidence of carcinogenicity or teratogenicity with quercetin has been reported, even when fed at dietary levels as high as 10%.[93] Oral administration of 20 mg/kg doses of resveratrol for 28 d was also not toxic to rats.[219] Others reported that 300 mg/kg/d was the maximum no-effect level seen.[220]

A study in Portugal observed a dose-dependent relationship between red wine consumption and incidence of gastric cancer.[221] However, it is not known if this observation is related to the ethanol, red wine polyphenols, or their interaction with other risk factors. Free radicals have been identified in red wines and their grape source but have not been detected in white wine.[222] Although their significance is not clear, phenolic compounds, including those found in red wine, have been shown to be mutagenic and genotoxic in bacterial and mammalian mutagenicity tests.[223, 224] This may also be due to the concomitant production of hydrogen peroxide of phenolics during their autoxidation in a process that is dependent on divalent metal ions. In general, flavonoids can also express pro-oxidant effects in the presence of Cu or NO.[225–227] Tea catechins can also generate hydrogen peroxide and the hydroxyl radical to different degrees in the pressure of Cu^{+2} or H_2O_2 in vitro.[228,229] This is similar to the prooxidant effect of vitamin C observed in the presence of metal salts involving the direct reduction of chelated Fe^{3+} to Fe^{2+} and succeeding radical generation, i.e., metal-induced oxidation. Haliwell reported that plant phenolics may show an oxidant effect against proteins and DNA.[163] Conditions where phenolic compounds act as prooxidants have been described by Decker[230] and Laughton et al.[231]

In general, the double-edged nature of polyphenols has added to the concerns over toxicity. For example, quercetin could induce DNA damage in a lymphocyte test at low concentrations, but at concentrations greater than 100 μM, DNA damage was inhibited.[232,233] Others have observed flavonoid-induced cytotoxicity in cultured human or rat cells, particularly at concentrations exceeding 150 μM,[234–236] but the effects may be cell specific. For the most part, whereas these compounds may express mutagenicity in test systems, they appear to be safe when ingested at modest doses associated with drinking wine or tea.

The safety of the interaction of polyphenols with other dietary supplements has been little investigated. In one study, 1 g/d supplement of grape seed polyphenols taken with 500 mg/dl vitamin C for 6 weeks raised blood pressure ~5mHg in human volunteers suggesting caution in the use of polyphenols in hypertensive patients.[237] Certainly, additional work in this area is needed.

VII. CONCLUSIONS

A. Significance of Polyphenols in CVD and Health

The results from the studies summarized here indicate that the polyphenols present in wines and teas possess antioxidant activity, may modify plasma cholesterol and lipoprotein concentrations, inhibit blood coagulation and inflammatory processes, and have vasorelaxant effects, all of which may potentially modify certain risk factors associated with the development of atherosclerosis or ischemic heart disease in susceptible individuals. The majority of these effects have been expressed in vitro, but the reproducibility of these effects in vivo has been less stellar. These differences may simply reflect low rates of absorption of the pharmacologically active compounds, differences in methodologies employed by the various investigators, sensitivity of certain cell types in vitro, or other factors. It is also realized that wines and teas are complex mixtures, and although techniques have improved to quantitate the various polyphenols in these drinks, investigators have attributed their observations to the substances they can measure, which may not be the most biologically active. As an example, Widlansky et al. observed a good connection between total polyphenol intake from tea and endothelial function in 66 volunteers, but could not link the results to the catechins in tea.[238] Even in studies where specific polyphenols are studied, the results have not always been consistent. In studies where red wine is reportedly superior to white wine, the differences most likely merely reflect the higher polyphenol concentrations in red than white wine, rather than differences in the potencies of the polyphenols in both wines. It has also been recognized that the polyphenols in red wine are rather uniform, but the absolute amounts may vary among different varieties or wines from different regions. Also, different processes are modified to produce the various teas in countries throughout the world, so the uniformity of polyphenols in similar teas is unknown. In addition, although studies may attempt to control the amount of tea solids used, brewing times have rarely been reported. Previous reports indicate that 84% of the antioxidant content of tea is extracted in the first 5 min of brewing, with an additional 13% extracted over the next 5 min.[131]

With respect to atherosclerosis and heart disease, in studies that have reported increased antioxidant potential in plasma after wine or tea consumption, the changes have been transient and disappear a few hours after drinking. In the platelet aggregation studies, results have been reported for only 1 or 2 time points after drinking, and aggregation may change in response to one agonist, but not another, making the overall physiologic significance difficult to interpret. Thus it remains to be established whether these results would be sustained after continued consumption. Insight into the long-term significance of these effects awaits comparisons of these variables in human populations who consume wine or tea frequently to populations where consumption of these beverages is less frequent or very little.

B. DIETARY RECOMMENDATIONS

As mentioned in earlier text, polyphenols are also present in a variety of common fruits and vegetables.[39,47,73] A number of studies have touted the potential health benefits of consuming diets rich in fruits and vegetables, e.g., protection from heart disease and cancer. As it is unclear which of the polyphenols offers the most health-promoting advantage, it would seem premature and inappropriate to recommend consuming wine or tea polyphenols specifically in an attempt to raise an individual's plasma antioxidant status as a means to reduce risk of CVD. Even in the case where wine may contain a particular polyphenol not generally found in other common foods, such as resveratrol, the evidence that it possesses any specific protective effects against CVD *in vivo* is insufficient. At present, data are insufficient to conclude that alcohol itself conveys health-promoting activity. It also remains unknown to what extent alcohol may improve the bioavailability of certain polyphenols in wine. On the other hand, there is sufficient information to suggest that, for adults, consuming one to two glasses of wine with meals, or moderate amounts of decaffeinated tea, should not be harmful.[239] In addition, the best evidence to date suggests that it would require at least 8 to 10 cups of tea/day to achieve a significant change in plasma antioxidant status.[131]

In summary, the available data to date indicate that wine and tea polyphenols, as well as the complex beverage, possess biologic activity that may potentially modify certain risk factors associated with atherogenesis and CVD. Unfortunately, the data are too slim to suggest convincingly that wine or tea may offer long-term protection from these diseases. Epidemiologic studies suggest that the population that may most benefit from these polyphenolic compounds is probably those of 30 to 65 or 70 years of age. However, before making definitive recommendations for consumption, as many polyphenols are also present in fruits and vegetables, one must always keep in mind the well-known health effects and consequences of ethanol abuse or the effects and risks of acute inebriation before making a blanket recommendation for wine consumption.[11,131,240,241] There is also no definitive evidence that wine or tea consumption should be recommended in an attempt to overcome the adverse health consequences of smoking or consuming a diet high in saturated fat. As the best polyphenols to promote health are not known, it is premature to recommend dietary supplements containing individual compounds or complexes. Currently, based on an individual's preference and available evidence, there is nothing to suggest that adding a glass of wine to the meal or drinking tea would be harmful. Both beverages should be enjoyed for themselves. As usual, eating or drinking "in moderation" should remain the best recommendation.

REFERENCES

1. Hennekens, C., Buring, J., Manson, J. et al., Lack of effect of long-term supplementation with beta carotene on the incidence of malignant neoplasms and cardiovascular disease, *N Engl J Med*, 334(18): 1145–1149, 1996.
2. Garcia-Palmieri, M., Sorlie, P., Tillotson, J., Costas, Jr., R., Cordero, E., and Rodriguez, M., Relationship of dietary intake to subsequent coronary heart disease incidence: the Puerto Rico Heart Health Program, *Am J Clin Nutr*, 33(8): 1818–1827, 1980.
3. Hegsted, D. and Ausman, L.M., Diet, alcohol and coronary heart disease in men, *J Nutr*, 118(10): 1184–1189, 1988.
4. St. Leger, A., Cochrane, A.L., and Moore, F., Factors associated with cardiac mortality in developed countries with particular reference to the consumption of wine, *Lancet* (8124): 1017–1020, 1979.
5. Nanji, A., Alcohol and ischemic heart disease: wine, beer or both? *Int J Cardiol*, 8(4): 487–489, 1985.
6. Hein, H., Suadicani, P., and Gyntelberg, F., Alcohol consumption, serum low-density lipoprotein cholesterol concentration, and risk of ischaemic heart disease: six year follow up in the Copenhagen male study, *Br Med J*, 312(7033): 736–741, 1996.
7. Klatsky, A., Armstrong, M., and Friedman, G., Red wine, white wine, liquor, beer, and risk for coronary artery disease hospitalization, *Am J Cardiol*, 80(4): 416–420, 1997.
8. Kushi, L., Lenart, E., and Willett, W., Health implications of Mediterranean diets in light of contemporary knowledge. 2. Meat, wine, fats, and oils, *Am J Clin Nutr*, 61(6 Suppl.): 1416S–1427S, 1995.
9. Schneider, J., Kaffarnik, H., and Steinmetz, A., Alcohol, lipid metabolism and coronary heart disease, *Herz*, 21(4): 217–226, 1996.
10. Hein, H.O., Suadicani, P. and Gyntelberg, F. Alcohol consumption, S-LDL-cholesterol and risk of ischemic heart disease: 6-year follow-up in The Copenhagen Male Study, *Ugeskr Laeger*, 159(26): 4110–4116, 1997.
11. Zakhari, S. and Gordis, E. Moderate drinking and cardiovascular health, *Proc Assoc Am Physicians*, 111(2): 148–158, 1999.
12. Camargo, C., Jr., Stampfer, M., Glynn, R. et al., Moderate alcohol consumption and risk for angina pectoris or myocardial infarction in U.S. male physicians, *Ann Intern Med*, 126(5): 372–375, 1997.
13. Gronbaek, M., Deis, A., Sorensen, T., Becker, U., Schnohr, P., and Jensen, G., Mortality associated with moderate intakes of wine, beer, or spirits, *Br Med J*, 310(6988): 1165–1169, 1995.
14. Yuan, J., Ross, R., Gao, R., Henderson, B., and Yu, M., Follow up study of moderate alcohol intake and mortality among middle aged men in Shanghai, China, *Br Med J*, 314(7073): 18–23, 1997.
15. Doll, R., Peto, R., Hall, E., Wheatley, K., and Gray, R., Mortality in relation to consumption of alcohol: 13 years' observations on male British doctors, *Br Med J*, 309(6959): 911–918, 1994.
16. Constant, J., Alcohol, ischemic heart disease, and the French paradox, *Clin Cardiol*, 20(5): 420–424, 1997.
17. Castelli, W., How many drinks a day? *JAMA*, 242(18): 2000, 1979.
18. Calabrese, E., Hormesis: from marginalization to mainstream: a case for hormesis as the default dose-response model in risk assessment, *Toxicol Appl Pharmacol*, 197(2): 125–136, 2004.
19. Castelli, W., Doyle, J., Gordon, T. et al., Alcohol and blood lipids, The cooperative lipoprotein phenotyping study, *Lancet*, 2(8030): 153–155, 1977.
20. Willett, W., Hennekens, C., Siegel, A., Adner, M., and Castelli, W., Alcohol consumption and high-density lipoprotein cholesterol in marathon runners, *N Engl J Med*, 303(20): 1159–1161, 1980.
21. Contaldo, F., D'Arrigo, E., Carandente, V. et al., Short-term effects of moderate alcohol consumption on lipid metabolism and energy balance in normal men, *Metabolism*, 38(2): 166–171, 1989.
22. Wolfort, F.G., Pan, D., and Gee, J., Alcohol and preoperative management, *Plast Reconstr Surg*, 98(7): 1306–1309, 1996.

23. Renaud, S. and de Lorgeril, M., Wine, alcohol, platelets, and the French paradox for coronary heart disease, *Lancet*, 339(8808): 1523–1526, 1992.
24. Drewnowski, A., Henderson, S., Shore, A., Fischler, C., Preziosi, P., and Hercberg, S., Diet quality and dietary diversity in France: implications for the French paradox, *J Am Diet Assoc*, 96(7): 663–669, 1996.
25. Renaud, S. and. Ruf, J., The French paradox: vegetables or wine, *Circulation*, 90(6): 3118–3119, 1994.
26. Criqui, M. and Ringel, B., Does diet or alcohol explain the French paradox? *Lancet*, 344(8939–8940): 1719–1723, 1994.
27. Cleophas, T., Tuinenberg, E., van der Meulen, J., and Zwinderman, K., Wine consumption and other dietary variables in males under 60 before and after acute myocardial infarction, *Angiology*, 47(8): 789–796, 1996.
28. Burr, M.L., Explaining the French paradox, *J R Soc Health*, 115(4): 217–219, 1995.
29. Law, M. and Wald, N., Why heart disease mortality is low in France: the time lag explanation, *Br Med J*, 318(7196): 1471–1476, 1999.
30. Hertog, M., Feskens, E., Hollman, P., Katan, M., and Kromhout, D., Dietary antioxidant flavonoids and risk of coronary heart disease: the Zutphen Elderly Study, *Lancet*, 342(8878): 1007–1011, 1993.
31. Keli, S., Hertog, M., Feskens, E., and Kromhout, D., Dietary flavonoids, antioxidant vitamins, and incidence of stroke: the Zutphen study, *Arch Intern Med*, 156(6): 637–642, 1996.
32. Knekt, P., Jarvinen, R., Reunanen, A., and Maatela, J., Flavonoid intake and coronary mortality in Finland: a cohort study, *Br Med J*, 312(7029): 478–481, 1996.
33. Stensvold, I., Tverdal, A., Solvoll, K., and Foss, O., Tea consumption: relationship to cholesterol, blood pressure, and coronary and total mortality, *Prev Med*, 21(4): 546–553, 1992.
34. Imai, K., and Nakachi, K., Cross sectional study of effects of drinking green tea on cardiovascular and liver diseases, *Br Med J*, 310(6981): 693–696, 1995.
35. Mukamal, K., Maclure, M., Muller, J., Sherwood, J., and Mittleman, M., Tea consumption and mortality after acute myocardial infarction, *Circulation*, 105(21): 2476–2481, 2002.
36. Brown, C., Bolton-Smith, C., Woodward, M., and Tunstall-Pedoe, H., Coffee and tea consumption and the prevalence of coronary heart disease in men and women: results from the Scottish Heart Health Study, *J Epidemiol Community Health*, 47(3): 171–175, 1993.
37. Loktionov, A., Bingham, S., Vorster, H., Jerling, J., Runswick, S., and Cummings, J., Apolipoprotein E genotype modulates the effect of black tea drinking on blood lipids and blood coagulation factors: a pilot study, *Br J Nutr*, 79(2): 133–139, 1998.
38. Sharp, D., When wine is red, *Lancet*, 341(8836): 27–28, 1993.
39. Ferro-Luzzi, A. and Serafini, M., Polyphenols in our diet: do they matter? *Nutrition*, 11(4): 399–400, 1995.
40. Goldberg, D., Does wine work? *Clin Chem*, 41(1): 14–16, 1995.
41. Hollman, P., Feskens, E., and Katan, M., Tea flavonols in cardiovascular disease and cancer epidemiology, *Proc Soc Exp Biol Med*, 220(4): 198–202, 1999.
42. Dreosti, I., Bioactive ingredients: antioxidants and polyphenols in tea, *Nutr Rev*, 54(11 Pt. 2): S51–S58, 1996.
43. Graham, H., Green tea composition, consumption, and polyphenol chemistry, *Prev Med*, 21(3): 334–350, 1992.
44. Ahmad, N. and Mukhtar, H., Green tea polyphenols and cancer: biologic mechanisms and practical implications, *Nutr Rev*, 57(3): 78–83, 1999.
45. King, A. and Young, G., Characteristics and occurrence of phenolic phytochemicals, *J Am Diet Assoc*, 99(2): 213–218, 1999.
46. Croft, K., The chemistry and biological effects of flavonoids and phenolic acids, *Ann N Y Acad Sci*, 854: 435–442, 1998.
47. Bravo, L., Polyphenols: chemistry, dietary sources, metabolism, and nutritional significance, *Nutr Rev*, 56(11): 317–333, 1998.
48. Frankel, E., Waterhouse, A., and Teissedre, P., Principal phenolic phytochemicals in selected California wines and their antioxidant activity in inhibiting oxidation of human low-density lipoproteins, *J Agric Food Chem*, 43: 890–894, 1995.
49. Cook, N. and Samman, S., Flavonoids: chemistry, metabolism, cardioprotective effects, and dietary sources, *J Nutr Biochem*, 7: 66–76, 1996.

50. Harborne, J. and Baxter, H., *Phytochemical Dictionary: A Handbook of Bioactive Compounds from Plants*, Washington, D.C.: Taylor and Francis, 1998.

51. Pietta, P., Flavonoids in medicinal plants, in *Flavonoids in Health and Disease*, C. Rice-Evans and L. Packer, Eds., Marcel Dekker: New York, 1998.

52. Salah, N., Miller, N., Paganga, G., Tijburg, L., Bolwell, G., and Rice-Evans, C., Polyphenolic flavanols as scavengers of aqueous phase radicals and as chain-breaking antioxidants, *Arch Biochem Biophys*, 322(2): 339–346, 1995.

53. Formica, J. and Regelson, W., Review of the biology of quercetin and related bioflavonoids, *Food Chem Toxicol*, 33(12): 1061–1080, 1995.

54. Soleas, G., Diamandis, E., and Goldberg, D., Resveratrol: a molecule whose time has come? And gone? *Clin Biochem*, 1997. 30(2): 91–113.

55. Soleas, G., Diamandis, E., and Goldberg, D., Wine as a biological fluid: history, production, and role in disease prevention, *J Clin Lab Anal*, 11(5): 287–313, 1997.

56. Hertog, M., Hollman, P., and van de Purtte, B., Content of potentially anticarcinogenic flavonoids of tea infusions, wines, and fruit juices, *J Agric Food Chem*, 41: 1242–1246, 1993.

57. Lanningham-Foster, L., Chen, C. Chance, D.S., and Loo, G., Grape extract inhibits lipid peroxidation of human low-density lipoprotein, *Biol Pharm Bull*, 18(10): 1347–1351, 1995.

58. Das, D., Sato, M., Ray, P., Maulik, G., Engelman, R., Bertelli, A., and Bertelli, A., Cardioprotection of red wine: role of polyphenolic antioxidants, *Drugs Exp Clin Res*, 25(2–3): 115–120, 1999.

59. Belguendouz, L., Fremont, L., and Linard, A., Resveratrol inhibits metal ion-dependent and independent peroxidation of porcine low-density lipoproteins, *Biochem Pharmacol*, 53(9): 1347–1355, 1997.

60. Hao, H.D. and He, L.R., Mechanisms of cardiovascular protection by resveratrol, *J Med Food*, 7(3): 290–298, 2004.

61. Solease, G. and Goldberg, D.M., Analysis of antioxidant wine polyphenols by gas chromatography mass spectrometry, *Methds Enzymol*, 229: 137–151, 1999.

62. Frankel, E.N., Waterhouse, A., and Kinsella, J., Inhibition of human LDL oxidation by resveratrol, *Lancet*, 341(8852): 1103–1104, 1993.

63. Brouillard, R., George, F., and Fougerousse, A., Polyphenols produced during red wine ageing, *Biofactors*, 6(4): 403–410, 1997.

64. Goldberg, D., Tsang, E., Karumanchiri, A., Diamandis, E., Soleas, G., and Ng, E., Method to assay the concentrations of phenolic constituents of biological interest in wines, *Anal Chem*, 68(10): 1688–1694, 1996.

65. Graham, H., Green tea composition, consumption, and polyphenol chemistry, *Prev Med*, 21(3): 334–350, 1992.

66. Makimura, M., Hirasawa, M., Kobayashi, K., Indo, J., Sakanaka, S., Taguchi, T., and Otake, S., Inhibitory effect of tea catechins on collagenase activity, *J Periodontol*, 64(7): 630–636, 1993.

67. Beecher, G., Warden, B., and Merken, H., Analysis of tea polyphenols, *Proc Soc Exp Biol Med*, 220(4): 267–270, 1999.

68. Mazur, W., Wahala, K., Rasku, S., Salakka, A., Hase, T., and Adlercreutz, H., Lignan and isoflavonoid concentrations in tea and coffee. *Br J Nutr*, 79(1): 37–45, 1998.

69. Vinson, J., Flavonoids in foods as in vitro and in vivo antioxidants, *Adv Exp Med Biol*, 439: 151–164, 1998.

70. Steele, V., Bagheri, D. Balentine, D. et al., Preclinical efficacy studies of green and black tea extracts, *Proc Soc Exp Biol Med*, 220(4): 210–212, 1999.

71. Manach, C., Scalbert, A., Morand, C., Remesy, C., and Jimenez, L. Polyphenols: food sources and bioavailability, *Am J Clin Nutr* 79: 727–747, 2004.

72. Kuhnau, J., The flavonoids: a class of semi-essential food components: their role in human nutrition, *World Rev Nutr Diet*, 24: 117–191, 1976.

73. Hertog, M., Hollman, P., Katan, M., and Kromhout, D., Intake of potentially anticarcinogenic flavonoids and their determinants in adults in The Netherlands, *Nutr Cancer*, 20(1): 21–29, 1993.

74. Clydesdale, F., Quercetin. *Crit. Rev. Food Sci. Nutr*, 235–244, 1999.

75. Paganga, G. and Rice-Evans, C., The identification of flavonoids as glycosides in human plasma, *FEBS Lett*, 401(1): 78–82, 1997.

76. Lee, M.J., Wang, Z.Y., Li, H., Chen, L., Sun, Y., Gobbo, S., Balentine, D.A., and Yang, C.S., Analysis of plasma and urinary tea polyphenols in human subjects, *Cancer Epidemiol Biomarkers Prev*, 4(4): 393–399, 1995.

77. Griffiths, L.A. and Barrow, A., Metabolism of flavonoid compounds in germ-free rats, *Biochem J*, 130(4): 1161–1162, 1972.

78. Bravo, L., Abia, R., Eastwood, M.A., and Saura-Calixto, F., Degradation of polyphenols (catechin and tannic acid) in the rat intestinal tract. Effect on colonic fermentation and faecal output, *Br J Nutr*, 71(6): 933–946, 1994.

79. Day, A., DuPont, M., Ridley, S., Rhodes, M., Rhodes, M.J., Morgan, M., and Williamson, G., Deglycosylation of flavonoid and isoflavonoid glycosides by human small intestine and liver beta-glucosidase activity, *FEBS Lett*, 436(1): 71–75, 1998.

80. Ader, P., Grenacher, B., Langguth, P., Scharrer, E., and Wolffram, S. Cinnamate uptake by rat small intestine: transport kinetics and transepithelial transfer, *Exp Physiol* 81: 943–955, 1996.

81. Gee, J., Du Pont, M., Rhodes, M., and Johnson, I., Quercein glucosides interact with the intestinal glucose transport pathway, *Free Radic Biol Med* 25: 19–25, 1998.

82. Rasmussen, S., Frederiksen, H., Krogholm, K., and Poulsen, L., Dietary proanthocyanidins: occurrence, dietary intake, bioavailability, and protection against cardiovascular disease, *Mol Nutr Food Res* 49: 159–174, 2005.

83. Halliwell, B., Zhao, K., and Whiteman, M., The gastrointestinal tract: a major site of antioxidant action? *Free Radic Res,* 33: 819–830, 2000.

84. Manach, C., Regerat, F., Texier, O., Agullo, G., Demigne, C., and Remesy, C., Bioavailability, metabolism, and physiological impact of 4-oxo-flavonoids, *Nutr. Res.*, 16: 517–544, 1996.

85. Manach, C., Morand, C., Texier, O. et al., Quercetin metabolites in plasma of rats fed diets containing rutin or quercetin, *J. Nutr.*, 125: 1911–1922, 1995.

86. Ueno, I., Nakano, N., and Hirono, I., Metabolic fate of [14C] quercetin in the ACI rat, *Jpn J Exp Med*, 53(1): 41–50, 1983.

87. de Vries, J.H., Hollman, P., Meyboom, S., Buysman, M., Zock, P., van Staveren, W., and Katan, M., Plasma concentrations and urinary excretion of the antioxidant flavonols quercetin and kaempferol as biomarkers for dietary intake, *Am J Clin Nutr*, 68(1): 60–65, 1998.

88. van het Hof, K., Kivits, G., Weststrate, J., and Tijburg, L., Bioavailability of catechins from tea: the effect of milk, *Eur J Clin Nutr*, 52(5): 356–359, 1998.

89. Hollman, P.C., vd Gaag, M,. Mengelers, M., van Trijp, J., de Vries, J., and Katan, M., Absorption and disposition kinetics of the dietary antioxidant quercetin in man, *Free Radic Biol Med*, 21(5): 703–707, 1996.

90. Bertelli, A., Giovannini, L., Stradi, R., Bertelli, A., and Tillement, J., Plasma, urine and tissue levels of trans- and cis-resveratrol (3,4,5-trihydroxystilbene) after short-term or prolonged administration of red wine to rats, *Int J Tissue React*, 18(2–3): 67–71, 1996.

91. Clifford, A.J., Ebeler, S., Ebeler, J., Bills, N., Hinrichs, S., Teissedre, P., and Waterhouse, A., Delayed tumor onset in transgenic mice fed an amino acid-based diet supplemented with red wine solids, *Am J Clin Nutr*, 64(5): 748–756, 1996.

92. Maiani, G., Serafini, M., Salucci, M., Azzini, E., and Ferro-Luzzi, A., Application of a new high-performance liquid chromatographic method for measuring selected polyphenols in human plasma, *J Chromatogr B Biomed Sci Appl*, 692(2): 311–317, 1997.

93. Clydesdale, F., Epigallocatechin and epigallocatechin-3-gallate, *Crit. Rev. Food Sci. Nutr.*, 39: 215–226, 1999.

94. van het Hof, K., Wiseman, S., Yang, C., and Tijburg, L., Plasma and lipoprotein levels of tea catechins following repeated tea consumption, *Proc Soc Exp Biol Med*, 220(4): 203–209, 1999.

95. Gugler, R., Leschik, M., and Dengler, H., Disposition of quercetin in man after single oral and intravenous doses, *Eur J Clin Pharmacol*, 9(2–3): 229–234, 1975.

96. Bourne, L. and Rice-Evans, C., Detecting and measuring bioavailability of phenolics and flavonoids in humans: pharmacokinetics of urinary excretion of dietary ferulic acid, *Methods Enzymol*, 299: 91–106, 1997.

97. Galijatovic, A., Walle, U., and Walle, T. Induction of UDP-glucuronosyl-transferase by the flavonoids chrysin and quercetin in Caco-2-cells, *Pharm Res* 17: 21–26, 2000.

98. Orzechowski, A., Ostaszewski, P., Jank, M., and Berwid, S.J.B., Bioactive substances of plant origin in food — impact on genomics, *Reprod Nutr Dev* 42: 461–477, 2002.

99. Ciolino, H., Daschner, P., and Yeh, G., Dietary flavonols quercetin and kaempferol are ligands of the aryl hydrocarbon receptor that effect cyp 1 alpha 1 transcription differentially, *Biochem J* 340: 715–722, 1999.

100. Hertog, M., Kromhout, D., Aravanis, C. et al., Flavonoid intake and long-term risk of coronary heart disease and cancer in the seven countries study, *Arch. Intern. Med*, 155: 381–386, 1995.

101. Hertog, M., Feskens, F., and Kromhout, D., Antioxidant flavonols and coronary heart disease risk, *Lancet*, 349(9053): 699, 1997.

102. Rimm, E., Katan, M., Ascherio, A., Stampfer, M., and Willett, W., Relation between intake of flavonoids and risk for coronary heart disease in male health professionals, *Ann Intern Med*, 125(5): 384–389, 1996.

103. Mennen, L., Sapinho, I., de Bree, A., Arnault, N., Bertrais, S., Galan, P., and Hercberg, S., Consumption of foods rich in flavonoids is related to a decreased cardiovascular risk in apparently healthy French women, *J Nutr*, 134(4): 923–926, 2004.

104. Lagiou, P., Samoli, E., Lagiou, A. et al., Intake of specific flavonoid classes and coronary heart disease — a case-control study in Greece, *Eur J Clin Nutr*, 58(12): 1643–1648, 2004.

105. Arts, I., Hollman, P., Feskens, E., Bueno de Mesquita, H., and Kromhout, D., Catechin intake might explain the inverse relation between tea consumption and ischemic heart disease: the Zutphen Elderly Study, *Am J Clin Nutr*, 74(2): 227–232, 2001.

106. Sesso, H., Gaziano, J., Liu, S., and Buring, J., Flavonoid intake and the risk of cardiovascular disease in women, *Am J Clin Nutr*, 77(6): 1400–1408, 2003.

107. Sesso, H.D., Paffenbarger, R., Jr., Oguma, Y., and Lee, I., Lack of association between tea and cardiovascular disease in college alumni, *Int J Epidemiol*, 32(4): 527–533, 2003.

108. Hertog, M., Sweetnam, P., Fehily, A., Elwood, P., and Kromhout, D., Antioxidant flavonols and ischemic heart disease in a Welsh population of men: the Caerphilly study, *Am J Clin Nutr*, 65(5): 1489–1494, 1997.

109. Steinberg, D., Parthasarathy, S., Carew, T., Khoo, J., and Witztum, J., Beyond cholesterol. Modifications of low-density lipoprotein that increase its atherogenicity, *N Engl J Med*, 320(14): 915–924, 1989.

110. Hansson, G., Inflammation, atherosclerosis, and coronary artery disease, *N Engl J Med*, 352(16): 1685–1695, 2005.

111. Lavy, A., Fuhrman, B., Markel, A., Dankner, G., Ben-Amotz, A., Presser, D., and Aviram, M., Effect of dietary supplementation of red or white wine on human blood chemistry, hematology and coagulation: favorable effect of red wine on plasma high-density lipoprotein, *Ann Nutr Metab*, 38(5): 287–294, 1994.

112. Klurfeld, D. and Kritchevsky, D., Differential effects of alcoholic beverages on experimental atherosclerosis in rabbits, *Exp Mol Pathol*, 34(1): 62–71, 1981.

113. Kono, S., Shinchi, K., Ikeda, N., Yanai, F., and Imanishi, K., Green tea consumption and serum lipid profiles: a cross-sectional study in northern Kyushu, Japan, *Prev Med*, 21(4): 526–531, 1992.

114. Unno, T., Tago, M., Suzuki, Y. et al., Effect of tea catechins on postprandial plasma lipid responses in human subjects, *Br J Nutr*, 93(4): 543–547, 2005.

115. Tijburg, L., Wiseman, S., Meijer, G., and Weststrate, J., Effects of green tea, black tea and dietary lipophilic antioxidants on LDL oxidizability and atherosclerosis in hypercholesterolaemic rabbits, *Atherosclerosis*, 135(1): 37–47, 1997.

116. Yamakoshi, J., Saito, M., Kataoka, S., and Kikuchi, M., Safety evaluation of proanthocyanidin-rich extract from grape seeds, *Food Chem Toxicol*, 40(5): 599–607, 2002.

117. Green, M. and Harari, G., Association of serum lipoproteins and health-related habits with coffee and tea consumption in free-living subjects examined in the Israeli CORDIS Study, *Prev Med*, 21(4): 532–545, 1992.

118. Xu, R., Yokoyama, W., Irving, D., Rein, D., Walzem, R., and German, J., Effect of dietary catechin and vitamin E on aortic fatty streak accumulation in hypercholesterolemic hamsters, *Atherosclerosis*, 137(1): 29–36, 1998.

119. Chan, P., Fong, W., Cheung, Y., Huang, Y., Ho, W., and Chen, Z., Jasmine green tea epicatechins are hypolipidemic in hamsters (*Mesocricetus auratus*) fed a high fat diet, *J Nutr*, 129(6): 1094–1101, 1999.

120. Sharpe, P., McGrath, L., McClean, E., Young, I., and Archbold, G., Effect of red wine consumption on lipoprotein (a) and other risk factors for atherosclerosis, *QJM*, 88(2): 101–108, 1995.
121. Harris, E., Lipoprotein[a]: a predictor of atherosclerotic disease, *Nutr Rev*, 55(3): 61–64, 1997.
122. Goldberg, D., Garovic-Kocic, V., Diamandis, E., and Pace-Asciak, C., Wine: does the colour count? *Clin Chim Acta*, 246(1–2): 183–193, 1996.
123. Moreno, D., Ilic, N., Poulev, A., Brasaemle, D., Fried, S., and Raskin, I., Inhibitory effects of grape seed extract on lipases, *Nutrition*, 19(10): 876–879, 2003.
124. Rice-Evans, C., Miller, N., and Paganga, G., Structure-antioxidant activity relationships of flavonoids and phenolic acids, *Free Radic Biol Med*, 20(7): 933–956, 1996.
125. Juan, S., Cheng, T., Lin, H., Chu, Y., and Lee, W., Mechanism of concentration-dependent induction of heme oxygenase-1 by resveratrol in human aortic smooth muscle cells, *Biochem Pharmacol*, 69(1): 41–48, 2005.
126. Chow, J., Shen, S., Huan, S., Lin, H., and Chen, Y., Quercetin, but not rutin and quercitrin, prevention of H_2O_2-induced apoptosis via anti-oxidant activity and heme oxygenase 1 gene expression in macrophages, *Biochem Pharmacol*, 69(12): 1839–1851, 2005.
127. Kerry, N. and Rice-Evans, C., Inhibition of peroxynitrite-mediated oxidation of dopamine by flavonoid and phenolic antioxidants and their structural relationships, *J Neurochem*, 73(1): 247–253, 1999.
128. Maxwell, S., Cruickshank, A., and Thorpe, G., Red wine and antioxidant activity in serum, *Lancet*, 344(8916): 193–194, 1994.
129. Campos, A. and Lissi, E., Total antioxidant potential of Chilean wines, *Nutr. Res.*, 16: 385–389, 1996.
130. Halder, J. and Bhaduri, A., Protective role of black tea against oxidative damage of human red blood cells, *Biochem Biophys Res Commun*, 244(3): 903–907, 1998.
131. Prior, R. and Cao, G., Antioxidant capacity and polyphenolic components of teas: implications for altering in vivo antioxidant status, *Proc Soc Exp Biol Med*, 220(4): 255–261, 1999.
132. Vinson, J. and Dabbagh, Y., Tea phenols: antioxidant effectiveness of teas, tea components, tea fractions and their binding with lipoproteins, *Nutr. Res.*, 18: 1067–1075, 1998.
133. Serafini, M., Ghiselli, A., and Ferro-Luzzi, A., Red wine, tea, and antioxidants, *Lancet*, 344(8922): 626, 1994.
134. Echeverry, C., Blasina, F. Arredondo, F. et al., Cytoprotection by neutral fraction of tannat red wine against oxidative stress-induced cell death, *J Agric Food Chem*, 52(24): 7395–7399, 2004.
135. Whitehead, T., Robinson, D., Allaway, S., Syms, J., and Hale, A., Effect of red wine ingestion on the antioxidant capacity of serum, *Clin Chem*, 41(1): 32–35, 1995.
136. Durak, I., Koseoglu, M., Kacmaz, M., Buyukkocak, S., Cimen, B., and Ozturk, H., Black grape enhances plasma antioxidant potential, *Nutr. Res.*, 19, 1999.
137. Nigdikar, S., Williams, N., Griffin, B., and Howard, A., Consumption of red wine polyphenols reduces the susceptibility of low-density lipoproteins to oxidation in vivo, *Am J Clin Nutr*, 68(2): 258–265, 1998.
138. Serafini, M., Maiani, G., and Ferro-Luzzi, A., Alcohol-free red wine enhances plasma antioxidant capacity in humans, *J Nutr*, 128(6): 1003–1007, 1998.
139. Struck, M., Watkins, T., Tomeo, A., Halley, J., and Bierrenbaum, M., Effect of red and white wine on serum lipids, platelet aggregation, oxidation products and antioxidant: a preliminary report, *Nutr. Res.*, 14: 1811–1819, 1994.
140. Rodrigo, R., Castillo, R., Carrasco, R., Huerta, P., and Moreno, M., Diminution of tissue lipid peroxidation in rats is related to the in vitro antioxidant capacity of wine, *Life Sci*, 76(8): 889–900, 2005.
141. Day, A. and Stansbie, D., Cardioprotective effect of red wine may be mediated by urate, *Clin Chem*, 41(9): 1319–1320, 1995.
142. Nyyssonen, K., Porkkala-Sarataho, E., Kaikkonen, J., and Salonen, J., Ascorbate and urate are the strongest determinants of plasma antioxidative capacity and serum lipid resistance to oxidation in Finnish men, *Atherosclerosis*, 130(1–2): 223–233, 1997.
143. Cao, G., Russell, R., Lischner, N., and Prior, R., Serum antioxidant capacity is increased by consumption of strawberries, spinach, red wine or vitamin C in elderly women, *J Nutr*, 128(12): 2383–2390, 1998.
144. Fenech, M., Stockley, C., and Aitken, C., Moderate wine consumption protects against hydrogen peroxide-induced DNA damage, *Mutagenesis*, 12(4): 289–296, 1997.

145. Wickramasinghe, S., Hasan, R., and Khalpey, Z., Differences in the serum levels of acetaldehyde and cytotoxic acetaldehyde-albumin complexes after the consumption of red and white wine: in vitro effects of flavonoids, vitamin E, and other dietary antioxidants on cytotoxic complexes, *Alcohol Clin Exp Res*, 20(5): 799–803, 1996.

146. Rah, D., Han, D., Baek, H., Hyon, S., and Park, J., Prevention of reactive oxygen species-induced oxidative stress in human microvascular endothelial cells by green tea polyphenol, *Toxicol Lett*, 155(2): 269–275, 2005.

147. Klaunig, J., Xu, Y., Han, C. et al., The effect of tea consumption on oxidative stress in smokers and nonsmokers, *Proc Soc Exp Biol Med*, 220(4): 249–254, 1999.

148. Pannala, A., Rice-Evans, C., Halliwell, B., and Singh, S., Inhibition of peroxynitrite-mediated tyrosine nitration by catechin polyphenols, *Biochem Biophys Res Commun*, 232(1): 164–168, 1997.

149. Pannala, A., Razaq, R., Halliwell, B., Singh, S., and Rice-Evans, C., Inhibition of peroxynitrite dependent tyrosine nitration by hydroxycinnamates: nitration or electron donation? *Free Radic Biol Med*, 24(4): 594–606, 1998.

150. Cestaro, B., Simonetti, P., Cervato, G., Brusamolino, A., Gatti, R., and Testolin, G., Red wine effects on peroxidation indexes of rat plasma and erythrocytes, *Int J Food Sci Nutr*, 47(2): 181–189, 1996.

151. Keaney, J., Jr., Simon, D., and Freedman, J., Vitamin E and vascular homeostasis: implications for atherosclerosis, *FASEB J*, 13(9): 965–975, 1999.

152. Nardini, M., Natella, F., Gentili, V., Di Felice, M., and Scaccini, C., Effect of caffeic acid dietary supplementation on the antioxidant defense system in rat: an in vivo study, *Arch Biochem Biophys*, 342(1): 157–160, 1997.

153. Pietta, P. and Simonetti, P., Dietary flavonoids and interaction with endogenous antioxidants, *Biochem. Mol. Biol. Int.*, 44: 1069–1074, 1998.

154. Belguendouz, L., Fremont, L., and Gozzelino, M., Interaction of transresveratrol with plasma lipoproteins, *Biochem Pharmacol*, 55(6): 811–816, 1998.

155. Ishikawa, T., Suzukawa, M., Ito, T. et al., Effect of tea flavonoid supplementation on the susceptibility of low-density lipoprotein to oxidative modification, *Am J Clin Nutr*, 66(2): 261–266, 1997.

156. Caldu, P., Hurtado, I., Fiol, C., Gonzalo, A., and Minguez, S., White wine reduces the susceptibility of low-density lipoprotein to oxidation, *Am J Clin Nutr*, 63(3): 403–404, 1996.

157. Rifici, V., Stephan, E., Schneider, S., and Khachadurian, A., Red wine inhibits the cell-mediated oxidation of LDL and HDL, *J Am Coll Nutr*, 18(2): 137–143, 1999.

158. Frankel, E., Kanner, J., German, J., Parks, E., and Kinsella, J., Inhibition of oxidation of human low-density lipoprotein by phenolic substances in red wine, *Lancet*, 1993. 341(8843): 454–457.

159. Aviram, M. and Fuhrman, B., Polyphenolic flavonoids inhibit macrophage-mediated oxidation of LDL and attenuate atherogenesis, *Atherosclerosis*, 137 Suppl.: S45–S50, 1998.

160. Hayek, T., Fuhrman, B., Vaya, J. et al., Reduced progression of atherosclerosis in apolipoprotein E-deficient mice following consumption of red wine, or its polyphenols quercetin or catechin, is associated with reduced susceptibility of LDL to oxidation and aggregation, *Arterioscler Thromb Vasc Biol*, 17(11): 2744–2752, 1997.

161. Lanningham-Foster, L., Chen, C., Chance, D., and Loo, G., Grape extract inhibits lipid peroxidation of human low-density lipoprotein, *Biol Pharm Bull*, 18(10): 1347–1351, 1995.

162. Miyagi, Y., Miwa, K., and Inoue, H., Inhibition of human low-density lipoprotein oxidation by flavonoids in red wine and grape juice, *Am J Cardiol*, 80(12): 1627–1631, 1997.

163. Abu-Amsha, R., Croft, K., Puddey, I., Proudfoot, J., and Beilin, L., Phenolic content of various beverages determines the extent of inhibition of human serum and low-density lipoprotein oxidation in vitro: identification and mechanism of action of some cinnamic acid derivatives from red wine, *Clin Sci (Lond)*, 91(4): 449–458, 1996.

164. Halliwell, B., Antioxidants in wine, *Lancet*, 341(8859): 1538, 1993.

165. Seingneur, M., Bonnet, J., Dorian, B. et al., Effect of the consumption of alcohol, white wine, and red wine on platelet function and serum lipids, *J. Appl. Cardiol.*, 5: 215–222, 1990.

166. Fuhrman, B., Lavy, A., and Aviram, M., Consumption of red wine with meals reduces the susceptibility of human plasma and low-density lipoprotein to lipid peroxidation, *Am J Clin Nutr*, 61(3): 549–554, 1995.

167. de Rijke, Y., Demacker, P., Assen, N., Sloots, L., Katan, M., and Stalenhoef, A., Red wine consumption and oxidation of low-density lipoproteins, *Lancet*, 345(8945): 325–326, 1995.

168. Crawford, R., Kirk, E., Rosenfeld, M., LeBoeuf, R., and Chait, A., Dietary antioxidants inhibit development of fatty streak lesions in the LDL receptor-deficient mouse, *Arterioscler Thromb Vasc Biol*, 18(9): 1506–1513, 1998.

169. Nagao, T., Komine, Y., Soga, S., Meguro, S., Hase, T., Tanaka, Y., and Tokimitsu, I., Ingestion of a tea rich in catechins leads to a reduction in body fat and malondialdehyde-modified LDL in men, *Am J Clin Nutr*, 81(1): 122–129, 2005.

170. O'Reilly, J., Mallet, A., McAnlis, G., Young, I., Halliwell, B., Sanders, T., and Wiseman, H., Consumption of flavonoids in onions and black tea: lack of effect on F2-isoprostanes and autoantibodies to oxidized LDL in healthy humans, *Am J Clin Nutr*, 73(6): 1040–1044, 2001.

171. Otero, P., Viana, M., Herrera, E., and Bonet, B., Antioxidant and prooxidant effects of ascorbic acid, dehydroascorbic acid and flavonoids on LDL submitted to different degrees of oxidation, *Free Radic Res*, 27(6): 619–626, 1997.

172. Rankin, S., de Whalley, C., Hoult, J., Jessup, W., Wilkins, G., Collard, J., and Leake, D., The modification of low-density lipoprotein by the flavonoids myricetin and gossypetin, *Biochem Pharmacol*, 45(1): 67–75, 1993.

173. Ndiaye, M., Chataigneau, T., Andriantsitohaina, R., Stoclet, J., and Schini-Kerth, V., Red wine polyphenols cause endothelium-dependent EDHF-mediated relaxations in porcine coronary arteries via a redox-sensitive mechanism, *Biochem Biophys Res Commun*, 310(2): 371–377, 2003.

174. de Moura, R.S., Miranda, D.Z., Pinto, A.C. et al., Mechanism of the endothelium-dependent vasodilation and the antihypertensive effect of Brazilian red wine, *J Cardiovasc Pharmacol*, 44(3): 302–309, 2004.

175. Duarte, J., Andriambeloson, E., Diebolt, M., and Andriantsitohaina, R., Wine polyphenols stimulate superoxide anion production to promote calcium signaling and endothelial-dependent vasodilatation, *Physiol Res*, 53(6): 595–602, 2004.

176. Fitzpatrick, D., Hirschfield, S., and Coffey, R., Endothelium-dependent vasorelaxing activity of wine and other grape products, *Am J Physiol*, 265(2 Pt. 2): H774–H778, 1993.

177. Keaney, J., Jr. and Vita, J., Atherosclerosis, oxidative stress, and antioxidant protection in endothelium-derived relaxing factor action, *Prog Cardiovasc Dis*, 38(2): 129–154, 1995.

178. Perez-Vizcaino, F., Ibarra, M., Cogolludo, A. et al., Endothelium-independent vasodilator effects of the flavonoid quercetin and its methylated metabolites in rat conductance and resistance arteries, *J Pharmacol Exp Ther*, 302(1): 66–72, 2002.

179. Wallerath, T., Li, H., Godtel-Ambrust, U., Schwarz, P.M., and Forstermann, U., A blend of polyphenolic compounds explains the stimulatory effect of red wine on human endothelial NO synthase, *Nitric Oxide*, 12(2): 97–104, 2005.

180. Bradamante, S., Barenghi, L., Piccinini, F.,. Bertelli, A., De Jonge, R., Beemster, P., and De Jong, J., Resveratrol provides late-phase cardioprotection by means of a nitric oxide- and adenosine-mediated mechanism, *Eur J Pharmacol*, 465(1–2): 115–123, 2003.

181. van Acker, S., Tromp, M., Haenen, G., van der Vijgh, W., and Bast, A., Flavonoids as scavengers of nitric oxide radical, *Biochem Biophys Res Commun*, 214(3): 755–759, 1995.

182. Andriambeloson, E., Kleschyov, A., Muller, B., Beretz, A., Stoclet, J., and Andriantsitohaina, R., Nitric oxide production and endothelium-dependent vasorelaxation induced by wine polyphenols in rat aorta, *Br J Pharmacol*, 120(6): 1053–1058, 1997.

183. Hodgson, J., Burke, V., and Puddey, I., Acute effects of tea on fasting and postprandial vascular function and blood pressure in humans, *J Hypertens*, 23(1): 47–54, 2005.

184. Muller, C. and Fugelsang, K., Take two glasses of wine and see me in the morning, *Lancet*, 343(8910): 1428–1429, 1994.

185. Demrow, H., Slane, P., and Folts, J., Administration of wine and grape juice inhibits in vivo platelet activity and thrombosis in stenosed canine coronary arteries, *Circulation*, 91(4): 1182–1188, 1995.

186. Gorinstein, S., Zemser, M., Lichman, I. et al., Moderate beer consumption and the blood coagulation in patients with coronary artery disease, *J Intern Med*, 241(1): 47–51, 1997.

187. de Lange, D., Scholman, W., Kraaijenhagen, R., Akkerman, J., and van de Wiel, A., Alcohol and polyphenolic grape extract inhibit platelet adhesion in flowing blood, *Eur J Clin Invest*, 34(12): 818–824, 2004.

188. Gryglewski, R., Korbut, R., Robak, J., and Swies, J., On the mechanism of antithrombotic action of flavonoids, *Biochem Pharmacol*, 36(3): 317–322, 1987.

189. Ruf, J., Berger, J., and Renaud, S., Platelet rebound effect of alcohol withdrawal and wine drinking in rats. Relation to tannins and lipid peroxidation, *Arterioscler Thromb Vasc Biol*, 15(1): 140–144, 1995.

190. Casani, L., Segales, E., Vilahur, G., Bayes de Luna, A., and Badimon, L., Moderate daily intake of red wine inhibits mural thrombosis and monocyte tissue factor expression in an experimental porcine model, *Circulation*, 110(4): 460–465, 2004.

191. Blann, A.D., Williams, N.R., Lip, G.Y., Rajput-Williams, J., and Howard, A.N., Acute ingestion of red wine by men activates platelets but does not influence endothelial markers: no effect of white wine, *Blood Coagul Fibrinolysis*, 13(7): 647–651, 2002.

192. Pellegrini, N., Pareti, F.I., Stabile, F., Brusamolino, A., and Simonetti, P., Effects of moderate consumption of red wine on platelet aggregation and haemostatic variables in healthy volunteers, *Eur J Clin Nutr*, 50(4): 209–213, 1996.

193. Pace-Asciak, C.R., Rounova, O., Hahn, S.E., Diamandis, E.P., and Goldberg, D.M.,Wines and grape juices as modulators of platelet aggregation in healthy human subjects, *Clin Chim Acta*, 246(1–2): 163–182, 1996.

194. Pace-Asciak, C.R., Hahn, S., Diamandis, E.P., Soleas, G., and Goldberg, D.M., The red wine phenolics trans-resveratrol and quercetin block human platelet aggregation and eicosanoid synthesis: implications for protection against coronary heart disease, *Clin Chim Acta*, 235(2): 207–219, 1995.

195. Shanmuganayagam, D., Beahm, M.R., Osman, H.E., Krueger, C.G., Reed, J.D., and Folts, J.D., Grape seed and grape skin extracts elicit a greater antiplatelet effect when used in combination than when used individually in dogs and humans, *J Nutr*, 132(12): 3592–3598, 2002.

196. Sugatani, J., Fukazawa, N., Ujihara, K. et al., Tea polyphenols inhibit acetyl-CoA:1-alkyl-sn-glycero-3-phosphocholine acetyltransferase (a key enzyme in platelet-activating factor biosynthesis) and platelet-activating factor-induced platelet aggregation, *Int Arch Allergy Immunol*, 134(1): 17–28, 2004.

197. Lill, G., Voit, S., Schror, K., and Weber, A.A., Complex effects of different green tea catechins on human platelets, *FEBS Lett*, 546(2–3): 265–270, 2003.

198. Lou, F.Q., Zhang, M.F., Zhang, X.G., Liu, J.M., and Yuan, W.L., A study on tea-pigment in prevention of atherosclerosis, *Chin Med J (Engl)*, 102(8): 579–583, 1989.

199. Vorster, H., Jerling, J., Oosthuizen, W. et al., Tea drinking and haemostasis: a randomized, placebo-controlled, crossover study in free-living subjects, *Haemostasis*, 26(1): 58–64, 1996.

200. Kaul, D., Sikand, K., and. Shukla, A.R., Effect of green tea polyphenols on the genes with atherosclerotic potential, *Phytother Res*, 18(2): 177–179, 2004.

201. Fuhrman, B., Volkova, N., Coleman, R., and Aviram, M., Grape powder polyphenols attenuate atherosclerosis development in apolipoprotein E deficient (E0) mice and reduce macrophage atherogenicity, *J Nutr*, 135(4): 722–728, 2005.

202. Vinson, J.A., Teufel, K., and Wu, N., Green and black teas inhibit atherosclerosis by lipid, antioxidant, and fibrinolytic mechanisms, *J Agric Food Chem*, 52(11): 3661–3665, 2004.

203. Ralay Ranaivo, H., Diebolt, M., and Andriantsitohaina, R., Wine polyphenols induce hypotension, and decrease cardiac reactivity and infarct size in rats: involvement of nitric oxide, *Br J Pharmacol*, 142(4): 671–678, 2004.

204. Brookes, P., Digerness, S., Parks, D., and Darley-Usmar, V., Mitochondrial function in response to cardiac ischemia-reperfusion after oral treatment with Quercetin, *Free Radic Biol Med*, 32(11): 1220–1228, 2002.

205. Aneja, R., Hake, P., Burroughs, T., Denenberg, A., Wong, H., and Zingarelli, B., Epigallocatechin, a green tea polyphenol, attenuates myocardial ischemia reperfusion injury in rats, *Mol Med*, 10(1–6): 55–62, 2004.

206. Gohil, K., Functional genomics identifies novel and diverse molecular targets of nutrient in vivo, *Biol Chem* 385: 691–696, 2004.

207. Lin, S., Defossez, P., and Guarente, L., Requirement of NAD and Sir2 for life-span extension by calorie restriction in *Saccharomyces cerevisiae*, *Science* 289: 2126–2128, 2000.

208. Cohen, H., Miller, C., Bitterman, Y. et al., Calorie restriction promotes mammalian cell survival by inducing the SIRT1 deacetylase, *Science* 305: 390–392, 2004.

209. Morris, B., A forkhead in the road to longevity: the molecular basis of lifespan become clearer, *J Hypertens.* 23: 1285–1309, 2005.

210. Stewart, J., Ward, N., Ioannides, C., and O'Brian, C., Resveratrol preferentially inhibits protein kinase C-catalyzed phosphorylation of a cofactor-independent, arginine-rich protein substrate by a novel mechanism, *Biochemistry* 38: 13244–13251, 1999.

211. Delmas, D., Jannin, B., and Latruffe, N., Resveratrol: Preventing properties against vascular alterations and aging, *Mol Nutr Food Res* 49: 377–395, 2005.

212. Thurberg, B. and Collins, T., The nuclear factor-kappa B inhibitor of kappa B autoregulatory system and atherosclerosis, *Curr Opin Lipidol* 9: 387–396, 1998.

213. Jaeger, A., Walti, M., and Neftel, K., Side effects of flavonoids in medical practice, *Prog Clin Biol Res*, 280: 379–394, 1988.

214. Bruene, M., Hoolman, P., and van de Putte, B., Content of potentially anticarcinogenic flavonoids of tea infusions: wines and fruit juices, *J Agric Food Chem*, 40: 2379–2383, 1993.

215. Prystai, E., Kies, C., and Driskell, J., Calcium, copper, iron, magnesium, and zinc utilization of humans as affected by consumption of black, decaffeinated black and green teas, *Nutr. Rev*, 19: 167–177, 1999.

216. Sakamoto, Y., Mikuriya, H., Tayama, K. et al., Goitrogenic effects of green tea extract catechins by dietary administration in rats, *Arch Toxicol*, 75(10): 591–596, 2001.

217. Ray, S., Bagchi, D., Lim, P., Bagchi, M., Gross, S., Kothari, S., Preuss, H., and Stohs, S., Acute and long-term safety evaluation of a novel IH636 grape seed proanthocyanidin extract, *Res Commun Mol Pathol Pharmacol*, 109(3–4): 165–197, 2001.

218. Yamaguchi, Y., Hayashi, M., Yamazoe, H., and Kunitomo, M., Preventive effects of green tea extract on lipid abnormalities in serum, liver and aorta of mice fed an atherogenic diet, *Nippon Yakurigaku Zasshi*, 97(6): 329–337, 1991.

219. Juan, M., Vinardell, M., and Planas, J., The daily oral administration of high doses of trans-resveratrol to rats for 28 days is not harmful, *J Nutr*, 132(2): 257–260, 2002.

220. Crowell, J., Korytko, P., Morrissey, P., Booth, R., and Levine, T., Resveratrol-associated renal toxicity, *Toxicol Sci*, 82(2): 614–619, 2004.

221. Falcao, J., Dias, J., Miranda, A., Leitao, C., Lacerda, M., and da Motta, L., Red wine consumption and gastric cancer in Portugal: a case-control study, *Eur J Cancer Prev*, 3(3): 269–276, 1994.

222. Troup, G., Hutton, D., Hewitt, D., and Hunter, C., Free radicals in red wine, but not in white? *Free Radic Res*, 20(1): 63–68, 1994.

223. Stadler, R., Markovic, H., and Turesky, R., In vitro anti- and pro-oxidative effects of natural polyphenols, *Biol Trace Elem Res*, 47(1–3): 299–305, 1995.

224. Arizza, R. and Pueyo, C., The involvement of reactive oxygen species in the direct-acting mutagenicity of wine, *Mutat Res*, 251(1): 115–121, 1991.

225. Cao, G., Sofic, E., and Prior, R., Antioxidant and prooxidant behavior of flavonoids: structure-activity relationships, *Free Radic Biol Med*, 22(5): 749–760, 1997.

226. Ohshima, H., Yoshie, Y., Auriol, S., and Gilibert, I., Antioxidant and pro-oxidant actions of flavonoids: effects on DNA damage induced by nitric oxide, peroxynitrite and nitroxyl anion, *Free Radic Biol Med*, 25(9): 1057–1065, 1998.

227. Furukawa, A., Oikawa, S., Murata, M., Hiraku, Y., and Kawanishi, S., (-)-Epigallocatechin gallate causes oxidative damage to isolated and cellular DNA, *Biochem Pharmacol*, 66(9): 1769–1778, 2003.

228. Hayakawa, F., Ishizu, Y., Hoshino, N., Yamaji, A., Ando, T., and Kimura, T., Prooxidative activities of tea catechins in the presence of Cu^{2+}, *Biosci Biotechnol Biochem*, 68(9): 1825–1830, 2004.

229. Elbling, L., Weiss, R., Teufelhofer, O., Uhl, M., Knasmueller, S., Schulte-Hermann, R., Berger, W., and Micksche, M., Green tea extract and (-)-epigallocatechin-3-gallate, the major tea catechin, exert oxidant but lack antioxidant activities, *FASEB J*, 19(7): 807–809, 2005.

230. Decker, E., Phenolics: prooxidants or antioxidants? *Nutr Rev.* 55(11 Pt. 1): 396–398, 1997.

231. Laughton, M., Halliwell, B., Evans, P and Hoult, J., Antioxidant and pro-oxidant actions of the plant phenolics quercetin, gossypol and myricetin: effects on lipid peroxidation, hydroxyl radical generation and bleomycin-dependent damage to DNA, *Biochem Pharmacol*, 38(17): 2859–2865, 1989.

232. Choi, E., Lee, B., Lee, K., and Chee, K., Long-term combined administration of quercetin and daidzein inhibits quercetin-induced suppression of glutathione antioxidant defenses, *Food Chem Toxicol*, 43(5): 793–798, 2005.

233. Yen, G., Duh, P., Tsai, H., and Huang, S., Pro-oxidative properties of flavonoids in human lymphocytes, *Biosci Biotechnol Biochem*, 67(6): 1215–1222, 2003.

234. Matsuo, M., Sasaki, N., Saga, K., and Kaneko, T., Cytotoxicity of flavonoids toward cultured normal human cells, *Biol Pharm Bull*, 28(2): 253–259, 2005.

235. Fan, P. and Lou, H., Effects of polyphenols from grape seeds on oxidative damage to cellular DNA, *Mol Cell Biochem*, 267(1–2): 67–74, 2004.

236. Watjen, W., Michels, G., Steffan, B. et al., Low concentrations of flavonoids are protective in rat H4IIE cells whereas high concentrations cause DNA damage and apoptosis, *J Nutr*, 135(3): 525–531, 2005.

237. Ward, N., Hodgson, J., Croft, K., Burke, V., Beilin, L., and Puddey, I., The combination of vitamin C and grape-seed polyphenols increases blood pressure: a randomized, double-blind, placebo-controlled trial, *J Hypertens*, 23(2): 427–434, 2005.

238. Widlansky, M., Duffy, S., Hamburg, N. et. al., Effects of black tea consumption on plasma catechins and markers of oxidative stress and inflammation in patients with coronary artery disease, *Free Radic Biol Med*, 38(4): 499–506, 2005.

239. Meister, K., Moderate Alcohol Consumption and Health, American Council on Science and Health report, 1999.

240. Dufour, M. and Caces, F., Epidemiology of the medical consequences of alcohol, *Alcohol Health Res. World*, 17: 265–271, 1993.

241. Rubin, E., The chemical pathogenesis of alcohol-induced tissue injury, *Alcohol Health Res. World*, 17: 272–278, 1998.

242. Price, K., Rhodes, M., and Barnes, K., The chemical pathogenesis of alcohol-induced tissue injury, *J. Agric. Food Chem.*, 46: 2517–2522, 1998.

6 Dietary Fiber and Coronary Heart Disease

Thunder Jalili, Denis M. Medeiros, and Robert E.C. Wildman

CONTENTS

I. DIETARY FIBER CLASSIFICATION AND FOOD SOURCES

Fiber is generally described as plant material that is resistant to human digestive enzymes. Most of these plant materials fall into the category of non-starch polysaccharides, with the exception of plant lignins, which are actually polyphenolic by nature. Table 6.1 provides the percentage of the total weight of select foods that is attributable to fiber.

Fiber is typically subdivided into two groups based on solubility in water. Soluble (water) fibers include pectin (pectic substances), gums, and mucilages, whereas the insoluble fibers include cellulose, hemicellulose, lignin, and modified cellulose. Table 6.2 presents these classes of fiber and lists some food sources for each type. Some of the better food sources of soluble fibers are fruit, legumes, oats, and some vegetables. Meanwhile, those foods known to be richer sources of insoluble fibers include cereals, grains, legumes, and vegetables. The amount of fiber present within the human diet can vary geographically. In more industrially developed countries, such as the U.S., fiber consumption is relatively lower than in other societies. For example, the average intake of fiber in the U.S. is only about 12–15 g daily. This consumption falls well below current recommendations of the World Health Organization of 25–40 g of fiber daily. The American diet tends to derive less than half of its dietary carbohydrate intake from fruit, vegetables, and whole grains. On the other hand, the people of some African societies are known to eat as much as 50 g of fiber daily.

Digestible polysaccharides in plant foods such as starch, and, to a much lesser degree, glycogen in meats, have repeating monosaccharide units bonded by 1–4 linkages (Figure 6.1). These bonds are readily digested by amylase in both salivary and pancreatic secretions. Branch points in the starch and glycogen chains are joined through 1–6 linkages that are hydrolyzed by the enzyme 1–6 dextrinase (isomaltase) in pancreatic secretions. On the contrary, 1–4 linkages are formed by plants instead of 1–4 linkages between monosaccharides in fibrous polysaccharides (Figure 6.1). Both salivary and pancreatic amylases are unable to hydrolyze 1–4 covalent bonds efficiently. This

TABLE 6.1
Fiber Content of Select Foods

Food	Fiber (% Weight)
Almonds	3
Apples	1
Lima beans	2
String beans	1
Broccoli	1
Carrots	1
Flour, whole wheat	2
Flour, white wheat	<1
Oat flakes	2
Pears	2
Pecans	2
Popcorn	2
Strawberries	1
Walnuts	2
Wheat germ	3

Source: Adapted from Wildman, R.E.C. and Medeiros, D.M., *Carbohydrates in Advanced Human Nutrition*, CRC Press, Boca Raton, FL, 2000. With permission.

TABLE 6.2
Fiber Types and Characteristics, Food Sources, and Bacterial Degradation

Types of Fiber	Characteristics	Food Sources	Degradation[a]
	Soluble		
Pectins	Rich in galacturonic acid, rhamnose, arabinose, galactose; characteristic of middle laminae and primary wall	Whole grains, legumes, cabbage, root vegetables, apples	+
Gums	Composed mostly of hexose and pentose monomers	Oatmeal, dried beans, other legumes	+++
Mucilages	Synthesized by plant cells and can contain glycoproteins	Food additives	+++
	Insoluble		
Cellulose	Structural basis for cell wall; only monomer is glucose	Whole grains, bran, cabbage family, peas, beans, apples, root vegetables	+
Hemicellulose	Component of primary and secondary cell walls; different types vary in monomer content	Bran, cereals, whole grains	+
Lignin	Composed of aromatic alcohols; cements, other cell wall components	Vegetables, wheat	0

[a] Denotes the degree of bacterial fermentation.

Source: Adapted from Wildman, R.E.C., and Medeiros, D.M., *Carbohydrates in Advanced Human Nutrition*, CRC Press, Boca Raton, FL, 2000. With permission.

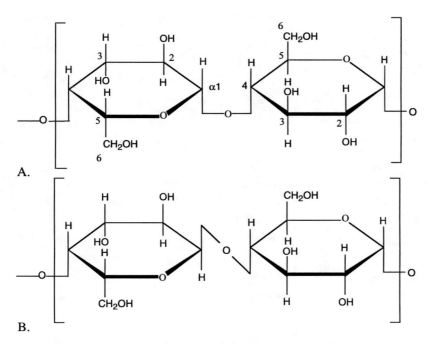

FIGURE 6.1 (A) The $\alpha 1$–4 bond between glucose monomers of starch and glycogen and (B) the $\beta 1$–4 linkage between glucose units in cellulose.

renders such polysaccharides resistant to human digestive action. However, bacteria inhabiting the large intestine can indeed metabolize some polysaccharide fibers and create short-chain fatty acids (acetic, propionic, and butyric acids) as metabolites. These short-chain fatty acids, often referred to as volatile fatty acids (VFA), are a potential energy substrate for the mucosal cells of the large intestine. Therefore, perhaps the notion that dietary fiber is not an energy source may need to be reconsidered. However, this point may only be significant in principle as the energy contribution would be very small.

Cellulose is known to be the most abundant organic molecule on Earth. The molecular structure is similar to amylose in that it is made up of repeating units of the hexose glucose. However, again, the linkages will be 1–4 by nature. Cellulose is produced as a component of the plant cell wall by an enzyme complex called cellulose synthase. Once cellulose chains are formed, they quickly assemble with other cellulose molecules and form microfibrils that strengthen the cell wall. Cellulose, along with certain other fibers (hemicellulose and pectin) and proteins, is found within the matrix between the cell wall layers. This concept is somewhat similar to the connective tissue matrix found within bones, tendons, and ligaments in humans. Hemicellulose is different from cellulose because its monomers are heterogeneous. Hemicellulose contains varied amounts of pentoses and hexoses covalently bound in a 1–4 linkage, as well as some branching side chains. Some of the more common and familiar monosaccharides in hemicelluloses are xylose, mannose, and galactose (Figure 6.2). Other monosaccharide subunits include arabinose and 4-O-methyl glucuronic acids.

Lignin is a unique fiber because it is not a carbohydrate; yet it is considered an insoluble dietary fiber. Lignin is made up of aromatic polymers of chemicals from plant cell walls and provides plants with their "woody" characteristics. Lignin molecules are highly complex and variable polymers and are composed of three major aromatic alcohols: coumaryl, coniferyl, and sinapyl. In plants, lignins provide structure and integrity, thus allowing the plant to maintain its form. A typical lignin monomer is presented in Figure 6.3.

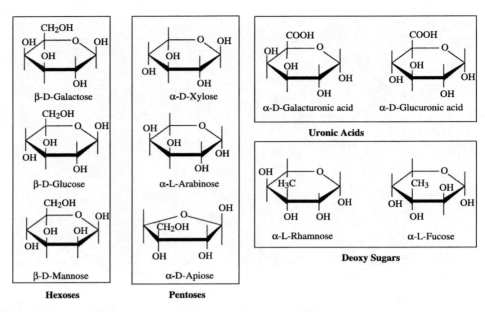

FIGURE 6.2 Carbohydrate monomers common to polysaccharide fibers.

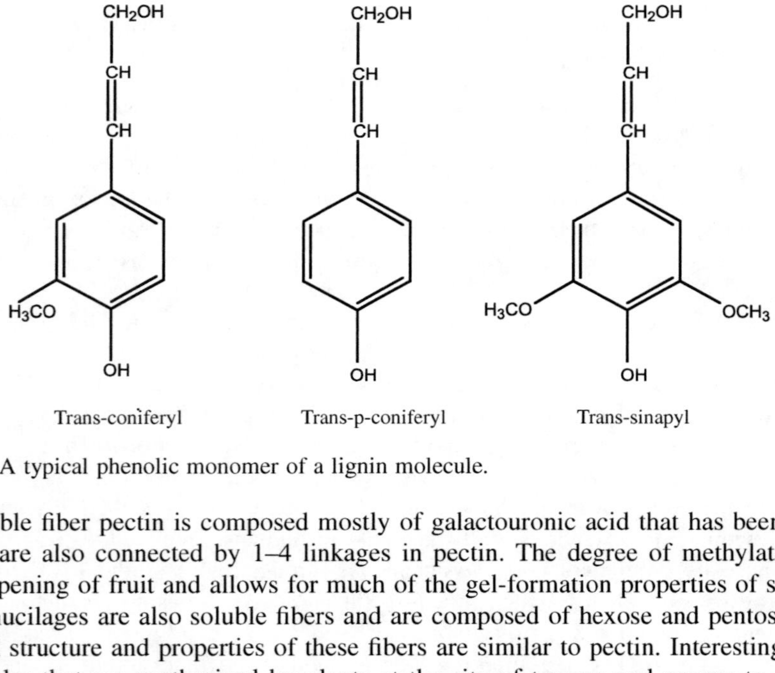

CH₂OH
CH
CH

H₃CO

OH

Trans-coniferyl

CH₂OH
CH
CH

OH

Trans-p-coniferyl

CH₂OH
CH
CH

H₃CO   OCH₃

OH

Trans-sinapyl

FIGURE 6.3 A typical phenolic monomer of a lignin molecule.

The soluble fiber pectin is composed mostly of galactouronic acid that has been methylated. These units are also connected by 1–4 linkages in pectin. The degree of methylation increases during the ripening of fruit and allows for much of the gel-formation properties of soluble fibers. Gums and mucilages are also soluble fibers and are composed of hexose and pentose monomers. The physical structure and properties of these fibers are similar to pectin. Interestingly, gums are polysaccharides that are synthesized by plants at the site of trauma and appear to function in a manner similar to scar tissue in humans. Meanwhile, mucilages are produced by plant secretory cells to prevent excess loss of water through transpiration.

II. PHYSICAL AND PHYSIOLOGICAL PROPERTIES OF FIBER

The physiological attributes of fibers largely depend upon their physical characteristics, namely, the molecular design and solubility. Although the physiological influences of dietary fibers were

TABLE 6.3
Changes in Fecal Bulk due to Different Dietary Fiber Sources

Food Item	% Increase in Fecal Weight
Bran	127
Cabbage	69
Carrots	59
Apple	40
Guar Gum	20

Source: Adapted from Wildman, R.E.C. and Medeiros, D.M., *Carbohydrates in Advanced Human Nutrition*, CRC Press, Boca Raton, FL, 2000. With permission.

once thought to be limited to the intestinal lumen, which is anatomically exterior, newer evidence suggests that derivatives of intestinal fiber metabolism can influence internal operations as well. The physical characteristics of dietary fiber can produce various gastrointestinal responses depending upon the segment of the digestive tract. Among these responses are gastric distention, the rate of gastric emptying, and enhancement of residue quantity (feces bulk) and moisture content. Furthermore, dietary fiber can influence fermentation by bacteria in the colon as well as the turnover of specific bacteria species. The bacterial population will likely increase due to fiber fermentation. Bacterial presence may contribute as much as 45% to the fecal dry weight. The influence of fiber upon fecal mass is presented in Table 6.3.

Different fiber molecules are subject to varying levels of bacterial degradation in the colon (Table 6.4). For instance, pectin, mucilages, and gums seem to be almost completely fermented. Meanwhile, cellulose and hemicellulose are only partly degraded and the noncarbohydrate nature of lignin allows it to go virtually unfermented. The physical structure of the plant itself may be associated with the degree of degradation of food fibers by intestinal bacteria. As an example, fibers derived from fruits and vegetables appear to be, in general, more fermentable than those from cereal grains. VFAs, namely, acetic acid (2:0), proprionic acid (3:0), and butyric acid (4:0), are among the products of bacterial fermentation. As mentioned earlier, these fatty acids can be oxidized for ATP production in mucosal cells of the colon wall. Furthermore, these fatty acids are fairly water-soluble and can be absorbed into the portal circulation. Other products of bacterial fermentation of dietary fibers include hydrogen gas (H_2), carbon dioxide (CO_2), and methane (CH_4). These

TABLE 6.4
Some Physical Properties of Different Fiber Types

Fiber Type	Action
Cellulose	Holds water, reduces colonic pressure, reduced transit time of digestion
Hemicellulose	Holds water, increases stool bulk, may bind bile acids, reduced colonic pressure, reduces transit time
Pectins, gums, mucilages	Slow gastric emptying, bind bile acids, increase colonic fermentation
Lignin	Holds water, may bind trace minerals and increase excretion, may increase fecal steroid levels

Source: Adapted from Wildman, R.E.C. and Medeiros, D.M., *Carbohydrates in Advanced Human Nutrition*, CRC Press, Boca Raton, FL, 2000. With permission.

products can lead to occasional uncomfortable gas buildup in the colon that may occur with high fiber consumption. The presence of H_2 in the breath (hydrogen breath test) is often used clinically as an estimation of bacterial fermentation. Once produced, H_2 dissolves into the blood and circulates to the lungs.

Among some of their more interesting physical properties is the water-holding capacity or the hydration of fiber. The ability of different fibers to associate with water molecules is largely attributable to the presence of sugar residues that have free polar groups (i.e., OH, COOH, SO, and C=O groups). These polar groups allow for the formation of hydrogen bonds with adjacent water molecules. It seems that pectic substances, mucilages, and hemicellulose have the greatest water-holding capacity. Cellulose and lignin can also hold water but not to the extent of other fibers. However, as soluble fibers are generally more fermentable, the associated water is liberated and absorbed in the colon. Thus, it is the insoluble fibers that hold onto water throughout the total length of the intestinal tract and give the fecal mass greater water content.

In the small intestine, the hydration of fiber will allow for the formation of a gel matrix. Theoretically, the formation of a gel in the small intestine could increase viscosity of the food-derived contents and slow the rate of absorption of nutrients. It has been suggested that this mechanism may slow the rate of carbohydrate absorption and decrease the magnitude of the postprandial spike in blood glucose. This notion may then be applicable to individuals with diabetes mellitus, as discussed in this chapter.

III. RELATIONSHIP BETWEEN CHOLESTEROL LEVELS AND CHD

Coronary heart disease (CHD) is the leading cause of death in the Western world after cancer according to the American Heart Association's 2005 Biostatistical Fact Sheet and reports from numerous medical organizations in Europe.[1] In contrast to popular belief, CHD is a leading cause of death among women as well.[2,3] Many risk factors can influence CHD, such as smoking, age, male sex, menopause, diabetes, serum cholesterol levels, and hypertension. Some of these risk factors are modifiable, such as smoking and serum cholesterol levels, and some are not, such as male sex or menopause. Among the most important risk factors that may be controlled are serum cholesterol levels. Many studies have established that high total-cholesterol levels and low-density lipoprotein (LDL) cholesterol levels are risk factors for CHD and mortality.[4–6] The well-known Framingham Study was among the first to establish a statistical relationship between serum lipo-proteins and CHD.[6] Other important studies using very large cohorts from the Multiple Risk Factor Intervention Trial (MRFIT) and from various countries have since strengthened the notion that serum cholesterol is a risk factor for CHD.[4,5,7]

Elevated serum cholesterol levels can result from a variety of influences. Severely high serum cholesterol is usually due to familial hypercholesterolemia, a condition characterized by genetic defects in LDL-receptor activity that result in accumulation of LDL cholesterol in the blood. Elevated serum cholesterol may also occur as a secondary effect of disorders such as diabetes, hypothyroidism, and alcoholism. More commonly, cholesterol disorders are characterized by mild or moderate hypercholesterolemia and are generally dietary in origin. Intake of saturated fats, trans fatty acids can also increase plasma LDL levels by decreasing LDL-receptor synthesis.

A. ROLE OF FIBER IN REDUCING SERUM CHOLESTEROL

Fiber has been implicated in reducing the risk for CHD. Many large epidemiological studies, such as the Nurses' Health Study and the Scottish Heart Health Study, have demonstrated a reduced risk for CHD in both men and women who consume higher amounts of dietary fiber.[8–10] Soluble fibers, in particular, are thought to exert a preventative role against heart disease as they appear to have the ability to lower serum cholesterol levels. A recent meta-analysis examining soluble fiber sources from pectin, oat bran, guar gum, and psyllium reported a small but significant reduction in serum cholesterol levels.[11] Many other studies have found that a high intake of soluble fiber results in decreased serum cholesterol levels.[12–19] These studies generally report a decrease in total cholesterol and LDL cholesterol with no changes in high-density lipoprotein (HDL) or triglycerides. Indeed, it is now recognized that soluble fiber is a viable intervention to reduce serum cholesterol levels by clinically significant amounts, thereby reducing a known risk factor for CHD.[20]

Oat bran, in particular, has received a great deal of attention as a fiber source with an appreciable level of soluble fiber that has been shown to reduce plasma cholesterol levels under controlled conditions.[14] Early studies examining the role of oats in reducing plasma cholesterol focused on supplementing oats without a great deal of dietary fat modification. In 1963, DeGroot and colleagues published a study that supplemented rolled oats in the form of bread to be consumed daily by 21 male volunteers between the ages of 30 and 50.[21] Over a 3-week period, an 11% reduction in serum cholesterol was observed. Another early study by Anderson et al. compared oat bran to fiber from beans in their ability to lower serum cholesterol.[22] This study was conducted in a metabolic ward and did not use a low-fat diet. After consuming 17 g of soluble fiber per day for 3 weeks, a 19% decrease in total cholesterol and a 23% decrease in LDL cholesterol were observed. In more recent years, scientists have been assessing the response of serum cholesterol to oat bran intake in conjunction with a low-fat diet. It has been found that a low-fat diet in conjunction with a high-fiber (soluble) intake reduces cholesterol beyond the levels associated with a low-fat diet alone.[23]

A review of the literature demonstrates that oat bran has been repeatedly proved to play a role in reducing serum cholesterol levels and is generally recommended by the nutrition and medical community as an important part of the diet. A meta-analysis done by Ripsin and colleagues reviewed results from ten trials and concluded that a significant amount of cholesterol reduction occurred when at least 3 g of soluble fiber from oat bran was consumed daily.[23] Furthermore, researchers observed that subjects who had the most dramatic decrease in cholesterol levels were those who had the highest initial serum cholesterol concentrations to begin with. In spite of the wealth of data supporting the role of oat bran in decreasing serum cholesterol, an issue that remains ambiguous for the typical American consumer is the amount of oat bran needed to reduce serum cholesterol levels by clinically significant amounts. The lay public must realize that several servings of oat bran are required daily to reduce plasma cholesterol by an appreciable amount. Indeed, many of the studies that report significant decreases in serum cholesterol levels use very high intakes of soluble oat bran fiber. Most studies have used anywhere from 3.4 to 17 g of soluble oat bran fiber to achieve total cholesterol and LDL-cholesterol reductions with the most severe declines observed with the highest use of soluble fiber. When one considers that the typical serving of instant oatmeal (0.5 cups) contains 1 to 2 g of soluble fiber, the reality of the dietary change involved becomes more apparent. In practice, it may be difficult for the average individual to consume levels of soluble fiber equivalent to the highest amounts used in certain studies. However, with moderate dietary changes it is possible to consume enough oat bran to fall in the lower range of experimental amounts previously used, which would result in a statistically significant reduction in serum cholesterol.

The long-term interest in oat bran has led to the identification of β-glucan as the active compound responsible for for LDL reduction.[16] In addition to oat bran, yeast has also been identified as a concentrated source of β-glucan and is currently under investigation for its potential as a commercial additive in a variety of food products.[16] A relatively new product that is known by the patented name Fibercel® is composed of purified β-glucan derived from the yeast *Saccharomyces cerevisiae,* the species found in baker's and brewer's yeast. This product is currently under investigation in clinical trials to establish its efficacy in treating individuals with high cholesterol levels. If proved successful, it could be used as an additive in foods such as salad dressing, frozen desserts, and cream cheese.

Recent studies using Konjac-mannan fiber (a highly soluble fiber also known as glucomannan) have also yielded very promising results by reducing risk factors for CHD. Subjects supplemented with a daily average of 23 g of Konjac-mannan in the form of biscuits experienced a lower total HDL cholesterol ratio and LDL cholesterol, lower systolic blood pressure, and improved their glycemic control.[24] These results were significantly better than those achieved with an identical diet using wheat bran instead of Konjac-mannan diet, thereby demonstrating the effectiveness of the soluble fiber in influencing not only cholesterol, but other CHD risk factors, as well. Konjac-mannan fiber is well known for having among the highest viscosity of all the soluble fiber types. The use of Konjac-mannan fiber may also lead one to speculate that highly soluble fibers, such as Konjac-mannan, may be more effective at reducing cholesterol levels than other soluble fibers. It must be remembered, however, that the use of Konjac-mannan entails supplementation in existing foods, such as breads or biscuits, rather than eating an actual product such as oatmeal cereal. This may have practical relevance as it is far simpler for the typical consumer to buy instant cereal and eat it daily for breakfast than to buy Konjac-mannan fiber and supplement it in baked goods on a daily basis.

Other types of soluble fibers have been extensively studied for their ability to lower serum cholesterol amounts. Psyllium has received attention over the years as a soluble fiber that can reduce cholesterol levels. Psyllium plant stalks contain tiny seeds, also called *psyllium*, covered by husks, which is the source of the fiber. There is a great deal of soluble fiber in psyllium; in fact, 71% of the weight of psyllium is derived from soluble fiber. In contrast, only 5% of oat bran by weight is made of soluble fiber; in other words, the soluble fiber in 1 tablespoon of psyllium is equal to 14 tablespoons of oat bran. The active fraction of psyllium seed husks that is thought to be responsible for the cholesterol-lowering effects is a highly branched arabinoxylan that is composed of a xylose backbone with arabinose-and xylose-containing side chains.[25] Interestingly, arabinoxylan from psyllium is not fermented by colonic bacteria, apparently due to still unidentified structural features of the molecule.

A number of animal studies have demonstrated that rats fed controlled diets supplemented with psyllium fiber experience a significant decrease in serum cholesterol levels.[26–28] A study done by Anderson et al. even found reductions of up to 32% in cholesterol levels in rats fed 6% dietary psyllium.[26] Many studies in humans have also found psyllium to be an effective agent.[12,13,18] Supplementation of 10.2 g of psyllium per day for 8 weeks in men consuming a 40% fat diet has resulted in a 14.8% reduction in total cholesterol and 20.2% reduction in LDL cholesterol.[19] Another study using higher amounts of dietary psyllium (15 g/d) observed a change of LDL cholesterol from 184 mg/dl to 169 mg/dl.[29] Another study has demonstrated that men with Type II diabetes supplemented with 10.2 g of psyllium daily for 8 weeks also experienced an 8.9% drop in total cholesterol and a 13% decline in LDL cholesterol.[30] This group of men with Type II diabetes displayed an improvement in glycemic control as well. Indeed, the results of a large-scale meta-analysis done recently that examined 12 published and unpublished studies has concluded that consumption of dietary psyllium is linked with reductions in serum total and LDL cholesterol.[12] Even though psyllium has not achieved as much attention in the popular press compared with oat bran, there is evidence that it may actually be more effective as a dietary agent to lower cholesterol levels. Anderson et al. compared ten different dietary fiber types in the rat model and found psyllium to be the most effective at lowering serum cholesterol levels.[26] A study in humans using psyllium and oat bran demonstrated an equivalent reduction in total and LDL cholesterol when psyllium was used in half the amount of oat bran. These studies could lead one to conclude that psyllium fiber may actually be more effective at reducing cholesterol levels and, therefore, could be consumed in lesser amounts to achieve desirable results. In fact, in 1998, the FDA approved labels on cereals supplemented with psyllium stating that regular consumption of psyllium as part of a low-fat diet can reduce cholesterol levels.

B. Mechanisms for Lowering of Serum Cholesterol by Fiber

There are several possible mechanisms by which soluble fiber is thought to reduce serum cholesterol levels; many are related to the ability of soluble fibers to form viscous gels in the intestinal tract. Among these potential mechanisms are reduced cholesterol absorption in the presence of soluble fiber, increased excretion of bile acids, an alteration of bile-acid type present in the gut, and possible influences of short-chain fatty-acid production by intestinal flora upon cholesterol synthesis.

It has been proposed that soluble fiber reduces plasma cholesterol through its ability to bind bile acids in the gastrointestinal tract. As soluble fibers bind bile acids in the intestinal tract, micelle formation is altered and reabsorption of bile acids is subsequently impaired, resulting in the excretion of the fiber–bile complex through the feces. There are two classes of bile acids, primary and secondary. Primary bile acids (cholic and chenodeoxycholic acid) are those synthesized directly from the liver, whereas secondary bile acids (deoxycholic and lithocholic acid) are produced after modification of primary bile acids by bacterial action in the colon. It has been demonstrated that consumption of oat bran doubles the loss of bile acids and specifically increases the loss of deoxycholic acid (secondary bile acid) by 240% in human subjects.[31] It was also concluded that the pool of bile acids was not decreased, even though bile-acid excretion is increased.[31] Another human study done with soluble fiber from psyllium found increased bile-acid turnover of both primary bile acids as well.[29] These studies point to the fact that bile excretion is increased when high amounts of soluble fiber are eaten. Usually, bile is reabsorbed in the large intestine and reused in emulsification of fats. However, because a constant pool is required, the excreted bile must be replaced to keep bile levels adequate for digestive needs. Theoretically, this would indicate that bile-acid synthesis would be increased under these conditions and, indeed, an increase in bile-acid synthesis has also been observed in individuals consuming high amounts of soluble fiber.[29] Specifically, the synthesis of deoxycholic acid has been found to increase with consumption of a high-fiber diet. This may have further beneficial effects as deoxycholic acid has been shown to decrease absorption of dietary cholesterol.[32]

Replacement of bile can be achieved in two ways: (1) more hepatic cholesterol can be dedicated for bile synthesis instead of being exported in the circulation as very low-density lipoprotein (VLDL) and (2) increased hepatic cholesterol demand will upregulate synthesis and activity of LDL receptors, allowing for greater amounts of VLDL remnants and LDL to be removed from circulation. The overall effect of these alterations is a reduction in LDL and total cholesterol levels. With regard to the first point, data from animal studies demonstrate an increased rate of cholesterol synthesis in the livers of psyllium-fed hamsters.[28] Specifically, the enzymatic activity of HMG CoA reductase, the rate-limiting enzyme for hepatic cholesterol synthesis, is observed to be increased three- to fourfold in hamsters fed soluble fiber.[33] This effect is thought to be transcriptionally mediated as mRNA levels have been found to be similarly increased in the same model.[33]

Alterations of LDL-receptor activity are also possible under the influence of psyllium fiber; however, this has been found to occur in experimental animals fed high-fat and high-cholesterol diets. Usually consumption of a high-fat diet tends to depress LDL receptor activity, but hamsters fed high-fat and high-cholesterol diets in conjunction with high dietary soluble fiber demonstrate a restoration of LDL receptor expression to normal levels.[33]

Examination of the effects of oat-bran consumption reveals a divergence in the mechanism of action between soluble fiber from oats vs. that of psyllium. Both have the ability to bind to bile acids and facilitate their excretion; however, they differ in their secondary influence on hepatic cholesterol synthesis. As mentioned above, psyllium fiber fed to animals has been found to increase hepatic cholesterol synthesis. Paradoxically, soluble fiber from oat bran has been found to depress hepatic cholesterol synthesis.[34] Bacterial fermentation of soluble fiber from oats results in the production of short-chain fatty acids, specifically propionate, that are absorbed in the colon and travel to the liver via the portal vein. Data from *in vitro* studies demonstrate an inhibition of hepatic cholesterol and fatty-acid synthesis under the influence of propionate.[34] The apparent paradox of psyllium fiber increasing cholesterol synthesis and oat fiber decreasing cholesterol synthesis may be explained by the fact that psyllium is very poorly fermented by bacteria in the colon; hence, little propionate is produced to decrease hepatic cholesterol synthesis.

In the final analysis, it seems that oat bran may be able to reduce cholesterol levels in a dual manner increasing bile loss and decreasing endogenous hepatic cholesterol synthesis, thus resulting in a shift of serum cholesterol for bile synthesis. Psyllium may reduce serum cholesterol levels through only one relevant mechanism: the loss of bile acids. Furthermore, in spite of the increase in HMG CoA reductase activity and cholesterol synthesis under the influence of psyllium, hepatic cholesterol content continues to be markedly reduced in animals fed a high-psyllium diet.[33] Therefore, it seems that this upregulation is barely enough to meet the demands of bile-acid synthesis, and obviously not enough to contribute significantly to VLDL exportation and, hence, LDL cholesterol levels. As one can conclude after careful consideration of the cited studies in this section, even though the net effect of soluble fiber consumption is well established, the specific biochemical events that occur in cholesterol metabolism are still incompletely understood and require more thorough testing.

C. Other Relevant Considerations for Fiber and CHD Risk

Fiber has also been implicated in reducing risk for CHD through mechanisms other than plasma-cholesterol modification. One such example is through modification of blood-clotting ability. An enhanced clotting ability coupled with atherosclerosis increases the risk of developing an occlusion in the coronary arteries and subsequent myocardial infarction. The ability of the blood to clot is dependent upon fibrinogen levels and the quality of the resulting fibrin network. Pectin has been found to influence the concentration and quality of fibrin networks in the blood and reduce the tensile strength of these networks. Pectin supplements have been shown to decrease the strength and quality of fibrin networks. These types of networks are thought to be less atherogenic than fibrin networks under normal conditions and thus may represent another vehicle for reducing risk for CHD.[35]

It was demonstrated that individuals consuming 18.5 g or more of dietary fiber had a 42% risk for elevated plasma C-reactive protein than those consuming 8.5 g or less. Similar findings were reported after analysis of survey data from the National Health and Nutrition Examination data as well. Using this data, a 41% lower risk of elevated C-reactive protein was found in individuals consuming high-fiber diets, after adjusting for smoking, BMI, physical activity, total energy, and fat intake.[36] Given the recent focus on C-reactive protein as a plasma marker of inflammation, and the emerging role of inflammation in the pathogenesis of atherosclerosis, it is noteworthy that dietary fiber may act in ways beyond its cholesterol-lowering ability.

Since the 1980s, it has also become evident that LDL particle size plays an important role in increasing risk of coronary heart disease. It has been reported that smaller LDL particles are strong indicators of CHD risk in middle-aged men.[37] Soluble fiber has been shown to significantly reduce the levels of small, dense LDL particles. In a study that gave 14 g fiber per day from oat cereal to overweight-middle aged men, overall LDL levels were reduced by 5%, but, more importantly, levels of small LDL particles were reduced by 17%.[38] Such a reduction is thought to contribute to an overall lower risk of coronary heart disease. In contrast, however, a dietary portfolio containing fiber, nuts, phytosterols, and vegetable protein did not demonstrate a greater reduction in small LDL particles compared to overall LDL levels.[39] Given the limited number of studies published thus far, more research is needed to define the role of fiber effects on small LDL particle content.

Whole grains have also been shown to be protective against CHD as demonstrated by an inverse relationship between whole-grain-consumption CHD.[40–42] However, it still remains unclear whether this association is due to the fiber content of whole grains or other components of whole grains such as phytochemicals, antioxidants, folate, vitamin B_6, monounsaturated fatty acids, or 3 poly-unsaturated fatty acids that may act to reduce CHD risk. In spite of a certain degree of confusion regarding the individual contribution of whole-grain-derived fiber in reducing CHD risk, the overall beneficial effect of whole grains, in general, should not be overlooked.

D. Fiber as Adjunct Therapy to Statin Medication

Current medical practice is to use statin drugs to reduce elevated plasma-cholesterol levels. There are many types of statin drugs used today, but they all share the common feature of inhibiting the hepatic enzyme HMG CoA reductase. As dietary fiber is thought to reduce cholesterol levels through other mechanisms in addition to HMG CoA inhibition, it has been proposed that combining fiber therapy with medication may be an effective approach to reduce cholesterol. A recent study examined the precise role of dietary fiber as adjunct therapy to statin medication and found that hypercholesterolemic patients taking 10 g of psyllium per day along with a 10 mg dose of simvastatin had the same degree of cholesterol reduction as those taking 20 mg of simvastatin alone.[43] These data demonstrate that dietary fiber can reduce the statin dosage required to meet cholesterol targets. The benefits to patients who employ such strategies are reduced medication cost and reduced drug burden on the liver.

IV. HEALTH CLAIMS ASSOCIATED WITH FIBER AND CHD

The U.S. Food and Drug Administration (FDA) allows food manufacturers to use certain health claims related to the link between dietary fiber and a reduced risk of heart disease. For example, upon review of the research literature, the FDA recognizes the relationship between fruits, vegetables, and grain products that contain fiber, particularly soluble fiber, and a reduced risk of CHD. Foods that apply for related health claims would include fruits, vegetables, and whole-grain breads and cereals. To qualify, foods must meet criteria for low saturated fat, low fat, and low cholesterol. The foods must contain, without fortification, at least 0.6 g of soluble fiber per reference amount, and the soluble fiber content must be listed on the label. The health claim must use the terms *fiber, dietary fiber, some types of dietary fiber, some dietary fibers,* or *some fibers and coronary heart disease* or *heart disease* in discussing the nutrient–disease link. The term *soluble fiber* may be added. A sample health claim may read:

> Diets low in saturated fat and cholesterol and rich in fruits, vegetables, and grain products that contain some types of dietary fiber, particularly soluble fiber, may reduce the risk of heart disease, a disease associated with many factors.

More specific to soluble fiber, the FDA has to date reviewed and authorized two sources of soluble fiber (whole oats and psyllium) to be eligible for use of a health claim with regard to a reduction in the risk of CHD (Table 6.5). In doing so, the FDA acknowledges that in conjunction with a low-saturated-fat and low-cholesterol diet, certain soluble fiber foods may favorably influence blood lipid levels, such as total cholesterol, and thus lower the risk of heart disease. Some foods that fall in this category include: oatmeal muffins, cookies, breads, and other foods made with rolled oats, oat bran, or whole oat flour; hot and cold breakfast cereals containing whole oats or

TABLE 6.5
Total and Soluble Fiber Content of Selected Cereal Brans

Crude Bran Source (100 g)	Total Dietary Fiber (g)	Soluble Fiber (g)
Wheat bran (1 2/3 cups)	42	3
Oat bran (2/3 cups)	16	7
Rice bran (1 cup)	22–24	3–9
Corn bran (1 1/4 cups)	85	2–3

Source: Adapted from Wildman, R.E.C. and Medeiros, D.M., *Carbohydrates in Advanced Human Nutrition*, CRC Press, Boca Raton, FL, 2000. With permission.

psyllium seed husk; and dietary supplements containing psyllium seed husk. Once again, in order for a food manufacturer to use such a health claim on a food label, the food must meet criteria for "low saturated fat," "low cholesterol," and "low fat." The food must provide whole oats in at least 0.75 g of soluble fiber per serving. Foods that contain psyllium seed husk must contain at least 1.7 g of soluble fiber per serving. In addition, a claim must indicate the daily dietary intake of the soluble-fiber source necessary to reduce the risk of heart disease. The claim must also indicate the contribution that one serving of the product will make toward that intake level. Further still, the soluble-fiber content must be stated in the nutrition label. In the health claim, the food manufacturer must state soluble fiber qualified by the name of the eligible source of soluble fiber and heart disease or coronary heart disease in describing the nutrient–disease association. A model claim is as follows:

Soluble fiber from foods such as [name of soluble fiber source, and, if desired, name of food product], as part of a diet low in saturated fat and cholesterol, may reduce the risk of heart disease. A serving of [name of food product] supplies __ grams of the [necessary daily dietary intake for the benefit] soluble fiber from [name of soluble fiber source] necessary per day to have this effect.

REFERENCES

1. Pyorala, K., DeBacker, G., Graham, I., Poole-Wilson, P., and Wood, D., Prevention of coronary heart disease in clinical practice: recommendations of the Task Force of the European Society of Cardiology, European Atherosclerosis Society and European Society of Hypertension, *Atherosclerosis*, 110: 121–161, 1994.
2. Eaker, E.D., Chesebro, J.H., Sacks, F.M., Wenger, N.K., Whisnant, J.P., and Winston, M., Cardiovascular disease in women, *Circulation*, 88: 1999–2009, 1993.
3. Rich-Edwards, J.W., Manson, J.E., Hennekens, C.H., and Buring, J.E., The primary prevention of coronary heart disease in women, *N. Engl. J. Med.*, 332: 1758–1766, 1995.
4. Martin, M.J., Hulley, S.B., Browner, W.S., Kuller, L.H., and Wentworth, D., Serum cholesterol, blood pressure, and mortality: implications from a cohort of 361,662 men, *Lancet*, 2: 933–936, 1986.
5. Simons, L.A., Interrelations of lipids and lipoproteins with coronary artery disease mortality in 19 countries, *Am. J. Cardiol.*, 57: 5G–10G, 1986.
6. Kannel, W.B., Gordon, T., and Castelli, W.P., Role of lipids and lipoprotein fractions in atherogenesis: the Framingham Study, *Prog. Lipid Res.*, 20: 339–348, 1981.
7. Stamler, J., Wentworth, D., and Neaton, J.D., Is relationship between serum cholesterol and risk of premature death from coronary heart disease continuous and graded? Findings in 356,222 primary screenees of the Multiple Risk Factor Intervention Trial (MRFIT), *JAMA*, 256: 2823–2828, 1986.
8. Anderson, J.W. and Hanna, T.J., Impact of nondigestible carbohydrates on serum lipoproteins and risk for cardiovascular disease, *J. Nutr.*, 129: 1457S–1466S, 1999.
9. Wolk, A., Manson, J.E., Stampfer, M.J., Colditz, G.A., Hu, F.B., Speizer, F.E., Hennekens, C.H., and Willett, W.C., Long-term intake of dietary fiber and decreased risk of coronary heart disease among women, *JAMA*, 281: 1998–2004, 1999.
10. Todd, S., Woodward, M., Tunstall-Pedoe, H., and Bolton-Smith, C., Dietary antioxidant vitamins and fiber in the etiology of cardiovascular disease and all-causes mortality: results from the Scottish Heart Health Study, *Am. J. Epidemiol.*, 150: 1073–1080, 1999.
11. Brown, L., Rosner, B., Willett, W.W., and Sacks, F.M., Cholesterol-lowering effects of dietary fiber: a meta-analysis, *Am. J. Clin. Nutr.*, 69: 30–42, 1999.
12. Olson, B.H., Anderson, S.M., Becker, M.P., Anderson, J.W., Hunninghake, J.B., Jenkins, D.J., LaRosa, J.C., Rippe, J.M., Roberts, D.C., Stoy, D.B., Summerbell, C.D., Truswell, A.S., Wolever, T.M.S., Morris, D.H., and Fulgoni, V.L., Psyllium-enriched cereals lower blood total cholesterol and LDL cholesterol, but not HDL cholesterol, in hypercholesterolemic adults: results of a meta-analysis, *J. Nutr.*, 127: 1973–1980, 1997.

13. Romero, A.L., Romero, J.E., Galaviz, S., and Fernandez, M.L., Cookies enriched with psyllium or oat bran lower plasma LDL cholesterol in normal and hypercholesterolemic men from Northern Mexico, *J. Am. Coll. Nutr.*, 17: 601–608, 1998.
14. Whyte, J.L., McArthur, R., Topping, D., and Nestel, P., Oat bran lowers plasma cholesterol levels in mildly hypercholesterolemic men, *J. Am. Diet. Assoc.*, 92: 446–449, 1992.
15. Gerhardt, A.L. and Gallo, N.B., Full-fat rice bran and oat bran similarly reduce hypercholesterolemia in humans, *J. Nutr.*, 128: 865–869, 1998.
16. Behall, K.M., Scholfield, D.J., and Hallfrisch, J., Effect of beta-glucan level in oat fiber extracts on blood lipids in men and women, *J. Am. Coll. Nutr.*, 16: 46–51, 1997.
17. Anderson, J.W., Floore, T.L., Geil, T.B., O'Neal, D.S., and Balm, T.K., Hypocholesterolemic effects of different bulk-forming hydrophilic fibers as adjuncts to dietary therapy in mild to moderate hypercholesterolemia, *Arch. Intern. Med.*, 151: 1597–1602, 1997.
18. Anderson, J.W., Zettwoch, N., Feldman, T., Tietyen-Clark, J., Oeltgen, P., and Bishop, C.W., Cholesterol-lowering effects of psyllium hydrophilic mucilloid for hypercholesterolemic men, *Arch. Intern. Med.*, 148: 292–296, 1988.
19. Coats, A.J., The potential role of soluble fibre in the treatment of hypercholesterolaemia, *Postgrad. Med. J.*, 74: 391–394, 1998.
20. DeGroot, A.P., Luyken, R., and Pikaar, N.A., Cholesterol lowering effects of rolled oats, *Lancet*, 2: 303–304, 1963.
21. Anderson, J.W., Story, L.S., Sieling, B., Chen, W.J.L., Pertro, M.S., and Story, J., Hypocholesterolemic effects of oat bran or beans intake for hypercholesterolemic men, *Am. J. Clin. Nutr.*, 40: 1146–1155, 1984.
22. Anderson, J.W., Garrity, T.F., Wood, C.L., Whitis, S.E., Smith, B.M., and Oeltgen, P.R., Prospective, randomized, controlled comparison of the effects of low-fat and low-fat plus high-fiber diets on serum lipid concentrations, *Am. J. Clin. Nutr.*, 56: 887–894, 1992.
23. Ripsin, C.M., Keenan, J.M., Jacobs, D.R., Elmer, P.J., Welch, R.R., Van Horn, L., Liu, K., Turnbull, W.H., Thye, F.W., Kestin, M. et al., Oat products and lipid lowering: a meta-analysis, *JAMA*, 267: 3317–3325, 1992.
24. Vuksan, V., Jenkins, D.J., Spadafora, P., Sievenpiper, J.L., Owen, R., Vidgen, E., Brighenti, F., Josse, R., Leiter, L.A., and Bruce-Thompson, C., Konjac-mannan (glucomannan) improves glycemia and other associated risk factors for coronary heart disease in type 2 diabetes. A randomized controlled metabolic trial, *Diabetes Care*, 22: 913–919, 1999.
25. Judith A. Marlet and Milton H. Fischer. Session: physiological aspects of fibre. The active fraction of psyllium seed husk. *Proc. Nutr. Soc.* 62: 207–209, 2003.
26. Anderson, J.W., Jones, A.E., and Riddell-Mason, S., Ten different dietary fibers have significantly different effects on serum and liver lipids of cholesterol-fed rats, *J. Nutr.*, 124: 78–83, 1994.
27. Kritchevsky, D., Tepper, S.A., and Klurfeld, D.M., Influence of psyllium preparations on plasma and liver lipids of cholesterol-fed rats, *Artery*, 21: 303–311, 1995.
28. Turley, S.D., Daggy, B.P., and Dietschy, J.M., Cholesterol-lowering action of psyllium mucilloid in the hamster: sites and possible mechanisms of action, *Metabolism*, 40: 1063–1073, 1991.
29. Everson, G.T., Daggy, B.P., McKinley, C., and Story, J.A., Effects of psyllium hydrophilic mucilloid on LDL-cholesterol and bile acid synthesis in hypercholesterolemic men, *J. Lipid Res.*, 33: 1183–1192, 1992.
30. Anderson, J.W., Allgood, L.D., Turner, J., Oeltgen, P.R., and Daggy, B.P., Effects of psyllium on glucose and serum lipid responses in men with type 2 diabetes and hypercholesterolemia, *Am. J. Clin. Nutr.*, 70: 466–473, 1999.
31. Marlett, J.A., Hosig, K.B., Vollendorf, N.W., Shinnick, F.L., Haack, V.S., and Story, J.A., Mechanism of serum cholesterol reduction by oat bran, *Hepatology*, 20: 1450–1457, 1994.
32. Leiss, O., von Bergmann, K., Streicher, U., and Strotkoetter, H., Effect of three different dihydroxy bile acids on intestinal cholesterol absorption in normal volunteers, Gastroenterology, 87: 144–149, 1984.
33. Horton, J.D., Cuthbert, J.A., and Spady, D.K., Regulation of hepatic 7 alpha-hydroxylase expression by dietary psyllium in the hamster, *J. Clin. Invest.*, 93: 2084–2092, 1994.
34. Wright, R.S., Anderson, J.W., and Bridges, S.R., Propionate inhibits hepatocyte lipid synthesis, *Proc. Soc. Exp. Biol. Med.*, 195: 26–29, 1990.

35. Veldman, F.J., Nair, C.H., Vorster, W.W., Vermaak, W.J., Jerling, J.C., Oosthuizen, W., and Venter, C.S., Dietary pectin influences fibrin network structure in hypercholesterolaemic subjects, *Thromb. Res.*, 86: 183–196, 1997.

36. Ajani U.A., Ford E.S., and Mokdad A.H., Dietary fiber and C-reactive protein: findings from national health and nutrition examination survey data. *J Nutr.* 134(5): 1181–5, 2004.

37. St. Pierre, A.C., Ruel, I.L., Cantin, B., Dagenais, G.R., Bernard, P.M., Despres, J.P., and Lamarche, B., Comparison of various electrophoretic characteristics of LDL particles and their relationship to the risk of ischemic heart disease. *Circulation* 104, 2295–2299, 2001.

38. Davy, B.M., Davy, K.P., Ho, R.C., Beske, S.D., Davrath, L.R., and Melby, C.L., High-fiber oat cereal compared with wheat cereal consumption favorably alters LDL-cholesterol subclass and particle numbers in middle-aged and older men. *Am J Clin Nutr.* 76(2): 351–8, 2002.

39. Lamarche, B., Desroches, S., Jenkins, D.J., Kendall, C.W., Marchie, A., Faulkner, D., Vidgen, E., Lapsley, K.G., Trautwein, E.A., Parker, T.L., Josse, R.G., Leiter, L.A., and Connelly, P.W., Combined effects of a dietary portfolio of plant sterols, vegetable protein, viscous fibre and almonds on LDL particle size, *Br J Nutr.* 92(4): 657–63. 2004.

40. Moreyra, A.E., Wilson, A.C., and Koraym, K., Effect of combining psyllium fiber with simvastatin in lowering cholesterol, *Arch Intern Med.* 2005;165:1161–1166.

41. Kushi, L.H., Meyer, K.A., and Jacobs, D.R., Jr., Cereals, legumes, and chronic disease risk reduction: evidence from epidemiologic studies, *Am. J. Clin. Nutr.*, 70: 451S–458S, 1999.

42. Jacobs, D.R., Jr., Meyer, K.A., Kushi, L.H., and Folsom, A.R., Whole-grain intake may reduce the risk of ischemic heart disease death in postmenopausal women: the Iowa Women's Health Study, *Am. J. Clin. Nutr.*, 68: 248–257, 1998.

43. Liu, S., Stampfer, M.J., Hu, F.B., Giovannucci, E., Rimm, E., Manson, J.E., Hennekens, C.H., and Willett, W.C., Whole-grain consumption and risk of coronary heart disease: results from the Nurses' Health Study, *Am. J. Clin. Nutr.*, 70: 412–419, 1999.

7 Omega-3 Fish Oils and Lipoprotein Metabolism

Sidika E. Kasim-Karakas

CONTENTS

I. INTRODUCTION

Although the overall effects of n-3 fish oils on plasma lipids have been well known for a long time, recent research has provided important information about the underlying mechanisms. Omega-3 fish oils consistently decrease plasma triglycerides (TG), raise low-density lipoprotein (LDL) cholesterol, and exert variable effects on high-density lipoprotein (HDL) cholesterol and apoprotein (apo) B levels. To better understand the effects of n-3 fish oils, a brief summary of the lipoprotein metabolism is provided.

II. LIPOPROTEIN METABOLISM

The major plasma lipids are TG, cholesterol, phospholipids, and nonesterified fatty acids (NEFA). Lipids are insoluble in the plasma. Therefore, NEFA are transported in the circulation by albumin; TG, cholesterol and phospholipids are carried in macromolecules called *lipoproteins*. Cores of the lipoproteins carry neutral lipids (TG and cholesterol ester), and the surfaces contain free cholesterol, phospholipids, and apoproteins.

There are five major classes of plasma lipoproteins: chylomicrons, very low-density lipoproteins (VLDL), intermediate density lipoproteins (IDL), LDL, and HDL. Chylomicrons and VLDL carry primarily TG, whereas LDL and HDL are the major cholesterol transporters. The IDL have approximately equal amounts of TG and cholesterol.

Chylomicrons are synthesized in the intestine, and VLDL are synthesized in the liver. The structural apoprotein of chylomicrons is apo B48 and that of VLDL is apo B100. These TG-rich lipoproteins are hydrolyzed by lipoprotein lipase (LpL) and converted into smaller lipoproteins called *remnants* and *IDL*, respectively. The remnants and IDL are cleared from the circulation by the liver through mechanisms involving LDL-receptor-related protein (LRP), which binds to apoE and hepatic lipase (HL). Although all the chylomicron remnants are cleared by the hepatic uptake, some of the IDL are further catabolized to LDL. During this process, the TG core is replaced by cholesterol ester; all of the apoproteins except apo B100 are removed.

Catabolism of LDL depends primarily on the receptor-mediated uptake. The LDL receptor binds the apo B100. The LDL and the LDL receptor are internalized and catabolized in the lysosomes, releasing free cholesterol. Free cholesterol inhibits the key enzyme of cholesterol synthesis (3-hydroxy 3-methyl glutaryl-CoA reductase), creating a feedback mechanism to prevent excessive cholesterol production. Simultaneously, LDL-receptor synthesis is decreased, and cholesterol esterification is stimulated. These feedback mechanisms tightly regulate the intracellular free cholesterol levels.

Metabolism of HDL is complicated. Nascent HDL containing only a bilayer of phospholipid and apoproteins is formed in the liver and the intestine.[1] These lipid-poor particles acquire cholesterol and phospholipids from peripheral tissues via ATP binding cassette transporter A1 (ABCA1) generating cholesterol-enriched particles. The enzyme lecithin cholesterol acyl transferase (LCAT), carried on HDL particles, esterifies the free cholesterol to form cholesteryl ester which migrates to the core of the HDL. These HDL particles change further through intravascular modeling by lipases and lipid transfer proteins. Cholesteryl ester transfer protein (CETP) facilitates the exchange of cholesteryl ester (CE) in HDL for the triglyceride in chylomicrons and VLDL. Phospholipid transfer protein (PLTP) mediates phospholipid transfer from chylomicrons and VLDL to HDL. These lipids are then delivered to the liver with the assistance of the hepatic lipase, which hydrolyzes the triglyceride in HDL and releases lipid-poor apoA-I HDL and the scavenger receptor (SR)-B1, which removes cholesterol.

III. EFFECTS OF N-3 FISH OILS ON LIPOPROTEINS

A. HEPATIC PRODUCTION OF VLDL

At the fasting state, elevated plasma triglyceride levels reflect the presence of excess amounts of VLDL in the circulation. Fish oils consistently decrease plasma concentration of triglycerides by decreasing VLDL-TG, VLDL-cholesterol, and VLDL-apoB (Figure 7.1). Kinetic studies in humans, nonhuman primates, and small animal models consistently demonstrate decreased VLDL-TG and VLDL apoB secretion rates.[2–5] The degree of suppression in TG relative to apoB influences the VLDL particle size. Although in general, fish oils decrease the secretion of TG more than apoB and lead to the production of smaller, lipid-poor particles, this response is modified by the genetic background.[4]

Fish oils regulate hepatic production of VLDL by inhibiting fatty-acid synthesis, increasing oxidation, decreasing triglyceride and cholesteryl ester production, and increasing the degradation of apoB. Recent research demonstrated that the effects of fish oils are mediated through the actions of several nuclear receptors such as peroxisome proliferator-activated receptor (PPAR), liver X receptors (LXR) and hepatic nuclear factor-4 (HNF4), and sterol regulatory element-binding proteins (SREBP).[6]

Fatty acid production: The major lipogenic enzyme in the liver is fatty acid synthase (FAS). The promoter of FAS has a SREBP response element. Thus, SREBP stimulates transcription of FAS. In turn, SREBP gene expression is regulated by the nuclear receptor LXR. Fish oils interfere with the binding of the ligand oxysterols to LXR, decrease SREBP availability, and consequently downregulate the transcription of FAS. Over-expression of the nuclear form of SREBP-1c overrides the suppressive effect of PUFA on lipogenic gene expression.[6–9] Thus, down-regulation of

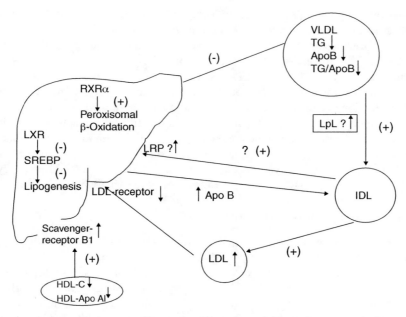

FIGURE 7.1 Effects of fish oil supplementation on lipoprotein metabolism.

the nuclear form of SREBP may account for many of the suppressive effects of fish oils on hepatic lipogenesis.

Fatty acid oxidation: Fish oils increase catabolism fatty acids by stimulating the hepatic enzymes to facilitate β-oxidation in the peroxisomes (acyl-CoA oxidase, AOX) and in the mitochondria (carnitine palmitoyltransferase, CPT). Fish oils mediate transcription of AOX through the nuclear receptor PPARα. The PPARα-deficient (PPARα –/–) mice do not increase liver AOX mRNA in response to fish oil.[10] Regulation of the rate-limiting enzyme of mitochondrial β-oxidation, the carnitine palmitoyltransferase 1 *(L-CPT 1)* gene, is not dependent on PPARα.[11]

Triglyceride and cholesteryl ester production: Fish oils are poor substrates for diacylglycerol acyltransferase, the last step in triglyceride synthesis.[12,13] They are also poor substrates for cholesterol esterification. Instead, they get preferentially incorporated into phospholipids.[14] *In vivo* studies show that fish oil feeding causes a 25% decrease in glycerol production from acyl CoA, a 15% decrease in the incorporation of DAG into the TG pool, and a 20% decrease in hepatic TG secretion.[15]

ApoB degradation: ApoB is the obligatory protein for VLDL assembly, which occurs in two steps[16]: During the first step, a small quantity of triglyceride becomes associated with apoB in the rough endoplasmic reticulum, forming a small, dense, VLDL precursor. This process is facilitated by the microsomal triacylglycerol transfer protein (MTP). During the second step, the VLDL-precursor joins with a triglyceride droplet and forms a large VLDL. A small GTP-binding protein that activates phospholipase D, ADP-ribosylation factor 1 (ARF-1), appears to facilitate the second step.

The apoB that cannot be lipidated during the first step is destroyed through endoplasmic reticulum-associated degradation and reuptake.[17] The apoB in the larger, lipid-enriched VLDL are degraded by a newly described pathway called post-ER presecretory proteolysis.[18] Fish oils reduce hepatic VLDL secretion primarily by increasing post-ER presecretory proteolysis of apoB.[18]

B. Intestinal Production of Chylomicrons

After a meal, the increase in plasma triglyceride levels reflects the amount of chylomicrons produced in the intestine. Effects of fish oils on chylomicron production have been addressed in humans and animal models by studying both the absorption characteristics of fish oils and the effects of long-term fish oil supplementation on chylomicron production from other fats. These studies show that in humans, fish oil-rich test meals increase plasma chylomicrons and triglycerides as much as olive oil-rich test meals. Fish oils given either as ethyl esters or triglycerides are equally well absorbed. The individual fatty acids in fish oils, EPA vs. DHA, have similar absorption rates.[19] All these findings suggest that a single load of fish oil does not affect chylomicron production in the human intestine. However, long-term fish oil supplementation can cause adaptive changes and blunt the increase in chylomicrons after oral fat loading. Furthermore, fish oil supplementation decreases the chylomicron remnants during the late postprandial phase.[20] These findings are in contrast with the results of animal studies that showed long-term fish oil feeding stimulated the enzymes that synthesize chylomicron lipids, acyl-CoA:cholesterol acyltransferase (ACAT and acyl-CoA:1,2-diacylglycerol acyltransferase (DGAT) and therefore increased chylomicron synthesis.[21]

C. Lipolysis of Triglyceride-Rich Lipoproteins

Both the VLDL-TG produced in the liver and the chylomicron-TG from the intestine are hydrolyzed in the peripheral tissues.

VLDL: A recent kinetic study demonstrated that fish oils increased the conversion rates of VLDL-apoB to IDL-apoB by 71% and to LDL-apoB by 93%.[2] One explanation for the accelerated conversion may be that the relatively TG-poor VLDL particles, produced during fish oil supplementation, can be lipolyzed more efficiently. However, the experimental evidence does not support this hypothesis. *In vitro*, when fish oil-enriched VLDL were hydrolyzed by using purified LpL and HL, both EPA-and DHA-enriched particles had lower rates of hydrolysis as compared with soy oil. Release of fatty acids from EPA-enriched particles was even slower than those of the DHA.[22] Fish-oil-enriched chylomicrons, treated with LpL, lipolyzed at a higher rate than the palm oil-rich particles, but at a comparable rate with olive oil-rich or corn oil-rich particles.[23] When accelerated lipolysis is induced *in vivo* by intravenous heparin infusion, there was no increase in the lipolysis of VLDL-TG during fish oil treatment as compared to the olive oil placebo.[24] Another explanation may be that although fish oils do not increase the susceptibility of the TG-rich lipoproteins to lipolysis *in vitro*, they can stimulate the activities of the lipolyzing enzymes LpL and HL *in vivo*. This hypothesis is supported by the findings that fish oils increased the heparin releasable LpL and HL in healthy subjects, and the post-heparin LpL in patients with hyperlipidemia.[24,25]

Chylomicron remnants and IDL: In humans, there is conflicting evidence about the effects of fish oils on the clearance of chylomicron remnants and IDL; both increased and unchanged rates have been observed. In patients with diabetes or hypertriglyceridemia, supplementation of fish oils or EPA-ethyl ester decreased the endogenous remnant-like particles in the circulation.[20,26] However, when remnant-like particles were injected intravenously in men treated with fish oils, their clearance rate was unchanged.[2] In rats, clearance of chylomicron remnants appears to be accelerated. Fish oil-rich remnants are taken up more efficiently by the isolated hepatocytes.[27,28] The biliary excretion of cholesterol from fish oil-rich chylomicrons is increased.[29] This may be partly due to the induction of 7α-hydroxylase, the rate-limiting enzyme of bile acid synthesis and cholesterol excretion, by fish oil.[30]

The hepatic uptake of chylomicron remnants can be facilitated by LDL receptor, LDL receptor-related protein (LRP), and hepatic lipase. ApoE is a ligand for the LRP. The current evidence suggests that the fatty acid composition of the chylomicron remnants influence their hepatic uptake. In addition, fish oil supplementation causes long-term adaptive changes in liver tissue. The response to the fatty acid composition is mediated primarily by the LDL receptor, whereas the long-term adaptation involves both the LDL receptor and the LRP.[27] Fish oils can modulate the LRP-mediated uptake also by increasing apoE levels.[31] However, the significance of this increase is not clear because in apoE*3-leiden transgenic mice model, which has decreased clearance of chylomicron and VLDL remnants, fish oils can still increase VLDL clearance.[32] Similarly, in apoE knockout

(Apoetm1Unc) mice, fish oil and n-3 fatty acid ethyl esters decrease triglyceride, cholesterol, and phospholipid levels and regulate the activity and mRNA levels of the hepatic enzymes involved in fatty acid oxidation and synthesis.[33] Finally, although hepatic lipase plays a role in chylomicron remnant clearance, the available evidence indicates that hepatic lipase does not mediate the effects of fish oils.[34]

D. Metabolism of LDL

Despite having beneficial effects on coronary artery disease,[35] fish oils do not decrease, and can even increase, the most atherogenic lipoproteins in the circulation: LDL. To explain this discrepancy, it was proposed that fish oils may increase the less atherogenic, large, buoyant LDL particles but not the more atherogenic, small, dense LDL particles. Recent research verified this in patients with combined hyperlipidemia[36] but not in patients with type 2 diabetes.[37] The increase in LDL is mostly due to increased conversion of VLDL apoB to LDL apoB,[2,38] but oversecretion of apoB into the IDL fraction also occurs.[38] Studies in animal models and cell cultures consistently demonstrate that n-3 fish oils decrease the number of LDL receptors.[39] However, kinetic studies in humans do not show a decreased fractional catabolic rate of LDL.[2,3]

E. Metabolism of HDL

Omega-3 fatty-acid supplementation has been associated with variable HDL cholesterol response. Recent research indicates that fish oils may preferentially increase the smaller, cholesterol-poor HDL particles, which may be more efficient in cholesterol uptake.[37] Fish oils may also increase the delivery of cholesterol from the HDL to the liver, the reverse cholesterol transport, by increasing scavenger receptor B-1 gene expression.[40] Plasma HDL is constantly remodeled by incorporation of cholesterol ester by LCAT, transfer of neutral lipids between lipoproteins by lipid transfer proteins and CETP, incorporation of surface lipids and apoproteins during the LpL-mediated lipolysis of TG-rich lipoproteins, removal of cholesterol ester and phospholipids by HL, and removal of cholesterol by scavenger receptor. Decreased LCAT,[41–43] increased as well as decreased CETP,[44,45] decreased lipid transfer protein,[41] and increased or unchanged LpL and HL activities[25,46] all have been reported.

IV. SPECIFIC EFFECTS OF INDIVIDUAL N-3 FATTY ACIDS

The recent availability of purified ethyl esters of EPA and DHA provided the opportunity to identify their specific actions on the lipid metabolism. Although earlier research showed a more potent triglyceride lowering effect of EPA[47] as compared to DHA, recent research disputes this finding.[31] Effects of fish oils have also been compared with those of flaxseed oil, which is rich in α-linolenic acid (18:3 n–3), the precursor of EPA and DHA. Flaxseed oil, unless given in very large amounts, does not lower plasma TG.[48,49]

V. POTENTIAL ADVERSE EFFECTS OF FISH OILS: LIPID PEROXIDATION

Oxidative modification of lipoproteins in the arterial wall is a significant step in atherosclerosis. The susceptibility of individual fatty acids to oxidation directly depends on their degree of unsaturation. Thus fish oils, with their five or six unsaturated double bonds, can be easily oxidized.[50] Recent research suggests that n-3 fatty acids are less susceptible to oxidation than the n-6 fatty acids that contain a similar number of double bonds;[51] fish oils may increase the HDL-bound antioxidant enzyme paraoxonase;[52] thus fish oils may not increase oxidation *in vivo*.[53] As an additional precaution, most fish oil supplements contain vitamin E.[54]

VI. FISH OILS AS COMBINATION THERAPY FOR HYPERLIPIDEMIA

Statins are the most effective therapeutic agents for LDL-cholesterol lowering while fibrates have potent triglyceride-lowering effects. Although these two classes of medicines can be used in combination, this increases the risk of myopathy. Therefore, fish oils have been combined with statins as an alternative to fibrates and provided additional triglyceride lowering.[55,56] Recently, a different class of LDL-lowering medicine that inhibits intestinal cholesterol absorption, ezetimibe, became available. To my knowledge, the effects of fish oil and ezetimibe in combination have not yet been tested.

VII. CONCLUSION

The potent triglyceride-lowering effects of fish oils have been known for a long time. In searching for the mechanisms, recent research highlighted the importance of fish oils in the regulation of nuclear receptors. It became evident that fish oils decreased lipogenesis by decreasing SREBP production by the LXR, and increased peroxisomal β-oxidation of the fatty acids by regulating PPARα. Currently, several studies are investigating the structural and functional properties of fish oils and their metabolic products as ligands for nuclear receptors. In addition, the gene-array technique is providing enormous information about the effects of fish oils on the mRNA abundance. These efforts are establishing the importance of fish oils, a readily available nutrient, as a significant modulator of important biochemical pathways.

REFERENCES

1. Lewis, G.F. and Rader, D.J. New insights into the regulation of HDL metabolism and reverse cho-lesterol transport. *Circ Res* 96: 1221–1232, 2005.
2. Chan, D.C., Watts, G.F., Mori, T.A., Barrett, P.H., Redgrave, T.G., and Beilin, L.J. Randomized controlled trial of the effect of n-3 fatty acid supplementation on the metabolism of apolipoprotein B-100 and chylomicron remnants in men with visceral obesity. *Am J Clin Nutr* 77: 300–307, 2003.
3. Harris, W.S., Connor, W.E., Illingworth, D.R., Rothrock, D.W., and Foster, D.M. Effects of fish oil on VLDL triglyceride kinetics in humans. *J Lipid Res* 31: 1549–1558, 1990.
4. Ko, C., O'Rourke, S.M., and Huang, L.S. A fish oil diet produces different degrees of suppression of apoB and triglyceride secretion in human apoB transgenic mouse strains. *J Lipid Res* 44: 1946–1955, 2003.
5. Parks, J.S., Johnson, F.L., Wilson, M.D., and Rudel, L.L. Effect of fish oil diet on hepatic lipid metabolism in nonhuman primates: lowering of secretion of hepatic triglyceride but not apoB. *J Lipid Res* 31: 455–466, 1990.
6. Ide, T., Shimano, H., Yoshikawa, T., Yahagi, N., Amemiya-Kudo, M., Matsuzaka, T., Nakakuki, M., Yatoh, S., Iizuka, Y., Tomita, S., Ohashi, K., Takahashi, A., Sone, H., Gotoda, T., Osuga, J., Ishibashi, S., and Yamada, N. Cross-talk between peroxisome proliferator-activated receptor (PPAR) alpha and liver X receptor (LXR) in nutritional regulation of fatty acid metabolism. II. LXRs suppress lipid degradation gene promoters through inhibition of PPAR signaling. *Mol Endocrinol* 17: 1255–1267, 2003.
7. Shimano, H., Yahagi, N., Amemiya-Kudo, M., Hasty, A.H., Osuga, J., Tamura, Y., Shionoiri, F., Iizuka, Y., Ohashi, K., Harada, K., Gotoda, T., Ishibashi, S., and Yamada, N. Sterol regulatory element-binding protein-1 as a key transcription factor for nutritional induction of lipogenic enzyme genes. *J Biol Chem* 274: 35832–35839, 1999.
8. Yahagi, N., Shimano, H., Hasty, A.H., Amemiya-Kudo, M., Okazaki, H., Tamura, Y., Iizuka, Y., Shionoiri, F., Ohashi, K., Osuga, J., Harada, K., Gotoda, T., Nagai, R., Ishibashi, S., and Yamada, N. A crucial role of sterol regulatory element-binding protein-1 in the regulation of lipogenic gene expression by polyunsaturated fatty acids. *J Biol Chem* 274: 35840–35844, 1999.

9. Yoshikawa, T., Ide, T., Shimano, H., Yahagi, N., Amemiya-Kudo, M., Matsuzaka, T., Yatoh, S., Kitamine, T., Okazaki, H., Tamura, Y., Sekiya, M., Takahashi, A., Hasty, A.H., Sato, R., Sone, H., Osuga, J., Ishibashi, S., and Yamada, N. Cross-talk between peroxisome proliferator-activated receptor (PPAR) alpha and liver X receptor (LXR) in nutritional regulation of fatty acid metabolism. I. PPARs suppress sterol regulatory element binding protein-1c promoter through inhibition of LXR signaling. *Mol Endocrinol* 17: 1240–1254, 2003.

10. Ren, B., Thelen, A.P., Peters, J.M., Gonzalez, F.J., and Jump, D.B. Polyunsaturated fatty acid suppression of hepatic fatty acid synthase and S14 gene expression does not require peroxisome proliferator-activated receptor alpha. *J Biol Chem* 272: 26827–26832, 1997.

11. Louet, J.F., Chatelain, F., Decaux, J.F., Park, E.A., Kohl, C., Pineau, T., Girard, J., and Pegorier, J.P. Long-chain fatty acids regulate liver carnitine palmitoyltransferase I gene (L-CPT I) expression through a peroxisome-proliferator-activated receptor alpha (PPARalpha)-independent pathway. *Biochem J* 354: 189–197, 2001.

12. Berge, R.K., Madsen, L., Vaagenes, H., Tronstad, K.J., Gottlicher, M., and Rustan, A.C. In contrast with docosahexaenoic acid, eicosapentaenoic acid and hypolipidaemic derivatives decrease hepatic synthesis and secretion of triacylglycerol by decreased diacylglycerol acyltransferase activity and stimulation of fatty acid oxidation. *Biochem J* 343(Pt. 1): 191–197, 1999.

13. Madsen, L., Rustan, A.C., Vaagenes, H., Berge, K., Dyroy, E., and Berge, R.K. Eicosapentaenoic and docosahexaenoic acid affect mitochondrial and peroxisomal fatty acid oxidation in relation to substrate preference. *Lipids* 34: 951–963, 1999.

14. Yeo, Y.K. and Holub, B.J. Influence of dietary fish oil on the relative synthesis of triacylglycerol and phospholipids in rat liver in vivo. *Lipids* 25: 811–814, 1990.

15. Moir, A.M., Park, B.S., and Zammit, V.A. Quantification in vivo of the effects of different types of dietary fat on the loci of control involved in hepatic triacylglycerol secretion. *Biochem J* 308 (Pt. 2): 537–542, 1995.

16. Gibbons, G.F., Wiggins, D., Brown, A.M., and Hebbachi, A.M. Synthesis and function of hepatic very-low-density lipoprotein. *Biochem Soc Trans* 32: 59–64, 2004.

17. Fisher, E.A. and Ginsberg, H.N. Complexity in the secretory pathway: the assembly and secretion of apolipoprotein B-containing lipoproteins. *J Biol Chem* 277: 17377–17380, 2002.

18. Pan, M., Cederbaum, A.I., Zhang, Y.L., Ginsberg, H.N., Williams, K.J., and Fisher, E.A. Lipid peroxidation and oxidant stress regulate hepatic apolipoprotein B degradation and VLDL production. *J Clin Invest* 113: 1277–1287, 2004.

19. Nordoy, A., Barstad, L., Connor, W.E., and Hatcher, L. Absorption of the n-3 eicosapentaenoic and docosahexaenoic acids as ethyl esters and triglycerides by humans. *Am J Clin Nutr* 53: 1185–1190, 1991.

20. Westphal, S., Orth, M., Ambrosch, A., Osmundsen, K., and Luley, C. Postprandial chylomicrons and VLDLs in severe hypertriacylglycerolemia are lowered more effectively than are chylomicron remnants after treatment with n-3 fatty acids. *Am J Clin Nutr* 71: 914–920, 2000.

21. Chautan, M., Charbonnier, M., Leonardi, J., Andre, M., Lafont, H., and Nalbone, G. Modulation of lipid chylomicron-synthesizing enzymes in rats by the dietary (n-6): (n-3) fatty acid ratio. *J Nutr* 121: 1305–1310, 1991.

22. Oliveira, F.L., Rumsey, S.C., Schlotzer, E., Hansen, I., Carpentier, Y.A., and Deckelbaum, R.J. Triglyceride hydrolysis of soy oil vs fish oil emulsions. *JPEN J Parenter Enteral Nutr* 21: 224–229, 1997.

23. Botham, K.M., Avella, M., Cantafora, A., and Bravo, E. The lipolysis of chylomicrons derived from different dietary fats by lipoprotein lipase in vitro. *Biochim Biophys Acta* 1349: 257–263, 1997.

24. Kasim-Karakas, S.E., Herrmann, R., and Almario, R. Effects of omega-3 fatty acids on intravascular lipolysis of very-low-density lipoproteins in humans. *Metabolism* 44: 1223–1230, 1995.

25. Harris, W.S., Lu, G., Rambjor, G.S., Walen, A.I., Ontko, J.A., Cheng, Q., and Windsor, S.L. Influence of n-3 fatty acid supplementation on the endogenous activities of plasma lipases. *Am J Clin Nutr* 66: 254–260, 1997.

26. Nakamura, N., Hamazaki, T., Kobayashi, M., Ohta, M., and Okuda, K. Effects of eicosapentaenoic acids on remnant-like particles, cholesterol concentrations and plasma fatty acid composition in patients with diabetes mellitus. *In Vivo* 12: 311–314, 1998.

27. Lambert, M.S., Avella, M.A., Berhane, Y., Shervill, E., and Botham, K.M. The fatty acid composition of chylomicron remnants influences their binding and internalization by isolated hepatocytes. *Eur J Biochem* 268: 3983–3992, 2001.

28. Lambert, M.S., Avella, M.A., Shervill, E., Berhane, Y., and Botham, K.M. Chylomicron remnants derived from fish oil are bound and internalised more rapidly by isolated hepatocytes than those derived from olive or palm oil. *Biochem Soc Trans* 26: S149, 1998.

29. Bravo, E., Ortu, G., Cantafora, A., Lambert, M.S., Avella, M., Mayes, P.A., and Botham, K.M. Comparison of the hepatic uptake and processing of cholesterol from chylomicrons of different fatty acid composition in the rat in vivo. *Biochim Biophys Acta* 1258: 328–336, 1995.

30. Berard, A.M., Dumon, M.F., and Darmon, M. Dietary fish oil up-regulates cholesterol 7alpha-hydroxylase mRNA in mouse liver leading to an increase in bile acid and cholesterol excretion. *FEBS Lett* 559: 125–128, 2004.

31. Buckley, R., Shewring, B., Turner, R., Yaqoob, P., and Minihane, A.M. Circulating triacylglycerol and apoE levels in response to EPA and docosahexaenoic acid supplementation in adult human subjects. *Br J Nutr* 92: 477–483, 2004.

32. van Vlijmen, B.J., Mensink, R.P., van't Hof, H.B., Offermans, R.F., Hofker, M.H., and Havekes, L.M. Effects of dietary fish oil on serum lipids and VLDL kinetics in hyperlipidemic apolipoprotein E*3-Leiden transgenic mice. *J Lipid Res* 39: 1181–1188, 1998.

33. Ide, T., Takahashi, Y., Kushiro, M., Tachibana, M., and Matsushima, Y. Effect of n-3 fatty acids on serum lipid levels and hepatic fatty acid metabolism in BALB/c.KOR-Apoeshl mice deficient in apolipoprotein E expression. *J Nutr Biochem* 15: 169–178, 2004.

34. Lambert, M.S., Avella, M.A., Berhane, Y., Shervill, E., and Botham, K.M. The differential hepatic uptake of chylomicron remnants of different fatty acid composition is not mediated by hepatic lipase. *Br J Nutr* 85: 575–582, 2001.

35. Harris, W.S. Are omega-3 fatty acids the most important nutritional modulators of coronary heart disease risk? *Curr Atheroscler Rep* 6: 447–452, 2004.

36. Calabresi, L., Donati, D., Pazzucconi, F., Sirtori, C.R., and Franceschini, G. Omacor in familial combined hyperlipidemia: effects on lipids and low density lipoprotein subclasses. *Atherosclerosis* 148: 387–396, 2000.

37. Petersen, M., Pedersen, H., Major-Pedersen, A., Jensen, T., and Marckmann, P. Effect of fish oil versus corn oil supplementation on LDL and HDL subclasses in type 2 diabetic patients. *Diabetes Care* 25: 1704–1708, 2002.

38. Fisher, W.R., Zech, L.A., and Stacpoole, P.W. Apolipoprotein B metabolism in hypertriglyceridemic diabetic patients administered either a fish oil- or vegetable oil-enriched diet. *J Lipid Res* 39: 388–401, 1998.

39. Harris, W.S. n-3 fatty acids and serum lipoproteins: animal studies. *Am J Clin Nutr* 65: 1611S–1616S, 1997.

40. le Morvan, V., Dumon, M.F., Palos-Pinto, A., and Berard, A.M. n-3 FA increase liver uptake of HDL-cholesterol in mice. *Lipids* 37: 767–772, 2002.

41. Abbey, M., Clifton, P., Kestin, M., Belling, B., and Nestel, P. Effect of fish oil on lipoproteins, lecithin: cholesterol acyltransferase, and lipid transfer protein activity in humans. *Arteriosclerosis* 10: 85–94, 1990.

42. Hatahet, W., Cole, L., Kudchodkar, B.J., and Fungwe, T.V. Dietary fats differentially modulate the expression of lecithin: cholesterol acyltransferase, apoprotein-A1 and scavenger receptor b1 in rats. *J Nutr* 133: 689–694, 2003.

43. Parks, J.S., Thuren, T.Y., and Schmitt, J.D. Inhibition of lecithin: cholesterol acyltransferase activity by synthetic phosphatidylcholine species containing eicosapentaenoic acid or docosahexaenoic acid in the sn-2 position. *J Lipid Res* 33: 879–887, 1992.

44. Bagdade, J.D., Ritter, M.C., Davidson, M., and Subbaiah, P.V. Effect of marine lipids on cholesteryl ester transfer and lipoprotein composition in patients with hypercholesterolemia. *Arterioscler Thromb* 12: 1146–1152, 1992.

45. de Silva, P.P., Agarwal-Mawal, A., Davis, P.J., and Cheema, S.K. The levels of plasma low density lipoprotein are independent of cholesterol ester transfer protein in fish oil fed F1B hamsters. *Nutr Metab (Lond)* 2: 8, 2005.

46. Kasim-Karakas, S.E., and Almario, R. Effects of omega-3 fatty acids on intravascular lipolysis of very low density lipoproteins in humans. *Metabolism* 44: 1223–1230, 1995.

47. Rambjor, G.S., Walen, A.I., Windsor, S.L., and Harris, W.S. Eicosapentaenoic acid is primarily responsible for hypotriglyceridemic effect of fish oil in humans. *Lipids* 31 Suppl.: S45–49, 1996.

48. Layne, K.S., Goh, Y.K., Jumpsen, J.A., Ryan, E.A., Chow, P., and Clandinin, M.T. Normal subjects consuming physiological levels of 18: 3(n-3) and 20: 5(n-3) from flaxseed or fish oils have characteristic differences in plasma lipid and lipoprotein fatty acid levels. *J Nutr* 126: 2130–2140, 1996.

49. Lucas, E.A., Wild, R.D., Hammond, L.J., Khalil, D.A., Juma, S., Daggy, B.P., Stoecker, B.J., and Arjmandi, B.H. Flaxseed improves lipid profile without altering biomarkers of bone metabolism in postmenopausal women. *J Clin Endocrinol Metab* 87: 1527–1532, 2002.

50. Pedersen, H., Petersen, M., Major-Pedersen, A., Jensen, T., Nielsen, N.S., Lauridsen, S.T., and Marckmann, P. Influence of fish oil supplementation on in vivo and in vitro oxidation resistance of low-density lipoprotein in type 2 diabetes. *Eur J Clin Nutr* 57: 713–720, 2003.

51. Napolitano, M., Bravo, E., Avella, M., Chico, Y., Ochoa, B., Botham, K.M., and Rivabene, R. The fatty acid composition of chylomicron remnants influences their propensity to oxidate. *Nutr Metab Cardiovasc Dis* 14: 241–247, 2004.

52. Calabresi, L., Villa, B., Canavesi, M., Sirtori, C.R., James, R.W., Bernini, F., and Franceschini, G. An omega-3 polyunsaturated fatty acid concentrate increases plasma high-density lipoprotein 2 cholesterol and paraoxonase levels in patients with familial combined hyperlipidemia. *Metabolism* 53: 153–158, 2004.

53. Tholstrup, T., Hellgren, L.I., Petersen, M., Basu, S., Straarup, E.M., Schnohr, P., and Sandstrom, B. A solid dietary fat containing fish oil redistributes lipoprotein subclasses without increasing oxidative stress in men. *J Nutr* 134: 1051–1057, 2004.

54. Suarez, A., Ramirez-Tortosa, M., Gil, A., and Faus, M.J. Addition of vitamin E to long-chain polyunsaturated fatty acid-enriched diets protects neonatal tissue lipids against peroxidation in rats. *Eur J Nutr* 38: 169–176, 1999.

55. Chan, D.C., Watts, G.F., Mori, T.A., Barrett, P.H., Beilin, L.J., and Redgrave, T.G. Factorial study of the effects of atorvastatin and fish oil on dyslipidaemia in visceral obesity. *Eur J Clin Invest* 32: 429–436, 2002.

56. Durrington, P.N., Bhatnagar, D., Mackness, M.I., Morgan, J., Julier, K., Khan, M.A., and France, M. An omega-3 polyunsaturated fatty acid concentrate administered for one year decreased triglycerides in simvastatin treated patients with coronary heart disease and persisting hypertriglyceridaemia. *Heart* 85: 544–548, 2001.

8 Omega-3 Fish Oils and Insulin Resistance

Sidika E. Kasim-Karakas

CONTENTS

I. CLINICAL INDICATIONS FOR N-3 FISH OILS IN DIABETES

It is important to note that fish oils do not lower blood glucose or exert any beneficial effects of glycemic control. The primary indication for fish oils in diabetes has been the treatment of coronary artery disease (CAD) risk factors. Diabetes increases the risk of coronary artery disease by 2.4 to 5.1 times. Although women develop CAD at a later age than men, diabetic women lose this relative protection. Recent research emphasizes the role of fish oils in the prevention and treatment of CAD, especially in diabetic women.[1] In a prospective study, Hu and colleagues[2] examined the association between intake of fish oils and risk of CAD mortality among 5103 female nurses with type 2 diabetes. The relative risk of CAD decreased from 1.0 to 0.36 as the fish intake increased from less than 1 serving per month to 5 or more servings per week. This inverse relationship was confirmed in another prospective cohort study of 229 postmenopausal women who participated in the Estrogen Replacement and Atherosclerosis trial.[3] This study used quantitative coronary angiography and showed that diabetic women who consumed more than 2 servings of fish per week had approximately 3 to 5% less increase in coronary artery stenosis than those women who rarely ate fish. Higher fish consumption was associated with smaller decreases in coronary artery diameter and also fewer new lesions.

It has been known for a long time that fish oils have potent triglyceride lowering effects.[4-7] As the CAD risk research expanded from the traditional risk factors such as hyperlipidemias and hypertension to the newer risk factors such as inflammation, lipid peroxidation, and arterial wall biology, effects of fish oils on these emerging risk factors were examined. Unfortunately, the research specific to diabetes is somewhat limited. Mori and colleagues[8] reported that both EPA and DHA reduced *in vivo* oxidant stress without changing inflammatory markers in hypertensive type 2 diabetic subjects. The same group also investigated changes in platelet aggregation, collagen-stimulated thromboxane release, tissue-type plasminogen activator, plasminogen activator inhibitor-1, von Willebrand factor and p-selectin levels, and flow-mediated and glyceryl-trinitrate-mediated dilatation of the brachial artery.[9] Relative to placebo, DHA but not EPA significantly reduced collagen aggregation and thromboxane release, whereas platelet aggregation, fibrinolysis, or vascular function did not change. It appeared that highly purified DHA might be a more effective antithrombotic agent than EPA. A report from Nomura and colleagues[10] indicated that EPA supplementation reduced monocyte activation markers, platelet activation markers, soluble adhesion molecule E-selectin and the autoantibodies directed against oxidized LDL. These findings suggest that fish oils reduce CAD risk through multiple mechanisms, above and beyond their beneficial effects on the plasma lipids. Unfortunately, it is not yet known whether these beneficial outcomes also occur in diabetic patients.

Another use for fish oils may be in the prevention of diabetes.[11] Suresh and Das[12] tested the effects of individual fatty acids on the development of alloxan induced diabetes in rats. Eicosapentanoic acid and DHA, administered either for 5 d prior to alloxan or along with alloxan, protected against diabetes. *In vitro* studies in a rat insulinoma cell line suggested that EPA and DHA rendered this protective effect by preventing alloxan-induced cytotoxicity. In humans, use of cod liver oil, but not other vitamin D supplements, during the first year of life was associated with a significantly lower risk of type-1 diabetes, suggesting possible protective effects of fish oils.[13]

Thus, patients who have diabetes or who are insulin resistant may be asked to supplement their diet with either fish or fish oils for several reasons. Because earlier studies indicated that fish oils may have adverse effects on glycemic control,[6,14] it is important to review the current information about the effects of fish oils on various aspects of diabetes.

II. MAINTENANCE OF GLUCOSE HOMEOSTASIS

Normal glucose homeostasis is achieved by a delicate balance among pancreatic insulin secretion, hepatic glucose production, and peripheral glucose utilization. A change in any one of these can be compensated for by an alteration in another. For example, impaired insulin action in the peripheral tissues or increased hepatic glucose output can be compensated for by increased pancreatic insulin secretion and hyperinsulinemia. In contrast, improvement in peripheral insulin action may result in decreased pancreatic insulin secretion.

Effects of fish oils on glucose homeostasis have been studied at various levels. Their overall effect on glycemic control is assessed by measuring blood glucose, glycosylated hemoglobin (Hgb A1C), and urine glucose excretion. Secretion of insulin from the pancreas is determined by measuring insulin and C-peptide responses to administration of oral or intravenous glucose, by mixed meal, and by hyperglycemic insulin clamp technique. Hepatic glucose production and peripheral insulin action are assessed by the euglycemic clamp technique and by simultaneous use of radioisotopes. All these assays and techniques have been adapted to animal models. Furthermore, *in vitro* studies were carried out to identify the cellular and molecular mechanisms of the effects of fish oils. In this chapter, the recent research about the effects of fish oils has been reviewed. The studies included in the earlier publication of this chapter[15] have been mentioned briefly.

III. EFFECTS OF N-3 FISH OILS ON GLYCEMIC CONTROL

Earlier clinical studies showed that fish oil supplementation caused either no change[16–19] or deterioration of glycemic control.[6,14] Two recent meta analyses[20,21] concluded that although fish oil supplementation increased fasting glucose by 5 to 7 mg/dl and HgBA1 by 0.15 to 0.2%, these changes were not statistically significant. An evidence-based review of the health effects of the fish oils also found similar elevations in blood glucose and HgBA1 levels, and agreed with the conclusion of the meta analyses that these changes were not significant (Figure 8.1 and Figure 8.2).[22] The studies included in these analyses showed a wide range of changes in fasting blood glucose levels, indicating that individual response to fish oil supplementation can be quite variable. All of the effects of fish oils were reversible after the discontinuation of the therapy.

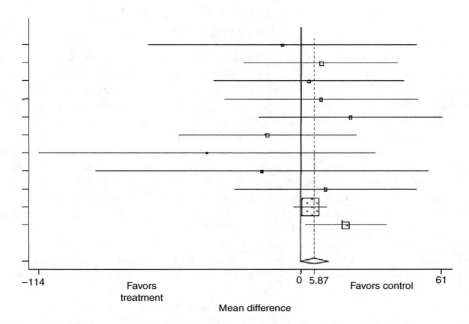

FIGURE 8.1 An evidence based review of the effects of fish oils on fasting blood glucose. (From Effects of omega-3 fatty acids on lipids and glycemic control in type II diabetes and the metabolic syndrome and on inflammatory bowel disease, rheumatoid arthritis, renal disease, systemic lupus erythematosus, and osteoporosis. *Evid Rep Technol Assess (Summ)*: 1–4, 2004. With permission.)

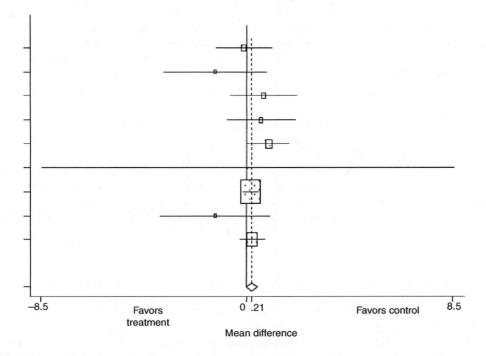

FIGURE 8.2 An evidence based review of the effects of fish oils on HgBA1 levels. (From Effects of omega-3 fatty acids on lipids and glycemic control in type II diabetes and the metabolic syndrome and on inflammatory bowel disease, rheumatoid arthritis, renal disease, systemic lupus erythematosus, and osteoporosis. *Evid Rep Technol Assess (Summ)*: 1–4, 2004. With permission.)

IV. EFFECTS OF N-3 FISH OILS ON PANCREATIC INSULIN SECRETION

Secretagogues such as glucose and arginine stimulate insulin secretion by acting at the β-cell surface receptors and modulating the concentrations of several second messengers, such as cyclic AMP, calcium, and diacylglycerol, which act through protein kinase (PK) A, calcium-calmodulin-dependent PK and PKC, respectively.[23,24] Specific secretagogues may use specific second messengers. Thus, insulin response to a glucose load may be different from the response to a mixed meal. Metabolic products of arachidonic acid and various prostaglandins modulate insulin secretion,[25–31] and fish oils may alter insulin secretion from the pancreas by interfering with the metabolism of arachidonic acid.

Consistent with this concept, several recent experimental studies show that fish oils alter insulin secretion. Studies in rats provided variable results, depending on the strain and gender of the animals and the duration of the supplementation. Holness and colleagues[32] investigated the acute effects of fish oils in female albino Wistar rats. After receiving a saturated fat enriched diet for four weeks, a subgroup of animals was fed a fish oil diet for 24 h. As expected, saturated fat diet caused insulin resistance and hyperinsulinemia. Although this short-term fish oil supplementation reversed the hyperinsulinemia, it failed to correct insulin resistance. Consequently, plasma glucose levels increased. Insulin secretion from the pancreatic islet cells mimicked the *in vivo* findings. When the fish oils were fed throughout the 4-week study, the long-term fish oil supplementation corrected the hyperinsulinemia and increased peripheral glucose disposal.[33] Fish oil feeding also completely reversed hyperinsulinemia in a rat model of sucrose-induced metabolic syndrome.[34] In other rat models of type-2 diabetes,[35] hypertension,[36] and a mouse model of obesity,[37] fish oil feeding improved glucose disposal and decreased plasma glucose but had variable effects on insulin levels. Several earlier studies described previously in detail[15] had reported variable effects of fish oils on insulin secretion.[38–40] In summary, studies in animal models suggest that fish oils acutely decrease insulin secretion from the pancreas and therefore increase plasma glucose. However, long-term administration of fish oils increases peripheral utilization of glucose and reverses the hyperglycemia.

In humans, earlier studies had reported that fish oil either decreased insulin secretion in response to a mixed meal or glucagon[41] oral glucose[42,43] and fructose,[44] or did not affect the insulin secretion.[19,45,46] Recent studies did not investigate the changes in insulin secretion specifically. To my knowledge, there is no evidence in humans to demonstrate that fish oils increase insulin secretion.

V. EFFECTS OF N-3 FISH OILS ON HEPATIC GLUCOSE PRODUCTION

In experimental animals, fish oils interfered with the suppression of hepatic glucose output by insulin.[33] In humans, earlier studies in patients with impaired glucose tolerance and type-2 diabetes reported that fish oil treatment either increased[41,47] or did not change[46,48] hepatic glucose output. A recent study investigating the effects of fish oil, both at rest and during exercise,[49] reported that at rest, fish oils did not affect hepatic glucose production; during exercise, fish oils blunted the increase in hepatic glucose production.

VI. EFFECTS OF N-3 FISH OILS ON PERIPHERAL INSULIN ACTION

As reviewed by Saltiel and Pesin,[50] glucose transport to the cell is accomplished through a series of events that are set into motion by binding of insulin to its receptor. The insulin receptor is a tyrosine kinase that undergoes autophosphorylation upon binding insulin. This increases kinase activity of the receptor for the intracellular insulin receptor substrate proteins (IRS). Once phosphorylated, the IRS proteins interact with phosphatidylinositol 3-kinase (PI3-K) and lead to the production of polyphosphoinositide phosphatidylinositol (3,4,5)-trisphosphate (PIP3), which in turn interacts with and localizes protein kinases such as phosphoinositide-dependent kinase 1 (PDK1).

These kinases then initiate a cascade of phosphorylation events, resulting in the activation of Akt and atypical protein kinase C (PKC), and stimulate the trafficking of Glut 4 vesicles to the plasma membrane, and consequently, transportation of glucose. In the sucrose-fed rat model of insulin resistance, fish oils restore Glut-4 protein quantity in adipocytes but not in muscle.[51] To my knowledge, there is no information about the effects of fish oils on the other steps of this cascade.

In humans, earlier studies showed that fish oils either did not affect[41,45,48] or increased peripheral glucose uptake.[46] A recent study demonstrated that fish oils failed to improve the insulin resistance caused by fructose-feeding in humans.[52] It was previously reported that diabetes decreases the polyunsaturated fatty acid content of adipocyte plasma membrane phospholipids, particularly arachidonic acid.[53] The decrease in the polyunsaturated and saturated fatty acid ratio results in decreased fluidity of the cell membrane and interferes with insulin-binding to the receptor. This can be reversed by increasing the polyunsaturated fat content of the membrane, which is accomplished by using either n-3 or n-6 polyunsaturated fatty acids, and the effect is not limited to n-3 fish oils.[54]

Recent research has demonstrated that in rats, fish oil treatment increased whole body glucose utilization and insulin-stimulated glucose disposal by increasing glucose storage in the skeletal muscle but not the oxidative pathway.[55] In the sucrose-fed insulin resistance model, fish oil reversed the decrease in whole body glucose utilization,[56,57] restored insulin induced glycogen and lipid accumulation in the muscle, and increased the active form of pyruvate dehydrogenase complex and the PDH kinase activities.[56] Similarly, in the high-fat fed rat model, fish oil treatment reversed the insulin resistance.[58] These results are in agreement with the findings of several earlier reports[59–61] described in detail in the previous version of this chapter.[15]

Interestingly, a synthetic metabolite of DHA has been found to have potent insulin sensitizer activity — similar to the thiazolidinedione drugs used for the treatment of diabetes.[62] However, so far, there is no evidence to suggest that fish oil supplementation can lead to the synthesis of such metabolites *in vivo*.

VII. EFFECTS OF N-3 FISH OILS ON ADIPOKINES

It was previously proposed that the effects of fish oils on glucose homeostasis may be related to their effects on the adipose tissue because fish oils caused less weight gain.[63] In recent years, it became clear that the adipose tissue produces and secretes several cytokines (adipokines) that have profound effects on glucose homeostasis. These are adiponectin, TNFα, leptin, and resistin.[64,65] Experimental data suggest that TNFα and resistin promote insulin resistance whereas adiponectin increases insulin sensitivity. There are conflicting data about the effects of leptin.[66] These adipokines may provide a link between obesity and insulin resistance. Obesity is associated with increased serum levels of leptin and TNFα, and reduced levels of adiponectin.[67] As fish oils have anti-inflammatory actions, it is conceivable they also affect the adipokines and therefore alter insulin action. Although there is a large body of literature related to fish oils and cytokines in the fields of infection and inflammation, there is not much information relating these changes to insulin action. In the sucrose-fed rat model of obesity and insulin resistance, both leptin and adiponectin levels are decreased. Here, fish oils decreased insulin resistance and increased plasma levels of adiponectin and leptin.[66,68] In a similar model, fish oils did not affect TNFα levels.[34] On the other hand, in a mouse model of insulin resistance, fish oils reduced TNFα levels but did not correct insulin resistance.[69] To my knowledge, there is no information about the effects of fish oils on resistin.

VIII. CONCLUSION

The primary use of fish oils in diabetic patients is aimed to reduce CAD risk, especially in women. The available evidence does not support a beneficial effect of fish oils on the glycemic control in diabetic patients. Although fish oils decrease insulin resistance and therefore may prevent progression of metabolic syndrome to type-2 diabetes, there is no evidence-based support for this hypothesis. The cytokines secreted by the adipose tissue have profound effects on the peripheral insulin resistance. Effects of fish oils and their metabolites on the adipokines are being studied.

REFERENCES

1. Connor, W.E. Will the dietary intake of fish prevent atherosclerosis in diabetic women? *Am J Clin Nutr* 80: 535–536, 2004.

2. Hu, F.B., Cho, E., Rexrode, K.M., Albert, C.M., and Manson, J.E. Fish and long-chain omega-3 fatty acid intake and risk of coronary heart disease and total mortality in diabetic women. *Circulation* 107: 1852–1857, 2003.

3. Erkkila, A.T., Lichtenstein, A.H., Mozaffarian, D., and Herrington, D.M. Fish intake is associated with a reduced progression of coronary artery atherosclerosis in postmenopausal women with coronary artery disease. *Am J Clin Nutr* 80: 626–632, 2004.

4. Connor, W.E. Importance of n-3 fatty acids in health and disease. *Am J Clin Nutr* 71: 171S–175S, 2000.

5. Harris, W.S., Ginsberg, H.N., Arunakul, N., Shachter, N.S., Windsor, S.L., Adams, M., Berglund, L., and Osmundsen, K. Safety and efficacy of Omacor in severe hypertriglyceridemia. *J Cardiovasc Risk* 4: 385–391, 1997.

6. Kasim, S.E., Stern, B., Khilnani, S., McLin, P., Baciorowski, S., and Jen, K.L. Effects of omega-3 fish oils on lipid metabolism, glycemic control, and blood pressure in type II diabetic patients. *J Clin Endocrinol Metab* 67: 1–5, 1988.

7. Kasim-Karakas, S.E., Herrmann, R., and Almario, R. Effects of omega-3 fatty acids on intravascular lipolysis of very-low-density lipoproteins in humans. *Metabolism* 44: 1223–1230, 1995.

8. Mori, T.A., Woodman, R.J., Burke, V., Puddey, I.B., Croft, K.D., and Beilin, L.J. Effect of eicosapentaenoic acid and docosahexaenoic acid on oxidative stress and inflammatory markers in treated-hypertensive type 2 diabetic subjects. *Free Radic Biol Med* 35: 772–781, 2003.

9. Woodman, R.J., Mori, T.A., Burke, V., Puddey, I.B., Barden, A., Watts, G.F., and Beilin, L.J. Effects of purified eicosapentaenoic acid and docosahexaenoic acid on platelet, fibrinolytic and vascular function in hypertensive type 2 diabetic patients. *Atherosclerosis* 166: 85–93, 2003.

10. Nomura, S., Kanazawa, S., and Fukuhara, S. Effects of eicosapentaenoic acid on platelet activation markers and cell adhesion molecules in hyperlipidemic patients with Type 2 diabetes mellitus. *J Diabetes Complications* 17: 153–159, 2003.

11. Delarue, J., LeFoll, C., Corporeau, C., and Lucas, D. N-3 long chain polyunsaturated fatty acids: a nutritional tool to prevent insulin resistance associated to type 2 diabetes and obesity? *Reprod Nutr Dev* 44: 289–299, 2004.

12. Suresh, Y. and Das, U.N. Long-chain polyunsaturated fatty acids and chemically induced diabetes mellitus: effect of omega-3 fatty acids. *Nutrition* 19: 213–228, 2003.

13. Stene, L.C. and Joner, G. Use of cod liver oil during the first year of life is associated with lower risk of childhood-onset type 1 diabetes: a large, population-based, case-control study. *Am J Clin Nutr* 78: 1128–1134, 2003.

14. Malasanos, T.H. and Stacpoole, P.W. Biological effects of omega-3 fatty acids in diabetes mellitus. *Diabetes Care* 14: 1160–1179, 1991.

15. Kasim-Karakas, S. *Omega-3 fatty acids and insulin resistance.* CRC Press, Boca Raton, FL, 2000.

16. Connor, W.E., Prince, M.J., Ullmann, D., Riddle, M., Hatcher, L., Smith, F.E., and Wilson, D. The hypotriglyceridemic effect of fish oil in adult-onset diabetes without adverse glucose control. *Ann N Y Acad Sci* 683: 337–340, 1993.

17. Sheehan, J.P., Wei, I.W., Ulchaker, M., and Tserng, K.Y. Effect of high fiber intake in fish oil-treated patients with non-insulin-dependent diabetes mellitus. *Am J Clin Nutr* 66: 1183–1187, 1997.

18. Sirtori, C.R., Paoletti, R., Mancini, M., Crepaldi, G., Manzato, E., Rivellese, A., Pamparana, F., and Stragliotto, E. N-3 fatty acids do not lead to an increased diabetic risk in patients with hyperlipidemia and abnormal glucose tolerance. Italian Fish Oil Multicenter Study. *Am J Clin Nutr* 65: 1874–1881, 1997.

19. Toft, I., Bonaa, K.H., Ingebretsen, O.C., Nordoy, A., and Jenssen, T. Effects of n-3 polyunsaturated fatty acids on glucose homeostasis and blood pressure in essential hypertension: a randomized, controlled trial. *Ann Intern Med* 123: 911–918, 1995.

20. Friedberg, C.E., Janssen, M.J., Heine, R.J., and Grobbee, D.E. Fish oil and glycemic control in diabetes: a meta-analysis. *Diabetes Care* 21: 494–500, 1998.

21. Montori, V.M., Farmer, A., Wollan, P.C., and Dinneen, S.F. Fish oil supplementation in type 2 diabetes: a quantitative systematic review. *Diabetes Care* 23: 1407–1415, 2000.

22. Effects of omega-3 fatty acids on lipids and glycemic control in type II diabetes and the metabolic syndrome and on inflammatory bowel disease, rheumatoid arthritis, renal disease, systemic lupus erythematosus, and osteoporosis. *Evid Rep Technol Assess (Summ)*: 1–4, 2004.

23. Corkey, B.E., Deeney, J.T., Yaney, G.C., Tornheim, K., and Prentki, M. The role of long-chain fatty acyl-CoA esters in beta-cell signal transduction. *J Nutr* 130: 299S–304S, 2000.

24. Deeney, J.T., Prentki, M., and Corkey, B.E. Metabolic control of beta-cell function. *Semin Cell Dev Biol* 11: 267–275, 2000.

25. Kowluru, A. Differential regulation by fatty acids of protein histidine phosphorylation in rat pancreatic islets. *Mol Cell Biochem* 266: 175–182, 2004.

26. Metz, S., VanRollins, M., Strife, R., Fujimoto, W., and Robertson, R.P. Lipoxygenase pathway in islet endocrine cells. Oxidative metabolism of arachidonic acid promotes insulin release. *J Clin Invest* 71: 1191–1205, 1983.

27. Metz, S.A., Fujimoto, W.Y., and Robertson, R.P. A role for the lipoxygenase pathway of arachidonic acid metabolism in glucose- and glucagon-induced insulin secretion. *Life Sci* 32: 903–910, 1983.

28. Metz, S.A., Fujimoto, W.Y., and Robertson, R.P. Oxygenation products of arachidonic acid: third messengers for insulin release. *J Allergy Clin Immunol* 74: 391–402, 1984.

29. Pareja, A., Tinahones, F.J., Soriguer, F.J., Monzon, A., Esteva de Antonio, I., Garcia-Arnes, J., Olveira, G., Ruiz de Adana, M.S. Unsaturated fatty acids alter the insulin secretion response of the islets of Langerhans in vitro. *Diabetes Res Clin Pract* 38: 143–149, 1997.

30. Robertson, R.P. Arachidonic acid metabolism, the endocrine pancreas, and diabetes mellitus. *Pharmacol Ther* 24: 91–106, 1984.

31. Robertson, R.P. Arachidonic acid metabolite regulation of insulin secretion. *Diabetes Metab Rev* 2: 261–296, 1986.

32. Holness, M.J., Smith, N.D., Greenwood, G.K., and Sugden, M.C. Acute omega-3 fatty acid enrichment selectively reverses high-saturated fat feeding-induced insulin hypersecretion but does not improve peripheral insulin resistance. *Diabetes* 53(Suppl. 1): S166–171, 2004.

33. Holness, M.J., Greenwood, G.K., Smith, N.D., and Sugden, M.C. Diabetogenic impact of long-chain omega-3 fatty acids on pancreatic beta-cell function and the regulation of endogenous glucose production. *Endocrinology* 144: 3958–3968, 2003.

34. Aguilera, A.A., Diaz, G.H., Barcelata, M.L., Guerrero, O.A., and Ros, R.M. Effects of fish oil on hypertension, plasma lipids, and tumor necrosis factor-alpha in rats with sucrose-induced metabolic syndrome. *J Nutr Biochem* 15: 350–357, 2004.

35. Minami, A., Ishimura, N., Sakamoto, S., Takishita, E., Mawatari, K., Okada, K., and Nakaya, Y. Effect of eicosapentaenoic acid ethyl ester v. oleic acid-rich safflower oil on insulin resistance in type 2 diabetic model rats with hypertriacylglycerolaemia. *Br J Nutr* 87: 157–162, 2002.

36. Ajiro, K., Sawamura, M., Ikeda, K., Nara, Y., Nishimura, M., Ishida, H., Seino, Y., and Yamori, Y. Beneficial effects of fish oil on glucose metabolism in spontaneously hypertensive rats. *Clin Exp Pharmacol Physiol* 27: 412–415, 2000.

37. Steerenberg, P.A., Beekhof, P.K., Feskens, E.J., Lips, C.J., Hoppener, J.W., and Beems, R.B. Long-term effect of fish oil diet on basal and stimulated plasma glucose and insulin levels in ob/ob mice. *Diabetes Nutr Metab* 15: 205–214, 2002.

38. Chicco, A., D'Alessandro, M.E., Karabatas, L., Gutman, R., and Lombardo, Y.B. Effect of moderate levels of dietary fish oil on insulin secretion and sensitivity, and pancreas insulin content in normal rats. *Ann Nutr Metab* 40: 61–70, 1996.

39. Lombardo, Y.B., Chicco, A., D'Alessandro, M.E., Martinelli, M., Soria, A., and Gutman, R. Dietary fish oil normalize dyslipidemia and glucose intolerance with unchanged insulin levels in rats fed a high sucrose diet. *Biochim Biophys Acta* 1299: 175–182, 1996.

40. Miura, T., Ohnishi, Y., Takagi, S., Sawamura, M., Yasuda, N., Ishida, H., Tanigawa, K., Yamori, Y., and Seino, Y. A comparative study of high-fat diet containing fish oil or lard on blood glucose in genetically diabetic (db/db) mice. *J Nutr Sci Vitaminol (Tokyo)* 43: 225–231, 1997.

41. Glauber, H., Wallace, P., Griver, K., and Brechtel, G. Adverse metabolic effect of omega-3 fatty acids in non-insulin-dependent diabetes mellitus. *Ann Intern Med* 108: 663–668, 1988.

42. Stacpoole, P.W., Alig, J., Ammon, L., and Crockett, S.E. Dose-response effects of dietary marine oil on carbohydrate and lipid metabolism in normal subjects and patients with hypertriglyceridemia. *Metabolism* 38: 946–956, 1989.

43. Zambon, S., Friday, K.E., Childs, M.T., Fujimoto, W.Y., Bierman, E.L., and Ensinck, J.W. Effect of glyburide and omega 3 fatty acid dietary supplements on glucose and lipid metabolism in patients with non-insulin-dependent diabetes mellitus. *Am J Clin Nutr* 56: 447–454, 1992.

44. Delarue, J., Couet, C., Cohen, R., Brechot, J.F., Antoine, J.M., and Lamisse, F. Effects of fish oil on metabolic responses to oral fructose and glucose loads in healthy humans. *Am J Physiol* 270: E353–362, 1996.

45. Annuzzi, G., Rivellese, A., Capaldo, B., Di Marino, L., Iovine, C., Marotta, G., and Riccardi, G. A controlled study on the effects of n-3 fatty acids on lipid and glucose metabolism in non-insulin-dependent diabetic patients. *Atherosclerosis* 87: 65–73, 1991.

46. Fasching, P., Ratheiser, K., Waldhausl, W., Rohac, M., Osterrode, W., Nowotny, P., and Vierhapper, H. Metabolic effects of fish-oil supplementation in patients with impaired glucose tolerance. *Diabetes* 40: 583–589, 1991.

47. Puhakainen, I., Ahola, I., and Yki-Jarvinen, H. Dietary supplementation with n-3 fatty acids increases gluconeogenesis from glycerol but not hepatic glucose production in patients with non-insulin-dependent diabetes mellitus. *Am J Clin Nutr* 61: 121–126, 1995.

48. Borkman, M., Chisholm, D.J., Furler, S.M., Storlien, L.H., Kraegen, E.W., Simons, L.A., and Chesterman, C.N. Effects of fish oil supplementation on glucose and lipid metabolism in NIDDM. *Diabetes* 38: 1314–1319, 1989.

49. Delarue, J., Labarthe, F., and Cohen, R. Fish-oil supplementation reduces stimulation of plasma glucose fluxes during exercise in untrained males. *Br J Nutr* 90: 777–786, 2003.

50. Saltiel, A.R. and Pessin, J.E. Insulin signaling pathways in time and space. *Trends Cell Biol* 12: 65–71, 2002.

51. Peyron-Caso, E., Fluteau-Nadler, S., Kabir, M., Guerre-Millo, M., Quignard-Boulange, A., Slama, G., and Rizkalla, S.W. Regulation of glucose transport and transporter 4 (GLUT-4) in muscle and adipocytes of sucrose-fed rats: effects of N-3 poly- and monounsaturated fatty acids. *Horm Metab Res* 34: 360–366, 2002.

52. Faeh, D., Minehira, K., Schwarz, J.M., Periasami, R., Seongsu, P., and Tappy, L. Effect of fructose overfeeding and fish oil administration on hepatic de novo lipogenesis and insulin sensitivity in healthy men. *Diabetes* 54: 1907–1913, 2005.

53. Clandinin, M.T., Cheema, S., Field, C.J., and Baracos, V.E. Dietary lipids influence insulin action. *Ann N Y Acad Sci* 683: 151–163, 1993.

54. Field, C.J., Ryan, E.A., Thomson, A.B., and Clandinin, M.T. Dietary fat and the diabetic state alter insulin binding and the fatty acyl composition of the adipocyte plasma membrane. *Biochem J* 253: 417–424, 1988.

55. D'Alessandro, M.E., Lombardo, Y.B., and Chicco, A. Effect of dietary fish oil on insulin sensitivity and metabolic fate of glucose in the skeletal muscle of normal rats. *Ann Nutr Metab* 46: 114–120, 2002.

56. D'Alessandro, M.E., Chicco, A., Karabatas, L., and Lombardo, Y.B. Role of skeletal muscle on impaired insulin sensitivity in rats fed a sucrose-rich diet: effect of moderate levels of dietary fish oil. *J Nutr Biochem* 11: 273–280, 2000.

57. Pighin, D., Karabatas, L., Rossi, A., Chicco, A., Basabe, J.C., and Lombardo, Y.B. Fish oil affects pancreatic fat storage, pyruvate dehydrogenase complex activity and insulin secretion in rats fed a sucrose-rich diet. *J Nutr* 133: 4095–4101, 2003.

58. Simoncikova, P., Wein, S., Gasperikova, D., Ukropec, J., Certik, M., Klimes, I., and Sebokova, E. Comparison of the extrapancreatic action of gamma-linolenic acid and n-3 PUFAs in the high fat diet-induced insulin resistance [corrected]. *Endocr Regul* 36: 143–149, 2002.

59. Zimmet, P., Alberti, K.G., and Shaw, J. Global and societal implications of the diabetes epidemic. *Nature* 414: 782–787, 2001.

60. Sebokova, E., Klimes, I., Moss, R., Mitkova, A., Wiersma, M., and Bohov, P. Decreased glucose transporter protein (GLUT4) in skeletal muscle of hypertriglyceridaemic insulin-resistant rat. *Physiol Res* 44: 87–92, 1995.

61. Mori, Y., Murakawa, Y., Katoh, S., Hata, S., Yokoyama, J., Tajima, N., Ikeda, Y., Nobukata, H., Ishikawa, T., and Shibutani, Y. Influence of highly purified eicosapentaenoic acid ethyl ester on insulin resistance in the Otsuka Long-Evans Tokushima Fatty rat, a model of spontaneous non-insulin-dependent diabetes mellitus. *Metabolism* 46: 1458–1464, 1997.

62. Yamamoto, K., Itoh, T., Abe, D., Shimizu, M., Kanda, T., Koyama, T., Nishikawa, M., Tamai, T., Ooizumi, H., and Yamada, S. Identification of putative metabolites of docosahexaenoic acid as potent PPARgamma agonists and antidiabetic agents. *Bioorg Med Chem Lett* 15: 517–522, 2005.

63. Hill, J.O., Peters, J.C., Lin, D., Yakubu, F., Greene, H., and Swift, L. Lipid accumulation and body fat distribution is influenced by type of dietary fat fed to rats. *Int J Obes Relat Metab Disord* 17: 223–236, 1993.

64. Grimble, R.F. Inflammatory status and insulin resistance. *Curr Opin Clin Nutr Metab Care* 5: 551–559, 2002.

65. Havel, P.J. Control of energy homeostasis and insulin action by adipocyte hormones: leptin, acylation stimulating protein, and adiponectin. *Curr Opin Lipidol* 13: 51–59, 2002.

66. Rossi, A.S., Lombardo, Y.B., Lacorte, J.M., Chicco, A.G., Rouault, C., Slama, G., and Rizkalla, S.W. Dietary fish oil positively regulates plasma leptin and adiponectin levels in sucrose-fed, insulin-resistant rats. *Am J Physiol Regul Integr Comp Physiol* 289: R486–R494, 2005.

67. Aldhahi, W. and Hamdy, O. Adipokines, inflammation, and the endothelium in diabetes. *Curr Diabetes Rep* 3: 293–298, 2003.

68. Peyron-Caso, E., Taverna, M., Guerre-Millo, M., Veronese, A., Pacher, N., Slama, G., and Rizkalla, S.W. Dietary (n-3) polyunsaturated fatty acids up-regulate plasma leptin in insulin-resistant rats. *J Nutr* 132: 2235–2240, 2002.

69. Muurling, M., Mensink, R.P., Pijl, H., Romijn, J.A., Havekes, L.M., and Voshol, P.J. A fish oil diet does not reverse insulin resistance despite decreased adipose tissue TNF-alpha protein concentration in ApoE-3*Leiden mice. *J Nutr* 133: 3350–3355, 2003.

9 Antioxidant Vitamin and Phytochemical Content of Fresh and Processed Pepper Fruit (*Capsicum annuum*)

Luke R. Howard and Robert E.C. Wildman

CONTENTS

I. INTRODUCTION

Capsicum species are a New World crop belonging to the Solanacae family. Chiles have been cultivated for thousands of years, and they are one of the oldest domesticated crops. Most cultivars grown in the U.S. belong to the species *C. annuum* and are typically classified according to fruit shape, flavor, and culinary uses. In addition to *C. annuum* species, *C. frutescens* (tabasco) and *C. chinense* (habanero) are commonly cultivated and used for culinary and medicinal purposes. The classification and varieties of peppers grown in the U.S.,[1,2] and the production, technology, chemistry, and quality of *Capsicum* spp., have been reviewed extensively.[3–7]

    Capsicum spp. exhibit great genetic diversity in terms of color, size, shape, and chemical composition. Researchers have recently recognized that *Capsicum* fruit also vary greatly in their content of antioxidant vitamins and phytochemicals. This information may be important for human health and nutrition as consumers incorporate more peppers into their diets. The goal of this chapter is to survey the antioxidant vitamin and phytochemical content of different *Capsicum* species, types, and cultivars, and to determine the effects of postharvest handling and processing on the levels of these important phytonutrients.

II. FRUITS AND VEGETABLES FOR DISEASE PREVENTION

Epidemiological studies indicate that antioxidants present in fruits and vegetables, including β-carotene and vitamins C and E, may be important in prevention of numerous degenerative conditions, including various types of cancer, cardiovascular disease, stroke, atherosclerosis, and cataracts.[8–10] Oxidative damage catalyzed by reactive oxygen species (ROS) has been implicated in over 100 degenerative conditions.[11] ROS cause damage to cellular membranes, proteins, and DNA, which increases the susceptibility of cells to chronic diseases. Oxidative damage in the body is exacerbated when the balance of ROS exceeds the amount of endogenous antioxidants. The human body has several enzymatic and nonenzymatic defense systems to regulate ROS *in vivo*, but these defense mechanisms are thought to deteriorate with aging. Consumption of fruits and vegetables that are rich in antioxidant nutrients may afford additional protection against ROS-mediated disorders. Scientists have recently recognized that fruits and vegetables are not only a good source of antioxidant vitamins but also an excellent source of other essential dietary phytochemicals that can retard the risk of degenerative diseases.[12] The potential health effects of phytochemicals are associated with numerous mechanisms, including prevention of oxidant formation, scavenging of activated oxidants, reduction of reactive intermediates, induction of repair systems, and promotion of apoptosis.[13]

Of interest is how and why fruits and vegetables generate nutraceutical compounds and for what purpose. With regard to peppers, the presence of different antioxidative enzymes and their corresponding metabolites in pepper peroxisomes implies that these organelles might be an important pool of antioxidants in fruit cells, where these enzymes could also act as modulators of signal molecules (O_2^-, H_2O_2) during fruit maturation.[14] In one study of the peroxisomal fractions of green and red pepper fruits (*Capsicum annuum* L., type Lamuyo), the quantity and activity of antioxidant enzyme systems was generally higher in green than in red fruits.[14]

In this work, the purification and characterisation of peroxisomes from fruits of a higher plant was carried out, and their antioxidative enzymatic and nonenzymatic content was investigated. Green and red pepper fruits (*Capsicum annuum* L., type Lamuyo) were used in this study. The analysis by electron microscopy showed that peroxisomes from both types of fruits contained crystalline cores that varied in shape and size, and the presence of chloroplasts and chromoplasts in green and red pepper fruits, respectively, was confirmed.

III. ASCORBIC ACID

Capsicum fruit have long been recognized as an excellent source of ascorbic acid, which is a required nutrient for humans. Svent-Gyorgyi isolated ascorbic acid from paprika fruit in the early 1930s, and subsequently identified the compound in 1933.[15] Ascorbic acid has strong reducing properties due to its enediol structure, which is conjugated with the carbonyl group in a lactone ring[16] (Figure 9.1). In the presence of oxygen, ascorbic acid is degraded to dehydroascorbic acid (DHA), which still retains vitamin C activity. However, upon further oxidation, the lactone ring of DHA is destroyed, resulting in formation of 2,3-diketogulonic acid and loss of vitamin activity. Ascorbic acid is required for collagen formation and prevention of scurvy. Researchers have postulated a role of ascorbic acid in the prevention of degenerative conditions, including cancer, heart disease, cataracts, and stimulation of the immune system.[17] Prevention of chronic diseases may be attributed to the ascorbate function as an aqueous reducing agent. Ascorbate can reduce superoxide, hydroxyl, and other ROS, which may be present in both intracellular and extracellular matrices. Ascorbate within cells participates as an electron donor, as part of the interaction between iron and ferritin. Extracellularly, ascorbate may act in concert with tocopherols in lipid membranes, to quench ROS and prevent lipid peroxidation. Thus, ascorbate may help prevent the oxidation of low-density lipoprotein (LDL), which is thought to be a major initiating step in the process of atherosclerosis. The role of ascorbate in cancer prevention may be attributed to its ability to block

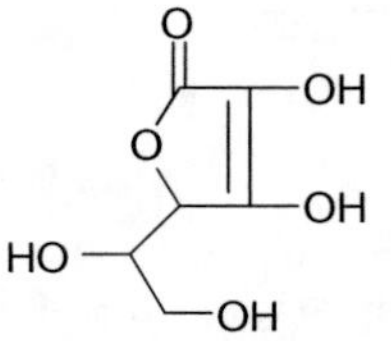

L-ascorbic acid

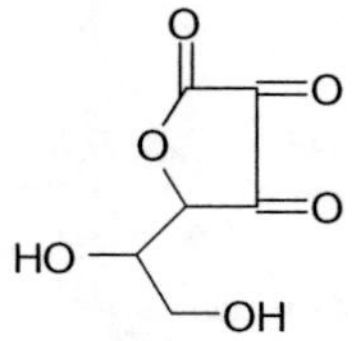

L-dehydroascorbic acid

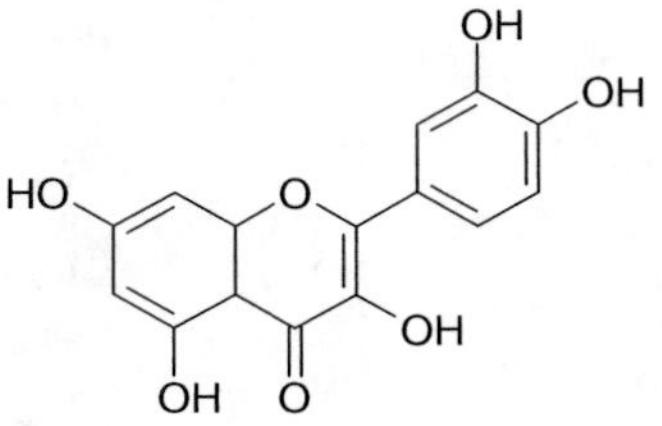

Quercetin

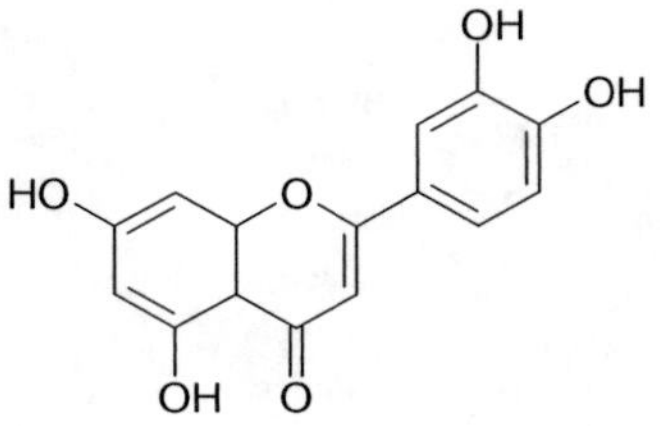

Luteolin

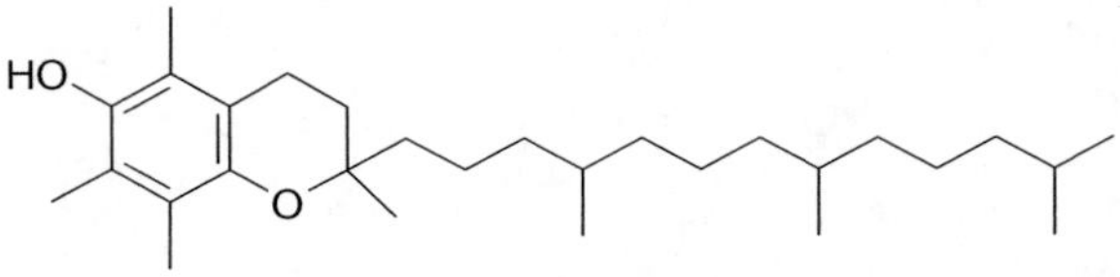

α-tocopherol

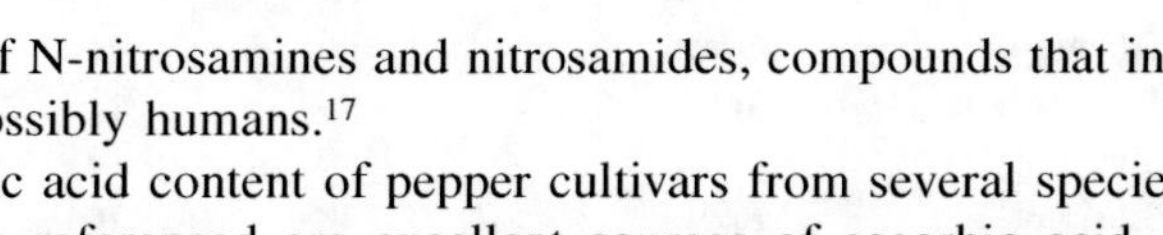

γ-tocopherol

FIGURE 9.1 Ascorbic acid, flavonoids, and tocopherols in *Capsicum* fruit.

the formation of N-nitrosamines and nitrosamides, compounds that induce cancer in experimental animals, and possibly humans.[17]

The ascorbic acid content of pepper cultivars from several species is shown in Table 9.1.[18–22] All the peppers referenced are excellent sources of ascorbic acid, with many of the cultivars contributing over 100% of the Recommended Daily Intakes (RDIs) in the U.S. The current RDI for vitamin C is 90 mg/d for adult men and 75 mg/d for adult women who are not pregnant or lactating. The only pepper cultivars that fail to meet at least 50% of the RDI for ascorbic acid are the chile-type cultivars NuMex RNaky, New Mexico, and B-18 at the green stage and the tabasco-type called *cv tabasco* at the green stage.

The ascorbic acid content of most of the pepper types increases during ripening, with much higher levels found in mature peppers at the final stage of ripening.[23–26] Higher levels of ascorbic acid observed during ripening may be related to light intensity and greater levels of glucose, the precursor of ascorbic acid.[27] Because total and reducing sugars increase during pepper fruit ripening, the elevated ascorbic acid levels in mature fruit may reflect greater synthesis due to the higher

TABLE 9.1
Ascorbic Acid Content of Fresh *Capsicum* Fruit

Species	Type	Cultivar	Maturity	mg/100 g Fresh Weight	%RDI[a] Male	%RDI[a] Female	Ref.
C.annuum	Ancho	San Luis Ancho	Green	168	187	224	18
	Bell	Dove	White	77	86	103	18
		Dove	Light Orange	103	114	137	18
		Ivory	White	89	99	119	18
		Ivory	Light Yellow	110	122	147	18
		Blue Jay	Purple	95	106	127	18
		Blue Jay	Orange	123	137	164	18
		Lilac	Purple	67	74	89	18
		Lilac	Orange	104	116	139	18
		Valencia	Green	119	132	159	18
		Valencia	Orange	73	81	97	18
		Oriole	Green	91	101	121	18
		Oriole	Orange	86	96	115	18
		Black Bird	Green	66	73	88	18
		Black Bird	Black	62	69	83	18
		Chocolate Beauty	Green	62	69	83	18
		Chocolate Beauty	Brown	100	111	133	18
		Cardinal	Green	102	113	136	18
		Cardinal	Brown	124	138	165	18
		King Arthur	Green	84	93	112	18
		King Arthur	Red	87	97	116	18
		Var. 862R	Green	88	98	117	18
		Var. 862R	Red	98	109	131	18
		Red Bell G	Green	95	106	127	18
		Red Bell G	Red	96	106	127	18
		Red Bell C	Green	72	80	96	18
		Red Bell C	Red	107	119	143	18
		Klondike Bell	Green	112	124	149	18
		Klondike Bell	Yellow	109	121	145	18
		Canary	Green	112	124	149	18
		Canary	Yellow	108	120	144	18
		Orobelle	Green	162	180	216	18
		Orobelle	Yellow	95	106	127	18
		Golden Bell	Green	106	118	141	18
		Golden Bell	Yellow	90	100	120	18
		Tam Bel-2	Green	109	121	145	20
		Tam Bel-2	Red	148	164	197	20
		Grande Rio-66	Green	98	109	131	20
		Grande Rio-66	Red	149	166	199	20
		Yellow Bell-47	Green	114	127	152	21
		Yellow Bell-47	Orange	135	150	180	21
	Cascabella	Peto Cascabella	Yellow	172	191	229	21
		Peto Cascabella	Red	202	224	269	21
	Cayenne	Mesilla	Green	63	70	84	21
		Mesilla	Red	102	113	136	21
	Chile	New Mexico-6	Green	141	157	188	20
		New Mexico-6	Red	205	228	273	20
		New Mexico-6	Green	130	144	173	18

TABLE 9.1 *(Continued)*
Ascorbic Acid Content of Fresh *Capsicum* Fruit

Species	Type	Cultivar	Maturity	mg/100 g Fresh Weight	%RDI[a] Male	Female	Ref.
		Tam Mild Chile	Green	155	172	207	20
		Tam Mild Chile	Red	233	259	311	20
		Green Chile	Green	122	136	163	18
		Sandia	Green	71	79	95	22
		Sandia	Breaker	220	244	293	22
		Sandia	Red	239	266	319	22
		New Mexico 6-4	Green	40	44	53	22
		New Mexico 6-4	Breaker	122	136	163	22
		New Mexico 6-4	Red	155	172	207	22
		NuMex RNaky	Green	28	31	37	22
		NuMex RNaky	Breaker	145	161	193	22
		NuMex RNaky	Red	164	182	219	22
		B-18	Green	15	17	20	22
		B-18	Breaker	91	101	121	22
		B-18	Red	186	207	248	22
	Jalapeno	Jalapeno-M	Green	173	192	231	20
		Jalapeno-M	Red	179	199	239	20
		Tam Veracruz	Green	101	112	135	20
		Tam Veracruz	Red	144	160	192	20
		Tam Veracruz	Green	72	80	96	18
		Tam Mild	Green	66	73	88	18
		Mitla	Green	49	54	65	18
		Jaloro	Yellow	131	146	175	18
		Sweet Jalapeno	Green	54	60	72	18
	Serrano	Hidalgo	Green	141	157	188	20
		Hidalgo	Red	263	292	351	20
	Yellow Wax	Hungarian Yellow	Yellow	114	127	152	18
		Long Hot Yellow	Yellow	114	127	152	18
		Gold Spike	Yellow	115	128	153	18
		Inferno	Yellow	92	102	123	21
		Inferno	Red	138	153	184	21
		Rio Grande Gold	Red	243	270	324	20
		Sante Fe Grande	Red	187	208	249	20
C. chinense	Habanero	Red Savina	Red	192	213	256	21
		Francisca	Orange	203	226	271	21
C. frutescens	Tabasco	McIhenny Tabasco	Green	15	17	20	21
		McIhenny Tabasco	Red	75	83	100	21

[a] Recommended daily intakes, adult males = 90 mg/100 g, adult females = 75 mg/100 g.

levels of sugar precursors.[22] In addition to maturation, variation in ascorbic acid content between pepper types and cultivars may be attributed to differences in genetics, fertilization practices, and environmental growing conditions. The effects of fertilization on ascorbic acid content of peppers have been studied. Ascorbic acid content of pepper fruits increased with increasing levels of phosphorus up to 48 kg/ha, at varying levels of nitrogen (0 to 100 kg/ha),[28] and applications including combinations of organic matter + nitrogen + phosphorus increased ascorbic acid content of capsicum fruit.[29] Application of bioregulators may also affect ascorbic acid content of peppers.

The ascorbic acid and citric acid contents of "bell" peppers increased with gibberellic acid treatment,[30] whereas in another study the ascorbic acid content of bell peppers was not affected by ethylene treatment.[31]

A. EFFECTS OF POSTHARVEST HANDLING AND PROCESSING ON ASCORBIC ACID CONTENT

The ascorbic acid content of peppers is influenced by postharvest handling, packaging, and processing. Fresh peppers are sensitive to chilling injury, so they should be stored at 8 to 12°C (46 to 54°F), at a relative humidity of 90 to 95%. Under optimum conditions, peppers may be stored for 2 to 3 weeks after harvest. However, the nutritional quality of peppers may change after harvest, handling, and transportation en route to various markets, especially under abusive handling conditions. The ascorbic acid content of sweet bell peppers from wholesale and retail markets and simulated consumer storage was reported to be similar, although a wide range of ascorbic acid was apparent among individual market samples.[32] Thus, it appears that the average concentration of ascorbic acid does not change appreciably from wholesale marketing to consumption. The ascorbic acid content of bell peppers was influenced by storage temperature but not by packaging in perforated films.[33] Ascorbic acid levels declined 10% after 4 d storage at 10°C (50°F), whereas a 25% loss occurred after 4 d storage at 20°C (68°F). In contrast, the ascorbic acid content of bell peppers was unaffected by storage temperature 2°C (35°F) and 8°C (46°F), varying levels of carbon dioxide (5, 10, 20%), or storage time (6, 9, and 12 d).[34] In another study, the ascorbic acid content of bell peppers increased with storage at 13°C (55°F), and with subsequent ripening at 20°C (68°F).[35] Meanwhile, fresh peppers (*Capsicum annuum* L., variety California) in their green and red ripe stages were stored at 20°C (68°F) for 7 and 19 d and the ascorbic acid content was noted to increase as both stages matured during storage.[25]

The ascorbic acid content of the Morron pepper of "Fresno de la Vega" (*Capsicum annuum* L.), a big, sweet variety cultivated in the province of Leon (northwestern Spain) increased as the peppers ripened.[23] For green mature, breaker and red peppers values of 107.3 ± 1.84, 129.6 ± 3.11, and 154.3 ± 7.56 mg/100 g edible portion were found. The vitamin C content for green mature and breaker peppers stored at room temperature (20°C, 68°F) increased up to 10 d of storage, reaching similar values as those obtained for red peppers direct from the plant. However, stored red ripe peppers showed a significant loss in vitamin C content, around 25%. Refrigeration at 4°C (39°F) for up to 20 d did not change the ascorbic acid content, except for red peppers, which showed losses around 15%.

Ascorbic acid content of fresh peppers may also be affected by postharvest chlorinated water treatments. Green bell peppers dipped in 50, 100, 150, and 200 μg/ml hypochlorite lost 6, 9, 10, and 18% of their initial total ascorbic acid concentrations, respectively.[36] It was recommended that chlorine concentrations of 50 to 100 μg/ml during a 20-min contact time could be used to control microbial spoilage without affecting overall quality of bell peppers.

Although the effects of modified-atmosphere storage on ascorbic acid retention in whole fresh bell peppers are conflicting, minimally processed peppers appear to benefit from modified atmosphere storage. Precut jalapeno peppers stored in modified-atmosphere packages (MAP, 5% O_2 and 4% CO_2) retained 85% of their ascorbic acid after 15 d storage at 13°C (55°F), whereas air-stored peppers retained only 56%.[37] The MAP treatment also retarded the conversion of L-ascorbic to dehydroascorbic acid. Similar results were reported for sweet blanched bell peppers stored in reduced-oxygen atmospheres.[38] Ascorbic acid levels were better retained in storage atmospheres of 2% O_2 and 4% O_2 than were samples stored in air. Conversion of ascorbic acid to dehydroascorbic acid was also retarded under reduced-oxygen storage.

Due to its water solubility, ascorbic acid is readily leached from pepper fruit during water blanching and pasteurization in salt–acid brines. The ascorbic acid content of the Morron pepper of "Fresno de la Vega" showed reductions of 12 and 20–25% during the water blanching and subsequent canning process.[23] Jalapeno peppers that were blanched prior to pasteurization lost 75% of their ascorbic acid,[20] whereas a 40% loss of ascorbic acid occurred during water blanching of green bell peppers, and a 15% loss occurred during steam blanching.[39] In another study, bell peppers blanched in water lost 24% of their ascorbic acid, though microwave blanched peppers lost only 15%.[40] Ascorbic acid content of unblanched "yellow banana" peppers declined substantially during pasteurization and storage, with only 10% remaining after 124 d.[41] Calcium chloride brine treatment did not affect ascorbic acid retention in pasteurized yellow banana peppers. In contrast, initial ascorbic acid levels were retained in jalapeno peppers after blanching and pasteurization.[42]

Blanching may also affect ascorbic acid retention in frozen peppers. Unblanched "padron" peppers lost 97% of their ascorbic acid within 1 month of freezing, whereas blanching resulted in a 28% loss, followed by an additional 10% loss after 12 months frozen storage.[43] In another study, average ascorbic acid losses of ten pepper cultivars that were blanched and stored for 12 months at −12°C (10°F) were 63%, while unblanched cultivars lost 71%.[44] Differences in ascorbic acid losses in these studies may be attributed to differences in pepper genetics, brine composition, blanching method, and pasteurization time and temperature.

Ascorbic acid content of dehydrated peppers is influenced by blanching and drying methods. Paprika fruit lost 63% of its ascorbic acid content when naturally dried, whereas losses of 4 to 54% were observed when freshly harvested and overripe fruit were dried using a forced-air method.[45] Other processing parameters may also influence ascorbic acid retention. A 40% loss of ascorbic acid in paprika powder was noted after centrifugation prior to drying, and a 73% loss occurred in carmelized paprika.[46] In another study, drying time and temperature did not affect the ascorbic acid content of dehydrated green bell peppers, but after 8 weeks of storage, blanched peppers dried for 8 h at 60°C (140°F) contained less ascorbic acid than unblanched peppers.[47] Unblanched peppers dried for 12 h at 49°C (120°F) contained more ascorbic acid than blanched peppers.

IV. FLAVONOIDS

Pepper fruit are particularly rich in flavonoids, a large class of compounds ubiquitous in plants, that exhibit antioxidant activity, depending on the number and location of hydroxyl groups present.[48] In addition to antioxidant function, flavonoids are reported to possess numerous biological, pharmacological, and medicinal properties, including vasodilatory, anticarcinogenic, immune-stimulating, antiallergenic, antiviral, and estrogenic effects, as well as inhibition of various enzymes involved in carcinogenesis.[49] In addition, many epidemiological studies indicate an inverse association between the intake of flavonols and flavones and the risk of coronary heart disease,[50–52] stroke,[53] and lung cancer.[54–55]

Much progress has been made over the past decade in the identification and quantification of flavonoids and phenolic acids in capsicum fruit due to advancements in HPLC, HPLC-mass spectrometry, and NMR techniques. Suskrano and Yeoman[56] identified three hydroxycinnamic acid derivatives: p-coumaroyl, caffeoyl, and 3,4-dimethoxycinnamoyl glycosides, and four flavonoid compounds, although only two were identified: quercetin 3-O-rhamnoside and luteolin 7-O-glucoside. Iorizzi and colleagues[57] identified three hydroxycinnamic acids in Capsicum annuum L. var. acuminatum fruit, cis-p-coumaric acid-β-D-glucoside, trans-sinapoyl β-D-glucoside, and vanilloyl β-D-glucoside, as well as one flavonoid, quercetin 3-O-rhamnoside. They also identified a unique lignan glycoside (icariside E_5) that possesses antioxidant properties. Materska and colleagues[58] identified nine compounds in pericarp tissue of hot pepper fruit (Capsicum annuum L., var. Bronowicka Ostra). The compounds identified included 3 hydroxycinnamic acid derivatives: trans-p-feruloylalcohol-4-)-(6-(2-methyl-3-hydroxypropionyl) glucoside, trans-p-feruoyl-β-D-glucoside, and trans-p-sinapoyl-β-D-glucoside, as well as six flavonoids: luteolin-7-O-(2-apiosyl-4-glucosyl-6-malonoyl)-glucoside, quercetin 3-O-α-L-rhamnoside-7-O-β-D-glucoside, luteolin 6-C-β-D-glucoside-8-C-α-L-arabinoside, apigenin 6-C-β-D-glucoside-8-C-L-arabinoside, luteolin 7-O-[2-((β-

D-apiosyl)-β-D-glucoside], and quercetin 3-O-α-L-rhamnoside. In a subsequent study, Materska and Perucka[59] evaluated 4 cultivars of *Capsicum annuum* L. fruit for phenolic content and antioxidant capacity and reported that sinapoyl and feruoyl glucosides were the predominant components in red pepper, ranging in concentration from 32 to 42 mg/100 g dry weight, and 15 to 36 mg/100 g dry weight, respectively, whereas quercetin 3-O-L-rhamnoside was the major component in green pepper, ranging in concentration from 33 to 99 mg/100 g dry weight. The antioxidant capacities evaluated by the β-carotene-linoleic acid and DPPH systems correlated highly with phenolic content in the fraction containing phenolic acids and flavonoids. Marin and colleagues[24] conducted a detailed characterization of sweet pepper phenolics (*Capsicum annuum* L., cv. Vergasa), and reported five hydroxycinnamic acid derivatives and 25 flavonoids in pericarp tissue. In addition to the hydroxycinnamic acid derivatives and flavonoids, previously identified by Materska and colleagues[58] in hot peppers, they identified several novel compounds including 4 flavonoid O-glycosides: luteolin 7-O-(2-apiosyl-6-acetyl) glucoside, chrysoeriol 7-O-(2-apiosyl-6-acetyl) glucoside, luteolin 7-O-(2-apiosyl-di-acetyl) glucoside, and luteolin 7-O-2-apiosyl-6-malonyl) glucoside. Additionally, 12 flavonoid glycosides were identified, which included 2 acylated derivatives, luteolin 6-C-(6-malonyl)-hexoside-8-C-hexoside, and luteolin 6-C-(6-malony)-hexoside-8-C-pentoside. Quercetin 3-O-rhamnoside and luteolin 7-O-(2-apiosyl-6-malonyl) glucoside were the predominant flavonoids present in red fruit, showing concentrations of 0.31 mg/100 g fresh weight and 0.39 mg/100 g fresh weight, respectively. The concentrations of total hydroxycinnamic acids and total flavonoids in red fruit were 0.44 mg/100 g fresh weight and 2.54 mg/100 g fresh weight, respectively.

The flavonoid content of different pepper types and cultivars is shown in Table 9.2.[60] Peppers contain both quercetin (a flavonol) and luteolin (a flavone). Quercetin has a hydroxyl group at C-3 in the aromatic ring, while luteolin does not (see Figure 9.1). The structural differences are important since the presence of a hydroxyl group at C-3 is reported to result in greater free radical-scavenging efficiency.[48] In plant cells, flavonoids occur as glycosides, with sugars bound typically at the C-3 position. Flavonoids are commonly quantified in the aglycone form after acid hydrolysis. Flavonoid levels vary greatly among pepper types and cultivars with total levels ranging from 1 to 852 mg/kg. Interestingly, *C. annuum* cultivars contain higher levels of flavonoids than *C. chinense* cultivars. Low levels of flavonoids in the pungent *C. chinense* peppers may indicate diversion of phenolic precursors from flavonoid to capsaicinoid synthesis. An exception is the *C. frutescens* cv. tabasco, which contains much higher levels of luteolin than the other *Capsicum* species and cultivars. It appears that fruit from different *Capsicum* species vary greatly in their genetic capacity for synthesizing specific flavonoids. Plant breeders and molecular biologists may take advantage of this genetic variability to increase the flavonoid content of *Capsicum* fruit. The exceptionally high flavonoid levels reported by Lee and colleagues[18] may be due to differences in genetics and environmental conditions in which the peppers were grown. Environmental stress during plant growth has been shown to stimulate the phenylpropanoid pathway and production of various phenolic compounds.

Increasing luteolin levels in pepper fruit may be important for prevention of coronary heart disease. A luteolin-rich artichoke extract was recently shown to protect LDL from oxidation *in vitro*, which may be due to its antioxidant function or ability to sequester prooxidant metal ions.[61] Additionally, luteolin does not complex with copper ions to produce oxidative damage to DNA, which contrasts with the prooxidant effect observed for quercetin.[62]

Total flavonoid content of pepper cultivars generally declines as fruit ripens and changes color. For instance, immature green pepper of sweet peppers (*Capsicum annuum* L.) cv. Vergasa had a very high phenolic content, but green, immature red, and red ripe peppers showed a four- to fivefold reduction.[24] Red fruit generally contain higher levels of hydroxycinnamic acids than green fruit, whereas green fruit contain higher levels of flavonoids than red fruit.[21,24,59] However, exceptions to this rule include the cayenne cv. Mesilla, in which the flavonoid content increased during maturation, and the "long yellow" cv. Inferno, and tabasco cv. Tabasco, in which no change in flavonoid content occurred during ripening.[21] In terms of antioxidant capacity, red fruit generally have greater radical scavenging capacity than green fruit, [21,57,59] which may be attributed to higher levels of hydroxy-

TABLE 9.2
Flavonoid Content of Fresh *Capsicum* Fruit

Species	Type	Cultivar	Maturity	Quercetin	Luteolin	Total Flavonoids	Ref.
				mg/kg Fresh Weight			
C. annuum	Ancho	San Luis Ancho	Green	276	34	310	18
	Bell	Yellow Bell	Green	22	11	33	21
		Yellow Bell	Orange	13	9	22	21
		Tam B-2	Green	44	9	53	60
		Romanian Sweet	Yellow	219	26	245	60
		YB 244	Yellow	81	10	91	60
		YB 126	Yellow	112	15	127	60
	Cascabella	Peto Cascabella	Yellow	42	16	58	21
		Peto Cascabella	Red	24	6	30	21
		Tam Cascabella	Yellow	67	30	97	60
	Cayenne	Mesilla	Green	25	17	42	21
		Mesilla	Red	11	6	17	21
	Chile	New Mexico-6	Green	126	51	177	18
		Green Chile	Green	210	52	262	18
	Jalapeno	Mitla	Green	40	14	54	18
		Tam Mild	Green	18	10	28	18
		Jaloro	Yellow	151	38	189	18
		Sweet Jalapeno	Green	45	6	51	18
		TAES Jaloro	Yellow	52	18	70	60
	Serrano	Hidalgo	Green	160	41	201	18
	Yellow Wax	Hungarian Yellow	Yellow	784	68	852	18
		Long Hot Yellow	Yellow	447	104	551	18
		Gold Spike	Yellow	288	37	325	18
		Inferno	Yellow	68	17	85	21
		Inferno	Red	65	17	82	21
		Short Sweet Yellow	Yellow	88	18	106	60
		Long Sweet Yellow	Yellow	56	9	65	60
		Short Hot Yellow	Yellow	62	14	76	60
		Long Hot Yellow	Yellow	78	15	93	60
		TAES Hot Yellow	Yellow	79	17	96	60
		Sweet Banana	Yellow	43	6	49	60
C. chinense	Habanero	Francisca	Orange	5	1	6	21
		Red Savina	Red	1	ND	1	21
C. frutescens	Tabasco	McIlhenny Tabasco	Green	2	44	46	21
		McIlhenny Tabasco	Red	1	36	37	21

cinnamic acid glycosides and capsaicinoids in the ripe fruit.[59] The loss of flavonoids observed during ripening of most cultivars is consistent with reported flavonoid losses that occur during maturation of *C. frutescens* fruit.[56] Flavonoid losses during ripening may reflect metabolic conversion of flavonoids to secondary phenolic compounds.[63] The oxidoreductase enzymes polyphenol oxidase[64] and peroxidase[65,66] may play a role in degradation of flavonols during maturation and senescence.

A. POSTHARVEST HANDLING AND EFFECT OF PROCESSING ON FLAVONOID CONTENT

Little information is available on the effects of postharvest handling and processing on flavonoid content of pepper fruit. The effect of pasteurization and storage on flavonoid content in yellow banana peppers has been studied.[41] Quercetin and luteolin contents declined 40 to 45% during 4 months' storage, whereas calcium chloride brine treatment did not affect flavonoid retention. Apparently, flavonoids are leached into the salt–acid brine during pasteurization and storage. Future studies should focus on methods to stabilize flavonoids during postharvest handling and processing.

V. TOCOPHEROLS

Capsicum fruit, especially in the dried form, are an excellent source of tocopherols. Vitamin E compounds including tocopherols and tocotrienols are well recognized for their effective inhibition of lipid oxidation in foods and biological systems.[67] The tocopherols are polyisoprenoid derivatives, which have a saturated C16 side chain (phytol), centers of asymmetry at the 2, 4′, and 8′ positions, and variable methyl substitution at R_1, R_2, and R_3[16] (see Figure 9.1). The antioxidant activity of tocopherols is due to their ability to donate their hydrogen ions to lipid free radicals, thereby neutralizing the radical and forming the tocopheroxy radical.

Tocopherols have been shown to be effective scavengers of peroxyl and superoxide radicals in lipid systems. Epidemiological and short-term intervention studies suggest that vitamin E may reduce the risk of coronary heart disease, some cancers, cataracts, and diabetes, and slow the progression of neurological diseases. The health effects of vitamin E may be related to numerous mechanisms, including protection of cells from oxidative damage; protection of LDL from oxidation; enhancement of the immune system; reduction of oxidative damage of specialized tissues such as the eye lens, nerve tissue, blood vessels, and cartilage; reduction of cholesterol synthesis by inhibition of the enzyme HMG-Co A reductase; and enhancement of the antioxidant status of the digesta.[68]

The α-tocopherol content of pepper types and cultivars is shown in Table 9.3.[69,70] γ-Tocopherol is found in pepper seeds, whereas α-tocopherol is found in pericarp tissue. Dried paprika and "New Mexico" type peppers used in the spice industry are a fair source of γ-tocopherol, and an excellent source of α-tocopherol. New Mexico type cultivars contain higher levels of γ-tocopherol in seeds than paprika cultivars.[22] At the red succulent stage, the γ-tocopherol content of seeds from four New Mexican pepper cultivars ranged from 35.2 to 47.5 mg/100 g.[22] These levels of γ-tocopherol would provide 2.3 to 3.2% of the RDI for adult males and females, per 1-g serving.

The α-tocopherol content of pericarp tissue in both paprika and New Mexico cultivars is exceptionally high, but the paprika cultivars are a better source of α-tocopherol. Per 100 g serving, paprika cultivars provide 107 to 1980% of the RDI for adult males and females, whereas the New Mexico type cultivars provide 13 to 207% of the RDI for adult males and females. Although small amounts of dried capsicum powders are typically used for food preparation, their exceptionally high levels of tocopherols may be an important source of vitamin E in the human diet. A 1-g serving of dried paprika would provide 1 to 20% of the RDI for adult males and females, whereas a similar serving of dried New Mexican peppers would provide only 0.1 to 2% of the RDI for adult males and females. Thus, dried peppers, especially paprika type, may be a significant source for vitamin E as people incorporate greater amounts of ethnic foods containing dried peppers into their diets.

The α- and γ-tocopherol content of pepper fruit is influenced by maturity. γ-Tocopherol content in seeds generally increases until the red succulent stage and then declines, while α-tocopherol content in pericarp tissue increases from the mature green to red fully dry stages.[22,46,69] The α-tocopherol content in pericarp tissue is dependent on lipid content, which varies according to ripening stage and variety.[69] A high correlation exists between oil content and α-tocopherol content in dry matter. The percentage of oil and α-tocopherol content is highest in red dried paprika fruit with 80% dry matter.

A. EFFECT OF PROCESSING ON TOCOPHEROL CONTENT OF PEPPERS

Color retention of dried paprika powder may be related to levels of γ-tocopherol in seeds,[71] but conflicting results are reported. Several studies[46,72] showed that color retention of paprika was

TABLE 9.3
Tocopherol Content of Fresh *Capsicum* Fruit

Species	Type	Cultivar	Maturity	α-Tocopherol[a] Pericarp (mg/100 g DW)	%RDI[b] M	F	Ref.
C. annuum	Paprika	Vandel	Green	16	107	200	69
		Vandel	Red	28	187	350	69
		Gamba	Green	17	113	410	69
		Gamba	Red	33	220	410	69
		Mild	Green	26	173	330	69
		Mild	Green-red	46	307	580	69
		Mild	Red	65	433	810	69
		Mild	Red-dried	68	453	850	69
		SZ-20	Ripe	47	313	590	70
		Mihalytelki	Ripe	33	220	410	70
		SZ-80	Ripe	38	253	480	70
		F-03	Ripe	61	407	760	70
		SZ-178	Ripe	56	380	710	70
		Km-622[c]	Green	17	113	210	46
		Km-622[c]	Breaker-1	48	320	606	46
		Km-622[c]	Breaker-2	85	567	1,060	46
		Km-622[c]	Faint red	92	613	1,150	46
		Km-622[c]	Deep red	109	727	1,360	46
		Km-622[d]	Green	34	227	430	46
		Km-622[d]	Breaker-1	35	233	440	46
		Km-662[d]	Breaker-2	43	287	540	46
		Km-622[d]	Faint red	48	320	606	46
		Km-622[d]	Deep red	115	767	1,440	46
		Mihalyteleki	Green	43	287	540	45
		Mihalyteleki	Breaker-1	39	260	490	45
		Mihalyteleki	Breaker-2	42	280	530	45
		Mihalyteleki	Faint red	38	253	480	45
		Mihalyteleki	Deep red	40	267	500	45
		K-50	Deep red	180	1200	2,250	45
		Km-622	Deep red	192	1280	2,400	45
		K-801	Deep red	161	1073	2,010	45
		Semi-Determ. 7/92	Deep red	297	1980	3,710	45
		SZ-80	Deep red	139	927	1,740	45
		K-V2	Deep red	205	1367	2,560	45
		K-90	Deep red	265	1767	3,310	45
		Strain-100	Deep red	141	940	1,760	45
		Mihalyteleki	Deep red	133	887	1,660	45
		SZ-20	Deep red	152	1013	1,900	45
		Bibor	Deep red	95	633	1,190	45
		Napfeny	Deep red	90	600	1,130	45
		Negral	Deep red	87	580	1,090	45
	New Mexico	Sandia	Green	5	33	60	22
		Sandia	Breaker	9	60	110	22
		Sandia	Red	17	113	210	22
		Sandia	Red-partially dry	10	67	130	22
		Sandia	Red-dried	19	127	240	22

Continued.

TABLE 9.3 *(Continued)*
Tocopherol Content of Fresh *Capsicum* Fruit

Species	Type	Cultivar	Maturity	α-Tocopherol[a] Pericarp (mg/100 g DW)	%RDI[b] M	%RDI[b] F	Ref.
		New Mexico 6-4	Green	6	40	80	22
		New Mexico 6-4	Breaker	6	40	80	22
		New Mexico 6-4	Red succulent	16	107	200	22
		New Mexico 6-4	Red-partially dry	12	80	150	22
		New Mexico 6-4	Red-dried	7	47	90	22
		Nu-Mex R-Naky	Green	3	20	40	22
		Nu-Mex R-Naky	Breaker	8	53	100	22
		Nu-Mex R-Naky	Red succulent	13	87	160	22
		Nu-Mex R-Naky	Red-partially dry	11	73	140	22
		Nu-Mex R-Naky	Red-dried	21	140	260	22
		B-18	Green	2	13	30	22
		B-18	Breaker	8	53	100	22
		B-18	Red succulent	24	160	300	22
		B-18	Red-partially dry	15	100	190	22
		B-18	Red-dried	31	207	390	22

[a] α-Tocopherol = 1.0 mg αTE.
[b] Recommended daily intakes, adult males and females = 15 mg αTE.
[c] Fruit harvested and analyzed in 1994.
[d] Fruit harvested and analyzed in 1995.

improved with the addition of seeds, though other studies[71,72] found that the color stability of paprika was unaffected by addition of seeds. Conflicting results obtained between the studies may be related to varying levels of α-tocopherol in the peppers studied. Tocopherol content of dried paprika powder may also be influenced by cultivar, maturity, and drying method.[45] Tocopherol retention was lower in naturally dried samples than in forced-air-dried paprika. The α-tocopherol content increased during natural drying, reaching a maximum concentration when the dry matter of the fruit was between 53 and 68%, whereas a decrease in tocopherol content was observed with fully dry fruits having a dry matter content of 89%. For forced-air-dried fruit, utilization of fresh fruit as the starting material resulted in substantial losses of α-tocopherol. The best retention of α-tocopherol was obtained by drying overripe fruit having 53 to 68% dry matter. Two cultivars evaluated (Km-622 and V-2) lost 12.4 and 41.2% of α-tocopherol, respectively, when their overripe fruits were dried by the forced-air method. Thus, genetic variation should be taken into account when investigating the processing quality of new paprika cultivars.

Tocopherol content is affected by additional processing parameters, including predrying centrifugation and carmelization during drying.[46] The α-tocopherol content of "paprika" fruit was highest in carmelized samples, indicating that carmelization of sugar afforded protection against tocopherol degradation during drying. The α-tocopherol content of centrifuged paprika was lower than values from noncentrifuged samples, indicating that it was removed from paprika fruit during the centrifugation step.

VI. CAROTENOIDS

Varying composition and concentration of carotenoids in capsicum are responsible for diversely colored fruit. Common carotenoids in capsicum fruits are shown in Figure 9.2. Capsicum species

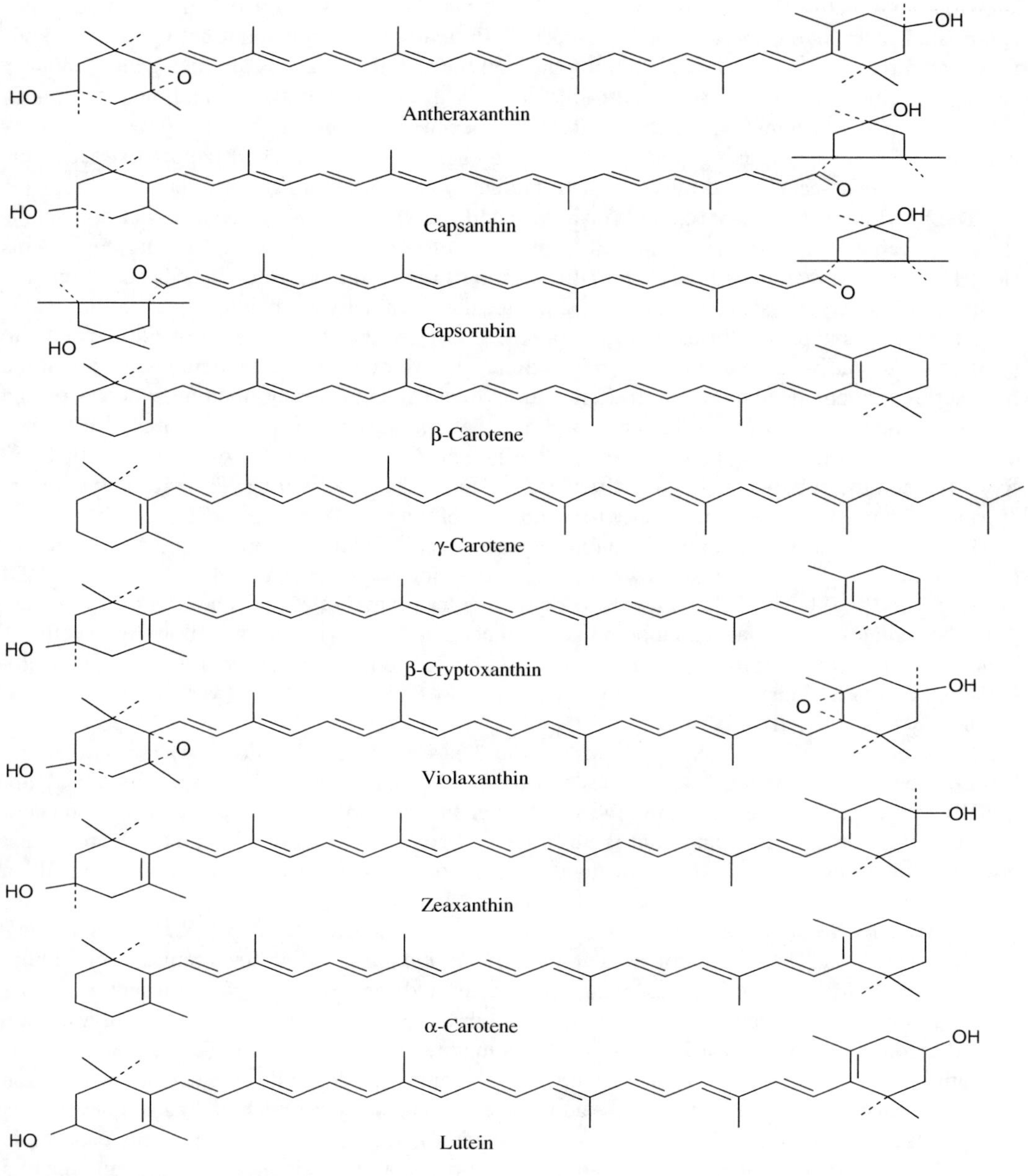

FIGURE 9.2 Major carotenoids in *Capsicum* fruit.

have been selectively bred to obtain fruit with various colors including white, green, yellow, orange, brown, black, and purple. The ketocarotenoids capsanthin and capsorubin contribute to red color, while α- and β-carotene, zeaxanthin, lutein, and β-cryptoxanthin are responsible for yellow-orange color. The carotenoids and additional pigments responsible for exotic colored brown and purple fruit have not been characterized.

The pepper carotenoids α- and β-carotene and β-cryptoxanthin contribute to provitamin A activity. However, pepper fruit are also a good source of oxygenated carotenoids, or xanthophylls, which vary considerably in composition and concentration due to differences in genetics and fruit maturation.[46,73] Oxygenated carotenoids, which do not possess provitamin A activity, have been shown to be effective free radical scavengers,[74] and may be important for prevention of advanced age-related macular degeneration and cataracts.[75] In addition to antioxidant activity, carotenoids may play a role in cancer chemoprevention through their ability to act as antimutagens,[76] enhance cell-to-cell communication,[77] act as anti-inflammatory and antitumor agents, and induce detoxification of enzyme systems.[78] Carotenoids present in pepper fruit may also be important in retarding changes associated with aging. Incorporation of a capsanthin-rich red bell pepper extract in the diet of senescence-accelerated mice resulted in amelioration of learning impairment.[79]

The provitamin A content (α- and β-carotene and β-cryptoxanthin) of fresh pepper cultivars is shown in Table 9.4.[80] Provitamin A values range from nondetectible to 502 retinal equivalents (RE)/100 g. The wide range of provitamin A carotenoids in the cultivars referenced is not surprising, as the cultivars vary greatly in visual color. Cultivars that terminally ripen at the green, light-yellow, or yellow stages typically have less provitamin A activity due to reduced genetic capacity to synthesize α- and β-carotene and β-cryptoxanthin.[73,81,82] Many studies have demonstrated that the β-, ε-series carotenoids in capsicum fruit, including lutein, decline during ripening, whereas α- and β-carotene increase, and other pigments, β-cryptoxanthin, capsanthin, and zeaxanthin are formed *de novo*.[46,73,82,83] However, some exceptions are notable. The bell cv. Yellow Bell contains 257 RE/100 g and the yellow wax cv. Rio Grande Gold contains 502 RE/100 g. These yellow cultivars apparently contain the genetic capacity to synthesize provitamin A carotenoids.

Pepper fruit that ripen to orange and red stages contain high levels of provitamin A carotenoids, contributing 3 to 52% of the RDI (900 µg RE/100 g) for adult males and 4 to 67% of the RDI (700 µg RE/100 g) for adult females. Pepper cultivars that contain >25% of the RDI of provitamin A for both males and females include bell cv. Grande Rio 66 (red), bell cv. Yellow Bell (yellow), chile cv. Tam Mild Chile (red), chile cv. New Mexico-6 (red), jalapeno cv. Tam Veracruz (red), serrano cv. TAES Hidalgo (red), yellow wax cv. Rio Grande Gold (yellow), and tabasco cv. McIlhenny tabasco (red).

Carotenoids in paprika cultivars have been studied extensively, because they are used in the form of powders and oleoresins as spices and food colorants. Dried paprika products are exceptionally rich in carotenoids, including the ketocarotenoids capsanthin and capsorubin, which occur only in red *Capsicum* fruit, and contribute to the red color and quality of paprika oleoresin and powder. Numerous studies have documented the composition and concentration of carotenoids in dried paprika products that vary greatly in color.[71,84–88]

Efforts have been made to increase the carotenoid content of dried paprika through plant-breeding programs. The total carotenoid content of *C. annuum* breeding lines ranged from 390 to 16,600 µg/g.[86] Most of the red pigments were esterified, and diesters were present at higher concentrations than monoesters. An important observation was that a narrow range of variation existed among the ratios of carotenoids present in the breeding lines. This indicates that the levels of synthesis and accumulation of various carotenoid pigments are controlled genetically by common regulatory genes. Plant breeders may take advantage of this genetic trait in breeding and developing new paprika cultivars with elevated levels of carotenoids, including the red pigments capsanthin and capsorubin, which affect the color and quality of paprika oleoresin and powder. One breeding line 4126 was identified,[86] which contained 240 mg of total carotenoids/100 g fresh weight, of which 20 mg was β-carotene. This level of β-carotene is comparable to levels found in carrots, but the total carotenoid content of this paprika breeding line is sixfold higher than levels found in carrots. Thus, breeding new pepper cultivars for elevated total carotenoid content appears to be feasible and may be beneficial for improving human health and nutrition.

In addition to genetics, the carotenoid content of peppers may be influenced significantly by environmental growing conditions. In a study involving five cultivars each of nonpungent and pungent pepper cultivars, grown in the field and a glasshouse, it was found that glasshouse grown peppers had much higher levels of carotenoids than those grown in the field.[83] The authors suggested that the more consistent and protected conditions in the glasshouse may have caused carotenoid levels to be increased, especially at the red stage.

TABLE 9.4
Provitamin A Content of Fresh *Capsicum* Fruit

Species	Type	Cultivar	Maturity	RE (µg)/100 g Fresh Weight	%RDIa Male	%RDIa Female	Ref.
C. annuum	Bell	Dove	White	16	2	2	19
		Dove	Light Orange	29	3	4	19
		Ivory	White	14	2	2	19
		Ivory	Light Yellow	46	5	7	19
		Blue Jay	White	22	2	3	19
		Blue Jay	Orange	59	7	8	19
		Lilac	Purple	17	2	2	19
		Lilac	Orange	86	10	12	19
		Valencia	Green	25	3	4	19
		Valencia	Orange	26	3	4	19
		Oriole	Green	37	4	5	19
		Oriole	Orange	99	11	14	19
		Black Bird	Green	32	4	5	19
		Black Bird	Black	41	5	6	19
		Chocolate Beauty	Green	38	4	5	19
		Chocolate Beauty	Brown	108	12	15	19
		Cardinal	Green	33	4	5	19
		Cardinal	Red	110	12	16	19
		King Arthur	Green	33	4	5	19
		King Arthur	Red	127	14	18	19
		Var. 862R	Green	38	4	5	19
		Var. 862R	Red	119	13	17	19
		Red Bell G	Green	44	5	6	19
		Red Bell G	Red	80	9	11	19
		Red Bell C	Green	35	4	5	19
		Red Bell C	Red	52	6	7	19
		Klondike Bell	Green	40	4	6	19
		Klondike Bell	Yellow	31	3	4	19
		Canary	Green	31	3	4	19
		Canary	Yellow	31	3	4	19
		Orobelle	Green	49	5	7	19
		Orobelle	Yellow	36	4	5	19
		Golden Bell	Green	37	4	5	19
		Golden Bell	Yellow	32	4	5	19
		Tam Bel 2	Green	33	4	5	19
		Tam Bel 2	Red	64	7	9	19
		Grande Rio-66	Green	81	9	12	19
		Grande Rio-66	Red	253	28	36	19
		Yellow Bell	Green	31	3	4	21
		Yellow Bell	Yellow	257	29	37	21
	Caribe	Caloro	Green	2	<1	<1	80
	Cascabella	Peto Cascabella	Yellow	4	<1	<1	21
		Peto Cascabella	Red	137	15	20	21
	Cayenne	Mesilla	Green	42	5	6	21
		Mesilla	Red	214	24	31	21
	Chile	New Mexico-6	Green	79	9	11	20

Continued.

TABLE 9.4 *(Continued)*
Provitamin A Content of Fresh *Capsicum* Fruit

Species	Type	Cultivar	Maturity	RE (μg)/100 g Fresh Weight	%RDIa Male	%RDIa Female	Ref.
		New Mexico-6	Red	259	29	37	20
		Tam Mild Chile	Green	69	8	10	20
		Tam Mild Chile	Red	470	52	67	20
	Jalapeno	Jalapeno-M	Green	56	6	8	20
		Jalapeno-M	Red	168	19	24	20
		Tam Veracruz	Green	64	7	9	20
		Tam Veracruz	Red	252	28	36	20
		Tam Mild Jalapeno	Green	44	5	6	20
		Tam Mild Jalapeno	Red	83	9	12	20
	Poblano	Ancho	Green	111	12	16	80
	Serrano	TAES Hidalgo	Green	141	16	20	20
		TAES Hidalgo	Red	263	29	38	20
		Tampiqueno 74	Green	87	10	12	80
	Yellow Wax	Rio Grande Gold	Yellow	502	56	72	20
		Sante Fe Gold	Yellow	27	3	4	20
		Inferno	Yellow	4	<1	<1	21
		Inferno	Red	104	12	15	21
	Verde	Anaheim	Green	30	3	4	80
C. chinense	Habanero	Francisca	Orange	ND	ND	ND	21
		Red Savina	Red	191	21	27	21
C. frutescens	Tabasco	McIlhenney Tabasco	Green	29	3	4	21
		McIlhenney Tabasco	Red	336	37	48	21

[a] Recommended daily intakes, adult males = 900 μg/RE, adult females = 700 μg/RE.

Dried paprika is an excellent source of vitamin A. A 1-g serving of freshly ground paprika provides 13 to 24% and 17 to 31% of the RDI for males and females, respectively.[45] Thus, dried paprika is an excellent source of various carotenoid pigments that may be important for prevention of chronic diseases.

The carotenoid content of fresh and dried paprika fruit is also affected by the ripening stage. The β-carotene content of the fresh paprika fruit cv. Mihalyteleki increased from 419 μg/g dry matter at the green stage to 468 μg/g at the deep red stage, whereas the β-carotene content of dried fruit increased from 610 μg/g at the green stage to 652 μg/g at the deep red stage.[45]

A. EFFECTS OF POSTHARVEST HANDLING AND PROCESSING ON CAROTENOID CONTENT

The carotenoid content of peppers is influenced by postharvest handling, storage time, and temperature. Green bell peppers obtained from a roadside market on the day of harvest had much greater levels of α- and β-carotene than peppers purchased from a supermarket, which incurred 7 to 14 d of storage and transportation.[89] Storage temperature may also influence carotenoid retention. Yolo Wonder green bell peppers stored for 7 and 14 d at 7.2° and 21°C (45 and 70°F) retained 94 and 78% of carotene, respectively.[90]

Major carotenoid losses may occur when peppers are physically wounded during minimal processing. A 32% loss of β-carotene and 48% loss of α-carotene occurred when jalapeno peppers were sliced into rings and stored in perforated packages for 12 d at 40°C (104°F), and an additional

3 d at 13°C (55°F).[37] Modified atmosphere storage (5% O_2 and 4% CO_2) protected against carotenoid degradation, with losses of 13 and 8% for β- and α-carotene, respectively, when pepper rings were stored under similar conditions as air-stored peppers. The beneficial effect of MAP storage on carotenoid retention may be due to inhibition of the enzymes peroxidase and lipoxygenase, which have been shown to cause destruction of β-carotene[91,92] or reduced chemical oxidation, due to the low oxygen levels inside the packages.

Carotenoids are better retained than ascorbic acid during pasteurization in salt-acid brines due to their hydrophobic properties, which prevent leaching into the brine solution. Pasteurization resulted in 13% reduction in β-carotene in mature green jalapenos and 31% reduction in mature red jalapenos,[20] whereas a 30% decrease in β-carotene occurred in pasteurized red bell peppers.[93] Loss of provitamin A in mature green jalapenos during pasteurization was 17%, and mature red jalapenos lost 33%.[20]

Carotenoid loss is recognized as the major cause of color degradation in dried red pepper products. Loss of the provitamin A carotenoids, β-carotene, and β-cryptoxanthin is associated with color loss during paprika processing. The red pigments capsorubin and capsanthin are more stable during drying and milling than the yellow pigments β-carotene and β-cryptoxanthin.[82] Esterified carotenoids show a greater degree of stability during processing than unesterified or free carotenoids. Thus, the ketocarotenoids capsanthin and capsorubin, which occur predominately in the diester form, are more stable than zeaxanthin, which occurs in the free, monoesterfied, or diesterified forms; β-cryptoxanthin, which occurs in only the free and monoesterified forms; and β-carotene, which occurs only in the free form. Greater susceptibility of free and monoesterified carotenoids to drying and milling results in provitamin A activity losses of 67 and 81% in the paprika varieties Agridulce and Bola, respectively.[82]

In addition to carotenoid composition and maturity, other factors influencing carotenoid stability in dried red peppers include levels of natural antioxidants, water activity, drying temperature and technique, particle size, package atmosphere, and storage atmosphere and temperature. Dehydration of fresh ripe paprika fruit by forced-air drying resulted in 8% loss of β-carotene, whereas overripe fruit dried using the same technique lost 53 to 55%.[45] Forced-air drying resulted in greater retention of β-carotene in dried paprika than naturally dried fruit. Higher drying temperatures are also detrimental to color stability of dried paprika.

The concentrations of natural antioxidants present in paprika have been shown to affect color and carotenoid stability. β-Carotene concentration in paprika fruit declined slightly during the first 2 months of storage, and then declined substantially during the next 2 months.[45] Loss of β-carotene paralleled ascorbic acid and α-tocopherol losses, which indicates that depletion of natural antioxidants accelerates β-carotene losses. It has been proposed that tocopherols provide a first oxidation barrier, whereas ascorbic acid is required for tocopherol regeneration, and the carotenoids function as a second barrier against lipid oxidation.[94] Because levels of natural antioxidants play an important role in prevention of carotenoid degradation and color stability, several researchers have investigated the efficacy of supplemental antioxidant treatments. Addition of pepper seeds, which are rich in γ-tocopherol, to paprika and New Mexican chile powders has been shown to prevent color and carotenoid degradation.[46,69,71,72] Other treatments that have been used successfully to prevent color degradation during dehydration and storage of dried peppers include the synthetic antioxidant ethoxyquin, δ-tocopherol, and ascorbic acid.[95,96] In addition to antioxidant treatments, removal of oxygen in the package atmosphere by nitrogen flushing has been shown to stabilize the color of dried red peppers.[94] Water activity and particle size of dried red pepper powders are also important considerations for carotenoid stability. It is recommended that coarse particles be used and powders dried to a water activity of 0.30.[97]

Chile powders are commonly treated with gamma irradiation as a microbial disinfection step. Color stability of dried red pepper powders was not affected by irradiation doses of 0, 1, 5, and 10 kGy, which indicates that carotenoids are relatively stable during irradiation.[98]

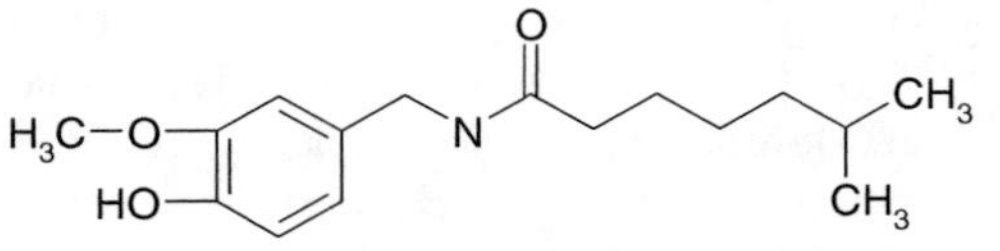

Nordihydrocapsaicin

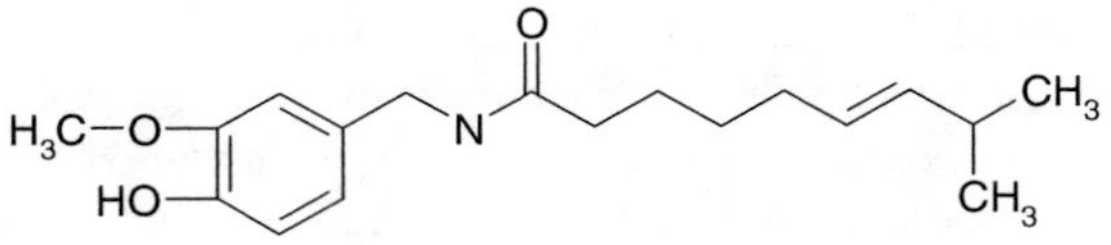

Capsaicin

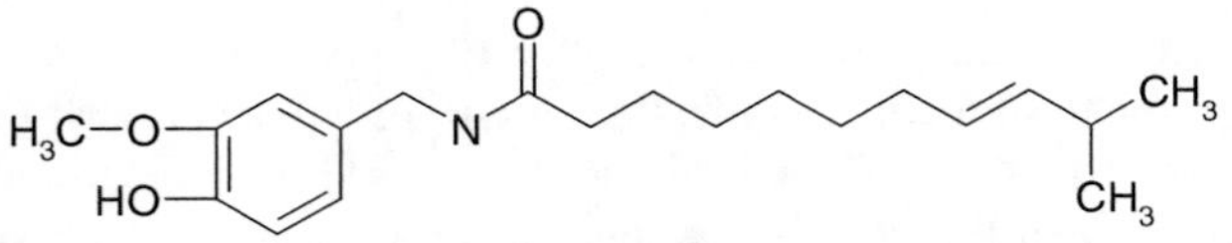

Dihydrocapsaicin

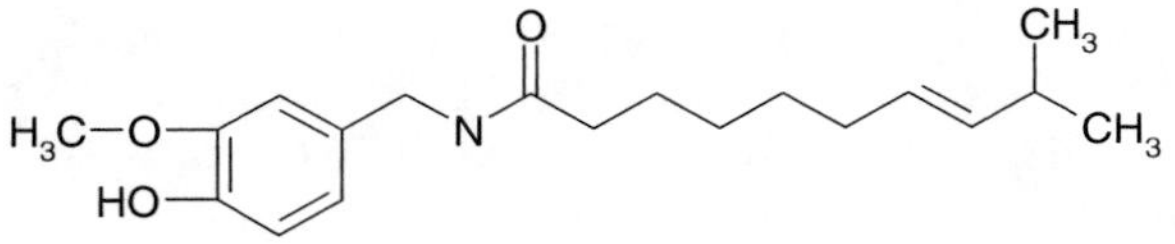

Homocapsaicin

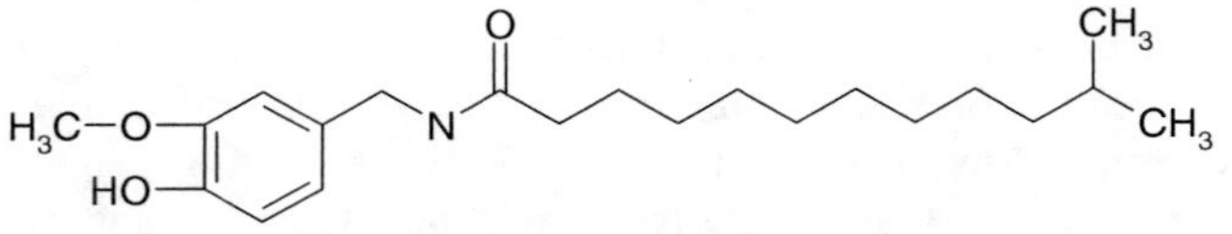

Homodihydrocapsaicin

FIGURE 9.3 Capsaicinoids in *Capsicum* fruit.

VII. CAPSAICINOIDS

Capsaicinoids are alkaloid compounds responsible for the hot flavor or pungency associated with consumption of *Capsicum* fruit. The hot flavor is due to structurally similar alkaloids or capsaicinoids (Figure 9.3). Capsaicin and dihydrocapsaicin are the major capsaicinoids commonly found in hot peppers, typically accounting for > 90% of the total capsaicinoids, whereas nordihydrocapsaicin, homocapsaicin, and homodihydrocapsaicin are present in lesser amounts.[99] The capaicinoids are synthesized primarily in the epidermal cells of placental tissue, with low levels found in the pericarp and seeds.[99,100,101] Two capsaicinoid-like substances, capsiate and dihydrocapsiate, the nonpungent ester analogues of capsaicin and dihydrocapsaicin were identified in fruit of a nonpungent cultivar of *Capsicum annuum* cv. CH-19 sweet.[102] The non-pungent capsainoids are reported to exhibit comparable antioxidant activity as their corresponding capsaicinoids (capsaicin and dihydrocapsaicin), indicating potential health benefits associated with consumption of sweet peppers.[103] Capsaicinoids are unique to the genus *Capsicum,* and their content varies greatly among species and cultivars due to differences in genetics, environmental growing conditions, and maturity.

Capsaicinoids are biosynthesized from L-phenylalanine and L-valine or L-leucine through vanillylamine and C_9 to C_{11} branch-chained fatty acids. The proposed pathway for synthesis of the vanillylamine moeity of capsaicinoids from L-phenylalanine is as follows: L-phenylalanine, *trans*-cinnamic acid, *trans-p*-coumaric acid, *trans*-caffeic acid, *trans*-ferulic acid, vanillin, and vanillylamine.[56] Unfortunately, many of the enzymes involved in capsaicinoid biosynthesis have yet to be identified.

Capsaicinoids are reported to possess numerous pharmacological and medicinal properties, which have been reviewed extensively.[7,104] Capsaicin is commonly used as a treatment for pain and inflammation. Its mode of action is related to its interaction with transgeminal nerve endings, which release a neurotransmitter called substance P. Repeated capsaicin ingestion or topical application results in increased release of substance P, which results in its depletion, rendering the nerve endings unresponsive to subsequent applications. Due to its ability to alleviate a variety of human pain disorders, capsaicin has been used to prevent or alleviate many medical conditions including postmastectomy syndrome, urticaria, psoriasis, diabetic neuropathy, arthritis, osteoarthritis, pruritis, apocrine, chromhidrosis, contact allergy, postsurgical neuromas, reflex sympathetic dystrophy syndrome, vascular vestibulitis, shingles (Herpes zoster), cluster headaches, and urological disorders.[104,105] Capsaicinoids may also exhibit anticarcinogenic and antimutagenic properties. Several studies have shown that capsaicinoids may inhibit the metabolism and mutagenicity of chemical carcinogens.[106] In addition, capsaicinoids also have antioxidant,[18,107–109] antiplatelet, and anti-inflammatory activities,[110,111] and have been shown to induce apoptosis, an important step in carcinogen removal.[112] Capsiate and dihydrocapsiate, the nonpungent analogues of capsaicin and dihydrocapsaicin also show promising chemopreventive potential due to their ability to modulate ROS, induce apoptosis, and disrupt mitochondrial transmembrane potential in tumoral cell lines.[113]

The capsaicinoid content of *Capsicum* fruit is largely influenced by genetics, as shown in Table 9.5.[114–116] It is difficult to classify pepper species and types according to heat level because of the wide variation in heat level observed between cultivars. Total capsaicinoid content ranges from 720 to 4360 ppm for cayenne cultivars, 1110 to 7260 ppm for jalapeno cultivars, and 81 to 2690 ppm for New Mexican cultivars. Chile peppers may be classified according to level of pungency with 0 to 47 ppm being nonpungent, 47 to 200 ppm being mildly pungent, 200 to 1667 ppm being moderately pungent, 1667 to 4667 being highly pungent, and >5333 ppm being very highly pungent. According to the literature, bell-type peppers are nonpungent, whereas all other pepper types listed in the table vary considerably in degree of pungency. The unknown cultivars of "Cascabel," New Mexican, and "Pasilla" are the only peppers that fall within the mildly pungent category. Moderately pungent peppers include most New Mexican cultivars, several jalapeno cultivars, cayenne cv. Cayenne Short, cherry cv. Hot Cherry Pepper, *C. baccatum* cv. unknown, *C. frutescens* cv. Tabasco, and *C. pubescens* cv. unknown. Highly pungent peppers include most cayenne cultivars, "DeArbol" cv. Chile DeArbol, several jalapeno cultivars, New Mexican cv. NewMex Centennial Chile, several serrano cultivars, and "yellow mushroom" and *C. Cardenasii* cv. unknown. *C. chinense* cultivars and one jalapeno cv. JM are considered to be very highly pungent.

In addition to genetics, pepper pungency is influenced by many factors, including fertilization practices, environmental growing conditions, application of bioregulators, and maturity. As demonstrated in Table 9.5, plant breeders have successfully developed pepper cultivars with varying levels of pungency. Genetic manipulation of pungency levels in peppers is important for various food and pharmaceutical applications. Development of heatless and mild jalapenos[117] has enabled processors of salsa and picante sauce to strictly control the pungency levels of their products. Mild, medium, and hot pungency levels in salsas are controlled through the addition of known amounts of capsaicinoid oleoresins. Conversely, plant breeders have developed pepper types with extremely high levels of capsaicinoids for use in skin ointments for pain relief and for manufacturing aerosol sprays designed to incapacitate aggressive criminals.

Environmental stresses incurred during growth including excessive variation in water, temperature, and fertility generally lead to increased capsaicinoid synthesis. Peppers grown in hot weather generally have higher capsaicinoid content than peppers grown in cool weather. Water deficit or excess will also induce stress and capsaicinoid synthesis. Extreme variation in capsaicinoid content may occur between plants grown in the same field due to differences in environmental conditions. New Mexican chile-type peppers grown in the same field in different plots differed by 400 ppm

TABLE 9.5
Capsaicinoid Content of Fresh *Capsicum* Fruit

Species	Type	Cultivar	Nordihydrocapsaicin	Dihydrocapsaicin	Homodihydrocapsaicin	Capsaicin	Total	Ref.
				ppm (dry weight)				
C. Annuum	Cascabel		7	42	—	88	137	114
	Cayenne	Cayenne Short	140	270	—	310	720	115
		Cayenne Long Thick	430	1,100	—	1,200	2,730	115
		Carolina Cayenne	380	1,100	—	1,900	3,380	115
		Ultra Cayenne (slim)	760	2,100	—	1,500	4,360	115
	Cherry	Hot Cherry Pepper	120	260	—	200	580	115
		Cubanella	55	291	18	834	1,198	114
	DeArbol	Chile DeArbol	280	620	—	1,100	2,000	115
	Jalapeno		107	595	28	1,307	2,037	115
		TAM	—			1,110	1,110	116
		TMJ	—			1,172	1,172	116
		T85	—			3,820	3,820	116
		JM	—			7,260	7,260	116
		M	360	1,200	—	1,900	3,460	116
		Early Jalapeno	190	840	—	770	1,800	116
	New Mexican	ND	42	ND	39	81	99	115
		Anaheim M	21	110	—	89	220	115
		Big Jim	14	100	—	160	274	115
		Sandia Hot	21	160	—	140	321	115
		Espanola Improved	28	190	—	250	468	115
		NewMex X Hot	54	480	—	640	1,174	115
		NewMex Cen. Chile	190	1,100	—	1,400	2,690	115
		Pasilla	18	144	7	195	364	114
	Serrano	Small Serrano	440	1,100	—	1,100	2,640	115
		Serrano	360	1,100	—	1,400	2,860	115
	Yellow Mushroom		92	627	34	1,196	1,949	114
C. baccatum			79	352	12	558	1,001	114
C. cardenasii			706	934	67	984	2,691	114
C. chinense	Habanero		279	3,002	60	10,951	14,292	114
		Dom	250	5,200	—	14,000	19,450	115
	Scotch bonnet		810	6,300	—	12,000	19,110	115
	Chocolate		20	1,600	—	7,000	8,620	115
C. frutescens	Tabasco		47	370	—	670	1,087	115
C. pubescens		Tabasco	300	487	14	401	1,202	114
			412	441	22	502	1,377	114

(6000 Scoville units) in total capsaicinoid content.[118] Fertilization practices have been shown to influence capsaicinoid content in pepper fruit. Plants receiving up to 48 kg/ha of phosphorus at varying levels of nitrogen (0, 80, 100 kg/ha) had elevated levels of capsaicinoids.[28] A combination of 100 kg/ha N and 48 kg/ha P resulted in the highest capsaicinoid content. In another study involving jalapeno peppers, cv Jalapa, increasing levels of N at the time of transplanting resulted in increased capsaicinoid content, with the highest level obtained at a rate of 15 mM.[119] Mineral supplementation of Padron peppers with 0.1 g of 13N–40P–13K during vegetative growth and 15N–11P–15K during flowering also resulted in increased capsaicinoid content.[120] Plant age also influences capsaicinoid content. Capsaicinoids typically reach maximum levels around 28 to 50 d after flowering, and then levels stabilize or decline gradually as fruit ripens.[99,121] Thus, immature fruit within the same plant may have higher capsaicinoid content and heat levels than more mature fruit. In *Capsicum annuum* cv. Padron fruit, the levels of capsaicin, dihydrocapsaicin, and soluble phenolics increase in concentration from the bottom to the top of the pepper, which may be associated with greater light intensity incurred by apical fruit.[122] In contrast to this study, Zewdie and Bosland[123] measured the pungency of fruits from different nodes of chile plants. They found that the most pungent fruits came from the lower or earliest nodes and suggested that the higher pungency was due to less fruit on the plant and that early fruits received most of the nutrients needed for capsaicinoid biosynthesis. Loss of capsaicinoids during pepper ripening may reflect increased peroxidase activity.[121] A peroxidase isoenzyme B6 was shown to oxidize phenolic precursors of capsaicin, indicating that phenylpropanoid intermediates of capsaicin biosynthesis may compete with capsaicin for synthesis of lignin-like substances in the cell wall.[124] Application of bioregulators may also affect capsaicinoid content. Ethephon applied at 1000 and 3000 µl/l increased capsaicinoid content of cayenne peppers by 50%.[125] However, the treatment does not appear to be commercially feasible due to fruit damage and yield loss.

A. EFFECTS OF POSTHARVEST HANDLING AND PROCESSING

Capsaicinoid content of pepper fruit is affected by food-processing conditions. Freezing and canning of jalapeno peppers resulted in total capsaicinoid losses of 43.8 and 33.1%, respectively, whereas cooking resulted in an increase of 19.2%.[126] Loss of capsaicinoids may be attributed to leaching during water blanching, residual enzyme activity, or liberation from complexed compounds during pasteurization. In another study, losses of capsaicin and dihydrocapsaicin in pasteurized yellow wax peppers after 4 months storage were 30 and 10%.[41] Calcium chloride brine treatment, which is commonly used as a firming agent, did not affect capsaicinoid losses in pasteurized yellow wax peppers stored for 4 months. In contrast, the capsaicinoid content of jalapeno peppers was unaffected by blanching and pasteurization steps.[42]

REFERENCES

1. Smith, P.G., Villalon, B., and Villa, P.L., Horticultural classification of pepper grown in the United States, *Hortic. Sci.,* 22: 11–13, 1987.
2. Bosland, P.W., Bailey, A.L., and Igleias-Olivas, J., Capsicum pepper varieties and classification, *New Mexico State Univ. Ext. Circ.,* 530, 1988.
3. Govindarajan, V.S., Capsicum-production, technology, chemistry and quality. Part I: History, botany, cultivation, and primary processing, *CRC Crit. Rev. Food Sci. Nutr.,* 22: 109–176, 1985.
4. Govindarajan, V.S., Capsicum-production, technology, chemistry, and quality. Part II. Processed products, standards, world production and trade, *CRC Crit. Rev. Food Sci. Nutr.,* 23: 207–288, 1986A.
5. Govindarajan, V.S., Capsicum-production, technology, chemistry, and quality. Part III. Chemistry of the color, aroma, and pungency stimuli, *CRC Crit. Rev. Food Sci. Nutr.,* 24: 245–355, 1986B.
6. Govindarajan, V.S., Rajalakshmi, D., and Chand, M., Capsicum-production, technology, chemistry, and quality. Part IV. Evaluation of quality, *CRC Crit. Rev. Food Sci. Nutr.,* 25: 185–283, 1987.

7. Govindarajan, V.S. and Sathyanarayana, M.N., Capsicum-production, technology, chemistry, and quality. Part V. Impact on physiology, pharmacology, nutrition, and metabolism; structure, pungency, pain, and desensitization sequences, *CRC Crit. Rev. Food Sci. Nutr.,* 29: 435–474, 1991.

8. Block, G. and Langseth, L., Antioxidant vitamins and disease prevention, *Food Technol.,* 48: 80–84, 1994.

9. Steinmetz, K.A. and Potter, J.D., Vegetables, fruit, and cancer prevention: a review, *J. Am. Diet. Assoc.,* 96: 1027–1039, 1996.

10. Van Poppel, G. and Van den Berg, H., Vitamins and cancer, *Cancer Lett.,* 114: 195–202, 1997.

11. Jacob, R.A., The integrated antioxidant system, *Nutr. Res.,* 15: 755–766, 1995.

12. Hasler, C.M., Functional foods: their role in disease prevention and health, *Food Technol.,* 52: 63–69, 1998.

13. German, J.B. and Dillard, C.J., Phytochemicals and targets of chronic disease, in *Phytochemicals: A New Paradigm,* Bidlack, W.R., Omaye, S.T., Meskin, M.S., and Jahner, D., Eds., Technomic Publishing Co., Lancaster, PA, 1998.

14. Mateos, R.M., Leon, A.M., Sandalio, L.M., Gomez, M., del Rio, L.A., and Palma, J.M., Peroxisomes from pepper fruits (*Capsicum annuum* L.): purification, characterisation and antioxidant activity, *J. Plant Physiol.,* 160: 1507–11516, 2003.

15. Haworth, W.N. and Svent-Gyorgyi, A., "Hexuronic acid" (ascorbic acid) as the antiscorbutic factor, *Nature,* 131: 24, 1933.

16. Tannenbaum, S.T., Young, V.R., and Archer, M.C., Vitamins and minerals, in *Food Chemistry,* Fennema, O.R., Ed., Marcel Dekker, New York, 1985.

17. Sauberlich, H.E., Pharmacology of vitamin C, *Annu. Rev. Nutr.,* 14: 371–391, 1994.

18. Lee, Y., Howard, L.R., and Villalon, B., Flavonoids and antioxidant activity of fresh pepper (*Capsicum annuum*) cultivars, *J. Food Sci.,* 60: 473–476, 1995.

19. Simmone, A.H., Simmone, E.H., Eitenmiller, R.R., Mills, H.A., and Green, N.R., Ascorbic acid and provitamin A contents in some unusually colored bell peppers, *J. Food Comp. Anal.,* 10: 299–311, 1997.

20. Howard, L.R., Smith, R.T., Wagner, A.B., Villalon, B., and Burns, E.E., Provitamin A and ascorbic acid content of fresh pepper cultivars (*Capsicum annuum*) and processed jalapenos, *J. Food Sci.,* 59: 362–365, 1994.

21. Howard, L.R., Talcott, S.T., Brenes, C.H., and Villalon, B., Changes in phytochemical and antioxidant activity of selected pepper cultivars (*Capsicum* species) as influenced by maturity, *J. Agric. Food Chem.,* 48: 1713–1720, 2000.

22. Osuna-Garcia, J.A., Wall, M.M., and Waddell, C.A., Endogenous levels of tocopherols and ascorbic acid during fruit ripening of New Mexican-type chile (*Capsicum annuum* L.), *J. Agric. Food Chem.,* 46: 5093–5096, 1998.

23. Martinez, S., Lopez, M., Gonzalez-Raurich, M., and Bernardo Alvarez, A., The effects of ripening stage and processing systems on vitamin C content in sweet peppers (*Capsicum annuum* L.), *Int. J. Food Sci. Nutr.,* 56: 45–51, 2005.

24. Marin, A., Ferreres, F., Tomas-Barberan, F.A., and Gil, M.I., Characterization and quantitation of antioxidant constituents of sweet pepper (*Capsicum annuum* L.), *J. Agric. Food Chem.,* 52: 3861–3869, 2004.

25. Jimenez, A., Romojaro, F., Gomez, J.M., Llanos, M.R., and Sevilla, F., Antioxidant systems and their relationship with the response of pepper fruits to storage at 20 degrees C, *J. Agric. Food Chem.,* 51: 6293–6299, 2003.

26. Gnayfeed, M.H., Daood, H.G., Biacs, P.A., and Alcaraz, C.F., Content of bioactive compounds in pungent spice red pepper (paprika) as affected by ripening and genotype, *J. Sci. Food Agric.,* 81: 1580–1585, 2001.

27. Mozafar, A., *Plant Vitamins: Agronomic, Physiological and Nutritional Aspects,* CRC Press, Boca Raton, FL, 1994.

28. Bajaj, K.L., Kaur, G., Singh, J., and Brar, J.S., Effect of nitrogen and phosphorous levels on nutritive values of sweet pepper (*Capsicum annuum*) fruits, *Qual. Plant Foods Hum. Nutr.,* 4: 287–292, 1979.

29. Das, R.C. and Mishra, B.N., Effect of NPK on growth, yield and quality of chilli, *Plant Sci.,* 4: 78–83, 1972.

30. Belakbir, A., Ruiz, J.M., and Romero, L., Yield and fruit quality of pepper (*Capsicum annuum* L.) in response to bioregulators, *Hortic. Sci.,* 33: 85–87, 1998.

31. Fox, A.J., Del Pozo-Insfran, D., Lee, J.H., Sargent, S.A., and Talcott, S.T., Ripening-induced chemical and antioxidant changes in bell peppers as affected by harvest maturity and postharvest ethylene exposure, *Hortic. Sci.,* 40: 732–736, 2005.

32. Hudson, D.E., Butterfield, J.E., and Lachance, P.A., Ascorbic acid, riboflavin, and thiamine content of sweet peppers during marketing, *Hortic. Sci.,* 20: 129–130, 1985.

33. Watada, A.E., Kim, S.D., Kim, K.S., and Harris, T.C., Quality of green beans, bell peppers and spinach stored in polyethylene bags, *J. Food Sci.,* 52: 163–171, 1987.

34. Cappellini, M.C., Lachance, P.A., and Hudson, D.E., Effect of temperature and carbon dioxide atmospheres on the market quality of green bell peppers, *J. Food Qual.,* 7: 17–25, 1984.

35. Wang, C.Y., Effect of CO_2 treatment on storage and shelf life of sweet peppers, *J. Am. Soc. Hortic. Sci.,* 102: 808–812, 1977.

36. Nunes, M.C. and Edmond, J.P., Chlorinated water treatments affects postharvest quality of green bell peppers, *J. Food Qual.,* 22: 353–361, 1999.

37. Howard, L.R. and Hernandez-Brenes, C., Antioxidant content and market quality of jalapeno pepper rings as affected by minimal processing and modified atmosphere packaging, *J. Food Qual.,* 21: 317–327, 1998.

38. Petersen, M.A. and Berends, H., Ascorbic acid and dehydroascorbic acid content of blanched sweet green pepper during chilled storage in modified atmospheres, *Z. Lebensm. Unters. Forsch.,* 197: 546–549, 1993.

39. Matthews, R.F. and Hall, J.W., Ascorbic acid, dehydroascorbic acid and diketogulonic acid in frozen green peppers, *J. Food Sci.,* 43: 532–534, 1978.

40. Ramesh, M.N., Wolf, W., Tevini, D., and Bognár, A., Microwave blanching of vegetables, *J. Food Sci.,* 67: 390–398, 2002.

41. Lee, Y. and Howard, L.R., Firmness and phytochemical losses in pasteurized yellow banana peppers (*Capsicum annuum*) as affected by calcium chloride and storage, *J. Agric. Food Chem.,* 47: 700–703, 1999.

42. Saldana, G. and Meyer, R., Effects of added calcium on texture and quality of canned jalapeno peppers, *J. Food Sci.,* 46: 1518–1520, 1981.

43. Oruna-Concha, M.J., Gonzalez-Castro, M.J., and Lopez-Hernandez, J.L., Monitoring of the vitamin C content of frozen green beans and padron peppers by HPLC, *J. Sci. Food Agric.,* 76: 477–480, 1998.

44. Rahman, F.M.N. and Buckle, K.A., Effects of blanching and sulphur dioxide on ascorbic acid and pigments of frozen capsicums, *J. Food Technol.,* 16: 671–682, 1981.

45. Daood, H.G., Vinkler, M., Makus, F., Hebshi, E.A., and Biacs, P.A., Antioxidant vitamin content of spice red pepper (paprika) as affected by technological and varietal factors, *Food Chem.,* 55: 365–372, 1996.

46. Markus, F., Daood, H.G., Kapitany, J., and Biacs, P.A., Change in the carotenoid and antioxidant content of spice red pepper (paprika) as a function of ripening and some technological factors, *J. Agric. Food Chem.,* 47: 100–107, 1999.

47. Kuzniar, A., Bowers, J.A., and Craig, J., Ascorbic acid and folic acid content and sensory characteristics of dehydrated green peppers, *J. Food Sci.,* 48: 1246–1249, 1983.

48. Rice-Evans, C.A., Miller, N.J., and Paganga, G., Structure-antioxidant activity relationships of flavonoids and phenolic acids, *Free Radical Biol. Med.,* 20: 933–956, 1996.

49. Hollman, P.C.H., Hertog, M.G.L., and Katan, M.B., Analysis and health effects of flavonoids, *Food Chem.,* 57: 43–46, 1996.

50. Hertog, M.G.L., Feskens, E.J.M., Hollman, P.C.H., Katan, M.B., and Krombout, D., Dietary antioxidant flavonoids and risk of coronary heart disease: the Zutphen study, *Lancet,* 342: 1007–1011, 1993.

51. Hertog, M.G.L., Kromhout, D., Aravanis, C., Blackburn, H., Buzina, F., Fidvanza, R., Giampli, S., Jansen, A., Menotti, A., Nedeljkovic, S., Pekkarinen, M., Simic, B.S., Toshima, H., Feskens, E.J.M., Hollman, P.C.H., and Katan, M.B., Flavonoid intake and the long-term risk of coronary heart disease and cancer in the Seven Countries Study, *Arch. Intern. Med.,* 155: 381–386, 1995.

52. Knekt, P., Jarvinen, R., Reunanen, A., and Maatela, J., Flavonoid intake and coronary mortality in Finland: a cohort study, *Br. Med. J.,* 312: 478–481, 1996.

53. Keli, S.O., Hertog, M.G.L., Feskens, E.J.M., and Kromhout, D., Dietary flavonoids, antioxidant vitamins and incidence of stroke, *Arch. Intern. Med.,* 156: 637–642, 1996.
54. Knekt, P., Jarvinen, R., Seppanen, R., Heliovaara, M., Teppo, L., Pukkala, E., and Aromaa, A., Dietary flavonoids and the risk of lung cancer and other malignant neoplasms, *Am. J. Epidemiol.,* 146: 223–230, 1997.
55. Garcia-Closas, R., Agudo, A., Gonzalez, C.A., and Riboli, E., Intake of specific carotenoids and flavonoids and the risk of lung cancer in women in Barcelona, Spain, *Nutr. Cancer,* 32: 154–158, 1998.
56. Sukrasno, N. and Yeoman, M., Phenylpropanoid metabolism during growth and development of *Capsicum frutescens* fruits, *Phytochemistry,* 32: 839–844, 1993.
57. Iorizzi, M., Lanzotti, V., De Marino, S., Zollo, F., Blanco-Molina, M., Mach, A., and Munoz, E., New glycosides from *Capsicum annuum* L. Var. *acuminatum.* Isolation, structure determination, and biological activity, *J. Agric. Food Chem.* 49: 2022–2029, 2001.
58. Materska, M., Piacente, S., Stochmal, A., Pizza, C., Oleszek, W. and Perucka, I., Isolation and structure elucidation of flavonoid and phenolic acid glycosides from pericarp of hot pepper fruit *Capsicum annuum* L, *Phytochemistry* 63: 893–898, 2003.
59. Materska, M. and Perucka, I., Antioxidant activity of the main phenolic compounds isolated from hot pepper fruit (*Capsicum annuum* L.), *J. Agric. Food Chem.* 53: 1750–1756, 2005.
60. Hernandez, C.H., Antioxidant Content and Market Quality of Pepper (*Capsicum annuum*) as Affected by Cultivar, Minimal Processing, Modified Atmosphere Packaging and Edible Coatings, Thesis, Texas A&M University, College Station, 1996.
61. Brown, J.E. and Rice-Evans, C.A., Luteolin-rich artichoke extract protects low density lipoprotein form oxidation in vitro, *Free Radical Res.,* 29: 247–255, 1998.
62. Yamashita, N., Tanemura, H., and Kawanishi, S., Mechanism of oxidative DNA damage induced by quercetin in the presence of Cu (II). *Mutat. Res.,* 425: 107–115, 1999.
63. Barz, W. and Hoesel, W., Metabolism and degradation of phenolic compounds in plants, *Phytochemistry,* 12: 339–369, 1977.
64. Jimenez, M. and Garcia-Carmona, F., Oxidation of the flavonol quercetin by polyphenol oxidase, *J. Agric. Food Chem.,* 47: 56–60, 1999.
65. Miller, E. and Schreier, P., Studies on flavonol degradation by peroxidase (donor:H_2O_2-oxidoreductase, EC 1.11.1.7). 1. Kaempferol, *Food Chem.,* 17: 143–154, 1985.
66. Miller, E. and Schreier, P., Studies on flavonol degradation by peroxidase (donor:H_2O_2-oxidoreductase, EC 1.11.1.7). 2. Quercetin, *Food Chem.,* 17: 301–317, 1985.
67. Kamal-Eldin, A. and Ake-Appelqvist, L., The chemistry and antioxidant properties of tocopherols and tocotrienols, *Lipids,* 31: 671–701, 1996.
68. Papas, A.M., Vitamin E: tocopherols and tocotrienols, in *Antioxidant Status, Diet, Nutrition, and Health,* Papas, A.M., Ed., CRC Press, Boca Raton, FL, 1999.
69. Kanner, J., Harel, S., and Mendel, H., Content and stability of -tocopherol in fresh and dehydrated pepper fruits (*Capsicum annuum* L.), *J. Agric. Food Chem.,* 27: 1316–1318, 1979.
70. Biacs, P.A., Czinkotai, B., and Hoschke, A., Factors affecting stability of colored substances in paprika powders, *J. Agric. Food Chem.,* 40: 363–367, 1992.
71. Biacs, P.A., Daood, H.G., Pavisa, A., and Hajdu, F., Studies on the carotenoid pigments of paprika (*Capsicum annuum* L. var Sz-20), *J. Agric. Food Chem.,* 37: 350–353, 1989.
72. Wall, M., Bosland, P., and Waddell, C., Postharvest color analyses of dehydrated red chile, *Proc. 12th Natl. Pepper Conf.,* Las Cruces, NM, 1994.
73. Davies, B.H., Matthews, S., and Kirk, J.T.O., The nature and biosynthesis of the carotenoids of different colour varieties of *Capsicum annuum*, *Phytochemistry,* 9: 797–805, 1970.
74. Matsufuji, H., Nakamura, H., Chino, M., and Takeda, M., Antioxidant activity of capsanthin and the fatty acid esters in paprika (*Capsicum annuum*), *J. Agric. Food Chem.,* 46: 3468–3472, 1998.
75. Seddon, J.M., Ajani, U.A., Sperduto, R.D., Hiller, R., Blair, N., Burton, T.C., Farber, M.D., Gragoudas, E.S., Haller, J., Miller, D.T., Yannuzzi, L.A., and Willet, W., Dietary carotenoids, vitamins A, C, and E, and advanced age-related macular degeneration, *JAMA,* 272: 1413–1420, 1994.
76. Gonzalez de Mejia, E., Quintanar-Hernandez, J.F., and Loarca-Pina, G., Antimutagenic activity of carotenoids in green peppers against some nitroarenes, *Mutat. Res.,* 416: 11–19, 1998.

77. Zhang, L.X., Cooney, R.V., and Bertram, J.S., Carotenoids enhance gap functional communication and inhibit lipid peroxidation in C3H/10T1/2 cells; relationship to their chemopreventative action, *Carcinogenesis,* 12: 2109–2114, 1991.

78. Khachik, F., Bertram, J.S., Mou-Tuan, H., Fahey, J.W., and Talalay, P., Dietary carotenoids and their metabolites as potentially useful chemoprotective agents against cancer, in *Antioxidant Food Supplements in Human Health,* Packer, L., Hiramatsu, M., and Yoshikawa, T., Eds., Academic Press, London, 1999.

79. Suganuma, H., Hirano, T., and Inakuma, T., Amelioratory effect of dietary ingestion with red bell pepper on learning impairment in senescence-accelerated mice (SAMP8), *J. Nutr. Sci. Vitaminol.,* 45: 143–149, 1999.

80. Mejia, L.A., Hudson, E., Gonzalez de Mejia, E., and Vasquez, F., Carotenoid content and vitamin A activity of some common cultivars of Mexican peppers (*Capsicum annuum*) as determined by HPLC, *J. Food Sci.,* 53: 1448–1451, 1988.

81. Matus, Z., Deli, J., and Szabolcs, J., Carotenoid composition of yellow pepper during ripening: isolation of β-cryptoxanthin 5,6-epoxide, *J. Agric. Food Chem.,* 39: 1907–1914, 1991.

82. Minguez-Mosquera, M.I. and Horneo-Mendez, D., Comparative study of the effect of paprika processing on the carotenoids in peppers (*Capsicum annuum*) of the Bola and Agridulce varieties, *J. Agric. Food Chem.,* 42: 1555–1560, 1994.

83. Russo, V.M. and Howard, L.R., Carotenoids in pungent and non-pungent peppers at various developmental stages grown in the field and glasshouse, *J. Sci. Food Agric.* 82: 615–624, 2002.

84. Almela, L., Lopez-Roca, J.M., Candela, M.E., and Alcazar, M.D., Carotenoid composition of new cultivars of red pepper for paprika, *J. Agric. Food Chem.,* 39: 1606–1609, 1991.

85. Deli, J., Matus, Z., and Szabolcs, J., Carotenoid composition in the fruits of black paprika (*Capsicum annuum* Variety longum nigrum) during ripening, *J. Agric. Food Chem.,* 40: 2072–2076, 1992.

86. Levy, A., Harel, S., Palevitch, D., Akiri, B., Menagem, E., and Kanner, J., Carotenoid pigments and β-carotene in paprika fruits (*Capsicum annuum* spp.) with different genotypes, *J. Agric. Food Chem.,* 43: 362–366, 1995.

87. Deli, J., Matus, Z., and Toth, G., Carotenoid composition in the fruits of *Capsicum annuum* cv. Szentesi Kosszarvu during ripening, *J. Agric. Food Chem.,* 44: 711–716, 1996.

88. Almela, L., Fernandez-Lopez, J.A., Candela, M.E., Egea, C., and Alcazar, M.D., Changes in pigments, chlorophyllase activity, and chloroplast ultrastructure in ripening pepper for paprika, *J. Agric. Food Chem.,* 44: 1704–1711, 1996.

89. Bushway, R.J., Yang, A., and Yamani, A.M., Comparison of alpha-and beta-carotene content of supermarket versus roadside stand produce, *J. Food Qual.,* 9: 437–443, 1986.

90. Matthews, R.F., Locasio, S.J., and Ozaki, H.Y., Ascorbic acid and carotene contents of peppers, *Proc. Fla. State Hortic. Soc.,* 88: 263–265, 1975.

91. Kanner, J., Mendel, H., and Budowski, P., Prooxidant and antioxidant effects of ascorbic acid and metal salts in a -carotene-linoleate model system, *J. Food Sci.,* 42: 60–64, 1977.

92. Cabibel, M. and Nicholas, J., Lipoxygenase from tomato fruit (*Lycopersicon esculentum* L.): partial purification, some properties and in-vitro cooxidation of some carotenoid pigments, *Sci. Aliments,* 11: 277–290, 1991.

93. Sweeney, J.P. and Marsh, A.C., Effect of processing on provitamin A in vegetables, *J. Am. Diet. Assoc.,* 59: 238–243, 1971.

94. Esterbauer, H., Role of vitamin E in preventing the oxidation of low-density lipoprotein, *Am. J. Clin. Nutr.,* 53: 314–321, 1991.

95. Osuna-Garcia, J.A., Wall, M.M., and Waddell, C.A., Natural antioxidants for preventing color loss in stored paprika, *J. Food Sci.,* 62: 1017–1021, 1997.

96. Carvajal, M., Remedios-Martinez, M., Martinez-Sanchez, F., and Alcaraz, C.F., Effect of ascorbic acid addition to peppers on paprika quality, *J. Sci. Food Agric.,* 75: 442–446, 1997.

97. Sun-Lee, D., Chung, S.K., and Yam, K.L., Carotenoid loss in dried red pepper products, *Int. J. Food Sci. Technol.,* 27: 179–185, 1992.

98. Chatterjee, S., Padwal-Desai, S.R., and Thomas, P., Effect of γ-irradiation on the colour power of tumeric (*Curcuma longa*) and red chilles (*Capsicum annuum*) during storage, *Food Res. Int.,* 31: 625–628, 1998.

99. Iwai, K., Suzuki, T., and Fujiwake, H., Formation and accumulation of pungent principles of hot pepper fruits, capsacin and its analogues, in *Capsicum annuum* L. var. annuum cv. Karayatsubusa at different growth stages after flowering, *Agric. Biol. Chem.,*43: 2493–2498, 1979.

100. Suzuki, T., Fujiwake, H., and Iwai, K., Intracellular localization of capsaicin and its analogues in *Capsicum* fruit I. Microscopic investigation of the structure of the placenta of *Capsicum annuum* var. *annuum* cv. Karayatsubusa, *Plant Cell Physiol.* 21: 839–853, 1980.

101. Ishikawa, K., Janos, T., Sakamoto, S., and Nunomura, O., The contents of capsaicinoids and their phenolic intermediates in various tissues of the plants of *Capsicum annuum* L, *Capsicum Eggplant News* 17: 222–225, 1998.

102. Kobata, K., Todo, T., Yazawa, S., Iway, K., and Watanabe, T., Novel capsaicinoid-like substances, capsiate and dihydrocapsiate, from the fruits of a nonpungent cultivar, CH-19 sweet, of pepper (*Capsicum annuum* L.), *J. Agric. Food Chem.* 46: 1695–1697, 1998.

103. Rosa, A., Deiana, M., Casu, V., Paccagnini, S., Appendino, G., Ballero, M., and Dessi, M.A., Anti-oxidant activity of capsinoids, *J. Agric. Food Chem.* 50: 7396–7401, 2002.

104. Palevitch, D. and Craker, L.E., Nutritional and medical importance of red pepper (*Capsicum* spp.), *J. Herbs Spices Med. Plants,* 3: 55–83, 1995.

105. Dasgupta, P. and Fowler, C.J., Chilies: from antiquity to urology, *Br. J. Urol.,* 80: 845–852, 1997.

106. Joon-Surh, Y., Lee, E., and Lee, J.M., Chemoprotective properties of some pungent ingredients present in red pepper and ginger, *Mutat. Res.,* 402: 259–267, 1998.

107. Fisher, C., Phenolic compounds in spices, in *Phenolic Compounds in Food and Their Effects on Health I*, Ho, C.T. and Lee, C.Y., Eds., American Chemical Society, Washington, D.C., 1992.

108. Nakatani, N., Natural antioxidants from spices, in *Phenolic Compounds in Food and Their Effects on Health II*, Ho, C.T. and Lee, C.Y., Eds., American Chemical Society, Washington, D.C., 1992.

109. Pulla-Reddy, A.C. and Lokesh, B.R., Studies on spice principles as antioxidants in the inhibition of lipid peroxidation of rat liver microsomes, *Mol. Cell. Biochem.,* 111: 117–124, 1992.

110. Wang, J.P., Hsu, M.F., and Teng, C.M., Antiplatelet effect of capsaicin, *Thromb. Res.,* 36: 497–507, 1984.

111. Wang, J.P., Hsu, M.F., Hsu, T.P., and Teng, C.M., Antihemostatic and antithrombotic effects of capsaicin in comparison with aspirin and indomethacin, *Thromb. Res.,* 37: 669–679, 1985.

112. Morre, D.J., Chueh, P.J., and Morre, D.M., Capsaicin inhibits preferentially the NADH oxidase and growth of transformed cells in culture, *Proc. Natl. Acad. Sci. U.S.A.,* 92: 1831–1835, 1995.

113. Macho, A., Lucena, C., Sancho, R., Daddario, N., Minassi, A., Munoz, E., and Appendino, G., Non-pungent capsaicinoids from sweet pepper, synthesis and evaluation of the chemopreventive and anticancer potential, *Eur. J. Nutr.,* 42: 2–9, 2003.

114. Collins, M.D., Wasmund, L.M., and Bosland, P.W., Improved method for quantifying capsaicinoids in Capsicum using high-performance liquid chromatography, *Hortic. Sci.,* 30: 137–139, 1995.

115. Thomas, B.V., Schreiber, A.A., and Weisskopf, C.P., Simple method for quantitation of capsaicinoids in peppers using capillary gas chromatography, *J. Agric. Food Chem.,* 46: 2655–2663, 1998.

116. Rowland, B., Villalon, B., and Burns, E., Capsaicin production in sweet bell and pungent jalapeno peppers, *J. Agric. Food Chem.,* 31: 484–487, 1983.

117. Villalon, B., "Tam Mild Jalapeno-1" pepper cultivars, *Capsicum annuum*, virus resistance, capsaicin, *Hortic. Sci.,* 18: 492–493, 1983.

118. Harvell, K.P. and Bosland, P.W., The environment produces a significant effect of pungency of chiles, *Hortic. Sci.,* 32: 1292, 1997.

119. Johnson, C.D. and Decoteau, D.R., Nitrogen and potassium fertility affects jalapeno pepper plant growth, pod yield, and pungency, *Hortic. Sci.,* 31: 1119–1123, 1996.

120. Estrada, B., Pomar, F., Diaz, J., Merino, F., and Bernal, M.A., Effects of mineral fertilizer supplementation on fruit development and pungency in "Padron" peppers, *J. Hortic. Sci. Biotechnol.,* 73: 493–497, 1998.

121. Contreras-Padilla, M. and Yahia, E.M., Changes in capsaicinoids during development, maturation, and senescence of chile peppers and relation with peroxidase activity, *J. Agric. Food Chem.,* 46: 2075–2079, 1998.

122. Estrada, B., Bernal, M.A., Diaz, J., Pomar, F., and Merino, F., Capsaicinoids in vegetative organs of *Capsicum annuum* L. in relation to fruiting, *J. Agric. Food Chem.,* 50: 1188–1191, 2002.

123   Zewdie, Y. and Bosland, P.W., Pungency of chile (*Capsicum annuum*) fruit is affected by node position, *Hortic. Sci.*, 35: 117 4, 2000.

124.   Bernal, M.A., Calderon, A.A., Ferrer, M.A., De Caceres, M., and Ros Barcelo, A., Oxidation of capsaicin and capsaicin phenolic precursors by the basic peroxidase isoenzyme B6 from hot pepper, *J. Agric. Food Chem.*, 43: 352–355, 1995.

125.   Krajayklang, M., Klieber, A., Wills, R.B.H., and Dry, P.R., Effects of ethephon on fruit yield, colour, and pungency of cayenne and paprika peppers, *Aust. J. Exp. Agric.*, 39: 81–86, 1999.

126.   Harrison, M.K. and Harris, N.D., Effects of processing treatments on recovery of capsaicin in jalapeno peppers, *J. Food Sci.*, 50: 1764–1765, 1985.

10 Osteoarthritis: Nutrition and Lifestyle Interventions

Dianne H. Volker and Peony Lee

CONTENTS

I. INTRODUCTION

Osteoarthritis (OA) is a common, chronic, musculoskeletal disorder. It is the most common form of arthritis and its prevalence increases with age. It is also referred to as degenerative-joint disease and is characterized by degeneration of the cartilage with reactive formation of new bone at the articular margins. This degeneration and new bone formation results in pain and stiffness of the affected joints.[1] OA was viewed traditionally as a passive process of joint wear and tear. However, it is now considered a metabolically active process with both anabolic and catabolic activity.[1] Joints commonly affected are the hands, knees, hips, and the cervical and lumbar spines, and OA is often associated with significant disability and an impaired quality of life. Risk factors include age, gender, ethnicity, genetic profile, hormonal status, bone-mineral density (BMD), and nutritional factors. Obesity, joint injury and deformity, sports participation, muscle weakness, and occupational factors are also associated with OA. There is no known cure.[1] The goals of management include reduction of pain and maintenance or improvement of joint function. The management of OA is broadly divided into pharmacological and non-pharmacological treatments. Exercise, patient education, telephone support, and weight reduction are safe nonpharmacological approaches. Pharmacological therapy includes paracetamol, NSAIDs, intra-articular therapy, and surgical treatment.[1] Nutritional health and lifestyle interventions do not receive sufficient attention.

II. OSTEOARTHRITIS

A. EPIDEMIOLOGY

OA is a major cause of pain and disability in the general population. According to the Australian Burden of Disease Study,[2] OA is the tenth leading cause of disease burden in Australia. It is also the fourth most common cause of years lost due to disability. According to the 1995 National Health Survey,[3] about 6.4% of the Australian population have OA. It is the ninth most prevalent long-term condition reported by Australian patients. According to the World Health Report 1997 of the World Health Organization,[4] up to 40% of people over 70 years of age suffer OA of the knee. Almost 80% of patients with OA have some degree of limitation of movement, and 25% cannot perform daily life activities.

B. PATHOGENESIS

OA is not a passive joint wear-and-tear process but a metabolically active process. Its pathogenesis involves both biomechanical and biochemical changes in cartilage and subchondral bone, resulting in cartilage destruction.[5] Cartilage is composed of water, collagen, and proteoglycans. Collagen provides strength and proteoglycans supply distensibility and adequate hydration. The cells of cartilage (chondrocytes) are responsible for the synthesis and catabolism of the extracellular matrix. In healthy cartilage, there is a dynamic balance between cartilage degradation by wear and its production by chondrocytes.[5] However, this process becomes disrupted in OA, leading to increased degenerative changes including disruption of collagen network and depletion of proteoglycans, leading to breakdown of cartilage.[5] This is accompanied by an abnormal bone-remodeling repair process, which then leads to formation of subchondral cysts and osteoaphytes. Synovial inflammation produces increased levels of cytokines such as interleukin 1 (IL-1) and tumor necrosis factor alpha (TNF-α) which stimulate the production of metalloproteinase and nitric oxide production inducing degradation of cartilage. Interleukin 6 (IL-6) in combination with mechanical stresses also induces cytokine receptors which bind to IL-1 and TNF-α within the cartilage causing further destruction.[5]

C. CLINICAL FEATURES

The main symptoms of OA are pain and joint stiffness which are exacerbated by exercise and relieved by rest. This may lead to a sedentary lifestyle, depression, and sleep problems, especially in the elderly.[6] The pain can range from poorly localized, asymmetric, and episodic pain in the early course of the disease to an increase in severity and frequency of pain as the disease progresses. Stiffness is common in the affected joints. It usually occurs in the morning or after inactivity.[6] Joint crepitus, swelling, inflammation, synovitis, and joint effusion may also be present but swelling, inflammation, and joint effusion are often seen in more advanced stages of OA. Inflammation, if present, is usually mild and localized to the affected joint. Eventually, joint mobility may be limited, which can lead to joint deformity.[6]

D. DIAGNOSIS

Diagnosis is based on a patient's history of symptoms, physical examination, and radiographic assessment. Physical findings include tenderness on pressure, bony enlargement, crepitus on motion, and limitation of range of motion. The radiographic changes associated with OA include joint-space narrowing, increased density of subchondral bone, and the presence of osteophytes.[7] However, the correlation between the clinical presentation of the disease and radiographic changes varies considerably among patients. Some patients with radiographic evidence of advanced joint degeneration have minimal symptoms, whereas other patients with minimal radiographic changes have severe symptoms. Blood tests are not useful for diagnosis because there are no associated laboratory test abnormalities for OA.[7]

III. RISK FACTORS

The development of OA is due to the interaction of both systemic factors and local biomechanical factors.[8] Systemic factors operate by influencing a person's predisposition to develop the disease, making the cartilage more vulnerable to daily injuries and less likely to repair whereas local biomechanical factors result in abnormal biomechanical loading at specific joint sites. Once systemic factors are in place, local biomechanical factors then begin to play a role in joint breakdown.[8] Systemic factors include age, gender, ethnicity, genetic profile, hormonal status, bone-mineral density (BMD), and nutritional factors. Age, gender, ethnicity, and genetic profile are unchangeable although hormonal status, BMD, and nutritional factors are alterable. Local biomechanical factors include obesity, joint injury and deformity, sports participation, muscle weakness, and occupational factors. They are potentially preventable. Ultimately, all these factors will determine the site and severity of OA and can influence either the development of OA or its subsequent progression.[9]

A. Age and Gender

The prevalence of OA is based on age and gender. OA increases with age and women show a higher prevalence than men. Before 50 years of age, men have a higher prevalence than women, but after 50, women have a greater prevalence and incidence of OA than men. This gender difference in prevalence increases with age. Incidence and prevalence of OA then level off or decline in both genders at about 80 years.[9] The ageing process increases the propensity for osteoarthritis through cartilage calcification, reduced chondrocyte function, reduced joint proprioception, and increased laxity around the joints.[9]

B. Obesity

Obesity is the strongest modifiable risk factor for OA. Literature has shown that being overweight is strongly and positively associated with the development of knee OA.[10–13] Moreover, being overweight increases the risk of progression of knee OA.[14,15] However, the increased risk for knee OA among overweight persons is greater in women than men.[11,15] The relationship between obesity and hip OA is inconsistent.[8] Some studies show no relationship.[16–18] They do reveal that the load on the hip with excess weight is substantially lower than the load on the knee.[6] Obesity may act by increasing mechanical stress in weight-bearing joints and increases the risk of developing progressive OA.[19]

C. Bone-Mineral Density

An inverse relationship between osteoporosis and OA has been discovered in which persons with osteoporosis have a decreased occurrence of OA, and persons with OA have a reduced occurrence of osteoporosis. Cross-sectional studies have linked OA with high bone density.[20] In the Study of Osteoporotic Fractures,[21] women with hip OA had an 8% to 12% increase in bone density compared with women without OA. Women with knee OA also appear to have relatively high bone density.[22] Furthermore, a study found that women with knee OA maintained or increased their bone-mineral density over 3 years of follow-up when compared with women without knee OA.[23] However, although high bone-mineral density increases the risk for development of OA, it may be a protective factor for the progression of established OA mainly due to its effect on reducing the risk of joint-space loss.[24]

D. HORMONES

The high incidence of OA in women after age 50, which is about the age of menopause, suggests that estrogen loss may play a role in causing the disease.[6] However, the literature regarding hormone-replacement therapy and OA is contradictory.[25] Several studies have reported a reduction in the risk of knee and hip OA with hormone-replacement therapy (HRT).[26–30] All five studies demonstrated an inverse relationship between HRT and the prevalence of OA. Moreover, the incidence of knee and hip OA is significantly reduced among long-term users in both the Framingham Study[27] and the Study of Osteoporotic Fractures.[26] In contradiction, HRT leads to higher bone density which can increase the risk for knee and hip OA. Studies have also reported a positive association between OA and estrogen use.[13,31] This indirect effect of estrogen could counteract the protective effect of estrogen on OA suggested by other studies. Thus, these conflicting reports of estrogen suggest the need for additional research to elucidate the mechanisms involved.

E. OCCUPATIONAL FACTORS

A systematic review of occupational risk factors and knee and hip OA was published in 1997.[32] Of the 123 studies conducted on risk factors for OA, 17 studies provided a comparison group and related OA to occupational factors. This review has the following conclusion: (1) a consistently positive relationship exists between occupational exposure and knee OA in men, (2) the evidence suggesting a relationship between knee OA and occupational exposure in women was inconclusive, (3) a consistently positive but weak relationship exists between occupational exposure and hip OA in men,[32] and there is a significant relationship between occupational kneeling and osteoarthritis.[33,34]

From 1994 onwards, five studies were identified.[33–37] The characteristics of the studies are shown in Table 10.1. Three studies concerned the knee, one concerned the hip, and one concerned both joints. Four studies were case-control studies and one study was a cross-sectional study. The results of the studies demonstrated a positive association between several physical activities with joint exposures and OA. However, the results differed somewhat between the genders. Two studies found that kneeling and squatting were risk factors for knee OA in men.[33,35] Climbing stairs was found to be a risk factor for knee OA in men in two studies.[33,36] For women, one study found that kneeling, squatting, and walking were risk factor for knee OA.[33] Climbing stairs was also found to be a risk factor for knee OA in women in three studies.[33,35,36] Two studies found that lifting heavy objects was a risk factors for knee OA in both men and women.[35,36] Two studies found that floorlayers, construction workers, forestry workers, and farmers were more likely to develop knee OA.[34,35] For hip OA, one study found that climbing stairs was a risk factor in men and lifting heavy objects was a risk factor in women.[36] Another study found that lifting heavy objects was also a risk factor and that sitting was a protective factor in women.[37] The results of these studies provide further evidence to support the role of occupational physical activities in the occurrence and progression of OA.

F. SPORTS PARTICIPATION AND TRAUMA

Participation in certain competitive sports increases the risk of OA.[9] Sports activities that demand high-intensity, acute, direct joint impact as a result of contact with other participants, playing surfaces, or equipment can increase the risk of OA, such as football and soccer. Men with a history of knee injury were 5–6 times more likely to develop OA.[33] OA develops at a younger age and is likely to lead to lengthy disability and unemployment.[33]

TABLE 10.1
Assessment of Occupational Exposure and Osteoarthritis Treatment

Study	Case/Control	Site of OA	Criteria for OA	Assessment of Occupational Exposure	Results: Odds Ratio (95% confidence intervals)
Coggon et al., 2000 [33]	518/518	Knee	Patients listed for joint-replacement surgery	Structured interview	Kneeling or squatting: 1.9 (1.3-2.8); Walking >2 miles/d: 1.9 (1.4-2.8); Regular lifting ≥ 25kg: 1.7 (1.2-2.6)
Jensen et al., 2000 [34]	Nil	Patients with radiologic confirmed OA	Other subjects from cross-section without other joint diseases	Self-administered questionnaire	Prevalence, age ≥ 50: Floor layers 34% (20%-50%), Carpenters 9% (2%-26%), Compositors 9% (3%-28%)
Sandmark et al., 2000 [35]	625/548	Knee	Patients who had joint replacement due to primary OA	Telephone interview and self-administered questionnaire	Men: Farmers: 3.2 (2.0-5.2) Construction workers: 3.1 (1.5-6.4) Forestry workers: 2.1 (1.0-4.6) Standing: 1.7 (1.0-2.9) Lifting 3.0 (1.6-5.5) Squatting/knee bending: 2.9 (1.7-4.9) Kneeling: 2.1 (1.4-3.3) Jumping: 2.7 (1.7-4.1) Women: Farmers: 2.4 (1.4-4.1) Standing: 1.6 (1.0-2.8) Lifting: 1.7 (1.0-2.9) Kneeling: 1.5 (0.9-2.4)

Continued.

TABLE 10.1 (*Continued*)
Assessment of Occupational Exposure and Osteoarthritis Treatment

Study	Case/Control	Site of OA	Criteria for OA	Assessment of Occupational Exposure	Results: Odds Ratio (95% confidence intervals)
Lau et al., 2000 [36]	138/414	Knee and hip	Patients who attended an orthopedic clinic	Structured interview	Hip, men: Climbing stairs: 12.5 (1.5-104.3) Lifting heavy weight: 3.1 (0.7-14.3) Hip, women: Climbing stairs: 2.3 (0.8-6.1) Lifting heavy weight: 2.4 (1.1-5.3) Knee, men: Climbing stairs: 2.5 (1.5-6.4) Lifting heavy weight: 5.4 (2.4-12.4) Knee, women: Climbing stairs: 5.1 (2.5-10.2) Lifting heavy weight: 2.0 (1.2-3.1)
Yoshimura et al., 2000 [37]	114/114	Hip	Patients listed for joint-replacement surgery	Structured interview	Regular lifting 25kg in first job: 3.6 (1.3-9.7) Regular lifting 50kg in main job: 4.0 (1.1-14.2) Sitting >2 h/d in first job: 0.5 (0.3-0.9)

G. MUSCLE WEAKNESS

Quadriceps muscle weakness is common in patients with knee OA.[9] It is generally thought to be the result of disuse and atrophy as a result of minimum use of the painful limb. However, in patients with knee OA who have no joint pain and whose quadriceps muscle mass is not diminished, quadriceps weakness can be evident even if the quadriceps muscle mass is normal or increased.[9]

H. GENETICS AND ETHNICITY

There are many genes linked to OA, and children of parents with early-onset OA are at a higher risk of developing it themselves.[9,11] Twin studies suggest that there is a strong genetic susceptibility to the disease. OA is more common in Europeans than in Asians, and OA of the hand is more common in European women than in women of Afro-Caribbean descent.[9]

I. NUTRITIONAL FACTORS — VITAMIN SUPPLEMENTS

There are multiple mechanisms by which nutrients can affect either the initiation or progression of OA. Various nutritional factors may influence OA in at least four ways: protection from excessive oxidative damage, modulation of the inflammatory response, cellular differentiation, and biological actions related to bone and collagen synthesis.[38] Antioxidants including vitamin A, C, and E have been identified as having a potential for antioxidant activity in OA. Vitamin D may also play an important role in OA through bone mineralization, cellular differentiation, and proprioception responses. There have been very few studies of nutritional factors in OA and none have demonstrated any influence on incident knee OA.[38]

There is no protective association between dietary or supplemental retinal or β-carotene on either incident OA or progression of OA reported in the literature.[38] In the longitudinal Framingham Knee OA Cohort Study,[39] a threefold reduction in risk of OA progression was observed in participants in the middle tertile (adjusted OR = 0.3, 95% confidence interval [95% CI] 0.1–0.8) and highest tertile (adjusted OR = 0.3, 95% CI 0.1–0.6) of vitamin C intake. Participants in the highest tertile of vitamin C intake also had a reduced risk of developing knee pain (adjusted OR = 0.3, 95% CI 0.1–0.8) during the course of the study. A reduction in risk of OA progression was also seen for β-carotene (adjusted OR = 0.4, 95% CI 0.2–0.9) and vitamin E intake (adjusted OR = 0.7, 95% CI 0.3–1.6) but was less consistent, in that the β-carotene association diminished substantially after adjustment for vitamin C, and the vitamin E effect was seen only in men. However, no significant association was observed for incident knee OA and vitamin C.[39]

Again, in the longitudinal Framingham Knee OA Cohort Study,[40] the risk for progression of knee OA increased from threefold to fourfold for participants in the middle and lower tertiles for both vitamin D intake (odds ratio for the lower compared with the upper tertile, 4.0 [95% CI, 1.4–11.6]) and serum levels of vitamin D (odds ratio for the lower compared with the upper tertile, 2.9 [CI, 1.0–8.2]). However, no effect was observed for vitamin D status on the risk of incident knee OA. The authors concluded that low serum concentration and low intake of vitamin D both seem to be associated with an increase in the risk of knee OA progression.[40] A few years later, Lane and colleagues found a threefold increase in the risk of incident hip OA in participant subjects in the middle (odds ratio [OR] 3.21, 95% CI 1.06, 9.68) and lowest (OR 3.34, 95% CI 1.13, 9.86) tertiles for serum level of 25-vitamin D, providing further evidence that vitamin D status may protect against osteoarthritis.[41] Vitamin D deficiency is an independent predictor of falls in older people and is linked to fragility fractures.[42]

There have been few clinical studies of vitamin E activity in relation to OA. A study randomly assigned 29 OA patients to treatment with either tocopherol 600 mg/d for 10 d or a placebo.[43] The authors found that 52% of those receiving vitamin E had significant reduction in pain compared with 4% of those receiving placebo. Unfortunately nutritional modalities are underutilized in the

OA-management algorithm. There is a need for a number of large, well-designed clinical nutritional studies to determine the mechanisms involved.

IV. MANAGEMENT

There is no known cure for OA. The goals of OA management are mainly reduction of pain, maintenance or improvement of joint function, and overall improvement in health-related quality of life.[44] OA management includes a combination of non-pharmacological, pharmacological, and complementary therapies.

A. NONPHARMACOLOGICAL TREATMENTS

Nonpharmacological treatment is the essential component of OA management and should be maintained throughout the treatment period, according to the American College of Rheumatology.[45] These treatment paradigms include *exercise, patient education* and *support, weight loss, mechanical aids*, and *acupuncture.* Nonpharmacological and complementary therapies should be utilized before commencement of pharmacological treatment.

Exercise should be the leading nonpharmacological intervention for arthritis patients. Exercise is the most effective and inexpensive intervention in OA.[46] The goals of an exercise program are to maintain range of motion, muscle strength, and general health.[7] Therefore, there are three categories of therapeutic exercise: range of motion and flexibility exercise, muscle conditioning and strengthening exercise, and aerobic cardiovascular exercise.[44] Aerobic exercises such as swimming, walking, and water aerobics can improve cardiovascular fitness, the sense of well-being and mental function, and reduce disability, depression and anxiety. Resistance exercise that increases muscle strength can improve joint function and mobility. Recently, the American Geriatrics Society published recommendations on exercise prescription for older adults with OA pain.[47] Maintenance of quadriceps strength is important in knee OA.[6] Quadriceps weakness is commonly found in knee OA, suggesting that the weakness may be due to muscle dysfunction and that weakness may be a risk factor for disease progression.[48] Therefore, exercise directed toward increasing quadriceps strength and strengthening the quadriceps muscles is beneficial.

A systematic review of randomized controlled trials on the effectiveness of exercise therapy in patients with hip or knee OA concluded that exercise therapy was effective in these patients.[49] Eleven trials were reviewed.[50–58] The characteristics of the studies are summarized in Table 10.2. Pain, self-reported disability, observed disability in walking, and the patient's global assessment of effect were used as outcome measures. The result of the review demonstrated beneficial short-term effects of exercise therapy in patients with knee OA and, to a lesser extent, in patients with hip OA (one study). There was a small beneficial effect of exercise therapy on both self-reported disability and observed disability in walking, small-to-moderate beneficial effect on pain, and moderate-to-great beneficial effect according to patients' global assessment of effect. However, there was no information available on long-term effects of exercise therapy. Comparison of the effectiveness of different exercise programs remained inconclusive.[49]

Recently, a number of studies have demonstrated the effectiveness of exercise therapy for the treatment of OA, and the results of some of them are quite interesting and worth reviewing.[50–64] The characteristics of these studies are also shown in Table 10.2. One study found that low-intensity cycling (40% of heart rate reserve (HRR) for 10 weeks was as effective as high-intensity cycling (70% of HRR) in improving function and gait, decreasing pain, and increasing aerobic capacity in older subjects.[59] Cycling did not increase acute pain in either group. Another study[58] randomly allocated elderly patients (mean age, 73 years) with knee OA to a progressive, home-based exercise program, including resistance and strengthening, or to a control program of range-of-motion exercises without resistance. Both groups were given a standard dosing of NSAIDs and allowed escape analgesia with paracetamol. Although both groups improved from baseline during the 8-

TABLE 10.2
Assessment of Exercise Experiences and Osteoarthritis Treatment

Study	(N)/Site of OA	Intervention	Control	Duration	Outcome Measurements	Results
Chamberlain et al., 1982 [50]	36, knee	T1: exercise at hospital T2: exercise at home	No control	4 weeks	Self-reported pain and physical function — VAS Range of movement at knee joint Maximum weight lift Endurance	Both groups showed decreased pain and increased function, maximum weight lift and endurance. There was no difference between the groups.
Minor et al., 1989 [51]	80, knee or hip	T1: walking T2: aquatics	Exercise	12 weeks	Self-reported pain and physical function — AIMS Aerobic capacity Physical performance 50-foot walk time	Walking and aquatics groups showed significant improvement over control group in aerobic capacity, 50-foot walking time, depression, anxiety and physical activity.
Jan et al., 1991 [52]	61, knee	T1: ultrasound therapy T2: shortwave diathermy T3: ultrasound + exercise T4: shortwave + exercise	No control	10 weeks	FIS Muscle strength	All patients had significant improvement in both functional capacity and muscle peak torque. No significant difference in treatment effect between ultrasound and shortwave diathermy. Exercise did promote treatment effect.
Kovar et al., 1992 [53]	92, knee	Walking + patient education	Usual care	8 weeks	Self-reported pain and physical function — AIMS 6-min walk distance	Walking group had significant improvement of 18% in walking distance, 39% in functional status, and 27% of decrease in pain.
Borjesson et al., 1996 [54]	68, knee	Exercise to increase strength	No treatment	5 weeks	Muscle strength Physical performance	Exercise group had significant improvement of perceived knee status and in descending steps.
Schilke et al., 1996 [55]	20, knee	Muscle-strengthening exercise	No exercise	8 weeks	50-foot walk time Range of motion at knee joint Knee-muscle strength Self-reported pain and mobility — AIMS	Exercise group had significant improvements in pain, stiffness, mobility, arthritis activity and more improvement in strength measures.

Continued.

TABLE 10.2 (Continued)
Assessment of Exercise Experiences and Osteoarthritis Treatment

Study	(N)/Site of OA	Intervention	Control	Duration	Outcome Measurements	Results
Ettinger et al., 1997 [56]	365, knee	T1: walking T2: strength exercise	Health education	18 months	Self-reported pain and physical disability — Likert scale Aerobic capacity Knee-muscle strength Knee X-rays Physical performance 6-min walk distance	Both aerobic exercise group and resistance exercise group had modest improvements in self-reported pain and disability score and better scores on physical performance measures compared with health education group.
Bautch et al., 1997 [57]	30, knee	Exercises, low-intensity walking + education	Education	12 weeks	Self-reported pain and physical function — AIMS Pain — VAS	Exercise group had significant decrease in pain.
Van Baar et al., 1998 [58]	191, knee or hip	Patient education + medication + exercise	Patient education + medication	12 weeks	Pain — VAS Use of NSAID Observed disability	Exercise group had significant decrease of pain and observed disability. Effect sizes were medium (0.58) and small (0.28), respectively.
Rogind et al, 1998 [59]	23, knee	Exercise focused on lower extremity muscle strengthening, stretching and balance	No intervention	12 weeks	Self-reported pain and physical function — AFI and VAS for pain Muscle strength Physical performance Self-reported pain, visual analog scale	Improvement in muscle strength and walking speed and pain in exercise group.

Study	N, location	Intervention	Control	Duration	Outcomes measured	Results
Mangione et al., 1999 [60]	39, knee	Stationary cycling T1: high-intensity (70% HRR) T2: low-intensity (40% HRR)	No control	10 weeks	Overall pain assessment —AIMS Times chair rise Aerobic capacity 6-min walk distance Gait Acute pain assessment — VAS and WOMAC	Both groups improved significantly and similarly in timed chair rise, 6-min walk, walking speed, aerobic capacity and in the amount of overall pain relief. No between-group differences were found. Cycling did not increase acute pain in either group. Low-intensity cycling was as effective as high-intensity cycling.
Maurer et al., 1999 [61]	98, knee	Muscle-strengthening exercise	Patient education	8 weeks	Self-reported pain and physical function — AIMS, WOMAC, Likert scales Strength	Significant strength gains and functional outcomes for both group. Exercise group also had improvement in pain scores.
O'Reilly et al., 1999 [62]	180, knee	Strengthening exercises	No intervention	24 weeks	Self-reported pain and physical function —WOMAC Strength	More improvement in pain scores and physical function scores in exercise group than control group.
Deyle et al., 2000 [63]	69, knee	T: manual therapy and supervised knee exercise program (stretching, ROM, and strengthening exercises)	Placebo: subtherapeutic ultrasound	4 weeks	Self-reported pain, stiffness and physical function — WOMAC 6-min walk distance	Significant improvement in 6-min walk and WOMAC score at 4 wk, 8 wk and 1 year in exercise group. By 1 year, patients in placebo group had significantly more knee surgeries than patients in exercise group.
Petrella et al., 2000 [64]	179, knee	Home-based ROM, resistance and strengthening exercise	Range of motion exercise	8 weeks	Self-reported pain, stiffness and physical function — WOMAC and VAS Physical function Physical activity level	Significant improvement from baseline in pain, physical function and physical activity level for both groups. Greater change in the exercise group.

Note: AFI = arthritis functional index; AIMS = arthritis impact measurement scale; FIS = functional incapacity score; HRR = heart rate reserve; T = training; VAS = visual analog scale; WOMAC, Western Ontario and McMaster Universities Osteoarthritis Index.

week study, those with the progressive exercise program using common items in the home showed greater reduction in activity-related pain and greater improvement in mobility and walking measures. There appears to be a beneficial short-term effect of exercise therapy in patients with knee OA and, to a lesser extent, in patients with hip OA. Further research is needed to study the long-term effectiveness of exercise therapy, effectiveness of exercise therapy in patients with hip OA, and comparison of effectiveness of different exercise programs.[49]

Patient education is important for patients with OA and their families so that they develop an understanding of the disease and how to avoid major disability by slowing disease progression. Psychological support is essential.[65] Patient education has been shown in randomized controlled trials to be cost-effective and associated with reduced pain and improved quality of life.[66–71] Table 10.3 shows the characteristics of the randomized controlled trials of patient education in management of OA. A meta-analysis comparing the effects of patient-education interventions and NSAIDs treatment on pain and functional disability in patients with OA identified ten controlled trials.[72] The authors concluded that patient education provided additional benefits that are 20 to 30% as great as the effects of NSAID treatments for pain relief in OA. The Arthritis Foundation Self-Management Program is one such program. These programs include information about disease processes, medications, and their actions and reactions, together with goal setting for exercises and pain-management strategies.[73]

Telephone support is another cost-effective non-pharmacological approach for patients with OA.[45] Telephone support has been shown to benefit reducing pain and improving functional status without a significant increase in costs.[74–78] Social support through telephone counseling demonstrated significant improvements in functional status, reduced health care costs, total health status as measured by the Arthritis Impact Measurement Scales (AIMS), Sickness Impact Profile (SIP), and Life Change Events (LCE).[74–78]

Weight loss is an important strategy as weight gain is an important modifiable risk factor for knee OA. The ACR guidelines recommend that overweight patients with hip or knee OA lose weight.[45] Studies have shown that weight loss can slow progression and show improvement in symptoms of knee OA.[79–81] The Framingham study demonstrated that modest weight loss reduced the risk of developing symptomatic OA of the knee in women.[11] In the management of OA, weight reduction should play a key role as should exercise. Pain and disability can preclude regular exercise, thus weight loss can also be accomplished through dietetic consultation, food diaries, cognitive behavior modification, and reduced energy intake.

Mechanical aids such as shock-absorbing footwear reduce the impact of load on the knee joint. Proprioception is improved and pain is reduced by heel wedging, and walking sticks can provide safe and functional assistance on movement.[82] Unfortunately, there is only anecdotal and historical evidence of benefit because of the paucity of well-designed studies. Physiotherapy and occupational therapy assessment is recommended for functional limitations.[82]

Acupuncture is a component of the Chinese health care system that can be traced back at least 2000 years. The general theory of acupuncture is based on the premise that there are patterns of energy flow through the body that are essential for health. Acupuncture is believed to correct the imbalances in the flow of this energy.[83] The result of a systematic review[84] on the effectiveness of acupuncture as a complementary treatment for OA is inconclusive. The characteristics of some of the studies[85–90] are summarized in Table 10.4. If only the evidence from randomized controlled trials is considered, the following conclusion can be drawn. Acupuncture is not superior to sham-needling (sham-needling is the needling of nonacupuncture points and represents the attempt to find a credible 'placebo' for acupuncture) in reducing pain from OA. Both reduce pain with similar effects. This could either mean sham-needling has specific effects similar to those of acupuncture or that both methods are associated with considerable and similar nonspecific effects.[84]

A more recent systematic review on the effectiveness of acupuncture for knee OA identified seven trials.[91] These trials demonstrated that there was strong evidence that real acupuncture was more effective than sham acupuncture for knee OA pain. However, from a practical viewpoint,

TABLE 10.3
Patient Education Effects and Osteoarthritis Treatment

Study	N	Interventions	Control	Duration	Outcome measurement	Results
Lorig et al., 1985 [66]	190	Education	Usual care	4 months	Knowledge, exercise, relaxation, pain (VAS), disability, no. of visits to physician	Improvement in pain for the intervention group.
Lorig et al., 1989 [67]	543	Education	Usual care	20 months	VAS, HAQ, BID Physician visits	Improvement in pain by 20%, depression by 14%, and visit to physicians by 35%.
Weinberger et al., 1989 [68]	439	Education by telephone	Usual care	1 year	AIMS	Improvement in physical health, pain and psychological health in intervention group.
Calfas et al., 1992 [69]	40	Cognitive behavior modification	Traditional education	1 year	QWB, AIMS, BDI	No difference between groups. But improvement compared to baseline for both groups.
Lorig et al, 1993 [70]	44	Education	Usual care	4 years	VAS, HAQ, BDI Physician visits	Decrease in pain by 20%, visits to physicians by 40% in intervention group.
Mazzuca et al., 1997 [71]	165	Education	Attention-control	1 year	HAQ, DDS, VAS, QWB	Significant improvement in disability and resting knee pain in intervention group.

Note: AIMS = arthritis impact measurement scale; BDI = Beck depression inventory; DDS = disability and discomfort scale; HAQ = health assessment questionnaire; QWB = quality of well-being; VAS = visual analog scale.

TABLE 10.4
Acupuncture Studies in Osteoarthritis Treatment

Study	(N)/OA Site	Intervention Group	Control	Duration	Outcome Measurements	Results
Gaw et al., 1975 [85]	40/various sites	Standard acupuncture	Sham acupuncture	8 sessions	Tenderness, subjective report of pain	All outcomes significantly improved in both groups from baseline, no significant differences for between-group result.
Thomas et al., 1991 [86]	44/cervical spine	Standard acupuncture	Sham acupuncture	Not mentioned	Pain by VAS	Both groups significantly reduced pain from baseline, between-group analysis found that acupuncture was not significantly more effective than sham acupuncture in reducing pain.
Christensen et al., 1992 [87]	29/knee	Standard acupuncture	No treatment	3 weeks	Analgesic use, pain function	All outcomes improved significantly from baseline. Improvements were maintained with monthly acupuncture treatments.
Takeda et al., 1994 [88]	40/knee	Standard acupuncture	Sham acupuncture	3 weeks	2 validated pain-rating scales, pain threshold at knee	All outcomes significantly improved in both groups, no between-group results were significant.
Berman et al., 1995 [89]	12/knee	Electro-acupuncture	No control	8 weeks	WOMAC Lequesne score 50-ft walk time	All outcomes improved significantly from baseline.
Berman et al., 1999 [90]	73/knee	Electro-acupuncture	Standard care	8 weeks	WOMAC Lequesne score	Significant improvement on WOMAC, global disability, and pain scores for acupuncture plus standard care compared with standard care alone.

Note: VAS = visual analog scale; WOMAC = Western Ontario and McMaster Universities Osteoarthritis Index.

there was inconclusive evidence that real acupuncture was more effective than sham acupuncture.[91] Therefore, there is moderately strong evidence from controlled trials to support the use of acupuncture as an adjunctive therapy for OA.

B. PHARMACOLOGICAL TREATMENTS

Pain is the primary symptom of OA, and multiple medications are available to relieve pain and improve function. In 2000, both the American College of Rheumatology (ACR)[45] and the European League of Associations of Rheumatology (EULAR) [92] published recommendations for the use of pharmacological treatment for hip and knee OA. Since then, an updated systematic review, epidemiologic studies, and clinical trials have been published. The results of these reviews, studies, and trials raise issues regarding the validity of the ACR and EULAR recommendations. Pharmacological treatments include paracetamol, NSAIDs, topical analgesics, COX-2 inhibitors, intra-articular therapies, and surgical treatments.

Paracetamol is the preferred initial treatment, with doses of up to 1 g four times a day. It is safe and well tolerated by older age groups. Both the ACR and the EULAR guidelines recommend it as initial therapy.[45,92] Many elderly patients have common comorbidities that place them at risk of side effects and drug interactions from other medications. Paracetamol at the therapeutic dosage mentioned has an excellent safety record. It has a narrow therapeutic and toxicity range so that a modest overdose may be associated with hepatic toxicity.[93] Other studies suggest that paracetamol is preferred to nonsteroidal anti-inflammatory drugs (NSAIDs) in treating patients with chronic liver disease. Paracetamol is thought to inhibit central cyclo-oxygenase (COX) with only a weak effect on peripheral prostaglandin synthesis. [94, 95]

Nonsteroidal anti-inflammatory drugs (NSAIDs) have been found to have equal efficacy to paracetamol in most patients. Both the ACR and EULAR recommendations stated that patients with OA who fail to respond to full doses of paracetamol should be considered as candidates for NSAIDs.[92,95,96] There is good evidence for the efficacy of NSAIDs compared to both paracetamol and placebos in patients with OA.[97–99] However, there is no consistent evidence suggesting that one NSAID is superior to another in relieving pain in patients with OA.[97–99] Traditional nonselective NSAIDs are associated with an increased risk for serious upper gastrointestinal complications, including bleeding and perforation; nephrotoxicity, including acute renal insufficiency; and congestive heart failure and adverse reproductive outcomes.[100]

The use of *topical analgesics,* such as capsaicin cream, is appropriate for persons with mild-to-moderate knee OA pain who do not respond to paracetamol and do not wish to take systemic therapy.[45] A thin film of capsaicin cream should be applied to the symptomatic joint four times daily. It generally requires consistent use over time to be effective.[101] Topical NSAIDs are used by patients who do not wish to use or cannot tolerate NSAIDs systemically. There is some systemic absorption but no excess risk of upper-GI bleeding.[101]

Cyclooxygenase-2 (COX-2) inhibitors celecoxib and refecoxib are drugs that should be used for OA patients who are at increased risk of serious upper gastrointestinal complications and where NSAIDs are contra-indicated. Both celecoxib and rofecoxib have been found to be more effective than placebos and comparable in efficacy to NSAIDs.[100] The results of two large long-term outcome studies, the Celecoxib Long-term Arthritis Safety Study (CLASS)[102] and the Vioxx Gastrointestinal Outcomes Research Study (VIGOR),[103] found that both celecoxib and rofecoxib are associated with a significantly lower risk for symptomatic and complicated gastroduodenal ulcers. These data suggest an advantageous safety profile in comparison with nonselective NSAIDs. Moreover, they appear to be better tolerated at doses recommended for treatment of OA and neither has a significant effect on platelet aggregation or bleeding time. Therefore, they are preferable to nonselective NSAIDs for OA patients with increased risk for upper gastrointestinal complications. However, as with nonselective NSAIDs, COX-2 inhibitors can cause renal toxicity.[104] An alternative to the use of COX-2 inhibitors is the use of nonselective NSAIDs with gastroprotective agents.[45] Because the adverse upper GI events attributed to NSAIDs in the elderly are dose-dependent, nonselective NSAIDs should be started in low, analgesic doses and increased to full anti-inflammatory doses only if lower doses do not provide adequate symptomatic relief. If the patient is at increased risk for a serious upper GI adverse event, gastroprotective agents should be used even if nonselective NSAIDs are given at low dosage. Regular monitoring of elderly patients taking COX-2 inhibitors is necessary for intercurrent illness, comorbidities, and new prescriptions that may reduce the safety of COX-2 inhibitors. COX-2 inhibitors are contraindicated for OA patients at risk of ischemic heart disease and stroke.[104]

Intraarticular therapy, in the form of injection of corticosteroids, is indicated for acute knee OA pain, especially in patients with signs of joint inflammation and joint effusion. Although it is effective in reducing pain, the effect is short-term.[45] Clinical trials have shown that the improvement of symptoms is marginally better than placebos and usually does not last more than a few weeks. However, there is the likelihood of infection and joint damage from repeated injections. Therefore, no more than four injections should be given in 1 year because of the possibility of joint damage.

Intraarticular injection of hyaluronan is used only for persons with knee OA. Hyaluronan is a substance found naturally in synovial fluid. In people with OA, there is a reduced concentration of hyaluronan, resulting in low-viscosity synovial fluid and an increase in cartilage loading. The viscous injections are intended to substitute for the hyaluronan normally found in the joint. The results of randomized controlled trials suggest superior pain relief to placebos and comparable with, or greater than, that with intraarticular corticosteroids injection but with a longer duration of action.[45]

Surgical treatment, such as total joint replacement, is indicated for patients with moderate-to-severe pain and functional impairment who have failed to respond to medical therapy.[45] In a study of the outcome of knee replacement, patients reported having significant and persistent relief of pain, improved physical function, and satisfaction for at least 2 to 7 years after surgery.[105] Knee-replacement procedures have also been shown to be cost effective.[106,107] However, timing of the surgery is important. A study found that subjects with poor functional status at the time of surgery had a worse outcome than subjects operated on at an earlier stage.[108]

C. COMPLEMENTARY THERAPIES

McAlindon and Felson have demonstrated that OA subjects whose diets are richer in antioxidants, such as vitamin C, vitamin D, and green tea, have slower progression of joint space narrowing on x-ray over long-term follow-up.[109] Whether these agents can alleviate the symptoms of arthritis or prevent joint damage is not clear. However, well-designed prospective randomized controlled studies are needed to develop an understanding of the mechanisms involved.

Omega-3 long-chain polyunsaturated fatty acids (n-3 LC PUFA) dietary supplements have been shown to significantly improve tender joint scores and duration of early-morning stiffness in OA.[110,111] The mechanism involved in n-3 LC PUFA supplementation is based on the fact that dietary n-6 and n-3 fatty acids are the primary modulators of the lipid composition of membrane phospholipids. Fatty acids in the membrane phospholipids are the precursors of prostaglandins and eicosanoids, which are important mediators of inflammation, cytokine synthesis, and cell communication.[112] The modern Western diet contains an excess of n-6 fatty acids and a low level of n-3 fatty acids.[113,114] Supplementation of n-3 LC PUFA in conjunction with a high dietary intake of n-6 fatty acids is not effective in increasing cellular levels of n-3 LCPUFA.[115,116] The key to supplementation is to limit the intake of n-6 fatty acids in the diet so that the n-6 to n-3 balance approaches 1.[117] There is considerable variation in activity of the prostaglandins and eicosanoids derived from n-6 fatty acids and n-3 LCPUFA. The n-6 derived eicosanoids exhibit proinflammatory activities, potent chemotactic activity, vasodilation, and increased vascular permeability.[112] The n-3 LC PUFA derived prostaglandins and eicosanoids are anti-inflammatory and much less active, as well as being poorly synthesized. Thus, n-3 LC PUFA supplementation can alter the balance of n-6 to n-3 prostaglandins and eicosanoids to produce decreased inflammatory activity.[117] Fish oil supplementation at the rate of 20 to 40 mg/kg body weight/day, in conjunction with a diet low in n-6 PUFA and saturated fat, leads to a significant incorporation of N-3 LC PUFA in membrane phospholipids.[110] n-3 LCPUFA in membrane phospholipids suppress the production of inflammatory cytokines such as IL-1 and TNF-α, which induce cartilage degradation and destruction.[112] This study suggests the need for further clinical trials in nutritional regimens in OA.

A systematic review of randomized controlled trials on the effectiveness of herbal medicines or symptomatic slow-acting drugs for OA (SYSODOA) in the treatment of OA[118] indicated 10 trials and 2 systematic reviews of 11 different herbal medicines. A summary of the studies is shown in Table 10.5. The review found promising evidence for the effective use of some herbal preparations in reducing pain and improving mobility, function, and disability in OA. There is moderately strong evidence for usage of capsaicin cream[119,120] for the relief of OA symptoms. There is promising evidence for avocado and soybean unsaponifiables (ASU).[121,122] There is weak evidence for Reumalex,[123] willow bark,[124] common stinging nettle,[125] and the ayurvedic herbal preparation Articulin-F.[126] However, there is no evidence for clinically significant benefits for ginger extract.[127] "Weak evidence" describes herbs with a single randomized controlled trial with significant results; "promising evidence" describes herbs with two favorable trials; "moderately strong evidence" describes herbs with three or more favorable trials.[118]

Capsaicin is derived from hot chili peppers. It is used as a topical analgesic for a variety of conditions characterized by pain. The results of a meta-analysis[119] and an RCT[120] for the treatment of OA with topically applied capsaicin have shown that capsaicin cream can significantly reduce the pain associated with OA.[118] Avocado and soybean unsaponifiables (ASU) is the extract of avocado and soya bean made of unsaponifiable fractions of avocado oil and soya bean oil. The results of two RCTs have shown that ASU could significantly improve hip or knee OA symptoms and reduce patients' NSAID consumption.[121,122] In addition, there is evidence suggesting that some herbal medicines reduce the consumption of NSAIDs[121] and the incidence of adverse effects for these herbal medicines was low, suggesting that they are relatively safe. In conclusion, some herbal medicines have proved to be effective for the treatment of OA and are relatively safe. Therefore, they may be employed to lower the consumption of NSAIDs and thus reduce the adverse effects of NSAIDs, particularly when comorbidities are involved.[118]

Glucosamine sulfate and Chondroitin sulfate are nutritional supplements available as over-the-counter preparations and are used to relieve musculoskeletal symptoms. Glucosamine is an amino sugar precursor to the glycosaminoglycans that form a component of the articular cartilage proteoglycans, and chondroitin sulfate is one of the glycosaminoglycans found in articular cartilage. A meta-analysis and quality assessment of 15 double-blind, randomized, placebo-controlled trials of glucosamine and chondroitin sulfate concluded that these supplements are likely to be effective for symptomatic management of OA. However, the authors were reluctant to draw any firm conclusions because of insufficient information about the study designs and potential for publication bias as most of the trials are industry supported.[128] The characteristics of the studies on glucosamine sulfate[129–136] and chondroitin sulfate[137–140] are summarized in Table 10.6. A systematic review studied 16 double-blind, randomized, controlled trials involving the use of glucosamine for the treatment of OA. The conclusion of this review was that glucosamine was effective and safe in OA. All but one of the 13 studies in which glucosamine was compared with placebos proved glucosamine to be superior in pain relief. The characteristics of the studies are shown in Table 10.6.[141]

A recently published randomized, double-blind placebo controlled trial study[142] is the first long-term study evaluating the efficacy of glucosamine sulfate on OA. It has shown that glucosamine has a beneficial effect in retarding generative joint changes and improving symptoms in patients with knee OA. This study followed 212 patients with knee OA for 3 years. They were randomly assigned to take either 1500 mg oral glucosamine sulfate or a placebo once daily for 3 years. Main outcome measures were joint-space width, assessed by radiographs and symptoms scored by the Western Ontario and McMaster Universities (WOMAC) Osteoarthritis Index. The 106 patients receiving glucosamine sulfate had a non-significant mean joint-space loss of 0.06 mm (95% CI,

TABLE 10.5
Herbal Medicine Usage in Osteoarthritis Treatment

Study	(N)/Time	Design	Intervention	Control	Primary Outcome Measures	Main Results
Zhang et al., 1994 [119]	70/4 weeks	Double-blind, placebo-controlled, parallel	Capsaicin cream (0.025%)	Placebo vehicle cream	Physician's and patient's global 5-point pain scores, pain severity (VAS)	Capsaicin significantly reduced pain
	14/4 weeks	Double-blind, placebo-controlled	Capsaicin cream (0.075%)	Placebo vehicle cream	Pain severity VAS, HAQ, TJS, SJS	Capsaicin significantly reduced tenderness (*P*>0.02) and OA pain (*P*>0.02)
	51/9 weeks	Double-blind, vehicle-controlled	Capsaicin cream (0.025%)	Placebo vehicle cream	Articular tenderness and pain (VAS)	Significant reduction in articular tenderness found with active compared with vehicle treatment
Altman et al., 1994 [120]	113/12 weeks	Double-blind, vehicle-controlled, parallel, MC	Capsaicin cream (0.025%)	Placebo vehicle cream	Physician's and patient's global score, VAS, TJS and range of motion	Capsaicin significantly reduced pain
Blotman et al., 1997 [121]	163/3 months	Double-blind, placebo-controlled, parallel, MC	ASU extract of avocado and soya (300 mg)	Placebo	Daily NSAIDs consumption	ASU significantly reduced NSAIDs consumption and delayed resumption
Maheu et al., 1998 [122]	164/6 months	Double-blind, placebo-controlled, parallel, MC	ASU extract of avocado and soya (300 mg)	Placebo	AIMS	ASU significantly improved pain and functional disability. Patients and physicians favoured ASU treatment

Mills et al., 1996 [123]	52/2 months	Double-blind, placebo-controlled, parallel	Reumalex herbal preparation 20–40 mg salicylic acid)	Placebo	AIMS	Reumalex had a significant mild analgesic effect
Schmid et al., 1998 [124]	78/2 weeks	Double-blind, placebo-controlled	Willow bark extract (1360 mg equivalent to 240 mg salicin)	Placebo	WOMAC pain index	Willow bark had a significant moderate analgesic effect
Randall et al., 2000 [125]	27/1 weeks	Double-blind, placebo-controlled crossover	Stinging nettle leaf	White deadnettle leaf	Pain (VAS) and disability (HAQ)	Pain and disability scores significantly lower after 1 week of treatment with stinging vs non-stinging nettles (deadnettle)
Kulkarni et al., 1991 [126]	42/6 months	Double-blind, crossover, placebo-controlled	Articulin-F (an ayurvedic herbomineral)	Placebo	Severity of pain (score), morning stiffness, joint score, grip strength, disability (score)	Articulin-F significantly improved pain severity and disability score
Bliddal et al., 2000 [127]	56/9 weeks	Double-blind, placebo-controlled, double-dummy, crossover	Ginger extract (1 capsule containing 170 mg)	Placebo	Pain (VAS)	A ranking for pain relief (VAS): ibuprofen>ginger extract>placebo. No significant differences between ginger extract and placebo

Note: AIMS = arthritis impact measurement score; ASU = avocado and soya unsaponifiables; HAQ = health assessment questionnaire; MC = multi-center; SJS = swollen joint score; TJS = tender joint score; VAS = visual analog scale.

TABLE 10.6
Glucosamine Sulfate and Chondroitin Sulfate Usage in Osteoarthritis Treatment

Study	(N)/GS/P	OA Site/Time	Treatment/P/NSAIDs	Administration Route	Outcome Measures	Result
Crolle et al., 1980 [129]	15/15	Not specified/ 3 weeks	400 mg injection/d (1 week); 1500 mg oral/d (2 weeks)	Parenteral, oral	Pain relief	GS group had more rapid and marked improvement.
Drovanti et al., 1980 [130]	40/40	Knee/4 weeks	1500 mg GS daily/placebo	Oral	Pain, restriction of movement, swelling	GS group had 72% reduction of sum of symptom scores compared with 36% for placebo group.*
Pujalte et al., 1980 [131]	10/10	Knee/6–8 weeks	1500 g daily/6–8 weeks	Oral	Pain relief	GS group had 80% improvement in pain compared with 20% for placebo group.
D'ambrosio et al., 1981 [132]	15/15	Not specified/ 3 weeks	400 mg injection (1 week); 1500 mg oral daily (2 weeks)	Oral	Pain relief	GS group had greater improvement at 1 wk compared with P* and improvement at 3 weeks.
Vajaradul et al., 1981 [133]	28/26	Knee/5 weeks	Intra-articular GS injection weekly/placebo	Parenteral	Pain scores, mobility, swelling	GS group had increased mobility and decreased pain scores.* No statistically significant decrease in swelling.
Vaz et al., 1982 [134]	18/20	Knee/8 weeks	1500 mg GS daily/1200 mg Ibuprofen	Oral	Pain relief	Ibuprofen group had more pain relief by 2 weeks; GS group had more gradual and sustained pain relief by 8 weeks.*

Study	n	Joint/Duration	Dose	Route	Outcome measures	Results
Muller-FasBender et al., 1994 [135]	100/99	Knee/4 weeks	1500 mg GS daily/1200 mg Ibuprofen	Oral	Lequesne Index	Both groups had improment in Lequesne Index; no inter-group differences.
Noack et al., 1994 [136]	126/126	Knee/4 weeks	1500 mg GS daily/placebo	Oral	Lequesne Index	Improvement in Lequesne Index: GS group 55% vs. placebo group 38%.*
Morreale et al., 1996 [137]	74/172	Knee/3 months	1200 mg CS/150 mg diclofenac	Oral	Lequesne Index, pain on load, paracetamol	Diclofenac group showed reduction in joint pain 10 d, which disappeared on treatment cessation. CS group improved at 30 d, which remained up to 3 months after treatment.
Bourgeois et al., 1998 [138]	40/44	Knee/6 months	1200 mg CS/placebo	Oral	Lequesne Index, spontaneous joint pain	CS group had significant reduction in both scores.*
Conrozier et al., 1998 [139]	104	Knee/1 year	800 mg CS/placebo	Oral	Lequesne Index	CS group, 50% decrease in Lequesne Index.
Bucsi et al., 1998 [140]	40/40	Knee/6 months	800 mg CS/placebo	Oral	Lequesne Index, joint pain, minimum time to walk 10 mi	CS group had statistically significant improvement over placebo group on all three parameters.* Acetaminophen use in CS group was significantly less than placebo group.

Note: CS = chondroitin sulfate; GS = glucosamine sulfate; P = placebo.

0.22–0.09). The 106 patients receiving placebos had progressive joint-space narrowing, with a mean joint space loss after 3 years of 0.31mm (95% CI, 0.48–0.13). Symptoms were significantly improved in the glucosamine sulfate group compared with the placebo group, with significant improvement in pain and physical function. The authors concluded that the long-term combined structure-modifying and symptom-modifying effects of glucosamine sulfate suggest that it could be a disease-modifying agent in OA.[142] Possible mechanisms of action of glucosamine and chondroitin sulfate include stimulating proteoglycans synthesis in articular cartilage and inhibiting the enzymes that destroy the cartilage. Therefore, glucosamine may act to relieve symptoms, increase cartilage production, and delay OA progression.[44]

V. LIFESTYLE AND NUTRITIONAL INTERVENTIONS — THE WHOLE PICTURE

OA is primarily a condition of an aging, overweight population and evidence suggests that increased body weight can cause and accelerate the development of OA. The prevalence of OA is likely to increase in Western societies as overweight people and obesity become more common. The association between obesity and the increased incidence of OA has been documented.[6–9] What is unclear is whether patients with OA are predisposed to obesity due to reduced physical activity or whether obesity contributes to the development of OA. Prospective longitudinal studies have demonstrated that being overweight or obese precedes the development of OA of the knee.[11,12]

In a recent descriptive cross-sectional study, 50% of subjects were obese (BMI >30) and 75% of subjects were assessed as being at moderate to high nutritional risk, despite their obesity. This assessment was made using the Australian Nutrition Screening Initiative (ANSI) tool. Approximately 33% of subjects reported eating alone, changes in eating habits causing weight change in the past 6 months, and 25% indicated that their OA interfered with shopping, preparing, and consuming food.[143] Overweight people and obesity are associated with greater risks of high blood pressure, coronary heart disease, type II diabetes mellitus, and some cancers. These comorbidities and the pharmaceutical load involved add to the problem of OA in the elderly. Important aspects of OA management should start with patient education, encouraging a well-balanced diet, weight loss, exercise, social interaction, and referral for routine nutritional assessment and advice (see Figure 10.1).[143]

Physical activity levels (PAL) involving joint-specific exercises reduce pain and improve function in patients with knee OA.[144] Exercise can involve joint-specific strength exercise, motion exercise, and general aerobic conditioning, which can be offered in group activities or by a home-based, self-directed program. The effectiveness of home-based exercise of knee OA has been demonstrated,[62,64] showing reduced pain scores and improved function. Aerobic and isokinetic exercise have been effective in reducing pain and improving gait and function.[60,61,63] Health-promotion campaigns exhort individuals to increase their PAL, lose weight, lead a healthy lifestyle, and avoid risky behavior. Research suggests that as weight increases, so do the health risks.[143] The promotion of healthy lifestyles and reduction of risky behavior can cause "risk fatigue" by asking too much of people in a climate where social trends run contrary to health messages, making compliance more difficult (see Figure 10.1).[143]

VI. CONCLUSIONS

For optimal results, management of OA requires a cohesive, multidisciplinary, and individualized approach. Patients need to be involved in their management plan, and as the disease progresses or comorbidities develop, the management plan may need to be revised. These patients may be at risk of poor nutritional health despite being overweight as obesity often masks nutritional risk. Weight loss can ameliorate the symptoms of OA and slow disease progression. Routine nutritional assess-

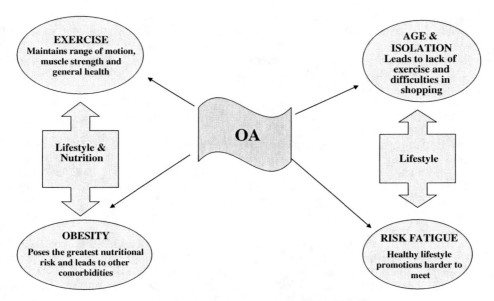

FIGURE 10.1 Osteoarthritis impacts, and effects of nutrition and lifestyle.

ment and dietary advice should be available to all OA patients. Continued research is needed to evaluate the efficacy of interventions to treat OA, particularly in the older population, which has varied responses to many of the current treatment paradigms.

REFERENCES

1. Jones, A. and Doherty, M. ABC of rheumatology: osteoarthritis, *Br. Med. J.*, 310(6977): 457–460, 1995.
2. Mathers, C.D., Vos, E.T., Stevenson, C.E., and Begg, S.J., The Australian Burden of Disease Study: measuring the loss of health from diseases, injuries and risk factors, *Med. J. Aust.*, 172: 592–596, 2000.
3. Australian Bureau of Statistics, National Health Survey, AGPS, Canberra, 2000.
4. World Health Organization, The World Health Report, 1997.
5. Hogue, J.H. and Mersfelder, T.L., Pathophysiology and first-line treatment of osteoarthritis, *Ann. Pharmacotherapy*, 36(4): 679–686, 2002.
6. Birchfield, P.C., Osteoarthritis overview, *Geriatr. Nurs.*, 22(3): 124–130, 2001.
7. Manek, N.J. and Lane, N.E., Osteoarthritis: current concepts in diagnosis and management, *Am Fam Physician*, 61(6): 1795–1804, 2000.
8. Felson, D.T. and Zhang, Y., An update on the epidemiology of knee and hip osteoarthritis with a view to prevention, *Arthritis Rheum.*, 41(8): 1343–1355, 1988.
9. Felson, D.T., Lawrence, R.C., Dieppe, P.A., Hirsch, R., Helmick, C.G,, Jordan, J.M., Kington, R.S., Lane, N.E., Nevitt, M.C., Zhang, Y., Sowers, M., McAlindon, T., Spector, T.D., Poole, A.R., Yanovski, S.Z,, Ateshian, G., Sharma, L., Buckwalter, J.A., Brandt, K.D., and Fries, J.F., Osteoarthritis: new insights. Part 1: the disease and its risk factors, *Ann. Intern. Med.*, 133(8): 635–646, 2000.
10. Manninen, P., Riihimaki, H., Heliovaara, M., and Makela, P., Overweight, gender and knee osteoarthritis, *Int. J. Obesity*, 20: 595–597, 1996.
11. Felson, D.T., Zhang, Y., Hannan, M.T., Naimark, A., Weissman, B., Aliabadi, P., and Levy, D., Risk factors for incident radiographic knee osteoarthritis in the elderly: the Framingham study, *Arthritis Rheum.*, 40(4): 728–733, 1997.
12. Spector, T.D., Hart, D.J., and Doyle, D.V., Incidence and progression of osteoarthritis in women with unilateral knee disease in the general population: the effect of obesity, *Ann. Rheum. Dis.*, 53: 565–568, 1994.

13. Sandmark, H., Hogstedt, C., Lewold, S., and Vingard, E., Osteoarthrosis of the knee in men and women in association with overweight, smoking, and hormone therapy, *Ann. Rheum. Dis.*, 58(3): 151–155, 1999.

14. Dougados, M., Gueguen, A., Nguyen, M., Thiesce, A., Listrat, V., Jacob, L., Nakache, J.P., Gabriel, K.R., Lequesne, M., and Amor, B., Longitudinal radiologic evaluation of osteoarthritis of the knee, *J. Rheumatol.*, 19: 378–383, 1992.

15. Schouten, J.S., van den Ouweland, F.A., and Valkenburg, H.A., A 12 year follow up study in the general population on prognostic factors of cartilage loss in osteoarthritis of the knee. *Ann. Rheum. Dis.*, 51: 932–937, 1992.

16. Saville, P.D. and Dickson, J., Age and weight in osteoarthritis of the hip, *Arthritis Rheum.*, 11: 635–644, 1968.

17. Tepper, S. and Hochberg, M.C., Factors associated with hip osteoarthritis: data from the First National Health and Nutrition Examination Survey (NHANES-1), *Am. J. Epidemiol.*, 137: 1081–1088, 1993.

18. Van Sasse, J.L., Vandenbroucke, J.P., van Romunde, K.J., and Valkenburg, H.A., Osteoarthritis and obesity in the general population: a relationship calling for an explanation, *J. Rheumatol.*, 15: 1152–1158, 1988.

19. Creamer, P. and Hochberg, M.C., Osteoarthritis, *Lancet*, 16: 350(9076): 503–508, 1997.

20. Kee, C.C., Osteoarthritis: manageable scourge of aging, *Nurs. Clin. N. Am.*, 35(1): 199–208, 2000.

21. Nevitt, M.C., Lane, N.E., Scott, J.C., Hochberg, M.C., Pressman, A.R., Genant, H.K., and Cummings, S.R., Radiographic osteoarthritis of the hip and bone mineral density. The Study of Osteoporotic Fractures Research Group, *Arthritis Rheum.*, 38: 907–916, 1995.

22. Hannan, M.T., Anderson, J.J., Zhang, Y., Levy, D. and Felson, D.T., Bone mineral density and knee osteoarthritis in elderly men and women: the Framingham study, *Arthritis Rheum.*, 36: 1671–1680, 1993.

23. Sowers, M., Lachance, L., Jamadar, D., Hochberg, M.C., Hollis, B., Crutchfield, M., and Jannausch, M.L., The associations of bone mineral density and bone turnover markers with osteoarthritis of the hand and knee in pre- and perimenopausal women, *Arthritis Rheum.*, 42: 483–489, 1999.

24. Zhang, Y., Hannan, M.T., Chaisson, C.E., McAlindon, T.E., Evans, S.R., Aliabadi, P., Levy, D., and Felson, D.T., Bone mineral density and risk of incident and progressive radiographic knee osteoarthritis in women: the Framingham study, *J. Rheumatol.*, 27: 1032–1037, 2000.

25. Sowers, M., Epidemiology of risk factors for osteoarthritis: systemic factors, *Curr. Opin. Rheumatol.*, 13(5): 447–451, 2001.

26. Nevitt, M.C., Cummings, S.R., Lane, N.E., Hochberg, M.C., Scott, J.C., Pressman, A.R., Genant, H.K., and Cauley, J.A., Association of estrogen replacement therapy with the risk of osteoarthritis of the hip in elderly white women, *Arch. Intern. Med.*, 156: 2073–2080, 1996.

27. Hannan, M.T., Felson, D.T., Anderson, J.J., Naimark, A., and Kannel, W.B., Estrogen use and radiographic osteoarthritis of the knee in women: the Framingham osteoarthritis study, Arthritis Rheum., 33: 525–532, 1990.

28. Samanta, A., Jones, A., Regan, M., Wilson, S., and Doherty, M., Is osteoarthritis in women affected by hormonal changes or smoking? *Br. J. Rheumatol.*, 32: 366–370, 1993.

29. Spector, T.D., Nandra, D., Hart, D.J., and Doyle, D.V., Is hormone replacement therapy protective for hand and knee osteoarthritis in women?: the Chingford study. *Ann. Rheum. Dis.*, 56: 432–434, 1997.

30. Vingard, E., Alfredsson, L., and Malchau, H., Lifestyle factors and hip arthrosis: a case referent study of body mass index, smoking and hormone therapy in 503 Swedish women. *Acta. Arthop. Scand.*, 68: 216–220, 1997.

31. Oliveria, S.A., Felson, D.T., Klein, R.A., Reed, J.I., and Walker, A.M., Estrogen replacement therapy and the development of osteoarthritis, *Epidemiology*, 7: 415–419, 1996.

32. Maetzel, A., Makela, M., Hawker, G., and Bombardier, C., Osteoarthritis of the hip and knee and mechanical occupational exposure: a systematic overview of the evidence. *J. Rheumatol.*, 24: 1599–1607, 1997.

33. Coggon, D., Croft, P., Kellingray, S., Barrett, D., McLaren, M., and Cooper, C., Occupational physical activities and osteoarthritis of the knee, *Arthritis Rheum.*, 43: 1443–1449, 2000.

34. Jensen, L.K., Mikkelsen, S., Loft, I.P., Eenberg, W., Bergmann, I., and Logager, V., Radiographic knee osteoarthritis in floorlayers and carpenters. *Scand. J. Work Environ. Health*, 26: 257–262, 2000.

35. Sandmark, H., Hogstedt, C., and Vingard, E., Primary osteoarthrosis of the knee in men and women as a result of lifelong physical load from work, *Scand. J. Work Environ. Health*, 26: 20–25, 2000.

36. Lau, E.C., Cooper, C., Lam, D., Chan, V.N., Tsang, K.K., and Sham, A., Factors associated with osteoarthritis of the hip and knee in Hong Kong Chinese: obesity, joint injury, and occupational activities, *Am. J. Epidemiol.*, 152: 855–862, 2000.

37. Yoshimura, N., Sasaki, S., Iwasaki, K., Danjoh, S., Kinoshita, H., Yasuda, T., Tamaki, T., Hashimoto, T., Kellingray, S., Croft, P., Coggon, D., and Cooper, C., Occupational lifting is associated with hip osteoarthritis: a Japanese case-control study, *J. Rheumatol.*, 27: 434–440, 2000.

38. Sowers, M.F. and Lachance, L., Vitamins and arthritis: the role of vitamins A, C, D and E, *Rheum. Dis. Clin. N. Am.*, 25: 315–332, 1999.

39. McAlindon, T.E., Jacques, P., Zhang, Y., Hannan, M.T., Aliabadi, P., Weissman. B., Rush, D., Levy, D., and Felson, D.T., Do antioxidant micronutrients protect against the development and progression of knee osteoarthritis? *Arthritis Rheum.*, 39(4): 648–56, 1996.

40. McAlindon, T.E., Felson, D.T., Zhang, Y., Hannan, M.T., Aliabadi, P., Weissman, B., Rush, D., Wilson, P.W., and Jacques, P., Relation of dietary intake and serum levels of vitamin D to progression of osteoarthritis of the knee among participants in the Framingham Study, *Ann. Intern. Med.*, 125(5): 353–359, 1996.

41. Lane, N.E., Gore, L.R., Cummings, S.R., Hochberg, M.C., Scott, J.C., Williams, E.N., and Nevitt, M.C., Serum vitamin D levels and incident changes of radiographic hip osteoarthritis: a longitudinal study. Study of Osteoporotic Fractures Research Group, *Arthritis Rheum.*, 42(5): 854–860, 1999.

42. Bischoff, H., Stahelin, H., Dick, W., Akos, R., Knecht, M., Salis, C., Nebiker, M., Theiler, R., Pfeifer, M., Begerow, B., Lew, R., and Conzelmann, M., Effects of vitamin D and calcium supplementation on falls: a randomized controlled trial, *J. Bone Miner. Res.*, 18: 343–351, 2003.

43. Machtey, I. and Ouaknine, L., Tocopherol in Osteoarthritis: a controlled pilot study, *J. Am. Geriatr. Soc.*, 26(7): 328–330, 1978.

44. Felson, D.T., Lawrence, R.C., Hochberg, M.C., McAlindon, T., Dieppe, P.A., Minor, M.A., Blair, S.N., Berman, B.M., Fries, J.F., Weinberger, M., Lorig, K.R., Jacobs, J.J., and Goldberg, V., Osteoarthritis: new insights, Part 2: Treatment approaches, *Ann. Intern. Med.*, 133: 726–737, 2000.

45. American College of Rheumatology Subcommittee on Osteoarthritis Guidelines, Recommendations for the medical management of osteoarthritis of the hip and knee, 2000 update, *Arthritis Rheum.*, 43: 1905–1915, 2000.

46. Puett, D.W. and Griffin, M.R., Published trials of nonmedicinal and noninvasive therapies for hip and knee osteoarthritis, *Ann. Intern. Med.*, 121: 133–140, 1994.

47. American Geriatrics Society Panel on Exercise and Osteoarthritis, Exercise prescription for older adults with osteoarthritis pain: Consensus practice recommendations, *J. Am. Geriatr. Soc.*, 49(6): 808–823, 2001.

48. Slemenda, C., Brandt, K.D., Heilman, D.K., Mazzuca, S., Braunstein, E.M., Katz, B.P., and Wolinsky, F.D., Quadriceps weakness and osteoarthritis of the knee, *Ann. Intern. Med.*, 127(2): 97–104, 1997.

49. Van Baar, M.E., Assendelft, W.J., Dekker, J., Oostendorp, R.A., and Bijlsma, J.W., Effectiveness of exercise therapy in patients with osteoarthritis of the hip or knee. A systematic review of randomized clinical trials, *Arthritis Rheum.*, 42: 1361–1369, 1999.

50. Chamberlain, M.A., Care, G. and Harfield, B., Physiotherapy in osteoarthrosis of the knees: a controlled trial of hospital versus home exercises, *Int. Rehabil. Med.*, 4(2): 101–106, 1982.

51. Minor, M.A., Hewett, J.E., Webel, R.R., Anderson, S.K., and Kay, D.R., Efficacy of physical conditioning exercise in patients with rheumatoid arthritis and osteoarthritis, *Arthritis Rheum.*, 32: 1396–1405, 1989.

52. Jan, M.H. and Lai, J,S., The effects of physiotherapy on osteoarthritic knees of females, *J. Formos. Med. Assoc.*, 90(10): 1008–1013, 1991.

53. Kovar, P.A., Allegrante, J.P., MacKenzie, C.R., Peterson, M.G., Gutin, B., and Charlson, M.E., Supervised fitness walking in patients with osteoarthritis of the knee, *Ann. Intern. Med.*, 116: 529–534, 1992.

54. Borjesson, M., Robertson, E., Weidenhielm, L., Mattsson, E., and Olsson, E., Physiotherapy in knee osteoarthrosis: effect on pain and walking, *Physiother. Res. Intern.*, 1: 89–97, 1996.

55. Schilke, J.M., Johnson, G.O., Housh, T.J., and O'Dell, J.R., Effects of muscle-strength training on the functional status of patients with osteoarthritis of the knee joint, *Nurs. Res.*, 45: 68–72, 1996.

56. Ettinger, W.H., Jr., Burns, R., Messier, S.P., Applegate, W., Rejeski, W.J., Morgan, T., Shumaker, S., Berry, M.J., O'Toole, M., Monu, J., and Craven, T., A randomized trial comparing aerobic exercise and resistance exercise with a health education program in older adults with knee osteoarthritis: the Fitness Arthritis and Seniors Trial (FAST), *JAMA*, 277: 25–31, 1997.

57. Bautch, J.C., Malone, D.G., and Vailas, A.C., Effects of exercise on knee joints with osteoarthritis: a pilot study of biologic markers, *Arthritis Care Res.*, 10: 48–55, 1997.

58. Van Baar, M.E., Dekker, J., Oostendorp, R.A., Bijl, D., Voorn, T.B., Lemmens, J.A., and Bijlsma, J.W., The effectiveness of exercise therapy in patients with osteoarthritis of the hip or knee: a randomized clinical trial, *J. Rheumatol.*, 25: 2432–2439, 1998.

59. Rogind, H., Bibow-Nielsen, B., Jensen, B., Moller, H.C., Frimodt-Moller, H., and Bliddal, H., The effects of a physical training program on patients with osteoarthritis of the knees, *Arch. Phys. Med. Rehab.*, 79(11): 1421–1427, 1998.

60. Mangione, K.K., McCully, K., Gloviak, A., Lefebvre, I., Hofmann, M., and Craik, R., The effects of high-intensity and low-intensity cycle ergometry in older adults with knee osteoarthritis, *J. Gerontol.*, 54: M184–M190, 1999.

61. Maurer, B.T., Stern, A.G., Kinossian, B., Cook, K.D., and Schumacher, H.R. Jr., Osteoarthritis of the knee: isokinetic quadriceps exercise versus an educational intervention, *Arch. Phys. Med. Rehab.*, 80(10): 1293–1299, 1999.

62. O'Reilly, S.C., Muir, K.R., and Doherty, M., Effectiveness of home exercise on pain and disability from osteoarthritis of the knee: a randomized controlled trial, *Ann. Rheum. Dis.*, 58: 15–19, 1999.

63. Deyle, G.D., Henderson, N.E., Matekel, R.L., Ryder, M.G., Garber, M.B., and Allison, S.C., Effectiveness of manual physical therapy and exercise in osteoarthritis of the knee: a randomized, controlled trial, *Ann. Intern. Med.*, 132: 173–181, 2000.

64. Petrella, R.J. and Bartha, C., Home based exercise therapy for older patients with knee osteoarthritis: a randomized clinical trial, *J. Rheumatol.*, 27: 2215–2221, 2000.

65. McCarberg, B.H. and Herr, K.A., Osteoarthritis. How to manage pain and improve patient function, *Geriatrics*, 56(10): 14–7, 20–2, 2001.

66. Lorig, K., Lubeck, D., Kraines, R.G., Seleznick, M., and Holman, H.R., Outcomes of self-help education for patients with arthritis, *Arthritis Rheum.*, 28: 680–685, 1985.

67. Lorig, K. and Holman, H.R., Long-term outcomes of an arthritis self-management study: effects of reinforcement efforts, *Soc. Sci. Med.*, 29(2): 221–224, 1989.

68. Weinberger, M., Tierney, W.M., Booher, P., and Katz, B.P., Can the provision of information to patients with osteoarthritis improve functional status — a randomised, controlled trial, *Arthritis Rheum.*, 32: 1577–1583, 1989.

69. Calfas, K.J., Kaplan, R.M., and Ingram, R.E., One-year evaluation of cognitive-behavioural intervention in osteoarthritis, *Arthritis Care Res.*, 5: 202–209, 1992.

70. Lorig, K.R., Mazonson, P.D., and Holman, H.R., Evidence suggesting that health education for self-management in patients with chronic arthritis has sustained health benefits while reducing health care costs, *Arthritis Rheum.*, 36: 439–446, 1993.

71. Mazzuca, S.A., Brandt, K.D., Katz, B.P., Chambers, M., Byrd, D., and Hanna, M., Effects of self-care education on the health status of inner city patients with osteoarthritis of the knee, *Arthritis Rheum.*, 40: 1466–1474, 1997.

72. Superio-Cabuslay, E., Ward, M.M., and Lorig, K.R., Patient education interventions in osteoarthritis and rheumatoid arthritis: a meta-analytic comparison with nonsteroidal antiinflammatory drug treatment, *Arthritis Care Res.*, 9: 292–301, 1996.

73. March, L.M. and Stenmark, J., Non-pharmacological approaches to managing arthritis, *Med. J. Aust.*, 175: S102–107, 2001.

74. Weinberger, M., Hiner, S.L., and Tierney, W.M., Improving functional status in arthritis: the effect of social support, *Soc. Sci. Med.*, 23: 899–904, 1986.

75. Rene, J., Weinberger, M., Mazzuca, S.A., Brandt, K.D., and Katz, B.P., Reduction of joint pain in patients with knee osteoarthritis who have received monthly telephone calls from lay personnel and whose medical treatment regimes have remained stable, *Arthritis Rheum.*, 35: 511–515, 1992.

76. Weinberger, M., Tierney, W.M., Cowper, P.A., Katz, B.P., and Booher, P.A., Cost-effectiveness of increased telephone contact for patients with osteoarthritis: a randomized, controlled trial, *Arthritis Rheum.*, 36: 243–246, 1993.

77. Maisiak, R., Austin, J., and Heck, L., Health outcomes of two telephone interventions for patients with rheumatoid arthritis or osteoarthritis, *Arthritis Rheum.*, 39(8): 1391–1399, 1996.
78. Cronan, T.A., Groessl, E., and Kaplan, R.M., The effects of social support and education interventions on health care costs, *Arthritis Care Res.*, 10(2): 99–110, 1997.
79. Toda, Y., Toda, T., Takemura, S., Wada, T., Morimoto, T., and Ogawa, R., Change in body fat, but not body weight or metabolic correlates of obesity, is related to symptomatic relief of obese patients with knee osteoarthritis after a weight control program, *J. Rheumatol.*, 25(11): 2181–2186, 1998.
80. Messier, S.P., Loeser, R.F., Mitchell, M.N., Valle, G., Morgan, T.P., Rejeski, W.J., and Ettinger, W.H., Exercise and weight loss in obese older adults with knee osteoarthritis: a preliminary study, *J. Am. Geriatr. Soc.*, 48(9): 1062–1072, 2000.
81. Williams, R.A. and Foulsham, B.M., Weight reduction in osteoarthritis using phentermine, *Practitioner*, 225: 231–232, 1981.
82. Keating, E., Faris, P., Ritter, M., and Kane, J., Use of lateral heel and sole wedges in the treatment of medical osteoarthritis of the knee, *Orthopaed. Rev.*, 22: 921–924, 1993.
83. Berman, B.M., Swyers, J.P., and Ezzo, J., The evidence for acupuncture as a treatment for rheumatologic conditions, *Rheum. Dis. Clin. N. Am.*, 26(1): 103–15, 2000.
84. Ernst, E., Acupuncture as a symptomatic treatment of osteoarthritis: a systematic review, *Scand. J. Rheum.*, 26(6): 444–447, 1997.
85. Gaw, A.C., Chang, L.W., and Shaw, L.C., Efficacy of acupuncture on osteoarthritic pain: a controlled, double-blind study, *N. Engl. J. Med.*, 293: 375–378, 1975.
86. Thomas, M., Eriksson, S.V., and Lundeberg, T., A comparative study of diazepam and acupuncture in patients with osteoarthritis pain: a placebo controlled study, *Am. J. Chin. Med.*, 19: 95–100, 1991.
87. Christensen, B.V., Iuhl, I.U., Vilbek, H., Bulow, H.H., Dreijer, N.C., and Rasmussen, H.F., Acupuncture treatment of severe knee osteoarthrosis: a long-term study, *Acta Anaesthesiol. Scand.*, 36: 519–525, 1992.
88. Takeda, W. and Wessel, J., Acupuncture for the treatment of pain of osteoarthritic knees, *Arthritis Care Res.*, 7: 118–122, 1994.
89. Berman, B.M., Lao, L., Greene, M., Anderson, R.W., Wong, R.H., Langenberg, P. and Hochberg, M.C., Efficacy of traditional Chinese acupuncture in the treatment of symptomatic knee osteoarthritis: a pilot study, *Osteoarthritis Cartilage*, 3(2): 139–142, 1995.
90. Berman, B.M., Singh, B.B., Lao, L., Langenberg, P., Li, H., Hadhazy, V., Bareta, J., and Hochberg, M.C., A randomized trial of acupuncture as an adjunctive therapy in osteoarthritis of the knee, *Rheumatology (Oxford)*, 38: 346–354, 1999.
91. Ezzo, J., Hadhazy, V., Birch, S., Lao, L., Kaplan, G., Hochberg, M.C., and Berman, B., Acupuncture for osteoarthritis of the knee: a systematic review, *Arthritis Rheum.*, 44(4): 819–825, 2001.
92. Pendleton, A., Arden, N., Dougados, M., Doherty, M., Bannwarth, B., Bijlsma, J.W., Cluzeau, F., Cooper, C., Dieppe, P.A., Gunther, K.P., Hauselmann, H.J., Herrero-Beaumont, G., Kaklamanis, P.M., Leeb, B., Lequesne, M., Lohmander, S., Mazieres, B., Mola, E.M., Pavelka, K., Serni, U., Swoboda, B., Verbruggen. A.A., Weseloh, G., and Zimmermann-Gorska, I., EULAR recommendations for the management of knee osteoarthritis: report of a task force of the Standing Committee for International Clinical Studies Including Therapeutic Trials (ESCISIT), *Ann. Rheum. Dis.*, 59: 936–944, 2000.
93. Eccles, M., Freemantle, N. and Mason, J., North of England evidence based guideline development project: summary guideline for non-steroidal anti-inflammatory drugs versus basic analgesia in treating the pain of degenerative arthritis, *Br. Med. J.*, 317(7157): 526–30, 1998.
94. Wolfe, F., Zhao, S., and Lane, N., Preference for nonsteroidal anti-inflammatory drugs over acetaminophen by rheumatic disease patients: a survey of 1,799 patients with osteoarthritis, rheumatoid arthritis, and fibromyalgia, *Arthritis Rheum.*, 43(2): 378–385, 2000.
95. Haq, I., Murphy, E., and Dacre, J., *Osteoarthritis, Postgrad. Med. J.*, 79: 377–383, 2003.
96. Garcia Rodriguez, L.A. and Hernandez-Diaz, S., The risk of upper gastrointestinal complications associated with nonsteroidal anti-inflammatory drugs, glucocorticoids, acetaminophen, and combinations of these agents, *Arthritis Res.*, 3(2): 98–101, 2001.
97. Gotzsche, P.C., Non-steroidal anti-inflammatory drugs, *Br. Med. J.*, 15: 320(7241): 1058–1061, 2000.
98. Watson, M.C., Brookes, S.T., Kirwan, J.R., and Faulkner, A., Non-aspirin, non-steroidal anti-inflammatory drugs for treating osteoarthritis of the knee, Cochrane Musculoskeletal Group, *Cochrane Database Syst. Rev.*, Issue 3, 2002.

99. Towheed, T., Shea, B., Wells, G., and Hochberg, M., Analgesia and non-aspirin, non-steroidal anti-inflammatory drugs for osteoarthritis of the hip, Cochrane Musculoskeletal Group, *Cochrane Database Syst. Rev.*, Issue 3, 2002.

100. Hochberg, M.C., What a difference a year makes: reflections on the ACR recommendations for the medical management of osteoarthritis, *Curr. Rheumatol. Rep.*, 3(6): 473–478, 2001.

101. Deal, C.L., Schnitzer, T.J., Lipstein, E., Seibold, J.R., Stevens, R.M., Levy, M.D., Albert, D., and Renold, F., Treatment of arthritis with topical capsaicin: a double-blind trial, *Clin. Ther.*, 13(3): 383–395, 1991.

102. Silverstein, F.E., Faich, G., Goldstein, J.L., Simon, L.S., Pincus, T., Whelton, A., Makuch, R., Eisen, G., Agrawal, N.M., Stenson, W.F., Burr, A.M., Zhao, W.W., Kent, J.D., Lefkowith, J.B., Verburg, K.M., and Geis, G.S., Gastrointestinal toxicity with celecoxib vs nonsteroidal anti-inflammatory drugs for osteoarthritis and rheumatoid arthritis: the CLASS study: a randomized controlled trial. Celecoxib Long-term Arthritis Safety Study, *JAMA*, 284(10): 1247–1255, 2000.

103. Bombardier, C., Laine, L., Reicin, A., Shapiro, D., Burgos-Vargas, R., Davis, B., Day, R., Ferraz, M.B., Hawkey, C.J., Hochberg, M.C., Kvien, T.K., and Schnitzer, T.J., VIGOR Study Group. Comparison of upper gastrointestinal toxicity of rofecoxib and naproxen in patients with rheumatoid arthritis. VIGOR Study Group, *N. Engl. J. Med.*, 343(21): 1520–1528, 2000.

104. Savage, R., Cyclo-oxygenase-2 inhibitors: when should they be used in the elderly? *Drugs Aging*, 22(3): 185–200,2005.

105. Hawker, G., Wright, J., Coyte, P., Paul, J., Dittus, R., Croxford, R., Katz, B., Bombardier, C., Heck, D., and Freund, D., Health-related quality of life after knee replacement, *J. Bone Joint Surg.*, 80(2): 163–173, 1998.

106. Dieppe, P., Basler, H.D., Chard, J., Croft, P., Dixon, J., Hurley, M., Lohmander, S., and Raspe, H., Knee replacement surgery for osteoarthritis: effectiveness, practice variations, indications and possible determinants of utilization, *Rheumatology*, 38(1): 73–83, 1999.

107. Chang, R.W., Pellisier, J.M., and Hazen, G.B., A cost-effectiveness analysis of total hip arthroplasty for osteoarthritis of the hip, *JAMA*, 275(11): 858–865, 1996.

108. Fortin, P.R., Clarke, A.E., Joseph, L., Liang, M.H., Tanzer, M., Ferland, D., Phillips, C., Partridge, A.J., Belisle, P., Fossel, A.H., Mahomed, N., Sledge, C.B., and Katz, J.N., Outcomes of total hip and knee replacement: preoperative functional status predicts outcomes at six months after surgery, *Arthritis Rheum.*, 42(8): 1722–1728, 1999.

109. McAlindon, T. and Felson, D.T., Nutrition: risk factors for osteoarthritis, *Ann. Rheum. Dis.*, 56: 397–402, 1997.

110. Volker, D.H., Katz, T., Shui, L., Quaggiotto, P., Garg, M., and Major, G., Nutrition in inflammatory disease: evidence for practice, *Asia Pac. J. Clin. Nutr.*, 24: 49, 2002.

111. Curtis, C., Rees, S., Cramp, J., Flannery, C., Hughes, C., Little, C., Williams, R., Wilson, C., Dent, C., Harwood, J., and Caterson, B., Effects of n-3 fatty acids on cartilage metabolism, *Proc. Nutr. Soc.*, 61: 381–389, 2002.

112. Miles, E.A. and Calder, P.C., Modulation of immune function by dietary fatty acids. *Proc. Nutr. Soc.* 57: 277–300, 1998.

113. National Research Council Committee on Diet and Health, *Diet and Health: Implications for Reducing Chronic Disease Risk*, 2nd ed., Washington, D.C., 1989.

114. Simopoulos, A.P., Omega-3 fatty acids in health and disease and in growth and development, *Am. J. Clin. Nutr.*, 54, 438–463, 1991.

115. Garg, M., Sebokova, E., Wierbicki, A., Thomson, A., and Clandinin, M., Differential effects of dietary linoleic acid and alpha linolenic acid on lipid metabolism in rat tissues, *Lipids*, 23: 847–852, 1988.

116. Hwang, D., Essential fatty acids and immune response, *FASEB*, 3: 2052–2061, 1989.

117. Whelan, J., Antagonistic effects of dietary arachidonic acid and n-3 polyunsaturated fatty acids, *J. Nutr.*, 126: 1086S–1091S, 1996.

118. Long, L., Soeken, K. and Ernst, E., Herbal medicines for the treatment of osteoarthritis: a systematic review, *Rheumatology*, 40(7): 779–793, 2001.

119. Zhang, W.Y. and Li Wan Po, A., The effectiveness of topically applied capsaicin: a meta-analysis, *Eur. J. Clin. Pharmacol.*, 46: 517–522, 1994.

120. Altman, R.D., Aven, A., and Ce, H., Capsaicin cream 0.025% as monotherapy for osteoarthritis: A double-blind study, *Sem. Arthritis Rheum.*, 23(Suppl.): 25–33, 1994.

121. Blotman, F., Maheu, E., Wulwik, A., Caspard, H., and Lopez, A., Efficacy and safety of avocado/soybean unsaponifiables in the treatment of symptomatic osteoarthritis of the knee and hip: a prospective, multicenter, three-month, randomized, double-blind, placebo-controlled trial, *Rev. Rheum. Engl. Ed.* 64: 825–834, 1997.

122. Maheu, E., Mazieres, B., Valat, J.P., Loyau, G., Le Loet, X., Bourgeois, P., Grouin, J.M. and Rozenberg, S., Symptomatic efficacy of avocado/soybean unsaponifiables in the treatment of osteoarthritis of the knee and hip: a prospective, randomized, double-blind, placebo-controlled, multicenter clinical trial with a six-month treatment period and a two-month follow-up demonstrating a persistent effect, *Arthritis Rheum.*, 41: 81–91, 1998.

123. Mills, S.Y., Jacoby, R.K., Chacksfield, M., and Willoughby, M., Effect of a proprietary herbal medicine on the relief of chronic arthritic pain: a double blind study, *Br. J. Rheumatol.*, 35: 874–878, 1996.

124. Schmid, B., Ludtke, R., Selbmann, H.K., Kotter, I., Tschirdewahn, B., Schaffner, W., and Heide, L., Efficacy and tolerability of a standardized willow bark extract in patients with osteoarthritis: randomized placebo-controlled, double blind clinical trial, *Phytother. Res.*, 15(4): 344–350, 2001.

125. Randall, C., Randall, H., Dobbs, F., Hutton, C., and Sanders, H., Randomized controlled trial of nettle sting for treatment of base-of-thumb pain., *J. R. Soc. Med.*, 93: 305–309, 2000.

126. Kulkarni, R.R., Patki, P.S., Jog, V.P., Gandage, S.G., and Patwardhan, B., Treatment of osteoarthritis with a herbomineral formulation: a double-blind, placebo-controlled, cross-over study, *J. Ethnopharmacol.*, 33: 91–95, 1991.

127. Bliddal, H., Rosetzsky, A., Schlichting, P., Weidner, M.S., Andersen, L.A., Ibfelt, H.H., Christensen, K., Jensen, O.N., and Barslev, J., A randomized, placebo-controlled, cross-over study of ginger extracts and ibuprofen in osteoarthritis, *Osteoarthritis Cartilage*, 8: 9–12, 2000.

128. McAlindon, T.E., LaValley, M.P., Gulin, J.P., and Felson, D.T., Glucosamine and chondroitin for treatment of osteoarthritis: a systematic quality assessment and meta-analysis, *JAMA*, 283: 1469–1475, 2000.

129. Crolle, G. and D'Este, E., Glucosamine sulfate for the management of arthrosis: a controlled clinical investigation, *Curr. Med. Res. Opin.*, 7(2): 104–109, 1980.

130. Drovanti, A., Bignamini, A.A. and Rovati, A.L., Therapeutic activity of oral glucosamine sulfate in osteoarthrosis: a placebo-controlled double-blind investigation, *Clin Ther.*, 3(4): 260–272, 1980.

131. Pujalte, J.M., Llavore, E.P., and Ylscupidez, F.R., Double-blind clinical evaluation of oral glucosamine sulfate in the basic treatment of osteoarthrosis, *Curr. Med. Res. Opin.*, 7(2): 110–114, 1980.

132. D'Ambrosio, E., Casa, B., Bompani, R., Scali, G., and Scali, M., Glucosamine sulfate: a controlled clinical investigation in arthrosis, *Pharmatherapeutica*. 2(8): 504–508, 1981.

133. Vajaradul, Y., Double-blind clinical evaluation of intra-articular glucosamine in outpatients with gonarthrosis, *Clin. Ther.*, 3(5): 336–343, 1981.

134. Vaz, A.L., Double-blind clinical evaluation of the relative efficacy of ibuprofen and glucosamine sulfate in the management of osteoarthrosis of the knee in out-patients, *Curr. Med. Res. Opin.*, 8(3): 145–149, 1982.

135. Muller-Fassbender, H., Bach, G.L., Haase, W., Rovati, L.C., and Setnikar, I., Glucosamine sulfate compared to ibuprofen in osteoarthritis of the knee, *Osteoarthritis Cartilage*, 2(1): 61–69, 1994.

136. Noack, W., Fischer, M., Forster, K.K., Rovati, L.C., and Setnikar, I., Glucosamine sulfate in osteoarthritis of the knee, *Osteoarthritis Cartilage*, 2(1): 51–59, 1994.

137. Morreale, P., Manopulo, R., Galati, M., Boccanera, L., Saponati, G., and Bocchi, L., Comparison of the antiinflammatory efficacy of chondroitin sulfate and diclofenac sodium in patients with knee osteoarthritis, *J. Rheumatol.*, 23(8): 1385–1391, 1996.

138. Bourgeois, P., Chales, G., Dehais, J., Delcambre, B., Kuntz, J.L., and Rozenberg, S., Efficacy and tolerability of chondroitin sulfate 1200 mg/day vs chondroitin sulfate 3 × 400 mg/d vs. placebo, *Osteoarthritis Cartilage*, 6(Suppl. A): 25–30, 1998.

139. Conrozier, T., Anti-arthrosis treatments: efficacy and tolerance of chondroitin sulfates, *Presse Med.*, 27(36): 1862–1865, 1998.

140. Bucsi, L. and Poor, G., Efficacy and tolerability of oral chondroitin sulfate as a symptomatic slow-acting drug for osteoarthritis (SYSADOA) in the treatment of knee osteoarthritis, Osteoarthritis Cartilage, 6(Suppl. A): 31–36, 1998.

141. Towheed, T.E., Anastassiades, T.P., Shea, B., Houpt, J., Welch, V., and Hochberg, M.C., Glucosamine therapy for treating osteoarthritis, *Cochrane Database Syst. Rev.*, Issue 2, 2002.

142. Reginster, J.Y., Deroisy, R., Rovati, L.C., Lee, R.L., Lejeune, E., Bruyere, O., Giacovelli, G., Henrotin, Y., Dacre, J.E., and Gossett, C., Long-term effects of glucosamine sulfate on osteoarthritis progression: a randomised, placebo-controlled clinical trial, *Lancet*, 357: 251–256, 2001.

143. Foley, A., Keogh, J., Miller, M., Halbert, J., and Crotty, M., Osteoarthritis: is more attention to nutritional health required? *Nutr. Diet.*, 60: 97–103, 2003.

144. Pennix, B., Messier, S., Rejeski, W., Williamson, J., DiBari, M., Cavazzini, C., Applegate, W., and Pahor, M., Physical exercise and the prevention of disability in activities of daily living in older persons with osteoarthritis, *Arch. Intern. Med.*, 116: 2309–2316, 2001.

11 Omega-3 Fatty Acids, Mediterranean Diet, Probiotics, Vitamin D, and Exercise in the Treatment of Rheumatoid Arthritis

Dianne H. Volker

CONTENTS

I. INTRODUCTION

Rheumatoid arthritis (RA) is a chronic, debilitating, and progressive condition that affects the physical, emotional, and social well-being of the RA patient and associated family members. The disease is primarily treated in an ambulatory care setting, and the clinical course of RA is characterized by highly variable periods of remission and relapse with some patients stabilized while others develop aggressive disease.[1] Patients with RA require continued drug treatment to alleviate symptoms and to delay disease progression. Most of the drugs used are expensive and have significant side effects which involve damage to the liver, kidneys, gastrointestinal tract, and eyes.[2] The physical and psychological implications are fatigue, lethargy, depression, and hand handicap, as well as modified appetite, nausea, vomiting, taste changes, and altered nutrient metabolism.[3–6] Changes such as these add to the detrimental effects of accepted RA pharmacologically based therapies. Chronic diseases such as cardiovascular disease and diabetes mellitus utilize a therapeutic dichotomy of drug therapy and dietary manipulation. This combination of therapies is not common practice in RA treatment modalities.

Rheumatologists are generally unwilling to embrace dietary manipulation, perhaps because of the abundance of fads and myths concerning dietary therapy and the willingness of RA patients to experiment with any regime that promises to improve quality of life. This negative response by rheumatologists squanders the limited available opportunities for conveying positive health messages and the encouragement of self-efficacy. Comorbidities have a significant effect on the outcome of RA, which is associated with increased morbidity and mortality from infection, neoplasm, renal disease, and iatrogenic consequences of the rheumatoid treatment.[7–9] Cardiovascular disease in RA patients occurs in a similar proportion to that of the general population; however, it is the most common cause of rheumatoid death. Patients with RA have a life expectancy of between two and 18 years less than the general population, with death from cardiovascular disease an important determinant of the excess mortality.[10,11] Traditional risk factors such as smoking, hypertension, hyperlipidemia, and diabetes are associated with 50% of all cardiovascular events, and inflammatory processes appear to be involved.[12,13] A chronic inflammatory response may promote the development of accelerated atherogenesis, thus active treatment is necessary to reduce the risk of cardiovascular disease complications.[14] Seropositivity for rheumatoid factor, late disease onset, and male gender all appear implicated in mortality and cardiovascular events.[10] Smoking and obesity are risk factors for all causes of ill health; however, smoking adversely influences the severity of RA and may be a risk factor in the development of *de novo* cases of RA.[12] The morbidity and mortality risk in the RA population is further exacerbated by lifestyle effects such as lack of exercise with associated obesity and poor diet, which often develops through progressive disability.

Lifestyle and behavioral changes are difficult for most people but particularly those with chronic diseases. The role of education and self-management is accepted and has been validated in the management of other chronic diseases such as diabetes and cardiovascular disease. Similar principles can be applied to rheumatic diseases, particularly RA, to enhance self-efficacy, and to reduce pain and disability.[13]

There is ample evidence in epidemiological, clinical, and mechanistic studies to support life-enhancing dietary advice for RA patients. Diet is a universal exposure for all people, and any improvement achieved by dietary manipulation of the RA patients' diet has the potential to reduce the required pharmacological therapies. Anti-inflammatory dietary regimens including omega-3 fatty acids, Mediterranean diet, probiotics, and vitamin D have demonstrated health enhancing benefits.[15–19]

II. RHEUMATOID ARTHRITIS

A. EPIDEMIOLOGY OF RA

Several incidence and prevalence studies of RA during the past decades suggest that there is considerable variation of the disease occurrence among different populations. Normally, disease occurrence can be determined through the measurement of incidence of RA (the rate of new cases arising in a given period) and prevalence (the number of existing cases). Both methods of measurement present difficulties because of the low overall incidence of RA, necessitating large sample sizes with prolonged follow-up times to ensure statistical precision. The incidence-rate trend suggests that the incidence and severity of RA is declining.[20] The annual incidence rate for RA cases diagnosed between 1950 and 1974 has been given as 0.5/1000 for females and 0.2/1000 for males, with an increasing incidence continuing into the seventh decade of life.[21] The use of the 1987/1991 ARC criteria to classify RA has resulted in a decrease in the annual incidence rate for females to 0.36/1000 and 0.14/1000 for males. The incidence for males increased with age whereas females plateaued between the ages of 45 to 70.[21] Symmons and coworkers claim that the prevalence in Caucasian, European, and North American populations ranges from 0.5% to 2.0% for those over 15 years of age, with age-specific prevalence rates increasing as RA patients age.[22] *Ipso facto,* the incidence and severity of RA may be declining over time; evidence suggests that the nature of this change is complex. Seropositive, erosive, and nodular disease in individuals with RA peaked in the 1960s and has declined since.[23,24]

There are a number of geographic variations observed world wide. The prevalence estimates for Europe, North America, Asia, and South Africa are quite similar at 0.5% to 1%. Some North American Indians have a disease prevalence of 5%, whereas other native North American Indian populations have a very low prevalence (<0.4%).[25] Solomon and colleagues maintained that the prevalence in urban black African populations suggests a rate similar to Europeans, whereas rural African populations show a very low prevalence.[26] Low prevalence rates have been reported from Chinese and Indonesian populations,[27,28] Schichikawa and colleagues reported a low prevalence in RA of 0.4% in Japan.[29] Roberts-Thomson and Roberts-Thomson found no evidence to suggest that RA in Australian aborigines occurred before and during the early stages of white settlement.[30] Comparisons of prevalence then become problematic if there is a change in the incidence and severity of RA; furthermore, it becomes difficult to determine whether global variations in prevalence are due to environmental or genetic factors.

B. PATHOGENESIS

RA is an autoimmune disease, characterized by a chronic inflammatory synovitis of unknown origin. The distinctive features of RA are chronic, symmetrical, and erosive arthritis of the peripheral joints. Previously, RA has been regarded as a benign, nonfatal disease; however, it is now accepted that RA reduces life expectancy by two to 18 years in both men and women.[11–13] Twice as many women as men are affected.[31] The peak onset of RA is in the fourth and fifth decade of life.[31] Mortality rates are higher in those patients who have more persistent joint inflammation, seropositivity for rheumatoid factor (RF), functional loss, and lower levels of education.[32] RA patients experience a range of lifestyle diseases, as do the general population; however, they die at a younger age.[9] The primary risk factors for reduced longevity are the greater number of involved joints, cardiovascular comorbidities, older age, lower education level, and poor functional status.[33] Care of patients with RA requires regular monitoring of disease progression and the effects of treatment. Both regular monitoring and the cost of pharmacological therapies, as well as the deleterious effect of these drugs, make expenditure on this group a major component of health care costs.[34] New treatment modalities are proving to be very expensive to develop and use.[35]

It is difficult to define RA because there is no single clinical, laboratory, or radiological marker that is specific for the disease. The difficulty posed by the need to classify RA results from the wide range of presentation modes in which RA presents as inactive, mild and self-limiting, or quite severe.[36] Additionally, there is a need to distinguish RA from a range of other destructive arthropathies to determine the use of appropriate pharmacological-based therapies.

C. CLINICAL FEATURES

The most common form of disease onset involves pain and joint swelling over a number of weeks. The usual presentation is that of polyarthritis affecting the small joints of the hands and feet and

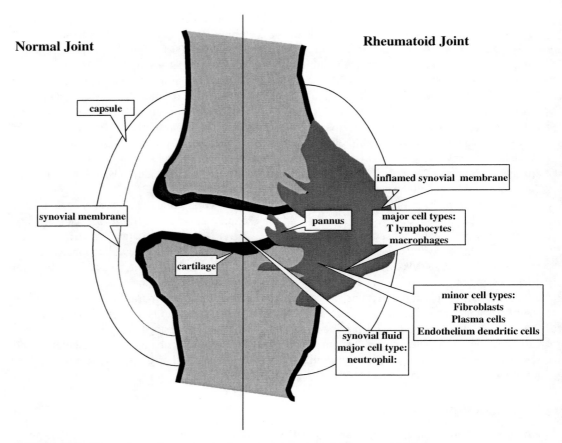

Normal Joint

Rheumatoid Joint

capsule

inflamed synovial membrane

synovial membrane

pannus

major cell types:
T lymphocytes
macrophages

cartilage

minor cell types:
Fibroblasts
Plasma cells
Endothelium dendritic cells

synovial fluid
major cell type:
neutrophil:

FIGURE 11.1 Comparison of structure in the normal joint and the rheumatoid joint.

one or more of the large joints[37,38] Inflammatory symptoms, such as pain, heat, swelling, and functional loss, are usually apparent on onset and are predominant in early RA.[39,40] If the inflammation and the resultant synovitis remain persistent and uncontrolled, joint damage ensues with deformity, malalignment, and instability (Figure 11.1). Other synovial sites that are commonly affected are the bursae and tendon sheaths.[41,42] The deterioration of tendons and their sheaths, as well as ligament laxity, leads to the typical rheumatoid deformity in hands and feet. Palpable thickening or nodality of tendons is common and may cause obstructive symptoms such as "locking." Tendon rupture can occur if the inflammatory tenosynovitis erodes through the tendon. Compressed nerves by synovitis are common and evident in the compression of the median nerve in the carpal tunnel.[43]

Typical rheumatoid deformities of the hand include the ulnar drift of the fingers, swan neck and boutonniere deformities in the fingers, and the Z deformity of the thumb. Tendon rupture of the extensor tendons of the thumb and third, fourth, and fifth fingers can occur. Rheumatoid involvement of the thoracic and lumbar spine is rare, but the cervical spine can be involved.[36] This may lead to compression of the spinal cord resulting in neck pain and stiffness, sensory loss, abnormal gait, and loss of bladder control. Herniation of the knee capsule posteriorly (Baker's cyst) can develop and rupture into the calf muscle. The most commonly involved joints of the feet and ankles are the metatarsophalangeal joints and the ankle joints.[36]

Extraarticular features of RA involve the skin, eyes, and cardiovascular system, and respiratory system, neurological, and hematological areas.[44] The systemic symptoms are usually weight loss, malaise, lethargy, and fatigue. Fever is not usually present. Many of the extraarticular features such as vasculitis, nodules, and lung disease correlate with the presence of RF and severe joint involvement. Rheumatoid nodules, although a characteristic of RA, occur in less than 50% of patients. Sicca symptoms (dry eyes) as a manifestation of Sjogren's syndrome are common. Interstitial lung disease and inflammatory pericarditis are frequently found at autopsy of 50% of rheumatoid patients.[45,46]

D. DIAGNOSIS

The diagnosis of RA is a clinical diagnosis.[36] There are no laboratory tests, historical, or x-ray images that indicate the definitive diagnosis. When RA is suspected a number of tests should be performed. RF is found in the serum of 80% of RA patients. Its presence supports the clinical diagnosis and has a prognostic value as its presence correlates with disease severity. Erythrocyte sedimentation rate (ESR) is usually elevated when RA is active; however, some patients may occasionally have a normal ESR.[1-20] C-reactive protein (CRP) is used to monitor the level of inflammation and the response to treatment. Radiography can detect the earliest changes in RA, such as soft-tissue swellings. Subsequently, x-rays can detect erosive disease.[47] RA diagnosis usually involves morning stiffness in and around the affected joints, generally lasting for at least 1 h, and at least three joint areas manifesting soft-tissue swelling or fluid accumulation. There are 14 possible affected joint areas: these are the right and left proximal interphalangeal joints, metacarpophalangeal joints, wrist, elbow, knee, ankle, and metatarsophalangeal joints.[48] Early diagnosis of RA is important if remission and prevention of joint destruction are to be achieved. These goals may be reached using the conventional disease modifying antirheumatic drugs (DMARDs), nonsteroidal anti-inflammatory drugs (NSAIDs), or biological agents. For RA with a severe prognosis, DMARDs or biological agents can be initiated as first line therapy.[49]

III. RISK FACTORS

A. AGE AND GENDER

Twice as many women as men are affected by RA and the peak onset of RA is in the fourth and fifth decade of life.[31] Mortality rates are higher in those patients who have more persistent joint inflammation and seropositivity for RF, functional loss, and lower levels of education.[50] There is some evidence that the incidence in Western populations may have fallen in young women during the 1960s and 70s. The peak age of incidence is now in the group older than 50 (postmenopausal), whereas previously peak age of incidence was younger (perimenopausal).[31] Estrogen and low testosterone levels appear to be implicated as risk factors for RA.[31-33]

B. GENETICS

Family genetic studies provide compelling evidence that there is a genetic influence in RA. Aho and his group maintain that twin studies can be prone to biased assessment.[51] However, when Silman and coworkers examined disease concordance rates between monozygotic twins of 12% to 14% and dizygotic twins of 4%, and compared them with the background disease prevalence of approximately 1% for nonrelatives, genetic factors appear to contribute to disease risk.[52] This twin and familial clustering provide some evidence for a genetic origin of RA. Nepom's group suggest that multiple genes are involved with the histocompatibility locus antigen (HLA) region on the chromosome.[53] On chromosome 6, the class II major histocompatibility complex (MHC) has a HLA–DR region that is located in the HLA DRB1 locus. DR4 is the serological marker associated with HLA DRB1 locus. The genetic susceptibility of Caucasians in North America and Europe has been identified by the presence of four DR4 positive alleles, Dw4, DR 1.1, DRw15, and Dw14.2. Gao and coworkers suggest that individuals who exhibit HLA–DRB/DR4 have a fivefold relative risk of developing RA compared to individuals in the general population.[54] According to Weyard's group, not all individuals exhibiting this genetic susceptibility develop RA.[55] The Japanese have a relatively high prevalence of HLA–DRw15 (which infers susceptibility) but paradoxically, display a low prevalence of RA.[29] Studies of the Hong Kong Chinese population suggest that PDCD1 polymorphisms and haplotypes are involved as a susceptibility gene for RA.[56]

C. ENVIRONMENTAL FACTORS

Spector's group claim that the strongest candidates for environmental triggers of RA are the sex hormones.[57] This is suggested by the marked female excess in both the incidence and prevalence of RA. It has been noted that the symptoms of RA often abate during pregnancy, with a subsequent flare in the postpartum period. The factors responsible for remission include estrogen levels and increased levels of pregnancy-associated glycoprotein. Spector's group also maintain that RA occurs less frequently in women taking the oral contraceptive pill (OCP), suggesting that the OCP may have a protective effect.[58] Studies on the effect of hormone replacement therapy (HRT) do not provide a clear association with risk.[59,60] In males, low testosterone levels are implicated with RA, however it is unknown whether the low testosterone levels occur as a result of the disease effect or before the initiation of RA.[61]

Researchers have postulated that RA is induced in genetically predisposed individuals by many different arthrogenic agents such as bacteria and viruses. The implicated viruses include retroviruses, Epstein-Barr virus, rubella virus, and parvovirus. Candidate bacteria are mycoplasma, mycobacteria, and some enteric organisms.[62–65] Additionally a number of studies have suggested a relationship between socioeconomic status, occupation, urban, industrialized environments, and RA. Data gathered from the Norfolk Arthritis Register suggests that there is no association between risk of RA and indicators of socioeconomic status.[22] A more generalized association between RA and urban, industrialized environments has been proposed but results appear to be in conflict.[66] Data on lifestyle factors provide conflicting information; however, increased risk of RA is associated with cigarette smoking according to studies conducted by Silman and coworkers.[67] Analysis by Pincus and his group contradicts Symmons' group by claiming that social conditions and self-management are the more powerful determinants of health.[22,68] It is possible that social conditions and self-management may reflect the lifestyle factors in the Silman studies.

D. INFLAMMATION

Inflammation in RA is not self-limiting as it is in generalized infection, it is a chronic inflammatory process.[69] Inflammation of the synovial membrane in RA is mediated by specialized cells necessary for an immune response.[70] The most prominent features are the accumulation of mononuclear phagocytes, lymphocytes, and leucocytes in the proliferating tissue.[70] Proinflammatory and proliferative signals are transmitted to bone marrow and synovial membranes with the resultant monoclonal stimulation of specific cell lines and synovial proliferation in the inflamed joint[70] (Figure 11.1). Angiogenesis, synovial hypertrophy, and increased perfusion facilitate the accumulation of inflammatory cells.[71] Proinflammatory signals are mediated by metabolites of arachidonic acid, an omega-6 fatty acid.[72] Eicosanoids such as prostaglandins, thromboxanes, and leukotrienes derived from arachidonic acid stimulate the formation and activity of adhesion molecules, cytokines, chemokines, and colony stimulating factors.[73] Dietary means to mitigate inflammation comprise the reduction of arachidonic acid and increase in the intake of eicosapentaenoic acid, an omega-3 fatty acid, as well as antioxidants.[74–76]

Manipulation of the inflammatory response by fatty acids is achieved through fatty acid conversion to eicosanoids.[73] These eicosanoids mediate platelet activation and inflammation and, more importantly, omega-6 and omega-3 fatty acids have quite different biological activities[73] (Figure 11.2). Eicosanoids derived from omega-6 fatty acids are referred to as the series 2 eicosanoids, which are proinflammatory, whereas the eicosanoids derived from omega-3 fatty acids are series 3 eicosanoids, which are anti-inflammatory or comparatively inactive. An example of the effect of

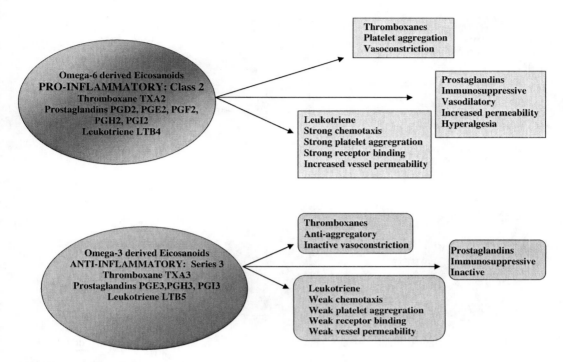

FIGURE 11.2 Dietary mitigation of inflammation.

omega-3 fatty acids on eicosanoids is the low incidence of myocardial infarction among Eskimos of Greenland and the Japanese, both of whom have a substantial fish intake. The preventative effect of a low omega-6 and high omega-3 dietary intake is apparent in the Japanese and again in the Eskimos with a low incidence and prevalence of RA.[75] Cytokines mediate protective immune responses and are responsible for harmful tissue destruction when produced in excessive amounts.[77] Cytokines are soluble proteins, produced by cells as a result of activation by specific stimuli. Cytokines influence the activity of cells, which express receptors to which they can bind. In binding to these receptors, cytokines are capable of acting in both a paracrine and autocrine manner.[77]

The proinflammatory cytokines that are implicated in RA are TNF-α, IL-1β, and IL-6. TNF-α is produced mainly by activated neutrophils, monocytes, and macrophages to initiate bacterial and tumor-cell killing, increase adhesion-molecule expression, stimulation of T and B cell function, upregulation of MHC antigens, and initiation of the production of IL-1β and IL-6.[78–80] TNF-α is the important link between the specific immune response and inflammation, through its action on both natural and acquired immunity. The production of TNF-α is beneficial in inflammation that is self-limiting; however, overproduction (as is the case in RA) can be problematic because of TNF-α involvement in endotoxic shock, adult respiratory stress syndrome, and other inflammatory conditions.[81] IL-1β shares many of the proinflammatory effects of TNF-α.[78] TNF-α. is produced mainly by activated monocytes and macrophages. IL-1β stimulates T and B lymphocyte proliferation and the release of other cytokines such as IL-2 and IL-6, as well as inducing hypotension, fever, weight loss, neutrophilia, and acute-phase response. IL-6 is produced mainly by activated monocytes and macrophages in response to IL-1 and TNF-α. IL-6 modulates T and B lymphocyte function and shares many of the TNF-α and IL-1 functions.[82]

An important, but often overlooked biochemical effect of omega-3 fatty acid dietary intake, is the significantly reduced expression of TNF-α and IL-1β by monocytes when stimulated *in vitro*.[83–85] This has been demonstrated in a number of human studies.[86–90] These results correlated with cellular levels of eicosapentaenoic acid (20:5n-3 and the competitor omega-6 form, arachi-

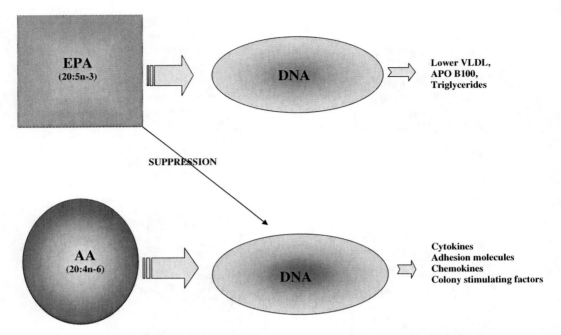

FIGURE 11.3 Biochemical effect of omega-3 fatty acid influence on functional activity of cells of the immune system.

donic acid (20:4n-6). Clearly, n-3 fatty acids do influence the functional activities of cells of the immune system, although a number of conflicting observations have been made. These fatty acids appear to alter the production of mediators involved in communications between cells of the immune system (eicosanoids, cytokines, NO).[91,92] Omega-3 fatty acids also appear to alter the expression of key cell-surface molecules involved in direct cell-to-cell contact (adhesion molecules).[93] The production of cytokines and NO is regulated by eicosanoids and, therefore, n-3 fatty acid-induced changes in the amount and types of eicosanoids produced could partly explain the effects of n-3 fatty acids. It is clear that the effects are exerted in an eicosanoid-dependent manner (Figure 11.3).[79,90]

E. COMORBIDITIES

Patients with RA exhibit a triad of conditions that are characterized as rheumatoid cachexia.[49,94–96] These conditions are lower than normal body-cell mass, elevated resting-energy expenditure, and elevated whole body-protein catabolism, which results in skeletal muscle wasting, reduced muscle strength, and reduced quality of life in RA patients.[97–99] Additionally, the loss of cell mass is accompanied by a trend toward higher fat mass, which has a detrimental effect on health.[95,100] The degree of disordered metabolism in patients with RA correlates with the level of TNF- and IL-1β produced.[95] Patients who have better control of inflammation exhibit protein and energy metabolism similar to those of healthy subjects.[96] Thus, RA patients with less control over inflammatory symptoms, despite the use of DMARDS, can do little to reverse rheumatoid cachexia.

The combination of decreased body-cell mass and physical activity levels is a powerful force in favor of fat accumulation, which leads to the problem of obesity and cardiovascular disease comorbidities. There is no evidence that the reduction in joint pain or the control of RA inflammatory activity can reverse the sedentary lifestyles of RA patients. Concern about obesity in RA is warranted because low muscle mass and increased fat mass can contribute to an increased risk of disability, as well as an increased risk of cardiovascular, metabolic, and osteoarthritic complications.[101]

Rheumatoid patients are at increased risk for cardiovascular disease (CVD), comorbidity, and death.[102,103] Comprehensive cardiovascular risk assessment comprises both determination of lipoprotein profiles in the individual patient and identification of other components of the metabolic syndrome.[104] In RA, the acute phase response is associated with low-density lipoprotein (LDL) and high-density lipoprotein (HDL), as well as insulin resistance (IR).[105–109] Subtle dyslipidemia predicts atherosclerosis in RA.[110] The acute phase response, body mass index (BMI), insulin resistance, HDL, triglycerides, and blood pressure interlink in RA in the same manner as the metabolic syndrome.[107,108] C-reactive protein (CRP) may directly contribute to atherosclerosis.[111] Disease-modifying antirheumatic drugs (DMARDs) may have an attenuating effect on CVD risk and death in RA.[112] Use of methotrexate in RA was associated with a 70% reduction in risk for cardiovascular death due to the action of methotrexate on inflammation.[113]

IV. MANAGEMENT

A. NONPHARMACOLOGICAL TREATMENT

Pain and decreased mobility associated with RA have a significant impact on quality of life in RA patients. These patients are far less active than the general population, so are at risk of additional conditions such as obesity, heart disease, diabetes mellitus, and hypertension.[114] Nonpharmacological treatments, including physiotherapy and occupational therapy, have been assigned a complementary role in the management of RA. Unfortunately, because of the dearth of research in the rheumatoid cohort there are still major challenges associated with these therapies, and they have not been considered as an automatic adjunct to pharmacological therapies. These challenges are the result of the lack of strong evidence associated with exercise and patient education. There is a lack of knowledge of models of nonpharmacological care, management of research, and the translation of research results to provide clinically useful evidence for treatment.[115]

RA disrupts physiological functions as well as musculoskeletal structures; this is evident in reduced muscle mass, strength, and BMD, which predisposes patients to falls and bone fractures.[116–119] Osteoporosis in RA patients is generalized and associated with decreased physical activity, impaired function, disease duration, and the inflammatory process itself.[118–122] Use of corticosteroids enhances the BMD decrease.[123] A vicious cycle of loss of muscle strength, functional capacity, and BMD in RA patients is further exacerbated by generalized fatigue, thus limiting physical activity. This results in the RA patient performing activities of daily living and professional duties at a higher percentage of their maximum physiological reserve.[124] Alternatively, poor physical fitness and a sedentary lifestyle are associated with increased morbidity and mortality.[125,126] Physiotherapy, occupational therapy, and rehabilitation applications significantly augment medical therapy by improving the management of RA and reducing handicaps in activities of daily living.[127] Physiotherapy modalities include cold/heat applications, electrical stimulation, and hydrotherapy. Rehabilitation treatment techniques for the RA patient comprise joint protection strategies, exercise, and patient education.[128]

Patient education programs have a modest but significant short-term benefit on patient knowledge and behavior.[129] The sociopsychological factors affecting the disease process, such as poor social relations, disturbance of communication patterns, unhappiness, and depression, are all common problems with RA patients. Patients who have participated in patient education programs have demonstrated improvement in disability associated with the disease, psychosocial interaction, and clinical prognosis.[130]

There is strong evidence that exercise for RA patients is an important factor in chronic disease development and subsequent quality of life issues.[114] However, the evidence to support the appropriate type of exercise and intensity in RA patients is lacking. Munneke demonstrated that the perceived benefit of exercise in the rheumatoid population is a significant predictor of exercise participation.[131] Perceived benefit by RA patients can be positively reinforced by physiotherapists and rheumatologists when research clarifies the appropriate exercise. Attending an educational-behavioral joint protection program significantly improves joint protection adherence and maintains functional ability long term.[132,133] Hydrotherapy of moderate intensity significantly improves muscle endurance in the upper and lower extremities in patients with RA.[134] Hydrotherapy increases range of movement (ROM), strengthens muscles, relieves painful muscle spasms, and improves quality of life.[135] Moderate or high intensity strength-training programs have better training effects on muscle strength in RA patients than lower intensity programs. The type of exercises, intensity, and frequency of training are key factors in the effectiveness of training, and it is essential to maintain the regime to obtain long-term benefits.[136–138]

Cold and hot application modalities are the most commonly used physical regimes in RA. Cold applications are used for acute stages of the disease, whereas hot applications are used in chronic disease stages. Heat applications can achieve analgesia and relieve muscle spasm.[139] Transcutaneous electrical nerve stimulation (TENS) is a short-acting therapy (6 to 24 h). The most beneficial frequency is 70 Hz. TENS cannot be used in every painful joint simultaneously, thus it is disadvantageous for patients with polyarticular involvement. Studies demonstrate TENS efficacy in analgesia, pain relief, swelling, and improvement in ROM.[140]

Rehabilitation techniques mainly involve rest and splinting, occupational therapy assistive devices, and adaptive equipment.[141] Various reports illustrate the benefit of wrist splints in the control of pain and inflammation, as well as the prevention of deformity development.[142,143] Patient compliance with splints can sometimes be an issue when orthoses are large or hard, generate heat, or interfere with ROM.[142–144] Occupational therapy improves the functional ability of RA patients. The assistive devices and adaptive equipment benefit joint protection and energy conservation in arthritic patients; they also reduce functional deficits, diminish pain, and maintain independence and self-efficacy.[145]

Therapeutic exercises are beneficial in RA patients when muscle weakness occurs as a result of immobilization or reduction in activities of daily living. Maintenance of normal muscle strength is important for physical function, joint stability, and injury prevention, particularly falls. The beneficial effects of therapeutic exercise develop through augmenting physical capacity rather than by ameliorating disease activity.[146] In establishing an exercise program for RA patients, consideration must be given to local or systemic joint involvement, stage of disease, age of the patient, compliance, and duration and severity of the exercise should be adjusted according to the patient needs. ROM exercises, stretching, strengthening, aerobic conditioning exercises, and activities of daily living can be used as components of the therapeutic exercise program.[146–147]

B. Pharmacological Treatment

1. Treatment Paradigms

Current therapies have various degrees of efficacy, but toxicity frequently limits long-term usage. Although the etiology of RA is still unknown, increasing knowledge and understanding of mechanisms underlying the pathogenesis of RA has facilitated selective targeting of the pathogenic elements of RA. These include cyclo-oxygenase type 2 inhibitors, adhesion molecules, T cells, B cells, cytokine receptors, chemokines, angiogenesis, oral tolerance antigens, costimulatory molecules, and new disease-modifying antirheumatic drugs. Improved efficacy is expected with more aggressive targeting of the pathogenic elements of the disease.[148]

The biomedical model has been successful in the treatment of infectious diseases; however, Engel suggested that this model had limited merit in the treatment of RA, a chronic noninfectious disease.[149] McCarty describes treatment choices as being nonsteroidal anti-inflammatory drugs (NSAIDs), including aspirin for 2 years, followed by another NSAID after 2 years of treatment, then gold after 2.5 years, antimalarials after 4.5 years, and immunosuppressive drugs after 8.5 years.[36] A reassessment of the traditional biomedical model for RA in the early 1980s caused a change from the paradigm based on the use of NSAIDs towards a strategy of early use of disease-modifying antirheumatic drugs (DMARDs).[29,150] The paradigm shift is based on the recognition that NSAIDs are more toxic than originally thought, and that NSAIDs do not reduce disability as effectively as DMARDs.[151] Some DMARDs (hydroxychloroquine and sulfasalazine) are less toxic than some NSAIDs; they reduce disability particularly if used in early treatment, and are more effective analgesics than NSAIDs over time.[150–154] Thus, the paradigm shift entails the early use of DMARDs before joint damage occurs, in conjunction with continual and/or serial use of one or a number of DMARDs, accompanied by careful monitoring and follow-up. DMARDs utilize a different mode of action from that of NSAIDs. DMARDs action takes from 4 to 12 weeks to influence symptoms; only then are they most effective in reducing abnormal levels of erythrocyte sedimentation rate (ESR), C-reactive protein (CRP), and rheumatoid factor (RF). DMARDs are classified according to toxicity and efficacy. Choice of DMARDs is usually determined by the severity of RA, presence of comorbidities, age, patient expectations, and lifestyle.[155,156]

Corticosteroid use in the treatment of RA is generally avoided. The use of this class of drug is controversial because of the long-term side effects that develop after prolonged use. Intravenous pulses of corticosteroids and intraarticular injections can improve the quality of life for some patients with RA. Corticosteroids are used in life-threatening complications of pericarditis and vasculitis. Kirwan recommends that they are used to reduce the rate of progression of early disease when combined with other treatments.[157] Surgical treatment for RA is usually indicated when loss of function is a major problem. Tendon rupture repair and joint replacement relieve pain and restore function.[158] Complete remission from RA is rare and generally necessitates the continued use of DMARDs and its associated monitoring.[159] Current treatments under trial are developing through the greater understanding of the pathogenesis of RA. Some of the immunological strategies are monoclonal antibodies to TNF-α, receptor antagonists, and antiinflammatory cytokines, which may enable a more successful approach to the treatment of RA to be developed. However, these are very expensive.[148,160]

Proactive attitudes to research are important in view of the current health policy, which is concerned with cost containment through limiting patient access to various services. Generally, rheumatological diseases are treated in ambulatory care settings; however, the high prevalence of the disease, the aging of patients, and the long duration of costly management makes cost an important consideration in the treatment of RA.[34,35,159] It makes sense to incorporate complementary therapies into the treatment regime to achieve additional amelioration of symptoms at a much reduced cost.

C. COMPLEMENTARY THERAPIES

Dietary supplementation using omega-3 fatty acid-based supplements is the most promising area of dietary manipulation in RA. Kremer and Bigaouette reviewed a number of studies and reported that fish oil supplementation reduces joint pain.[5] The mechanism of amelioration involves the inhibition of proinflammatory eicosanoids and cytokines.[161] Shapiro's group, in a well-designed population-based case control study in women, found that two or more servings of baked or broiled fish per week are protective in RA prevention.[162] A population study of a fish-eating society in the Faroe Islands reports the prevalence of RA was 1.1%.[163] The high functional capacity and lower occurrence of rheumatoid nodules and erosions, compared with previous studies in northern European societies, suggest that RA takes a milder course in the Faroe Islands population. An advantage of dietary manipulation is that the inclusion of two or more fish meals per week is an inexpensive modifier of eicosanoid production.[16,164]

The fundamental tenet of dietary manipulation in RA treatment modalities is that the Western diet is abundant in omega-6 fatty acids with minimal, often suboptimal levels of omega-3 fatty acids. This is particularly important in relation to risk of thrombotic vascular disease, arrhythmias, and inflammatory disorders.[15] The mechanism involved is based on the fact that dietary omega-6 and omega-3 fatty acids are the primary modulators of the lipid composition of membrane phospholipids. Fatty acids in the membrane phospholipids are the precursors of eicosanoids which are important mediators of inflammation, cytokine synthesis, and cell communication.[165] The modern Western diet contains an excess of total fat, omega-6 fatty acids and a low level of omega-3 fatty acids.[15,166,167] Dietary intake of omega-3 fatty acids, in conjunction with a high dietary intake of omega-6 fatty acids, does not appear to be effective in increasing cellular levels of omega-3 fatty acids.[168,169] The key to successful dietary intake is to limit the level of omega-6 fatty acids in the diet so that the omega-6 to omega-3 balance approaches 5:1, instead of the typical Western diet of 25:1.[16,169] This ratio is important because the dietary ratio of omega-6/omega-3 determines the eicosanoid series to be expressed in the inflammatory response.

The eicosanoids include entities such as prostaglandins, thromboxanes, and leukotrienes. There is considerable variation in activity of the eicosanoids derived from omega-6 and omega-3 fatty acids. The omega-6 derived eicosanoids exhibit proinflammatory activities, potent chemotactic activity, vasodilation, platelet aggregation, and increased vascular permeability.[165,170] The omega-3 derived eicosanoids are anti-inflammatory and much less active, as well as being poorly synthesized. Thus, omega-3 fatty acids, when omega-6 fatty acid intake is low, alter the balance of omega-6 to omega-3 derived eicosanoids to produce decreased inflammatory activity (Figure 11.2).[169]

In the past, pharmacological doses (1.0 to 7.1 g/d) of eicosapentaenoic acid (EPA) and docosahexaenoic acid (DHA) derived from 16 to 20 g/d of fat, either as a triglyceride or an ethyl ester, have been used in clinical trials with few recommendations concerning the quality of fat in the background diet. This is an important consideration because the omega-6 fatty acid, arachidonic acid (AA), is an EPA antagonist. Oils and spreads that are rich in the omega-9 nonessential fatty acids such as monounsaturated olive oil and the omega-3 precursor fatty acid α-linolenic acid (ALA) can be used to displace omega-6 fats from the diet without increasing the undesirable saturated fatty acids. These strategies demonstrate the ability to increase the incorporation of dietary omega-3 fatty acids into cell membranes.[76,171,172]

There is sufficient evidence in the literature to form the basis of a positive health message with the potential to reduce inflammation, cardiovascular disease, and increased mortality. This health message is to choose foods that are rich in omega-3 fatty acids (fish, products based on omega-3 rich seeds and vegetables) and to avoid foods that are very rich in omega-6 fatty acids (products based on omega-6 rich polyunsaturated oil, some nuts). Variety in omega-3 rich and/or omega-6-poor foods and food products has been developed to aid dietary change. Fish oil supplements can be utilized to provide an extra effect. The potential benefits of dietary manipulation and supplementation include the amelioration of RA symptoms and a reduction in health care costs. The most recent cost estimates of RA care (in the U.S.) for 6.5 million American RA sufferers is $14 billion/year.[35]

1. Dietary Regimens

Epidemiological studies from selected geographical regions support the hypothesis that a lifelong consumption of fish, olive oil, and cooked vegetables has an independent protective effect on the development and severity of RA.[162,173] RA in the Faroe Islands takes a milder form where the population diet is high in fish and whale meat.[163] RA prevalence is low in northwest Greece, where there is high olive oil consumption.[174] The Seven Countries Study demonstrated that the Mediterranean diet was a healthy, chronic-disease prevention diet.[175–177] Compared with Western diets, the Mediterranean diet, particularly the Cretan variant, contains less red meat, more fish, uses olive oil as the primary source of fat, and includes a moderate intake of wine.[173]

Rheumatologists noted that the consumption of the Cretan type of Mediterranean diet resulted in secondary prevention of coronary heart disease and was reported to reduce the recurrence rate of new cardiac events.[177] The effect of omega-3 fatty acids on eicosanoids may explain the low incidence of myocardial infarction in this instance as it does with Greenland Eskimos and Japanese populations, as both cultures have a substantial fish intake. Pathogenesis of atheromatosis involves inflammatory processes with obvious similarities to those of rheumatoid synovitis.[178] In the atherosclerotic plaque microenvironment, as in rheumatoid synovitis, macrophages are the principle inflammatory mediators with the ability to form numerous growth factors and cytokines.[178] RA patients can ameliorate rheumatoid activity and cardiac risk by the adoption of a dietary regimen that is rich in deep sea, omega-3-rich fish, low in red meat, uses olive oil as the primary fat source, and has ample supplies of fruit and vegetables accompanied by a moderate intake of wine.[173]

2. Vitamin D

Vitamin D has important functions that are unrelated to calcium and bone metabolism. This premise is supported by the presence of the vitamin D receptor (VDR) in various tissues that are not involved in calcium and bone metabolism.[19] These additional functions include effects on immunity, muscular strength, and coordination.[19,179] VDRs are found in significant concentrations in T lymphocytes and macrophage populations. The highest concentration of VDRs is found in immature immune cells of the thymus and the mature CD-8 T lymphocytes. The significant role of vitamin D compounds as selective immunosuppressants is illustrated by the ability of vitamin D to either prevent or suppress animal models of immune disease. Results demonstrate that 1,25-dihydroxyvitamin D3 can prevent or suppress experimental autoimmune RA, systemic lupus erythematosis, type 1 diabetes mellitus, and inflammatory bowel disease. Vitamin D hormone stimulates transforming growth factor (TGFβ-1) and IL-4, which in turn may suppress inflammatory T cell activity.[180–182] Vitamin D assists with neuromuscular function.[183] Vitamin D deficiency produces muscle weakness and there is a direct correlation between serum vitamin D levels and leg muscle strength in the elderly.[183] This is particularly relevant in RA, which occurs in the fifth and sixth decade of life, predominantly in females. Muscle strength and muscle mass decline in this cohort and are major factors contributing to falls.[179,183]

3. Probiotics

Altered bowel flora may play a role in RA.[18] Gastrointestinal tract (GIT) microflora are involved in the stimulation of the immune system, synthesis of B group and K vitamins, enhancement of GIT motility and function, digestion and nutrient absorption, inhibition of pathogens through colonization resistance, metabolism of plant compounds/drugs, and production of short chain fatty acids and polyamines.[184,185] Many factors can harm colonies of beneficial bacteria in the GIT flora. These include antibiotics, physiological and psychological stress, radiation, altered GIT peristalsis, and dietary changes.

Stress can induce significant changes in GIT microflora. These changes include a significant decrease in beneficial bacteria such as *Lactobacilli* and *Bifidobacteria,* and an increase in potential pathogenic micro-organisms such as *E. coli.* The cause of these changes may be the growth-enhancing effects of norepinephrine on gram negative micro-organisms or by stress-induced changes to GIT motility and secretions.[186]

The effect of the overall diet on the composition and metabolic activities of GIT microflora has been the subject of research for a number of years. The changing content of the diet (protein, carbohydrate, fat, fiber) may influence the quality and quantity of colonic flora; however, comparisons of developed and developing cultures' dietary patterns reveal only minor variations.[187] A recent study in animals to determine the effect of omega-3 fatty acid deficiency on rat intestinal structure and bacterial populations demonstrated that omega-3 fatty acid deficiency caused significant detrimental changes in ileum structure and bacterial populations.[188] Changes in bowel flora and activities are now considered to be contributing factors to many chronic degenerative diseases. There is considerable evidence in the current literature to suggest that dysbiosis is an important clinical entity.[189] Pharmacological agents, psychological stress, physical stress, and dietary factors

TABLE 11.1
Food Sources of n-3 Fatty Acids

Food	Serving Size (g)	Total n-3 (g)
Fresh raw salmon	100	3.0
Fresh raw tuna	100	1.17
Canned salmon	100	1.4
Canned sardines	100	1.74
Canned mackerel	100	1.4
Canned tuna	100	0.2
Omega eggs[a]	60	0.34
Regular eggs	60	0.06
Flaxseed oil	20	11.0
Canola™ [a]	20	2.0
Walnut oil	20	1.6
Wheatgerm oil	20	1.4
Soybean oil	20	1.4
Gold n Canola spread[a]	5	0.2
Gold n Canola lite[a]	5	0.15
Butter canola blend[a]	5	0.12
Linseeds	5	0.9
Walnuts	15	0.75
Pecans	15	0.16

[a] Functional foods.

contribute to dysbiosis. Diets can be manipulated, the effects of stress reduced, and pharmacological agents used sparingly in order to minimize the effects of these factors on intestinal flora and subsequent effect on quality of life for the rheumatoid patient.

4. Supplementation Strategies

The dietary imbalance of omega-6/omega-3 fatty acids is primarily due to a high intake of omega-6 rich vegetable oils and a limited intake of fish and other seafood. The correction of this dietary imbalance between omega-6 and omega-3 fatty acids may be achieved by the use of encapsulated fish oil, and dietary fortification with omega-3 fatty acids in combination with a background diet low in omega-6 fatty acids.[190–192] Dietary manipulation can be a process of selective intake and supplementation. In selective intake, foods that are rich sources of omega-6 fatty acids such as safflower, sunflower, corn, grape seed and blended oils, as well as spreads derived from these oils, are replaced with olive oil or canola oil and the associated spreads (Table 11.1). Dietary supplementation of omega-3 fatty acids can be achieved through fish oil capsules and increasing intake of omega-3 fatty acid-rich foods. Results from clinical studies suggest that the level of supplementation can be calculated as 40 mg of omega-3 fatty acids/kg body-weight per day in an active inflammatory state. This level of omega-3 fatty acid supplementation, with a background diet <10 g/d of omega-6 fatty acids, is sufficient to achieve significant levels of cellular incorporation of EPA.[76] Foods rich in omega-3 fatty acids are listed in Table 11.1.[193]

V. CONCLUSION

Evidence from these clinical and biochemical studies suggests that omega-3 fatty acids derived from fish oil do have a modest beneficial effect both for RA and CHD; however, rheumatologists are unwilling to recommend fish oil supplements to their patients with RA because of the confusion surrounding the amount to prescribe, the clinical effectiveness and efficacy, and the additional expense of a nonpharmacological remedy. There is a need to include dietary omega-3 fatty acids, a background Mediterranean diet, vitamin D, and probiotics to achieve an anti-inflammatory effect, to prevent CHD, and to reduce the development of chronic diseases in the rheumatoid cohort. In this climate of evidence-based treatment modalities there is a need to better define the overall therapeutic effect of fish oil; to place these dietary supplements in the appropriate niche in relation to NSAID and DMARD; to provide a formula relating to the balance of omega-3 fatty acid rich foods (and omega-6 poor foods) to include in the diet, and the omega-6 fatty acid-rich foods to exclude; to determine the level of fish oil supplementation related to body weight and concentration of EPA and DHA in a supplement; to monitor background diet for omega-6 competition at the cellular level, and to determine the critical variables that modulate the effects of dietary supplementation of omega-3 fatty acids on the mechanism of inflammation. This information should be made available to RA patients seeking advice on ways to improve their health by dietary means, with or without conventional medications.

REFERENCES

1. Hilliquin, P. and Menkes, C.J., Evaluation and management of early and established rheumatoid arthritis, *Practical Rheumatology*, Klippel, J.H. and Dieppe, P.M., Eds., Times Mirror International Publisher Limited, London, 1995.
2. Semple, E.L., Rheumatoid arthritis: New approaches for its evaluation and management, *Arch. Physical Med. Rehab.*, 76: 190–210, 1995.
3. Darlington, L.G., Jump, A. and Ramsey, N.W., Dietary treatment of rheumatoid arthritis, *The Practitioner*, 234: 456–460, 1990.
4. Ryan, S., Nutrition and the rheumatoid patient. *Br. J. Nurs.*, 4: 132–136, 1995.
5. Kremer, J.M. and Bigaouette, J., Nutrient intake of patients with rheumatoid arthritis is deficient in pyridoxine, zinc, copper and magnesium, *J. Rheumatol.*, 23: 990–994, 1996.
6. Brooks, P.M., Rheumatoid arthritis: pharmacological approaches. Dieppe, P.M. and Klippel, J.H., Eds., *Rheumatology*, Mosby Year Book Ltd., London, 1994.
7. Wolfe, F., Mitchell, D., Sibley, J., Fries, J.F., Block, D., Williams, C., Spitz, P., Haga, M., Kleinheksel, S., and Cathey, M., The mortality of rheumatoid arthritis, *Arthritis Rheum.*, 37: 481–494, 1994.
8. Mitchell, D., Splitz, P., Young, D., Block, D., McShane, D., and Fries, J.F., Survival, prognosis and cause of death in rheumatoid arthritis, *Arthritis Rheum.*, 29: 706–714, 1986.
9. Prior, P., Symmons, D.P.M., Scott, D. L., Brown, R., and Hawkins, C.F., Cause of death in rheumatoid arthritis, *Br. J. Rheumatol.*, 23: 92–99, 1984.
10. Walberg-Jonsson, S., Ohman, M.L., and Dahlqvist, S.R., Cardiovascular morbidity and mortality in patients with seropositive rheumatoid arthritis in northern Sweden, *J. Rheumatol.*, 26: 445–451, 1999.
11. Turesson, C., Jacobsson, I., and Bergstrom, U., Extra-articular rheumatoid arthritis: prevalence and mortality, *Rheumatology (Oxford)*, 38: 668–674, 1999.
12. Uhig, T., Hagen, R. and Kulen, T., Current tobacco smoking, formal education and the risk of rheumatoid arthritis, *J. Rheumatol.*, 26: 47–54, 1999.
13. Alderson, M., Starr, L., Gow, S., and Moreland, J., The program for rheumatic independent self management: A pilot evaluation, *Clin. Rheumatol.*, 18: 283–292, 1999.
14. Gonzalez-Gay, M., Gonzalez-Juanatey, C., and Martin, J., Rheumatoid arthritis: a disease associated with accelerated atherogenesis, *Sem. Arthritis Rheum.*, 35: 8–17, 2005.
15. Simopoulos, A.P., Omega-3 fatty acids in health and disease and in growth and development, *Am. J. Clin. Nutr.*, 54: 438–463, 1991.
16. Cleland, L.G. and James, M., Rheumatoid arthritis and the balance of dietary N-6 to N-3 essential fatty acids, *Br. J. Rheumatol.*, 36: 513–515, 1997.
17. Kjeldsen-Kragh, J., Mediterranean diet interventions in rheumatoid arthritis, *Ann. Rheum. Dis.*, 62: 193–195, 2003.

18. Peltonen, R., Nenonen, M., Helve, T., Hanninen, O., Toivanen, P., and Eerola, E., Faecal microbial flora and disease activity in rheumatoid arthritis during a vegan diet, *Br. J. Rheumatol.*, 36: 64–68, 1997.

19. De Luca, H.F., Overview of general physiologic features and functions of vitamin D, *Am. J. Clin. Nutr.*, 80: 1689S–1696S, 2004.

20. MacGregor, A.J., Classification criteria for rheumatoid arthritis, *Bailliere's Clin. Rheumatol.*, 9: 287–304, 1995.

21. Linos, A., Worthington, J.N., O'Fallon, W.M., and Kurland, L.T., The epidemiology of rheumatoid arthritis in Rochester, Minnesota: a study of the incidence, prevalence and mortality, *Am. J. Epidemiol.*, 111: 7–98, 1980.

22. Symmons, D.P.M., Barrett, E.M., Bankhead, C.K., Scott, D.G.I., and Silman, A. J., The occurrence of rheumatoid arthritis in the United Kingdom: results from the Norfolk Arthritis Register, *Br. J. Rheumatol.*, 33: 735–739, 1994.

23. Silman, A.J., Davies, P., Curry, H.L.F. and Evans, S.J.W., Is rheumatoid arthritis becoming less severe? *J. Chronic Dis.*, 36: 891–897, 1983.

24. Silman, A.J., Has the incidence of rheumatoid arthritis declined in the U.K.? *Br. J. Rheumatol.*, 27: 77–78, 1988.

25. O'Brien, W.M., Bennett, P.H., Burch, T.A. and Bunim, J.J., A genetic study in rheumatoid arthritis and rheumatoid factor in Blackfeet and Pima Indians, *Arthritis Rheum.*, 10: 163–179, 1967.

26. Solomon, L., Robin, G. and Valkenburg, H.A., Rheumatoid arthritis in South African Negro populations, *Ann. Rheum. Dis.*, 34: 128–135, 1975.

27. Lau, E.M.C., Symmons, D.P.M., MacGregor, A.J., Bankhead, C.K. and Donnan, S.P.B., Low prevalence of rheumatoid arthritis in the urbanised Chinese population of Hong Kong, *J. Rheumatol.*, 20: 1133–1137, 1993.

28. Darnawan, J., Muirden, K., Valkenburg, H.A., and Wigley, R.D., The epidemiology of rheumatoid arthritis in Indonesia, *Br. J. Rheumatol.*, 32: 537–540, 1993.

29. Shichikawa, K., Takenaka, Y., Maeda, A., Yoshino, R., Tsujimoto, M., Ota, H., Kashiwade, T., and Hongo, I., A longitudinal population survey of rheumatoid arthritis in a rural district in Wakayama, *The Ryumachi*, 21 Suppl.: 35–43, 1981.

30. Roberts-Thomson, R.A. and Roberts-Thomson, P.J., Rheumatic disease and the Australian Aborigine, *Ann. Rheum. Dis.*, 58: 266–270, 1999.

31. Harris, E.D.J., Rheumatoid Arthritis: pathophysiology and implications for therapy, *N. Engl. J. Med*, 322: 1277–1289, 1990.

32. Pincus, T., The paradox of effective therapies but poor long term outcomes in rheumatoid arthritis, *Sem. Arthritis Rheum.*, 21: 2–15, 1992.

33. Erhardt, C.C., Mumford, P.A., Venables, P.J.W. and Maini, R.N., Factors predicting a poor life prognosis in rheumatoid arthritis: an eight year prospective study, *Ann. Rheum. Dis.*, 48: 7–13, 1989.

34. Criswell, L.A., and Such, C.L., Cost effectiveness analysis of drug therapies for rheumatoid arthritis, *J. Rheumatol.*, 23: 52–55, 1996.

35. Lubeck, D.P., The economic impact of rheumatoid arthritis, *Rheumatoid Arthritis: Pathogenesis, Assessment, Outcomes and Treatment*, Wolfe, F. and Pincus, T., Eds., Marcel Dekker, New York, 1994.

36. McCarty, D.J., Clinical features of rheumatoid arthritis, in *Arthritis and Allied Health Conditions: A Textbook of Rheumatology*, 12th ed., McCarty, D.L. and Koopman, K.T., Eds., Lea and Febiger, Philadelphia, 1993.

37. Short, C.L., Bauer, W., and Reynolds, W., *Rheumatoid Arthritis*, Harvard University Press, Cambridge, MA, 1957.

38. Ropes, M.W., Bennett, G.A., Cobb, S., Jacox, R., and Jessar, R., Revision of diagnostic criteria for rheumatoid arthritis, *Bull. Rheum. Dis.*, 9: 175–176, 1958.

39. Feigenbaum, S.L., Masi, A.T., and Kaplan, S.B., Progress in rheumatoid arthritis: a longitudinal study of newly diagnosed younger adult patients, *Am. J. Med.*, 66: 377–384, 1979.

40. Sherrer, Y.S., The development of disability in rheumatoid arthritis, *Arthritis Rheum.*, 29: 494–5000, 1986.

41. Sokoloff, L., McCluskey, R.T. and Bunim, J.J., Vascularity of the early subcutaneous nodules of rheumatoid arthritis, *Arch. Pathol.*, 55: 475–481, 1953.

42. Wisnieski, J.J. and Askari, A.D., Rheumatoid nodulosis: a relatively benign rheumatoid variant, *Arch. Intern. Med.*, 141: 615–661, 1981.

43. Matteson, E.L., Cohen, M.D., and Conn, D.L., Clinical features of rheumatoid arthritis: systemic involvement, *Practical Rheumatology*, Klippel, J.H. and Dieppe, P.A., Eds., Mirror Times International, London, 1995.

44. Gordon, D.H., Steen, J.L., and Broder, I., The extra articular features of rheumatoid arthritis: a systematic analysis of 127 cases, *Am. J. Med.*, 54: 445–452, 1973.

45. Bonfiglio, T. and Atwater, E.C., Heart disease in patients with seropositive rheumatoid arthritis, *Arch. Intern. Med.*, 77: 837–843, 1969.

46. Franco, A., Levine, H.D., and Hall, A.P., Rheumatoid pericarditis: report of 17 cases diagnosed clinically, *Ann. Intern. Med.*, 77: 837–841, 1972.

47. Larsen, A., Dale, K., and Eek, M., Radiographic evaluation of rheumatoid arthritis and related conditions by standard reference films, *Acta Radiol. Diagn.*, 18: 481–491, 1977.

48. Arnett, F.C., Edworthy, S.M., Bloch, D., McShane, D.J., Fries, J.F., Cooper, N.S., Healy, L.A., Kaplan, S.R., Liang, M.H., and Luthra, H.S., The American Rheumatism Association 1989 revised criteria for the classification of rheumatoid arthritis, *Arthritis Rheum.*, 31: 315–324, 1988.

49. Morel, J. and Combe, B., How to predict prognosis in early rheumatoid arthritis, *Best Pract. Res. Clin. Rheumatol.*, 19: 137–146, 2005.

50. Pincus, T. and Callahan, L.F., Taking mortality in rheumatoid arthritis seriously — predictive markers, socioeconomic status and co-morbidities, *J. Rheumatol.*, 13: 841–845, 1986.

51. Aho, K., Koskenvuo, M., Touminen, J., and Kaprio, J., Occurrence of rheumatoid arthritis in a nationwide series of twins, *J. Rheumatol.*, 13: 899–902, 1986.

52. Silman, A.J., MacGregor, A.J., and Thomson, W., Twin concordance rates for rheumatoid arthritis: results from a nationwide study, *Br. J. Rheumatol.*, 32: 903–907, 1993.

53. Nepom, G.T. and Nepom, B.S., Prediction of susceptibility of rheumatoid arthritis by human leukocyte antigen genotyping, *Rheum. Dis. Clin. N. Am.*, 18: 785–792, 1992.

54. Gao, X., Olsen, N.J., Pincus, T., and Stastny, P., HLA-DR alleles with naturally occurring amino acid substitutions and risk of developing rheumatoid arthritis, *Arthritis Rheum.*, 33: 939–940, 1990.

55. Weyand, C.M., Hicok, K.C., Coll, D.L., and Goronozy, J.J., The influence of HLA-DRB1 genes in the disease severity of rheumatoid arthritis, *Ann. Intern. Med.*, 17: 801–809, 1992.

56. Kong, E., Prokunina-Olsson, L., Wong, W., Lau, C., Chan, T., Alarcon-Riquelme, M., and Lau, Y., A new haplotype and PDCD1 is associated with rheumatoid arthritis in Hong Kong Chinese, *Arthritis Rheum.*, 52: 1058–1062, 2005.

57. Spector, T.D., Roman, E., and Silman, A.J., The pill, parity and rheumatoid arthritis, *Arthritis Rheum.*, 33: 782–789, 1990.

58. Spector, T.D., Brennan, P., Haws, P., Studd, J.W., and Silman, A.J., Does estrogen replacement therapy protect against rheumatoid arthritis? *Arthritis Rheum.*, 50: 1472–1476, 1991.

59. Vanderbroucke, J.P., Witteman, J.C.M., Valkenburg, H.A., Boersma, J.W., and Cats, A., Non-contraceptive hormones and rheumatoid arthritis in peri-menopausal and post-menopausal women, *JAMA*, 255: 1299–1303, 1986.

60. Chander, C.L. and Spector, T.D., Oestrogens, joint disease and cartilage. *Ann. Rheum. Dis.*, 50: 139–140, 1991.

61. Spector, T.D., Perry, L.A., Tubb, G., Silman, A.J., and Huskisson, E.C., Low testosterone levels in males with rheumatoid arthritis, *Ann. Rheum. Dis.*, 49: 65–68, 1988.

62. Walker, D., Griffiths, I. and Madeley, R., Auto-antibodies and antibodies to micro-organisms in rheumatoid arthritis: Comparison of histocompatible siblings, *J. Rheumatol*, 14: 426–428, 1987.

63. Phillips, P.E., Evidence implicating infectious agents in rheumatoid arthritis and juvenile rheumatoid arthritis, *Clin. Exp. Med.*, 6: 87–94, 1988.

64. Wilder, R.L., and Crofford, L.J., Do infectious agents cause rheumatoid arthritis? *Clin. Orthopaed. Relat. Res.*, 265: 36–41, 1991.

65. Harjeer, A.H., MacGregor, A.J., Rigby, A.S., Ollier, W.E.R., Carthy, D., and Silman, A.J., Influence of previous exposure to human parvovirus B19 infection in explaining the susceptibility to rheumatoid arthritis: an analysis of disease discordant twin pairs, *Ann. Rheum. Dis.*, 53: 137–139, 1994.

66. MacGregor, A.J., Riste, L.K., Hazes, J.W.M., and Silman, A.J., Low prevalence of rheumatoid arthritis in Black-Caribbeans compared with whites in inner city Manchester, *Ann. Rheum. Dis.*, 53: 239–297, 1995.

67. Silman, A.J., Newman, J., and MacGregor, A.J., Cigarette smoking increases the risk of rheumatoid arthritis: results from a nationwide study of disease discordant twins, *Arthritis Rheum.*, 39: 732–735, 1996.

68. Pincus, T., Esther, R., DeWalt, D.A., and Callaghan, L.F., Social conditions and self-management are more powerful determinants of health than access to care, *Ann. Intern. Med.*, 129: 406–411, 1998.

69. Dieppe, P.A., Emphysema in rheumatoid arthritis, *Ann. Rheum. Dis.*, 34: 181–189, 1975.

70. Henderson, B., Revelle, P. and Edwards, J.W.C., Synovial cell hyperplasia in rheumatoid arthritis: dogma and fact, *Ann. Rheum. Dis.*, 47: 348–349, 1988.

71. Hara, K.S., Ballard, D., Ilstrup, D.M., Connolly, D.C. and Vollertsen, R.S., Rheumatic pericarditis: clinical features and survival, *Medicine*, 69: 81–89, 1990.

72. Wilkinson, L.S., Worrell, L.G., Sinclair, H.S. and Edwards, J.C.W., Immunohistochemical reassessment of accessory cell populations in normal and diseased synovium, *Br. J. Rheumatol.*, 29: 259–263, 1990.

73. Kelley, D.S., Modulation of human immune and inflammatory responses by dietary fatty acids, *Nutrition*, 17: 669–673, 2001.

74. Kremer, J.M., Lawrence, D.A., Petrillo, G.F., Litts, L.L., Mullaly, P.M., Rynes, R.I., Stocker, R.P., Parhami, N., Greenstein, N.S., Fuchs, B.R., Mathur, A., Robinson, D.R., Sperling, R.I., and Bigaouette, J., Effects of high-dose fish oil on rheumatoid arthritis after stopping nonsteroidal antiinflammatory drugs: Clinical and immune correlates, *Arthritis Rheum.*, 38: 1107–1114, 1995.

75. James, M. and Cleland, L.G., Dietary n-3 fatty acids and therapy for rheumatoid arthritis, *Sem. Arthritis Rheum.*, 27: 85–97, 1997.

76. Volker, D.H, FitzGerald, P.E.B., Major, G.A.C., and Garg, M.L., Efficacy of fish oil concentrate in the treatment of rheumatoid arthritis, *J. Rheumatol.* 27: 2343–2346, 2000.

77. Elliott, M., Maini, R., Feldmann, M., Fongfox, A., Charles, P., Katsikis, P., Brennan, F., Walker, J., Bijlh, H., Ghrayeb, J., and Woody, J., Treatment of RA with chimeric monoclonal antibodies to TNF-α, *Arthritis Rheum.*, 36: 1681–1690, 1993.

78. Kunkel, S.L., Remick, D.G., Spengler, M. and Chensue, S.W., Modulation of macrophage-derived interleukin-1 and tumour necrosis factor by prostaglandins E2, *Adv. Prostaglandin. Thromboxane Leukocyte Res.*, 9: 331–339, 1982.

79. Renz, H., Gong, J.H., Schmidt, D.T.A., Nain, M., and Gemsa, D., Release of tumor necrosis factor alpha from macrophages: Enhancement and suppression are dose dependently regulated by prostaglandin E2 and cyclic nucleotides, *J. Immunol.*, 141: 2388–2393, 1988.

80. Spinas, G.A., Bloesch, D., Keller, U., Zimmerli, W., and Cammisuli, S., Pretreatment with ibuprofen augments circulating tumour necrosis factor, IL-6 and elastase during acute endotoxaemia, *J. Infect. Dis.*, 163: 89–95, 1991.

81. Poubelle, P., Stankova, J., Grassii, J., and Rola-Pleszczynski, M., Leukotriene B4 upregulates IL-6 rather than IL-1 synthesis in human monocytes, *Agents Actions*, 34: 42–45, 1991.

82. Hopkins, S.J. and Meager, A., Cytokines in synovial fluid II: The presence of TNF alpha and IFN gamma, *Clin. Exp. Immunol.*, 72: 422–427, 1988.

83. Cooper, A.L., Gibbons, L., Horan, M.A., Little, R.A., and Rothwell, N.J., Effect of dietary fish oil supplementation on fever and cytokine production in human volunteers, *Clin. Nutr.*, 12: 312–328, 1993.

84. Endres, S., Ghorbani, R., Kelly, V., Georgilis, K., Lonnemann, G., van der Meer, J.M.W., Cannon, J.G., Rogers, T.S., Klempner, M.S., Weber, P.C., Schaeffer, E.J., Wolff, S.M., and Dinarello, C.A., The effect of dietary supplements with n-3 polyunsaturated fatty acids on the synthesis of interleukin-1 and tumor necrosis factor by mononuclear cells, *N. Engl. J. Med.*, 320: 265–271, 1989.

85. Endres, S., Meydani, S.N., Ghorbani, R., Schindler, R., and Dinarello, R.A., Dietary supplementation with n-3 fatty acids suppresses IL-2 production and mononuclear cell proliferation, *J. Leukocyte Biol.*, 54: 599–603, 1993.

86. Meydani, S.N., Endres, S., Woods, M.M., Goldin, B.R., Soo, C., Morill-Labrode, A., Dinarello, C.A., and Gorbach, S.L., Oral n-3 fatty acid supplementation suppresses cytokine production and lympho-cyte proliferation: comparison between younger and older women, *J. Nutr.*, 121: 547–555, 1991.

87. Meydani, S.N., Lichrestein, A.H., Cornwall, S., Meydani, S., Goldin, B.R., Rasmussen, H., Dinarello, C.A. and Schaefer, E.J., Immunologic effects of national cholesterol education panel step-2 diets with and without fish-derived n-3 fatty acid enrichment, *J. Clin. Invest.*, 92: 105–113, 1993.

88. Molvig, P., Pociot, F., Worsaae, H., Wogensen, L.D., Baek, L., Christensen, P., Mandrup-Poulsen, T., Andersen, K., Madsen, P., Dyerberg, J. and Nerup, J., Dietary supplementation with omega-3 poly-unsaturated fatty acids decreases mononuclear cell proliferation and interleukin 1 beta content but not monokine secretion in healthy and insulin independent diabetic individuals, *Scand. J. Immunol.*, 34: 399–410, 1991.

89. Caughey, G.E., Mantzioris, E., Gibson, R.A., Cleland, L.G., and James, M.J., The effect on human tumor necrosis factor alpha and interleukin 1 beta production of diets enriched in n-3 fatty acids from vegetable oil or fish oil, *Am. J. Clin. Nutr.*, 63: 116–122, 1996.

90. Caughey, G.E., Pouliot, M., Cleland, L.G., and James, M.J., Regulation of tumor necrosis factor-alpha and IL-1-beta synthesis by thromboxane A2 in nonadherent human monocytes, *J. Immunol*, 158: 351–358, 1997.

91. Harris, W.S., Rambjor, G.S., Windsor, S.L., and Diederich, D., n-3 fatty acids and urinary secretion of nitric oxide metabolites in humans, *Am. J. Clin. Nutr.*, 65: 459–464, 1997.

92. Clancy, R.M., Amin, A. R. and Abramson, S.B., The role of nitric oxide in inflammation and immunity, *Arthritis Rheum.*, 41: 141–1151, 1998.

93. Springer, T.A., Adhesion receptors in the immune system, *Nature*, 346: 425–433, 1990.

94. Gomez-Vaquero, C., Nolla, J., Fiter, J., Ramon, J., Concustell, R., Valverde, J., and Roig-Escofet, D., Nutritional status in patients with rheumatoid arthritis, *Joint Bone Spine*, 68: 403–409, 2001.

95. Roubenoff, R., Roubenoff, R.A., Cannon, J.G., Kehayias, J.J., Zhaung, H., Dawson-Hughes, B., Dinarello, C.A., and Rosenberg, I.H., Rheumatoid cachexia: cytokine driven hypermetabolism accompanying reduced body cell mass in chronic inflammation, *J. Clin. Invest.*, 93: 2379–2386, 1994.

96. Rall, L., Rosen, C., Dolnikowski, G., Hartman, W., Lundgren, N., Abad, L., Dinarello, C.A., and Roubenoff, R., Protein metabolism in rheumatoid arthritis and aging: effects of muscle strength training and tumor necrosis factor alpha, *Arthritis Rheum*, 39: 1115–1124, 1996.

97. Munro, R. and Capell, H., Prevalence of low body mass in rheumatoid arthritis: association with acute phase response, *Ann. Rheum. Dis.*, 56: 326–329, 1997.

98. Westhovens, R., Nijs, J., Faelman, V., and Dequeker, J., Body composition in rheumatoid arthritis, *Br. J. Rheumatol.*, 36: 444–448, 1997.

99. Roubenoff, R., Roubenoff, R.A., Ward, L., Holland, S., and Hellmann, D.B., Rheumatoid cachexia: depletion of lean body mass in rheumatoid arthritis: possible association with tumor necrosis factor, *J. Rheumatol.*, 19: 1505–1510, 1992.

100. Rall, R., Meydani, S., Kehayias, J., Dawson-Hughes, B. and Roubenoff, R., The effect of progressive resistance training in rheumatoid arthritis: increased strength without changes in energy balance or body composition, *Arthritis Rheum.*, 39: 415–426, 1996.

101. Lainer, L., Harris, T., Rumpel, C. and Madans, J., Body mass index, weight change and risk of mobility disability in middle aged and older women, *JAMA*, 271: 1093–1098, 1994.

102. Van Doornum, S., McColl, G. and Wicks, I.P., Accelerated atherosclerosis: An extra-articular feature of rheumatoid arthritis? *Arthritis Rheum.*, 46: 862–873, 2002.

103. Goodson, N., Coronary artery disease and rheumatoid arthritis, *Curr. Opin. Rheumatol.*, 14: 115–120, 2002.

104. Expert Panel on Detection, Evaluation and Treatment of High Blood Cholesterol in Adults: Executive summary of the third report to The National Cholesterol Education Program (NCEP) blood cholesterol in adults (Adult Treatment Panel III), *JAMA*, 285: 2486–2497, 2001.

105. Svenson, K.L., Lithell, H., Hallgren, R., Vessby, B., Serum lipoprotein in active rheumatoid arthritis and other chronic inflammatory arthrides, *Arch. Intern. Med.*, 147: 1917–1920, 1987.

106. Svenson, K.L., Pollare, T., Lithell, H., and Hallgren, R., Impaired glucose handling in active rheumatoid arthritis: relationship to peripheral insulin resistance, *Metabolism*, 37: 125–130, 1988.

107. Dessein, P.H., Joffe, B.I., Stanwix, A.E., Botha, A.S. and Moomal, Z., The acute phase response does not fully predict the presence of insulin resistance and dislipidaemia in inflammatory arthritis, *J. Rheumatol.*, 24: 462–466, 2002.

108. Dessein, P.H., Stanwix, A.E., and Joffe, B.I., Cardiovascular risk in rheumatoid arthritis versus osteoarthritis: acute phase response related to decreased insulin sensitivity and high-density lipoprotein cholesterol as well as clustering of metabolic syndrome features in rheumatoid arthritis, *Arthritis Res.*, 4: R5, 2002.

109. del Rincon, I., Williams, K., Stern, M.P., Freeman, G.L., and Escalante, A., High incidence of cardiovascular events in a rheumatoid arthritis cohort not explained by traditional cardiac risk factors, *Arthritis Rheum.*, 44: 2737–2745, 2001.

110. Wallberg-Jonsson, S., Backman, C., Johnson, O., Karp, K., Lundstrom, E., Sundqvist, K.-G., and Rantapaa-Dahlqvist, S., Increased prevalence of atherosclerosis in patients with medium term rheumatoid arthritis, *J. Rheumatol.*, 28: 2597–2602, 2001.

111. Pepys, M.B. and Berger, A., The renaissance of C reactive protein, *Br. Med. J.*, 322: 4–5, 2001.
112. Wallberg-Jonsson, S., Johansson, H., Ohman, M.L., and Rantapaa-Dahlqvist, S., Extent of inflammation predicts cardiovascular disease and overall mortality in seropositive rheumatoid arthritis: a retrospective cohort study from disease onset, *J. Rheumatol.*, 26: 2562–2571, 1999.
113. Choi, H.K., Hernan, M.A., Seeger, J.D., Robins, J.M., and Wolfe, F., Methotrexate and mortality in patients with rheumatoid arthritis: a prospective study, *Lancet*, 359: 1173–1177, 2002.
114. Kuritzky, L. and Weaver, A., Advances in rheumatology: coxibs and beyond, *J. Pain Symptom Manage.*, 25: S6–20, 2003.
115. Li, L.C., What else can I do but take drugs? The future of research in nonpharmacological treatment in early inflammatory arthritis, *J. Rheumatol.*, 72: 21–24, 2005.
116. Roubenoff, R., Exercise and inflammatory disease, *Arthritis Rheum.*, 15: 263–266, 2003.
117. Ekdahl, C. and Broman, G. Muscle strength, endurance and aerobic capacity in rheumatoid arthritis: a comparative study with healthy subjects, *Ann. Rheum. Dis.*, 51: 35–40, 1992.
118. Gough, A., Lilley, J., Ayre, S., Holder, R., and Smery, P., Generalised bone loss patients with early rheumatoid arthritis, *Lancet*, 344: 23–27, 1994.
119. Laan, R., Buijs, W., Verbeek, A., Draad, M., van de Putte, L. and van Riel, P., Bone mineral density in patients with recent onset rheumatoid arthritis: influence of disease activity and functional capacity, *Ann. Rheum. Dis.*, 52: 21–26, 1993.
120. Kroger, H., Honkanen, R., Saarikoski, S., and Alhava, E., Decreased axial bone mineral density in perimenopausal women with rheumatoid arthritis: a population based study, *Ann. Rheum. Dis.*, 53: 18–23, 1994.
121. Haugeberg, G., Uhlig, T., Falch, J., Halse, J., and Kvien, T.K., Bone mineral density and frequency of osteoporosis in female patients with rheumatoid arthritis: results from 394 patients in the Oslo County Rheumatoid Arthritis register, *Arthritis Rheum.*, 43: 522–530, 2000.
122. Martin, J.C., Munro, R., Campbell, M.K., and Reid, D.M., Effects of disease and corticosteroids on appendicular bone mass in postmenopausal women with rheumatoid arthritis: comparison with axial measurements, *Br. J. Rheumatol.*, 36: 43–49, 1997.
123. Butler, R.C., Davie, M.W., Worsfold, M., and Sharp, C.A., Bone mineral content in patients with rheumatoid arthritis: relationship to low-dose steroid therapy, *Br. J. Rheumatol.*, 30: 86–90, 1991.
124. Grady, M., Flether, J., and Ortiz, S., Therapeutic and physical fitness exercise prescription for older adults with joint disease: An evidence-based approach, *Rheum. Dis. Clin. N. Am.*, 26: 617–646, 2004.
125. Bacon, P.A. and Townend, J.N., Nails in the coffin: increasing evidence for the role of rheumatic disease in the cardiovascular mortality of rheumatoid arthritis, *Arthritis Rheum.*, 44: 2707–2710, 2001.
126. Del Rincon, I.D., Williams, K., Stern, M.P., and Escalante, A., High incidence of cardiovascular events in a rheumatoid arthritis cohort not explained by traditional risk factors, *Arthritis Rheum.*, 44: 2737–2745, 2001.
127. Sandy, B., Ganz, P.T., and Harriss, L.L., General overview of rehabilitation in the rheumatoid patient, *Rheum, Dis. Clin. N. Am.*, 24: 181–201, 1998.
128. Kavuncu, V. and Evcik, D., Physiotherapy in Rheumatoid Arthritis, *Medscape Gen. Med.*, 6: e44, 2004. www.medscape.com/viewarticle/474880.
129. Schrieber, L. and Colley, M., Patient education, *Best Pract. Res. Clin. Rheumatol.*, 18: 465–476, 2004.
130. Scholten, C., Brodowicz, T., Graninger, W., Gardavsky, I., Pils, K., Pesau, B., Eggl-Tyle, E., Wanivenhaus, A., and Zielinski, C.C., Persistent functional and social benefit 5 years after a multidisciplinary arthritis training program, *Arch. Phys. Med. Rehabil.*, 80: 1282–1287, 1999.
131. Munneke, M., de Jong, Z., Zwinderman, A.H., Ronday, H.K., van der Ende, C.H.M., Vlieland, T.P.M., and Hazes, J.M.W., High intensity exercise or conventional exercise for patients with rheumatoid arthritis? Outcome expectations of patients, rheumatologists and physiotherapists, *Ann. Rheum.*, 63: 804–808, 2004.
132. Hammond, A. and Freeman, K., The long-term outcomes from a randomized controlled trial of an educational-behavioural joint protection programme for people with rheumatoid arthritis, *Clin. Rehabil.*, 18: 520–528, 2004.
133. Munneke, M., de Jong, Z., Zwinderman, A.H., Ronday, H.K., van Schaardenburg, D., Dijkmans, B.A., Kroon, H.M., Vliet Vlieland, T.P.M., and Hazes, J.M.W., Effect of a high-intensity weight-bearing exercise program on radiologic damage progression of the large joints in sub-groups of patients with rheumatoid arthritis, *Arthritis Rheum.*, 53: 410–407, 2005.

134. Bilberg, A., Ahlmen, M. and Mannerkorpi, K., Moderately intensive exercise in temperate pool for patients with rheumatoid arthritis: a randomized controlled study, *Rheumatology (Oxford)*, 44: 502–508, 2005.

135. Becker, B.E., The biologic aspect of hydrotherapy, *J. Back Muscloskel., Rehabil.*, 4: 255–264, 1994.

136. Eurenius, E. and Stenstrom, C.H., Physical activity, physical fitness and general health perception among individuals with rheumatoid arthritis, *Arthritis Rheum.*, 53: 48–55, 2005.

137. de Jong, Z. and Vlieland, T.P., Safety of exercise in patients with rheumatoid arthritis, *Curr. Opin. Rheumatol.*, 17: 177–182, 2005.

138. Hakkinen, A., Effectiveness and safety of strength training in rheumatoid arthritis, *Curr. Opin. Rheumatol.*, 16: 132–137, 2004.

139. Abelson, K., Langley, G.B., Sheppeard, H., Vlieg, M. and Wigley, R.D., Transcutaneous electrical nerve stimulation in rheumatoid arthritis, *N. Z. Med.*, 96: 156–158, 1983.

140. Jarit, G.J., Mohr, K.J., Waller, R. and Glousman, R.E., The effects of home interferential therapy on post-operative pain, edema and range of motion of the knee, *Clin. J. Sport Med.*, 13: 16–20, 2003.

141. Steultjens, E., Dekker, J., Bouter, L., Schaardenburg, D., Kuyk, M. and Ende, C., Occupational therapy for rheumatoid arthritis. *Cochrane Database Syst. Rev.*, 1: CD003114, 2004.

142. Philips, C.A., Management of the patient with rheumatoid arthritis: the role of the hand therapist, *Hand Clin.*, 5: 291–309, 1989.

143. Ouellette, E.A., The rheumatoid hand: orthotics as preventive, *Sem. Arthritis Rheum.*, 2: 65–72, 1991.

144. Kjelen, I., Moller, G. and Kvien, T., Use of commercially produced elastic wrist orthosis in chronic arthritis: a controlled study, *Arthritis Care Res.*, 8: 108–113, 1995.

145. Neumann, D.A., Biochemical analysis of selected principles of hip protection, *Arthritis Care Res.*, 2: 146–155, 1989.

146. Van den Ende, C.H.M., Vliet Vieland, T.P.M., Munneke, M., and Hazes, J.M.W., Dynamic exercise therapy in rheumatoid arthritis: a systematic review, *Br. J. Rheumatol.*, 37: 677–678, 1998.

147. Lynberg, K.K., Ramsing, B.U., Nawrocki, A., Harreby, M., and Samsoe, B.D., Safe and effective isokinetic knee extension training in rheumatoid arthritis, *Arthritis Rheum.*, 37: 623–628, 1994.

148. Chen, O. and Wei, W., New therapeutic approaches for rheumatoid arthritis, *Assay Drug Dev. Technol.*, 3: 329–337, 2005.

149. Engel, G. L., The need for a new medical model: a challenge for biomedicine, *Science*, 196: 29–135, 1977.

150. Ad Hoc Committee, Guidelines for monitoring drug therapies in rheumatoid arthritis, *Arthritis Rheum.*, 39: 723–731, 1996.

151. Fries, J.F., Williams, C.A., Morfeld, D., Singh, G., and Sibley, J., Reduction in long term disability in patients with rheumatoid arthritis by DMARDs based treatment strategies, *Arthritis Rheum.*, 39: 616–623, 1996.

152. Edmonds, J.P., Scott, D.L., Furst, D.E., Brooks, P. and Paulus, H.E., Antirheumatic drugs: a proposed new classification, *Arthritis Rheum.*, 36: 336–339, 1993.

153. Simon, L.S. and Strand, V., Clinical response to NSAIDs, *Arthritis Rheum.*, 40: 1940–1943, 1997.

154. Rodriguez, L., NSAID, ulcers and risk: a collaborative meta-analysis, *Sem. Arthritis Rheum.*, 26: S16–S29, 1997.

155. Felson, D.T., Anderson, J., and Meenan, R.F., Use of short term efficacy/toxicity trade offs to select second line drugs in rheumatoid arthritis, *Arthritis Rheum.*, 35: 1117–1125, 1992.

156. Mottonen, T., Paimela, L., and Ahonen, J., Outcome in patients with early rheumatoid arthritis treated according to the "sawtooth strategy," *Arthritis Rheum.*, 39: 996–1005, 1996.

157. Kirwan, J.R., The effect of glucocorticoids on joint destruction in rheumatoid arthritis, *N. Engl. J. Med.*, 333: 142–146, 1995.

158. Harris, W.H. and Sledge, C.B., Total hip and total knee replacement I and II. *N. Engl. J. Med.*, 323: 725–731; 801–807, 1990.

159. Rothfuss, J., Mau, W., Zeidler, H., and Brennan, M., Socioeconomic evaluation of rheumatoid arthritis and osteoarthritis: A literature review, *Sem. Arthritis Rheum.*, 26: 771–779, 1997.

160. Brennan, F.M., Maini, R.N., and Feldmann, M., Cytokines in rheumatoid arthritis. *Cytokines in Autoimmunity*, Brennan, F.M. and Feldmann, M., Eds., Chapman and Hall, London, 1996.

161. Calder, P.C., Polyunsaturated fatty acids, inflammation and immunity, *Lipids*, 36: 1007–1024, 2001.

162. Shaperio, J.A., Koepsell, T.D., Voight, L., Dugawson, C.E., Kesten, M., and Nelson, J.L., Diet and rheumatoid arthritis in women: a possible preventative effect of fish consumption, *Epidemiology*, 7: 256–263. 1996.

163. Recht, L., Helin, P., Rasmussen, J.O., Jacobsen, J., Lithman, T., and Schersten, B., Hand handicap and rheumatoid arthritis in a fish-eating society (the Faroe Islands), *J. Intern. Med.*, 227: 49–55, 1990.

164. Siscovick, D.S., Lemaitre, R.N., and Mozaffarian, D., The fish story: a diet-heart hypothesis with clinical implications: n-3 polyunsaturated fatty acids, myocardial vulnerability and sudden death, *Circulation*, 107: 2632–2634, 2003.

165. Miles, E.A. and Calder, P.C., Modulation of immune function by dietary fatty acids, *Proc. Nutr. Soc.*, 57: 277–300. 1998.

166. World Health Organization, Diet, Nutrition and the Prevention of Chronic Diseases, World Health Org. Tech. Rep. Ser., 797, 1990.

167. The British Nutrition Foundation, Unsaturated fatty acids: Nutritional and physiological significance, The Report of the British Nutrition Foundation's Task Force, London, Chapman and Hall, 1992.

168. Hwang, D., Essential fatty acids and immune response, *FASEB J.*, 3: 2052–2061, 1989.

169. Whelan, J., Antagonistic effects of dietary arachidonic acid and n-3 polyunsaturated fatty acids, *J. Nutr.*, 126: 1086S–1091S, 1996.

170. Yam, D., Eleraz, A., and Berry, E.M., Diet and disease — the Israeli paradox: possible dangers of a high omega-6 polyunsaturated diet, *Isr. J. Med.*, 32: 1134–1143, 1996.

171. Cleland, L.G., James, M., Neumann, M., D'Angelo, M., and Gibson, R., Linolate inhibits EPA incorporation from dietary fish oil supplement in human subjects, *Am. J. Clin. Nutr.*, 55: 395–399, 1992.

172. Mantzioris, E., James, M., Gibson, R., and Cleland, L.G., Dietary substitution with an n-3 rich vegetable oil increases EPA levels in plasma and neutrophil phospholipids, *Am. J. Clin. Nutr.*, 59: 1304–1309, 1994.

173. Linos, A., Kaklamani, V., Kaklamani, E., Koumantaki, Y., Giziaki, E., and Papazoglou, S., Dietary factors in relation to rheumatoid arthritis: a role for olive oil and cooked vegetables? *Am. J. Clin. Nutr.*, 70: 1077–1082, 1999.

174. Drosos, A.A., Alamanos, I., Voulgari, P.V., Psychos, D.N., Katsaraki, A., Papadopoulos, I., Dimou, G., and Siozos, C., Epidemiology of adult rheumatoid arthritis in northwest Greece, 1987–1995, *J. Rheumatol.*, 24: 2129–2133, 1997.

175. Keys, A., *Seven Countries: A Multivariate Analysis of Diet and Coronary Heart Disease*, Harvard University Press, Cambridge, 1980.

176. Trichopoulou, A. and Vasilopoulou, E., Mediterranean diet and longevity, *Br. J. Nutr.*, 84: 205–209, 2000.

177. de Lorgeril, M., Renaud, S., Mamelle, N., Salen, P., Martin, J.-L., Monaud, I., Saqlen, P., and Toubol, P., Mediterranean alpha-linolenic acid rich diet in secondary prevention of coronary heart disease, *Lancet*, 343: 1454–1459, 1994.

178. Ross, R., The pathogenesis of atherosclerosis: a perspective for the 1990s, *Nature*, 362: 801–809, 1993.

179. Janssen, H.C., Samson, M.M., and Verhaar, H.J., Vitamin D deficiency, muscle function and falls in elderly people, *Am. J. Clin. Nutr.*, 75: 611–615, 2002.

180. Cantorna, M.T., Hayes, C.E., and De Luca, H.G., 1,25-Dihydroxycholecalciferol inhibits the progression of arthritis in murine models of human arthritis, *J. Nutr.*, 128: 68–72, 1998.

181. Lemire, J.M., Ince, A., and Takashima, M., 1,25-Dihydroxyvitamin D3, attenuates the expression of experimental murine lupus of MRL/1 mice, *Autoimmunity*, 12: 143–148, 1992.

182. Cantorna, M.T., Munsick, C., Bemiss, C., and Mahon, B.C., 1,25-Dihydroxycholecalciferol prevents and ameliorates symptoms of experimental murine inflammatory bowel disease, *J. Nutr.*, 130: 2648–2652, 2000.

183. Dhesi, J.K., Jackson, S.H., Bearne, L.M., Moniz, C., Hurley, M.V., Swift, C.G., and Allain, T.J., Vitamin D supplementation improves neuromuscular function in older people who fall, *Age Ageing*, 33: 589–595, 2004.

184. Gibson, G.R. and Roberfroid, M.B., Dietary modulation of human colonic microbiota: introducing the concept of prebiotics, *J. Nutr.*, 125: 1401–1412, 1995.

185. Hatakka, K., Martio, J., Korpela, M., Herranen, M., Poussa, T., Laasanen, T., Saxelin, M., Vapaatalo, H., Moilanen, E. and Korpela, R., Effects of probiotic therapy on the activity and activation of mild rheumatoid arthritis — a pilot study, *Scand. J. Rheumatol.*, 32: 211–215, 2003.

186. Lyte, M. and Bailey, M.T., Neuroendocrine-bacterial interactions in a neurotoxin-induced model of trauma, *J. Surg. Res.*, 70: 195–201, 1997.

187. Salminen, S., Isolauri, E., and Onnela, T., Gut flora in normal and disordered states, *Chemotherapy*, 41: 5–15, 1995.

188. Ralph, H.J., Volker, D.H., and Chin, J., Effects of omega-3 fatty acid deficiency on rat intestinal structure and microbiology, *Asia Pac. J. Clin. Nutr.*, 13: S79, 2004.

189. Hopkins, M.J., Sharp, R., and Macfarlane, G.T., Age and disease related changes in intestinal bacterial populations assessed by cell culture, 16S rRNA abundance and community cellular fatty acid profiles, *Gut,* 48: 198–205, 2001.

190. Sinclair, A.J., O'Dea, K., Dunstan, G., Ireland, P.D., and Naill, M., Effects on plasma lipids and fatty acid composition of very low fat diets enriched with fish or kangaroo meat, *Lipids*, 22: 523–529, 1987.

191. Sinclair, A.J. and O'Dea, K., Fats in human diets through history: is the western diet out of step? In *Reducing Fat in Meat Animals,* Wood, J.D. and Fisher, A.V. (Eds.), Elsevier Applied Science, London, 1990.

192. Sinclair, A.J., O'Dea, K., and Johnson, L., Estimation of n-3 status of a group of urban Australians by analysis of plasma phospholipids, *Aust. J. Nutr. Diet.*, 51: 53–56, 1994.

193. Sinclair, A.J., Oon, K., Lim, L., Lio, D., and Mann, N., The omega-3 fatty acid content of canned, smoked and fresh fish in Australia, *Aust. J. Nutr. Diet.*, 55: 116–120, 1998.

12 Skeletal Effects of Soy Isoflavones in Humans: Bone Mineral Density and Bone Markers

D. Lee Alekel

CONTENTS

I. INTRODUCTION

The purpose of this review is to highlight research findings on the skeletal effects of soy isoflavones or soy protein containing isoflavones in humans. Soybeans and their constituents have been extensively investigated for their role in preventing chronic disease, with particular focus on cardiovascular health and cancer protection. At this junction, the role of soy in bone health deserves further consideration. The observations suggesting that soybeans may contribute to bone health include the low rate of hip fracture in Asians originating from the Pacific Rim,[1,2] the effectiveness of the isoflavone-derivative ipriflavone to prevent and treat postmenopausal osteoporosis,[3,4] the *in vitro*[5] and *in vivo*[6] estrogenic activity of soy isoflavones, and the lower urinary calcium losses in soy vs. animal protein diets.[7] However, there are caveats to these findings that do not support the role of soy isoflavones in bone health. Thus, evidence suggesting a bone-protective effect of isoflavone-containing soy is intriguing and encouraging, but it is nonetheless speculative at this time.

This chapter focuses on prospective intervention trials, with references to observational studies. Animal and *in vitro* cell studies will not be reviewed in this chapter. Data from prospective studies have been published on the effect of soy isoflavones on bone mineral density (BMD) by dual-energy x-ray absorptiometry (DXA), and on biochemical markers of bone turnover measured in human blood or urine. Prior to the discussion on soy isoflavones, some background on osteoporosis and its currently approved treatments will be provided. Readers are referred to previously published reviews on the skeletal effects of soy isoflavones.[8–14]

Phytoestrogens include several classes of plant molecules, in particular isoflavones, lignans, and coumestans, which are structurally similar to mammalian estrogens and exert estrogenic activity in animal and human tissues.[15] Soy isoflavones (genistein, daidzein, glycitein), structurally similar to 17β-estradiol, are hypothesized to protect against chronic diseases like osteoporosis, breast cancer, and cardiovascular disease.[16] Phytoestrogens are extracted from soybeans and clover and put on the market in supplement form. However, this review focuses on soy isoflavones, because most of the studies have been conducted on the naturally occurring nonsteroidal isoflavones that are obtained primarily from soy foods. To date, maintenance of BMD has been found only in women (pre-, peri-, and postmenopausal), whereas studies in men have not yet been reported.

Dietary isoflavones are weakly estrogenic, particularly in the face of endogenous estrogen deficiency as occurs in postmenopausal women, and are thought to conserve bone through the estrogen receptor (ER)-mediated pathway. Isoflavones exert an estrogenic effect on the central nervous system, induce estrus, stimulate growth of the genital tract in female mice, and bind to ERs.[17] Isoflavones preferentially bind to ER-β,[18] implying their action is distinctly different from that of classical steroidal estrogens that preferentially bind to ER-α. Isoflavones are weak agonists of 17 β-estradiol in bone cells, but they may act as estrogen antagonists in reproductive tissues, indicating that the differential tissue response is due to different numbers of ER-α and ER-β in various cell types. Furthermore, the stronger affinity of isoflavones for ER-β compared to ER-α may be particularly important because ER-β has been identified in bone tissue.[19] Shutt and Cox[20] determined that the relative binding affinity of daidzein (0.1%) and genistein (0.9%) is weak compared with 17 β-estradiol. Genistein has a particular binding affinity for ER-β but removing one hydroxyl group (daidzein) leads to great loss in this affinity.[21] Thus, because some tissues contain predominantly ER-α or ER-β and different isoflavones exert various effects, isoflavones indeed may exert tissue-selective effects. Hence, isoflavones behave much like drugs known as selective estrogen receptor modulators (SERMs). Although further study is needed to determine which isoflavones *in vivo* inhibit bone resorption and which stimulate formation, *in vitro* studies indicate that isoflavones both suppress osteoclastic and enhance osteoblastic function.

II. EPIDEMIOLOGIC PERSPECTIVE

A. OVERVIEW OF OSTEOPOROSIS

Osteoporosis is a silent epidemic that afflicts 25 million, accounting for 1.5 million new fractures each year in the U.S. alone and countless millions worldwide.[22] Osteoporotic fractures are contributing to major increases in health-care costs and disability, with impending social implications worldwide.[23] Men typically develop fractures 5 years later than women,[24] but osteoporosis afflicts almost twice as many women as men.[22] The longer life expectancy of women amplifies their disease burden. Osteoporosis is estimated to cost our society $60 billion by the year 2020.[25] Many areas of the world are experiencing increases in hip fracture incidence, although it has stabilized in some countries.[26,27] The projected rise in the number of older adults could cause the number of hip fractures worldwide to increase from an estimated 1.7 million in 1990 to a projected 6.3 million in 2050, with the majority of the world's hip fractures occurring in Asia.[28] At present, the majority of hip fractures occur in Europe and North America, but enormous increases in the number of elderly in South America, Africa, and Asia will shift this burden of disease from the developed to the developing world.[29] Effective prevention strategies will need to be designed and disseminated in these parts of the world to prevent the expected increase in hip fractures.

Osteoporosis is defined as a "disease characterized by low bone mass and microarchitectural deterioration of bone tissue leading to enhanced bone fragility and a consequent increase in fracture incidence."[30] The World Health Organization (WHO) has developed an operational definition of osteoporosis based on the BMD of young adult Caucasian women.[31] Unfortunately, because of insufficient data on the relationship between BMD and fracture risk in men or nonwhite women, the WHO does not offer a definition of osteoporosis for groups other than Caucasian women.[32] The WHO defines osteoporosis as a BMD less than 2.5 standard deviations (SD) below the mean for young women. The WHO defines osteopenia as a BMD between 1 and 2.5 SD below the mean for young women (also referred to as a t-score). A t-score ranging from −1 SD below the mean, or any value greater than this indicates normal BMD. Based on these cut-offs, it is estimated that 54% of postmenopausal Caucasian women in the U.S. are osteopenic and 30% are osteoporotic.[33] For each SD below (−1 t-score) the mean, a woman's risk of fracture doubles. However, a limitation of using a cut-off is that the fracture risk varies directly and continuously with BMD,[32] with many risk factors being independent of BMD.[34] Peak bone mass is the maximum BMD achieved by early adulthood and is a key determinant of future risk of fracture. However, the age at which this occurs differs in various populations and differs with respect to skeletal site.

B. Caucasian vs. Asian Populations: Bone Density and Fractures

Ethnic and genetic differences in bone may make some groups more susceptible than others to osteoporotic fractures.[35] For example, Caucasian American women are at greater risk than African and Mexican Americans,[36] who have lower fracture rates.[37] Vertebral fracture incidence among Taiwanese[38] is comparable (18%) to that of Caucasian women, whereas hip fracture incidence among elderly Taiwanese[38] and those from mainland China[39] is lower. Despite 10 to15% lower femoral BMD than Caucasians, Taiwanese have lower hip fracture rates, which may be due to structural differences between racial/ethnic groups. Researchers have determined hip-axis length in premenopausal Chinese women living in Australia[40] and women originating from the Indian subcontinent[41] compared with their Caucasian counterparts, indicating that structural differences likely contribute to variations in hip fracture prevalence in distinct racial groups.[42] Investigators have also examined determinants of peak bone mass in Chinese women in China,[43] risk factors for hip fracture in Asian men and women,[44] and the contribution of anthropometric and lifestyle factors to peak bone mass in a multiethnic population.[45] Some differences in osteoporotic risk among ethnic groups are inexplicable but may be largely due to frame size differences that lead to size-related artifacts in BMD measurements[46,47] and to differences in hip-axis length.[48,49] Thus, when comparing BMD across ethnic groups, it is important to correct for frame size to accurately interpret spinal BMD values[50] and to consider hip geometry to accurately assess hip-fracture risk.[49] Differences in osteoporotic risk may also be related to culture-specific dietary and exercise-related factors, which is beyond the scope of this review.

C. Soy Intake, Bone Density, and Fractures

The low hip fracture rate among Asians has been credited to the beneficial effect of isoflavone-containing soybeans on bone health.[1,2] However, human studies found that isoflavone-rich soy protein (40 g/d) intake was associated with favorable effects on *spinal*[51,52] but not on *femoral* (hip) bone. Also, the amount of isoflavones (in aglycone form) consumed by subjects in the high isoflavone groups in these two studies (80 or 90 mg/d) was greater than what is typically consumed by either Chinese (39 mg/d)[53] or Japanese (23 mg/d)[54] women, or by women from a multiethnic population in Hawaii (ranged from 5 mg/d in Filipino to 38.2 mg/d in Chinese).[55] Nevertheless, it is possible that lower amounts of soy isoflavones consumed over the course of many years could have significant bone-sparing effects. Still, differences are not apparent in the spinal fracture rate,[56,57] or in lumbar spine BMD[47,58] of Asian compared with Caucasian women. In contrast, higher spine and hip BMD values have been reported in U.S.-born vs. Japan-born Japanese women.[59] Many factors may contribute to the lower hip fracture rate in Asians, notably the shorter hip-axis length of Asians originating from the Pacific Rim.[48,49] Other protective factors include the reduced propensity of Asians to fall[60] and the shorter stature of Asians,[44] although these unmodifiable factors have little practical importance in preventing hip fractures.

A few observational studies have published data on the relationship between soy intake and BMD, or fracture risk. Somekawa and colleagues[61] examined the relationship between soy isoflavone intake, menopausal symptoms, lipid profiles, and spinal BMD measured by DXA in 478 postmenopausal Japanese women. They reported that after adjusting BMD for weight and years since menopause, BMD values were significantly different among four isoflavone intake levels, ranging from 35 to 65 mg/d, in both the early ($p \leq 0.001$) and late ($p \leq 0.01$) postmenopausal groups. The women who consumed more soy isoflavones had higher BMD values. Differences were not significant in other characteristics (i.e., height, weight, years since menopause, lipid, or lipoprotein concentrations) across isoflavone intakes. Another study in midlife (40 to 49 years) Japanese women (N = 995) examined the relationship of various dietary factors (including soybean intake) to metacarpal BMD, as measured by computed x-ray densitometry.[62] Women who consumed soybeans at least twice per week had greater BMD than those who had soybeans once or 0 times per week, with this tendency ($p = 0.03$) remaining after controlling for age, height, weight, and weekly calcium intake. Likewise, baseline data analysis from the Study of Women's Health Across the Nation (SWAN), a U.S. community-based cohort study in women 42 to 52 years,[63] revealed that Japanese premenopausal women in the highest vs. lowest tertile of genistein intake had 7.7% and 12% greater spine and femoral neck BMD, respectively. Among the Chinese women, no association was found between genistein intake and BMD, probably because their median intakes (μg/d) were lower (3511) than those of the Japanese women (7151).

In the Netherlands, Kardinaal and colleagues[64] tested the hypothesis that the rate of postmenopausal radial bone loss, measured by single photon absorptiometry, is inversely related to urinary phytoestrogen excretion as a marker of long-term dietary intake. Contrary to their hypothesis, they reported that women with a relatively high rate (1.91 ± 0.08%) of yearly bone loss had higher urinary excretion of enterolactone (median = 838 vs. 1108 μg/g, respectively) than women with a low rate (0.27 ± 0.08%) of loss. Colonic bacteria synthesize enterolactone from precursors found in grains, legumes, seeds, and vegetables.[65] However, urinary genistein, daidzein, and equol concentrations did not differ between the two groups of bone losers. Further, this group of women had very low intakes of dietary isoflavones, similar to what Dutch women typically consume.

In contrast, a prospective study of soy food intake and fracture risk in approximately 75,000 postmenopausal Chinese women[66] indicated a protective effect of soy protein intake. After adjusting for age, BMI, energy, and calcium intake (as well as other dietary factors), lifestyle risk factors for osteoporosis, and socioeconomic status, the relative risk of fracture ranged from 0.63 to 1.00 in the highest to lowest quintiles of soy protein intake ($p < 0.001$), with a more pronounced inverse association among women in early menopause. These published studies differ with respect to the type and site of bone measured, as well as the amount of dietary isoflavones habitually consumed. Nonetheless, the evidence for an effect of soy-derived isoflavones on bone appears to be stronger for trabecular (i.e., spinal) than cortical (i.e., radial, metacarpal) bone, and is probably dependent upon habitual intakes, appearing to be more pronounced in the perimenopausal rather than the late postmenopausal years.

III. CURRENT AND POTENTIAL ALTERNATIVE TREATMENTS FOR OSTEOPOROSIS

A. ESTROGEN THERAPY/HORMONE THERAPY

The accelerated bone loss during the perimenopausal years has been attributed to estrogen deficiency due to ovarian failure. This bone loss contributes to 20 to 30% loss in cancellous (trabecular) bone and 5 to10% loss in cortical bone[67] and may continue for the next decade after menopause. Estrogen alone (estrogen therapy) or in combination with progestin (hormone therapy) prevents bone loss at the spine and hip[68] and reduces hip fracture rates.[69] Locally active growth factors and cytokines modulate the effects of estrogen on osteoblasts and osteoclasts,[70] leading to bone loss. Estrogen deficiency plays a key role in osteoporosis and other menopause-related chronic diseases, but hormone therapy is often accompanied by side effects[71] and increases the risks of endometrial cancer,[72] invasive breast cancer, and total cardiovascular (arterial and venous) disease.[73] Certainly, estrogen or hormone therapy alleviates vasomotor symptoms,[74] prevents bone loss,[75] and decreases the risk for colorectal cancer and hip fractures.[73] Yet, non-compliance is a major obstacle with traditional hormone therapies[76] because of adverse effects and the fear of cancer. Due to undesirable side effects, two thirds of women discontinue treatment within 5 years of initiation.[77] Treatment provided at the onset of menopause, continued for less than 10 years, but then discontinued, has little if any effect on fracture incidence by age 70.[69] Hence, when therapy is discontinued, bone loss ensues and is similar to what occurs following menopause.[78] Clinical guidelines recommend against hormone therapy as a first-line therapy for the prevention of postmenopausal osteoporosis.[79] Research has recently focused on alternatives to steroid hormones, with comparable skeletal and cardiovascular benefits, but without side effects. An overview of these alternatives to steroid hormones in preventing and treating osteoporosis is provided in the next four subsections.

B. BISPHOSPHONATES

Bisphosphonates, pyrophosphate derivates, are potent inhibitors of bone resorption[80] and the most effective class of bone-active agents. They have a strong affinity for bone,[80] increase BMD, and are safe and effective in treating and preventing osteoporosis,[81] including that which is corticosteroid-induced.[82] Alendronate (Fosamax®), risedronate (Actonel®), and etidronate (Didrocal®) are the three agents shown in prospective trials to reduce the risk of vertebral fractures.[83] Alendronate and risedronate have been shown to prevent hip fractures[84] and are more effective than etidronate. Alendronate and risedronate are FDA-approved to prevent bone loss in early postmenopausal women, to treat postmenopausal osteoporosis, and to manage glucocorticoid-induced bone loss.[81] Bisphosphonates combined with estrogen lead to greater gains in BMD than either agent alone, but it is not clear if fracture risk is lessened.[81]

C. CALCITONIN

Calcitonin is an FDA-approved antiresorptive agent to treat but not prevent osteoporosis.[85] The advantages of calcitonin are that it is bone-specific, may be used as an alternative to estrogen, has analgesic action, and may be used in men. Although its anabolic action has not been clearly demonstrated, and it does not appear to have long-term efficacy, a single dose of nasal calcitonin has been shown to decrease bone resorption by 15% as evidenced by biochemical markers of bone turnover.[86] Calcitonin does not affect nonvertebral (i.e., hip) BMD or fractures,[87] but reduces the risk of vertebral fractures by up to 40%.

D. Calcium and Vitamin D

Bone cells are dependent upon all nutrients for their cellular activity and hence nutrition plays an important role in the development, prevention, and treatment of osteoporosis. The reader is referred to an excellent overview of dietary components that affect bone,[88] since an in-depth review is beyond the scope of this chapter. Calcium and vitamin D have been shown to be effective as adjunctive therapies in preventing and treating osteoporosis, but are not effective therapies alone. However, they assume prominent roles in conjunction with antiresorptive agents such as estrogen, calcitonin, bisphosphonates, or SERMs. Adequate vitamin D status along with adequate calcium intake prevents bone loss and reduces fracture risk, particularly during the peri- and postmenopausal years,[89] and with advancing age.[90] Vitamin D and calcium requirements[91] change throughout life because of skeletal growth and age-related alterations in absorption and excretion. Recommended dietary reference intakes for vitamin D vary from 5 μg/d (200 IU) at birth through 50 years, to 15 μg/d (600 IU) after 70 years of age; for calcium they vary from 210 mg/d at birth to 1300 mg/d during adolescence. The North American Menopause Society[89] consensus opinion indicates that at least 1200 mg/d of calcium is required for most women, with 400 to 600 IU (10 to 15 μg)/d of vitamin D from dietary sources or supplements, in addition to sun exposure, to ensure adequate calcium absorption. The vast majority (50 of 52) of calcium intervention studies and 75% of 86 observational studies[92] indicate that high calcium intakes promote bone health. Estrogen therapy exhibits a considerably greater protective effect when coadministered with supplemental calcium than when taken alone.[93] Indeed, agents that increase bone density (i.e., fluoride, bisphosphonates) do not achieve their full effect when calcium is limited. Vitamin D facilitates osteoclastic resorption and normal mineralization, as well as calcium and phosphorus absorption. Vitamin D supplementation is particularly important in the elderly, who are often deficient, and assists in lowering elevated serum parathyroid hormone,[94,95] which leads to bone loss. Vitamin D repletion is associated with significant annual increases in BMD at the lumbar spine ($p \leq 0.0001$) and femoral neck ($p = 0.03$) in osteopenic patients.[96] Calcium and vitamin D supplementation alone is insufficient but is nevertheless a cornerstone in preventing and treating osteoporosis.

E. Selective Estrogen Receptor Modulators (SERMs)

Selective estrogen receptor modulators are comprised of a group of chemically diverse nonsteroidal compounds that bind to and interact with the estrogen receptor. These estrogen-like compounds exert tissue selectivity, such that a given SERM may act as an estrogen agonist in some tissues and an estrogen antagonist in others.[97] Structurally and pharmacologically similar to soy isoflavones, synthetic SERMs (such as ipriflavone, tamoxifen, and raloxifene) are effective in preventing or reducing bone loss. An isoflavone derivative of plant origin,[98] ipriflavone has been used to prevent and treat postmenopausal osteoporosis[3,4,99] and also in several models of experimental osteoporosis.[100,101] Ipriflavone also enhances the therapeutic bone response when combined with estrogen, above that of single therapy.[102] In contrast, a muticenter trial[103] revealed that ipriflavone did not prevent bone loss or affect bone turnover, casting doubt on its effectiveness. Tamoxifen is widely used in treating breast cancer but also has weak estrogenic effects on bone remodeling.[104] A randomized clinical trial indicated that whereas the placebo group lost 1% after one year, the tamoxifen[105] group increased spine BMD significantly (0.6%). These beneficial skeletal effects of tamoxifen have been borne out in other studies, but its major drawback is its endometrial stimulatory effect.[106] Unlike tamoxifen, raloxifene does not stimulate the endometrium[107] but prevents bone loss and remodeling[108]; hence, the FDA has approved raloxifene for preventing postmenopausal osteoporosis.[107] A drawback of raloxifene is that it may increase hot flushes in some women,[109] thus perhaps limiting its use to those who are well beyond the menopausal transition. Yet more recent research demonstrated that, in comparison with placebo, raloxifene did not increase the frequency or severity of hot flushes in women who discontinue hormone therapy.[110] Interestingly, a 24-week study found that isoflavone-rich soy had no adverse or favorable effects on vasomotor symptoms in perimenopausal women.[111] The purported mechanism of action for SERMs on bone is similar to that of estrogen in decreasing bone resorption. These potential beneficial effects of SERMs make them very appealing in preventing and treating osteoporosis, but naturally occurring soy isoflavones may be more acceptable to many menopausal women than the synthetic analogues.

F. SOY ISOFLAVONES: POTENTIAL ALTERNATIVE FOR OSTEOPOROSIS PREVENTION?

The most promising effect of isoflavones in menopausal women may be that of bone-sparing. Soy protein isolate with isoflavones has been shown to prevent femoral and lumbar bone loss in ovariectomised rats[112] and lumbar spine bone loss in humans in the short-term.[51] Animal research provides valuable information on potential mechanisms of action, but clinical trials ultimately must be conducted to confirm the long-term effects of soy isoflavones in humans. Numerous clinical trials from various parts of the world have examined the impact of soy foods, isolated soy protein, or isolated isoflavones on BMD or bone mineral content (BMC) and biochemical markers of bone in midlife women. First, we will consider the effects of isoflavone-containing soy protein on calcium metabolism, another purported mechanism by which soy isoflavones are thought to impact bone. The two sections following this first section will review key published studies on the response of BMD and biochemical markers of bone to soy isoflavones in humans.

1. Protein and Soy Isoflavone Intake in Relation to Calcium Homeostasis

Soy protein may protect against bone loss indirectly by mechanisms independent of its estrogenic effects. Similar to the estrogen-enhancing effects on calcium uptake *in vitro,*[113] isoflavones may improve calcium absorption. Yet, a recent human study found no evidence that fractional calcium absorption or net calcium retention was affected by either soy protein enriched with or devoid of isoflavones.[114] Based on kinetic modeling (N = 14), bone deposition was ~ 20% greater in the soy with isoflavones vs. soy diets devoid of isoflavones, but this was not statistically significant. However, urinary calcium excretion with soy intake (regardless of isoflavone content) was less ($p < 0.01$) compared with the control diet (casein-whey protein). Thus, diets high in soy compared to animal protein may reduce urinary calcium loss. Legumes, including soybeans, are somewhat lower in sulfur amino acids than meat.[115] Animal protein is more hypercalciuric than soy protein based on human studies,[7,116,117] perhaps due to the greater net renal acid excretion with high meat diets.[118] Intakes of milk whey (2.8 g methionine/100 g) and soy (1.3 g methionine/100 g) protein were compared acutely over a 24-h period.[116] After 4 h, the calcium:creatinine ratio in urine increased by 45% with the intake of milk whey, but increased by only 3% with a similar amount of soy as the primary source of protein. After 24 h, the calcium:creatinine ratio was 56% higher than baseline in the whey compared with 27% higher in the soy group.

A longer term two-week study[119] in subjects (N = 9) aged 22 to 69 years were fed protein (~ 80 g) derived primarily from either soybeans or chicken, but with similar amounts of calcium, phosphorus, magnesium, and sulfur. Compared to baseline values, urinary total titratable acid increased only 4% in the soy, but by 46% in the meat diet. Urinary calcium excretion was 169 mg in the soy vs. 203 mg in the meat diet, demonstrating that soy was less hypercalciuric than meat protein. Similarly, Breslau et al.[7] examined calcium metabolism in 15 subjects, 23 to 46 years of age, who consumed each of three diets in random order (crossover) for 12 d: soy protein (vegetarian), soy and egg protein (ovo-vegetarian), or animal (beef, chicken, fish, cheese) protein. Diets were kept constant in protein (75 g/d), calcium (400 mg), phosphorus (1000 mg), sodium (400 mg), and fluid (3 l), providing sufficient energy to maintain weight. They reported no difference in fractional[47] calcium absorption among the diets, but 24-h urinary calcium excretion increased ($p < 0.02$) from 103 ± 15 mg/d on the vegetarian to 150 ± 13 mg/d on the animal protein diet. Likewise, Pie and Paik[117] fed young Korean women (N = 6) a meat-based (71 g protein/d) followed by a soy-based

(83 g protein/d) diet for 5 d each. Despite similar dietary calcium (525 mg/d) intake, urinary and fecal calcium excretions, respectively, were higher ($p < 0.025$) while subjects consumed the meat- (127 and 467 mg/d) vs. the soy- (88 and 284 mg/d) based diet. Thus, overall calcium balance was more negative ($p < 0.001$) on the meat- (–65.4 mg/d) vs. soy- (155.3 mg/d) based diet. In contrast, daily substitution of meat protein with 25 g of soy protein in the context of a mixed diet for seven weeks did not improve or impair calcium retention or bone markers in healthy postmenopausal women.[120] Despite higher urinary pH and lower renal acid excretion (ammonium plus titratable acidity) in the soy protein vs. control group, there was no difference in urinary calcium excretion in this randomized crossover controlled-feeding study. Perhaps one explanation for seemingly contradictory findings in these studies is that the protein-associated hypercalciuria is due to enhanced intestinal calcium absorption (which is dependent upon many factors) rather than an increase in bone resorption.[121]

A related question is whether the calcium recommendation (age 50 +, 1200 mg/d) for Caucasians should apply to Asians who have a smaller skeletal size who typically consume ~ 500 mg/d.[122] Kung et al.[123] found in nonosteoporotic postmenopausal Chinese women that calcium absorption was 58% with a 600 mg supplement, 60% during the unmodified period, but rose to 71% during calcium deprivation (< 300 mg/d). These absorption values are twofold higher than what is reported in Caucasians.[124] Might this difference in calcium absorption be related to the high vegetable and soy intakes of Chinese,[125] which provide 41% of their calcium in contrast to < 10% of intake in the U.S.?[126] Further study is required to determine more precisely how soy- vs. animal-based diets affect bone and calcium homeostasis over the long term. The beneficial effect of soy foods on calcium excretion may be clinically relevant. If individuals consume two or three servings/d, substituting soy for animal protein over the long term, the balance could be tipped in favor of calcium retention.

2. Soy Isoflavones and Bone Mineral Density: Prospective Studies

Among the more notable prospective studies, six used either soy protein isolate[51,52,127,128] or a soy food[129,130] as the isoflavone source; two examined usual soy food intake among Asians[66,131] as the source of isoflavones; and three used extracted soy isoflavones.[132–134] One of these studies[66] examined the association between soy consumption and risk of fracture, and is reviewed in earlier text in section 2C. Two intervention studies[51,130] were designed specifically to examine bone as the primary outcome. Nine studies[51,52,127–133] are reviewed below because they illustrate the breadth of what we know to date about soy isoflavones and bone.

Dalais and coworkers[129] supplied daily 45 g soy grits (flour) containing 53 mg/d isoflavones, 45 g linseed (flaxseed with mammalian lignan precursors), or 45 g wheat kibble (control) to 44 postmenopausal women for 12 weeks using a crossover design. They found that total body BMC increased 5.2% ($p = 0.03$) in the soy, 5.2% (NS) in the linseed, and 3.8% (NS) in the wheat groups, whereas BMD did not change. The magnitude of this increase is implausible, but in addition, there were increases in BMC in the other two groups, one of which was a control. Thus, these results should be interpreted with caution. Another study,[52] designed to examine the lipid-related effects of soy protein, randomly assigned 66 hypercholesterolemic postmenopausal women to one of three treatments for six months: (1) casein + nonfat dry milk protein, (2) soy protein (40 g/d) isolate (SPI +) with 56 mg/d of isoflavones, or (3) SPI+ with 90 mg/d of isoflavones. The women were heterogeneous with respect to time since menopause, and age (49 to 83 years). Women in the high isoflavone group experienced an increase (~ 2%; $p < 0.05$), whereas those in the casein+milk-based protein had slight decreases, in lumbar spine BMD and BMC. Although women in the high isoflavone group began the study with lower BMD and BMC than the other two groups, baseline values were not taken into account. The effect of treatment on bone is typically greater in those with lower bone mass[135] and hence baseline BMD should be considered.

Nonetheless, the study by Alekel and coworkers[51] in 69 perimenopausal women is in general agreement with the previously described work. Women were randomized (double-blind) to treatment, with dose expressed as aglycone units: isoflavone-rich soy (SPI+, 80.4 mg/d; $n = 24$), isoflavone-poor soy (SPI, 4.4 mg/d; $n = 24$), or whey (control; $n = 21$) protein. No change was reported in the SPI+ (-0.2%, $p = 0.7$; $+0.6\%$, $p = 0.5$) or SPI (0.7%, $p = 0.1$; 0.6%, $p = 0.3$) groups, but loss ($p = 0.004$) occurred in controls (-1.3%, -1.7%) in the lumbar spine BMD and BMC, respectively, values. As baseline BMD and BMC ($p \leq 0.0001$) affected (negatively) percentage change in these outcomes, baseline values were taken into account in the analysis of covariance (ANCOVA) and regression analysis. Results of ANCOVA indicated that treatment had a significant effect on % change in BMC ($p = 0.021$), but not on % change in BMD ($p = 0.25$). Further, contrast coding using ANCOVA with BMD or BMC as the outcome revealed that isoflavones, not soy protein, exerted a positive effect. Taking various contributing factors into account, including weight gain, regression analysis indicated that SPI + had a positive effect on % change in both BMD (5.6%, $p = 0.023$) and BMC (10.1%, $p = 0.0032$). Body weight at baseline, rather than final weight or weight gain, was related to percentage change in BMD, suggesting that weight gain did not confound the effect of SPI+ on bone. Contrary to their hypothesis, the authors did not find an effect of endogenous reproductive hormones or estrogen status on bone loss. Soy (SPI–) or whey protein had no effect on the spine and treatment in general had no effect on bone sites other than the spine. These last two studies provide support for the contention that isoflavones are the bioactive component of soy with respect to bone.

Another study was designed to examine habitual soy intake and BMD in premenopausal Chinese women, 30 to 40 years of age, living in Hong Kong.[131] After adjusting for age and body size (height, weight, and bone area), researchers reported a positive effect of soy isoflavones on spinal BMD after an average follow-up time of 38.1 months. The mean percentage decline in spinal BMD in 116 women was greater ($p < 0.05$) in the lowest (-3.5%) vs. highest (-1.1%) quartile of soy isoflavone intake. Multiple regression revealed that soy isoflavone intake (along with lean body mass, physical activity, energy adjusted calcium intake, and follow-up time) accounted for 24% of the variance in spinal BMD in these women. This 3-year study indicated that soy isoflavone intake had a positive effect on maintaining spinal BMD in premenopausal women 30 to 40 years of age. In contrast, a study in 37 postmenopausal women supplemented with soy isoflavones (150 mg/d, but undefined) for 6 months did not produce a significant change in calcaneous BMD.[132] Because this study was conducted in Taiwanese women who habitually consume soy and there was no control group, interpretation is difficult. Alternatively, because the calcaneous (heel) is weight-bearing and has greater trabecular content[45] than vertebral bone, it may respond differently to isoflavone treatment than the lumbar spine. Chen and coworkers[133] conducted a double-blind, randomized clinical trial to examine the effect of soy-germ extract of isoflavones (40 or 80 mg/d), compared with placebo (corn starch) for 1 year, on bone loss in postmenopausal (48 to 62 years) Chinese women who habitually consume soy products. Univariate and multivariate analyses indicated that women in the high-dose group lost less BMC in the trochanter and total proximal femur than either the placebo or low-dose group, with or without adjusting for potential confounding factors. The positive effect of soy isoflavone supplementation was observed only among women with low baseline BMC values. Because the intervention of soy germ (relatively rich in glycitein) used in this study is different compared with other studies (products are typically relatively rich in genistein), this makes it difficult to compare results to other trials. Yet results of this study suggest that isoflavones may have a significant effect on cortical (proximal femur or hip) bone, or that appendicular bone responds differently from that of the axial (i.e., spine) skeleton.

Kreijkamp-Kaspers et al.[127] have reported a lack of effect of soy protein (25.6 g/d) isolate on cognitive function, BMD, and plasma lipids for one year in postmenopausal women. However, this trial included women considerably older (60 to 75 years) than most other trials reporting an effect of isoflavones. Their participants were advanced in age, heterogeneous in menopausal status, and they did not account for critical potentially confounding factors. The authors stated that "adjustment for smoking history and baseline BMD did not change the results," but current smoking status, baseline BMD (which appeared to differ between groups by ~ 3.5% for total hip and ~ 2.4% for lumbar spine, biologically important differences), and antihypertensive medication use should have been taken into account statistically. As acknowledged by the authors, those who had more recently transitioned through menopause experienced better results (both hip and spine) after one year of soy compared with placebo, although the interaction was not significant ($p = 0.07$ for total hip). This suggests that either time since menopause was critically important in dictating a treatment effect, and/or that the power was insufficient. Their assumption that "soy isoflavones (99 mg/d) are as effective as conventional hormone therapy" is not correct, perhaps resulting in insufficient power. These methodological limitations make interpretation difficult.

Reporting similar results, Gallagher and coworkers[128] examined the effect of soy protein isolate with isoflavones (96 or 52 mg/d) and without isoflavones (< 4 mg/d) on bone loss and lipids in postmenopausal women (N = 65; mean age of 55, and 7.5 years since menopause). Soy protein was provided for nine months, but participants were followed off-treatment for another six months. Soy supplements had no significant effect on BMD of the lumbar spine or femoral neck, whereas BMD increased significantly in the trochanter at nine months ($p = 0.02$) and at 15 months ($p < 0.05$) in the isoflavone-free soy group compared with the other two groups. These results are difficult to explain. In contrast to findings from the previous two studies, Lydeking-Olsen et al.[130] reported that postmenopausal (mean age of 58.2, maximum age of 75 years) women (N = 89) in the isoflavone-rich (76 mg/d) soy milk or transdermal progesterone (25.7 mg/d) group did not lose lumbar spine BMD, whereas the placebo control (isoflavone-poor soy milk plus progesterone-free cream; -4.2%, $p = 0.01$) and combination isoflavone-rich soy milk and progesterone (-2.8%, $p = 0.01$) groups had significant loss. Daily intake of two glasses of soy milk with 76 mg isoflavones prevented lumbar spine bone loss, but when combined with progesterone cream, lumbar spine BMD was inexplicably lost, although not as such as with the placebo. Equol-producer status was associated with a better bone response, but this did not reach statistical significance due to insufficient sample size.

Taken together, results of these human studies suggest that isoflavones may attenuate bone loss from the lumbar spine in estrogen-deficient women, who may otherwise be expected to lose 2 to 3% yearly. Such attenuation of loss, particularly if continued throughout the postmenopausal period, could translate into a decreased risk of osteoporosis. As a bone-remodeling cycle ranges from 30 to 80 weeks,[136] such short-term (1 year or less) preliminary studies cannot answer the question of whether these bone-sparing effects would be sustained over a longer period. From these results, we cannot determine whether the reported bone-sparing effect is due to treatment or is an artifact of the bone-remodeling transient,[136] although the longer-term study in Asian women[131] suggests true bone-sparing. A clinical trial for at least 2, and preferably 3 years, is necessary to determine whether soy isoflavones will affect the remodeling balance, tipping it in favor of bone formation rather than resorption. Such studies are underway in the U.S.

3. Biochemical Markers of Bone in Response to Soy Isoflavones

Biochemical markers of bone serve as indices of change in bone turnover, reflecting increases or decreases in rates of resorption and formation. Several markers are found either in blood or urine and can be measured by enzyme-linked immunosorbent assay (ELISA), high-pressure liquid chromatography (HPLC), or radioimmunoassay (RIA or IRMA) procedures. The advantages of biochemical markers of bone are that the method is noninvasive, may predict (albeit imperfectly) the rate of bone loss in menopausal women, may predict the response to some antiresorptive therapies[137] and may be performed more frequently than bone density scans. In a research setting, measurements of bone markers are typically made at baseline and again at one or more times during the course of treatment. In a clinical setting, bone markers may be measured at baseline and then a few weeks after the initiation of treatment to determine whether or not a patient has experienced a therapeutic response. The primary limitation of bone markers is that circadian rhythms affect circulating concentrations, and hence biologic variability is sufficiently great to necessitate large differences in the markers to detect a response to therapy.[137] Additional limitations are that some markers are not sensitive or specific (i.e., bone- vs. nonbone-derived biomarkers) enough to detect small changes; over time the renal clearance capacity of the patient greatly influences values for certain blood- and urine-derived markers; sample procurement and measurement should be standardized; and the overall metabolic status of the patient at the time of sample collection should be considered. Nevertheless, increasing concentrations of both formation and resorption markers are associated with more rapid bone loss and differences in these rates correspond to clinically significant differences in fracture risk.[138] Existing data indicate that biochemical markers can aid in determining which women are at greater risk of rapid bone loss and fracture.[139] The most valuable biomarkers[137] for bone formation are serum bone-specific alkaline phosphatase, osteocalcin, and the N-terminal propeptide of procollagen I; for bone resorption, they are serum N-telopeptide and C-telopeptide of type I collagen, and urinary pyridinoline and deoxypyridinoline collagen crosslinks. The reader is referred to a review by the International Osteoporosis Foundation on the use of biochemical markers of bone turnover in osteoporosis.[140]

Few studies have been published examining the response of biochemical markers of bone turnover to isoflavone-rich soy protein, or extracted isoflavones in humans. This first section will review studies using soy protein as the treatment and the next section will cover trials using extracted isoflavones, illustrating the somewhat inconsistent results in the biochemical markers. The first group to include a measure of bone turnover as part of a study designed to examine hot flushes was that of Murkies and coworkers.[141] Postmenopausal women had their diets supplemented with either wheat or soy flour (45 g/d) for 12 weeks. Urinary hydroxyproline, a nonspecific marker of bone resorption, increased over time in the wheat flour ($p < 0.05$) but not in the soy-flour group; however, the difference between groups was not significant ($p = 0.47$). Washburn et al.[142] reported on alkaline phosphatase activity in a study designed to examine the effects of soy protein on cardiovascular disease risk factors and menopausal symptoms. This randomized crossover (double-blind) trial had 51 subjects consume isocaloric supplements for 6 weeks each: (1) single dose of 20 g soy protein (34 mg isoflavones); (2) split (two) dose of 20 g soy protein (34 mg isoflavones); or (3) 20 g complex carbohydrate. Alkaline phosphatase (non-specific marker of bone formation) activity decreased ($p < 0.05$) in women on either soy diet compared with the carbohydrate-supplemented group. The authors suggest that this decline may have reflected a beneficial effect of soy, but these results are difficult to interpret because they did not measure any bone-resorption marker. Crossover designs have an inherent drawback due to the potential for carryover or contamination in the outcomes of interest.

In one of the studies described above, Alekel and coworkers[51] did not find a decline in bone resorption (using cross-linked N-telopeptides) during the course of 24 weeks of treatment in perimenopausal women (N = 69). Repeated ANCOVA measures indicated that treatment *per se* had no significant effect on either cross-linked N-telopeptides ($p = 0.12$) or bone-specific alkaline phosphatase ($p = 0.32$), but both time ($p < 0.005$) and baseline values ($p \leq 0.0001$) were significant. Yet, cohort (group of subjects that began the study at the same time) had a significant effect on N-telopeptides ($p = 0.0089$), but not on bone-specific alkaline phosphatase ($p = 0.56$), suggesting that cohort may reflect a seasonal influence on bone resorption. This study appears to corroborate findings in the rat model,[112,143] indicating that soy with isoflavones does not decrease bone turnover. Another study[144] examined the effect of consuming 25 g/d of soy protein (n = 35) in the form of foods vs. a comparative control diet (n = 27) on biochemical markers of bone in postmenopausal women. Both treatment groups experienced an increase in circulating bone-specific alkaline phosphatase, insulin-like growth factor-1 (IGF-1), and osteocalcin, but no change in urinary deoxypyridinoline or bone, indicating no effect of treatment. Similarly, Knight and colleagues[145] reported no differences in serum alkaline phosphatase (nonspecific bone formation marker) or pyridinoline cross-links (bone resorption marker) between the soy protein (40 g/d) with isoflavones (77.4 mg/d aglycone components) and casein-treated control groups in a randomized (double-blind) placebo-controlled 12-week study in 24 women.

Wangen and colleagues[146] conducted a randomized, crossover 3-month soy-protein (63 g/d) isolate study to examine the dose-response effect of isoflavones on bone markers in 14 premenopausal and 17 postmenopausal women. On a per kg body-weight basis, expressed as aglycone units, the daily dose was 10 ± 1.1, 64 ± 9.2, or 128 ± 16 mg/d in the premenopausal women, and was 7 ± 1.1, 65 ± 11, or 132 ± 22 mg/d in the postmenopausal women. There were no effects of treatment on osteocalcin in the premenopausal women, but during the early follicular phase, deoxypyridinoline crosslinks increased in both isoflavone diets; during the periovulatory phase, serum IGF-1 increased in the low (64 mg/d) compared with high (128 mg/d) isoflavone diets. In the postmenopausal women, the low (65 mg/d) and high (132 mg/d) isoflavone diets decreased bone-specific alkaline phosphatase. The high isoflavone group experienced a trend toward a decrease in osteocalcin and in IGF-I. Compared with baseline, all three diets increased bone-specific alkaline phosphatase, osteocalcin, and IGF-I, although the increases in the latter two markers were not statistically significant at the highest isoflavone dose. The authors suggest that although isoflavones modestly affected markers of bone turnover, the changes were small and not clinically relevant. Another study[147] examined the effect of consuming dietary whole soy foods (~ 60 mg/d) for 12 weeks on serum bone-specific alkaline phosphatase, osteocalcin, and urinary cross-linked N-telopeptides in 42 postmenopausal women. Serum bone-specific alkaline phosphatase did not change, whereas osteocalcin increased ($p < 0.03$) and N-telopeptides decreased ($p < 0.02$) from baseline to week 12. However, the lack of placebo control in this study makes interpretation difficult, given the biologic variability of bone turnover markers.

To determine the effects on early climacteric symptoms, Scambia and coworkers[148] randomly assigned subjects (N = 39) to a standardized soy extract (50 mg/d of isoflavones) or placebo treatment for 6 weeks and then provided conjugated equine estrogen (0.625 mg/d) for 4 weeks. They did not observe soy-related changes in serum osteocalcin (bone formation marker) and estrogen-related changes were not modified by soy extract. At 15 geographical sites, Upmalis and colleagues[149] used a soy isoflavone extract (50 mg/d of isoflavones), compared with placebo, to determine the effects on climacteric symptoms in postmenopausal women (N = 177). They reported no treatment effect, or change in either serum osteocalcin, or urinary N-telopeptides, but they found a reduction in the number and severity of hot flushes with soy. In contrast, Uesugi et al.[150] reported a reduction of urinary pyridinoline in the soy isoflavone-(62 mg/d) supplemented (n = 12) compared with placebo (n = 11) group after four weeks, but no change in serum osteocalcin in either group. Likewise, Harkness et al.[134] reported a significant decline in type 1 collagen α_1-chain helical peptide (bone-resorption marker) during isoflavone (110 mg/d) supplementation, and a significant difference in this marker when the isoflavone group was compared with the control group.

At this time, with apparent contradictory findings, it is difficult to draw conclusions about the effect of soy isoflavones or soy protein on bone turnover in humans. Some of this discrepancy is probably due to differences in study design that do not allow reasonable comparisons, and to the extreme variability of these markers, particularly in early menopausal women. Sources of variability include differences in the type or dose of soy isoflavones used but also the duration of the study and particular biochemical marker of bone examined. However, overall, some of the studies suggest that soy isoflavones may not have the same effect as estrogen or bisphosphonate therapy in decreasing bone resorption but may indeed prevent a decline at the very least in bone formation.

IV. SUMMARY AND CURRENT STATE OF UNDERSTANDING

Taken together, we have tentative evidence that soy protein containing isoflavones may favorably affect BMD, but these preliminary data must be substantiated. In contrast, we have little evidence as yet that extracted isoflavones impact bone in humans. We cannot state definitively at this time whether soy or its isoflavones stimulate bone formation or inhibit bone resorption. Although the actions of isoflavones may be distinct from that of estrogen, which has antiresorptive skeletal effects, we do have evidence that isoflavones exert estrogen-like effects in human cells due to their unique organic structure. Depending upon the tissue and species, isoflavones may act as weak estrogen agonists or as weak estrogen antagonists. We must await further studies to corroborate the skeletal effects of isoflavones and to determine how they spare bone tissue in the face of estrogen deficiency. Until such data are published and concurrence is reached, evidence-based medicine should not recommend isoflavones in supplement form to treat or prevent osteoporosis. Although we cannot recommend the use of soy foods as a substitute for estrogen or hormone therapy, health professionals should suggest that the public increase consumption of soy foods because of their excellent nutrient profile and other health benefits. It may be that in the future we can recommend to perimenopausal and early postmenopausal women the inclusion of dietary isoflavone-containing soy products as an adjunct to nonsteroidal osteoporosis treatment. The few studies that have reported a positive response suggest that perhaps 60 to 90 mg/d of isoflavones may be bone-protective, translating into ~ 2 to 3 servings of traditional soy foods. However, further data are needed to determine a dose-response for humans, as well as the long-term safety of isoflavone supplements.

V. GAPS IN KNOWLEDGE/FUTURE RESEARCH DIRECTIONS

A major gap in our knowledge relates to the interindividual biologic variability in response to the isoflavone preparations provided in studies. Some individuals apparently are high excretors and others are low excretors of isoflavones, likely corresponding to higher and lower isoflavone bio-availability, respectively.[151] Bioavailability is less for the aglycones than their corresponding β-glycosides,[152] which may be related to gut motility and gut microflora.[151] One explanation for the biologic variability is that an individual's intestinal microflora governs the capacity to convert daidzein to equol.[153] Another explanation is that dietary fat intake decreases the capacity of gut microflora to synthesize equol,[154] but that interindividual variation in equol excretion may also reflect different hormonal patterns.[155] Related to the issue of biologic variability is that of differences among various commercial soy isoflavone supplements[152] and the need to clearly define the isoflavone source in a given study. For example, the aglycones (genistein, daidzein, glycitein), unlike their corresponding β-glycosides (genistin, daidzin, glycitin), do not require hydrolytic cleavage prior to absorption and hence the former require less time (4 to 7 vs. 8 to 11 h) to attain peak plasma concentrations.[152] We do not know at this point whether or not soy isoflavones from food or from supplements will exert similar effects on the skeleton. Given the differences in pharmacokinetics and bioavailability among isoflavones, it cannot be assumed that all isoflavones are comparable. Studies must carefully define qualitatively and quantitatively the type of isoflavones provided to subjects.

Another gap relates to the estrogen status of study subjects, as circulating estrogens may influence the response to isoflavone treatment. Studies with postmenopausal women should include measures of circulating estrone and 17 β-estradiol; those with normal-cycling premenopausal women should include these measures at menses, at midcycle (near ovulation), and during the midluteal phase; those with men should also include circulating estrogens. In prospective studies, a reasonable approach would be to take circulating estrogen concentrations, as well as baseline BMD values, into account when monitoring response to treatment. As we have no information about the effects of soy isoflavones in elderly women or in men at risk for osteoporosis, long-term human studies in these groups using both soy foods and isolated isoflavones should be undertaken.

This leads to another major gap — that of unknown negative side-effects of long-term use of isolated isoflavones. Although data suggest that isoflavones are the primary bone-active components of soy, studies should be conducted on both soy foods and extracted isoflavones, particularly as the public has access to isoflavone supplements. It is easier to design and carry out long-term studies using extracted isoflavones because this intervention should not disturb eating habits and body weight, thus allowing better long-term compliance and less potential confounding by extraneous factors. However, dietary intake of soy protein itself may promote health benefits unrelated to bone. Clearly, long-term, dose-response randomized clinical trials in

humans designed to corroborate the findings reviewed herein and to examine potential mechanisms are needed. Not only should we examine potential mechanisms, we must try to understand
the effects of soy isoflavones on bone architecture or quality, not simply on bone density. Two-
and-three year clinical trials on soy isoflavones and bone are currently underway in the U.S. We
must also examine the effect of isoflavones on systems other than bone, such as the cardiovascular,
immune, and renal systems. If and when researchers confirm a favorable effect of soy isoflavones
on bone or other systems in midlife women, these results with specific recommendations should
be conveyed to the public.

REFERENCES

1. Ho, S.C., Bacon, E., Harris, T., Looker, A., Muggi, S. Hip fracture rates in Hong Kong and the United States, 1988 through 1989. *Am J Public Health* 83: 694–697, 1993.
2. Ross, P.D., Norimatsu, H., Davis, J.W., Yano, K., Wasnich, R.D., Fujiwara, S., Hosoda, Y., Melton, J., III. A comparison of hip fracture incidence among native Japanese, Japanese Americans, and American Caucasians. *Am J Epidemiol* 133: 801–809, 1991.
3. Fujita, T., Yoshikawa, S., Ono, K., Inoue, T., Orimo, H. Usefulness of TC-80 (ipriflavone) tablets in osteoporosis: multi-center, double-blind, placebo-controlled study. *Igaku Noayumi* 138: 113–141, 1986.
4. Agnusdei, D., Camporeale, A., Zacchei, F., Gennari, C., Baroni, M.C., Costi, D., Biondi, M., Passeri, M., Ciacca, A., Sbrenna, C., Falsettini, E., Ventura, A. Effects of ipriflavone on bone mass and bone remodeling in patients with established postmenopausal osteoporosis. *Curr Ther Res* 52: 81–92, 1992.
5. Markiewicz, L., Garey, J., Adlercreutz, H., Gurpide, E. In vitro bioassays of non-steroidal phytoestrogens. *J Steroid Biochem Mol Biol* 45: 399–405, 1993.
6. Song, T.T., Hendrich, S., Murphy, P.A. Estrogenic activity of glycitein, a soy isoflavone. *J Agric Food Chem* 47: 1607–1610, 1999.
7. Breslau, N.A., Brinkley, L., Hill, K.D., Pak, C.Y.C. Relationship of animal protein-rich diet to kidney stone formation and calcium metabolism. *J Clin Endocrinol Metabol* 66: 140–146, 1988.
8. Anderson, J.J.B., Alekel, D.L. Skeletal effects of phytoestrogens in humans: bone mineral density and bone markers. In *Phytoestrogens and Health*, Eds., Gilani, G.S., Anderson, J.J.B. American Oil Chemists' Society Press, Champaign, IL, 2002, pp. 341–353.
9. Anthony, M.S., Anderson, J.J.B., Alekel, D.L. Association between soy and/or isoflavones and bone: evidence from epidemiologic studies. In *Phytoestrogens and Health*, Eds., Gilani, G.S., Anderson, J.J.B. American Oil Chemists' Society Press, Champaign, IL, 2002. pp. 331–340.
10. Anderson, J.J.B., Garner, S.C. Phytoestrogens and bone. *Balliere's Clin Endocrinol Metab* 12: 1–15, 1998.
11. Messina, M., Gugger, E.T., Alekel, D.L. Soy protein, soybean isoflavones, and bone health: a review of the animal and human data. In *Handbook of Nutraceuticals and Functional Foods*, R.E.C. Wildman (Ed.), CRC Press, Boca Raton, FL, 2001, pp 77–98, chap. 5.
12. Arjmandi, B.H. The role of phytoestrogens in the prevention and treatment of osteoporosis in ovarian hormone deficiency. *J Am Coll Nutr* 20(Suppl. 5): 398S–402S, 417S–420S, 2001.
13. Scheiber, M.D., Rebar, R.W. Isoflavones and postmenopausal bone health: a viable alternative to estrogen therapy? *Menopause* 6: 233–241, 1999.
14. Doren, M., Samsioe, G. Prevention of postmenopausal osteoporosis with estrogen replacement therapy and associated compounds: update on clinical trials since 1995. *Hum Reprod Update* 6: 419–426, 2000.
15. Setchell, K.D., Cassidy, A. Dietary isoflavones: biological effects and relevance to human health. *J Nutr* 129: 758S–767S, 1999.
16. Kurzer, M.S., Xu, X. Dietary phytoestrogens. *Annu Rev Nutr* 17: 353–381, 1997.
17. Liberman, S. Are the differences between estradiol and other estrogens, naturally occurring or synthetic, merely semantical? *J Clin Endrocinol Metab* 81: 850, 1996.
18. Setchell, K.D.R. Non-steroidal estrogen of dietary origin: possible role in health and disease, metabolism and physiological effects. *Proc Nutr Soc N Z* 20: 1–21, 1995.
19. Vidal, O., Kindblom, L.-G., Ohlsson, C. Expression and localization of estrogen-receptor-β in murine and human bone. *J Bone Mineral Res* 14: 923–929, 1999.

20. Shutt, D.A., Cox, R.I. Steroid and phytoestrogen binding in sheep uterine receptors in vitro. *Endocrinology* 52: 299–310, 1972.

21. Kuiper, G.G., Lemmen, J.G., Carlsson, B., Corton, J.C., Safe, S.H., van der Saag, P.T., van der Burg, B., Gustafsson, J.A. Interaction of estrogenic chemicals and phytoestrogens with estrogen receptor-β. *Endocrinology* 139: 4252–4263, 1998.

22. Melton, L.J., III, Chrischilles, E.A., Cooper, C., Lane, A.W., Riggs, B.L. Perspective: how many women have osteoporosis? *J Bone Miner Res* 7: 1005–1010, 1992.

23. Cummings, S.R., Melton, L.J., III. Osteoporosis I: epidemiology and outcomes of osteoporotic fractures. *Lancet* 359: 1761–1767, 2002.

24. De Laet, C.E., van Hout, B.A., Burger, H., Hofman, A., Pols, H.A. Bone density and risk of hip fracture in men and women: cross sectional analysis. *Br Med J* 315: 221–225, 1997.

25. Tucci, J.R. Osteoporosis update. *Med Health R I* 81: 169–73, 1998.

26. Melton, L.J., III, Therneau, T.M., Larson, D.R. Long-term trends in hip fracture prevalence: the influence of hip fracture incidence and survival. *Osteoporos Int* 8: 68–74, 1998.

27. Rogmark, C., Sernbo, I., Johnell, O., Nilsson, J.-Å. Incidence of hip fractures Malmö, Sweden, 1992–1995. *Acta Orthopaed Scan* 70: 19–22, 1999.

28. Cooper, C., Campion, G., Melton, L.J., III. Hip fractures in the elderly: a world-wide projection. *Osteoporos Int* 2: 285–289, 1992.

29. Genant, H.K., Cooper, C., Poor, G., Reid, I., Ehrlich, G., Kanis, J., Nordin, B.E.C., Barrett-Connor, E., Black, D., Bonjour, J.-P., Dawson-Hughes, B., Delmas, P.D., Dequeker, J., Ragi Eis, S., Gennari, C., Johnell, O., Johnston, C.C., Jr., Lau, E.M.C., Liberman, U.A., Lindsay, R., Martin, T.J., Masri, B., Mautalen, C.A., Meunier, P.J., Miller, P.D., Mithal, A., Morii, H., Papapoulos, S., Woolf, A., Yu, W., Khaltaev, N. Interim report and recommendations of the World Health Organization Task-Force for Osteoporosis. *Osteoporos Int* 10: 259–264, 1999.

30. Melton, L.J., III, Riggs, B.L. Epidemiology of age-related fractures. In *The Osteoporotic Syndrome*, Ed., Avioli, A.V. New York, Grune and Stratton, 1983, pp. 45–72.

31. Melton, L.J., III. Who has osteoporosis? A conflict between clinical and public health perspectives. *J Bone Miner Res* 15: 2309–2314, 2000.

32. Kanis, J.A., Melton, L.J., III, Christiansen, C., Johnston, C.C., Khaltaev, N. Perspective: the diagnosis of osteoporosis. *J Bone Miner Res* 9: 1137–1141, 1994.

33. Melton, L.J., III. How many women have osteoporosis now? *J Bone Miner Res.*, 10: 175–177, 1995.

34. Cummings, S.R., Nevitt, M.C., Browner, W.S., Stone, K., Fox, K.M., Ensrud, K.E., Cauley, J., Black, D., Vogt, T.M. Risk factors for hip fracture in white women. Study of Osteoporotic Fractures Research Group. *N Engl J Med* 332: 767–773, 1995.

35. Anderson, J.J.B., Pollitzer, W.S. Ethnic and genetic differences in susceptibility to osteoporotic fractures. In *Advances in Nutritional Research*, Vol. 9, Ed., Harold H. Draper. Plenum Press, New York, 1994, chap. 8.

36. Looker, A.C., Orwoll, E.S., Johnston, C.C., Jr., Lindsay, R.L., Wahner, H.W., Dunn, W.L., Calvo, M.S., Harris, T.B., Heyse, S.P. Prevalence of low femoral bone density in older U.S. adults from NHANES III. *J Bone Miner Res* 12: 1761–1768, 1997.

37. Silverman, S.L., Madison, R.E. Decreased incidence of hip fracture in Hispanics, Asians, and Blacks: California hospital discharge data. *Am J Public Health* 78: 1482–1483, 1988.

38. Tsai, K.S. Osteoporotic fracture rate, bone mineral density, and bone metabolism in Taiwan. *J Formos Med Assoc* 96: 802–805, 1997.

39. Xu, L., Lu, A., Zhao, X., Chen, X., Cummings, S.R. Very low rates of hip fracture in Beijing, People's Republic of China, the Beijing Osteoporosis Project. *Am J Epidemiol* 144: 901–907, 1996.

40. Chin, K., Evans, M.C., Cornish, J., Cundy, T., Reid, I.R. Differences in hip axis and femoral neck length in premenopausal women of Polynesian, Asian and European origin. *Osteoporos Int* 7: 344–347, 1997.

41. Alekel, D.L., Mortillaro, E., Hussain, E.A., West, B., Ahmed, N., Peterson, C.T., Werner, R.K., Arjmandi, B.H., Kukreja, S.C. Lifestyle and biologic contributors to proximal femur bone mineral density and hip axis length in two distinct ethnic groups of premenopausal women. *Osteoporos Int* 9: 327–338, 1999.

42. Parker, M., Anand, J.K., Myles, J.W., Lodwick, R. Proximal femoral fractures: prevalence in different racial groups. *Eur J Epidemiol* 8: 730–732, 1992.

43. Ho, S.C., Wong, E., Chan, S.G., Lau, J., Chan, C., Leung, P.C. Determinants of peak bone mass in Chinese women aged 21–40 years. III. Physical activity and bone mineral density. *J Bone Miner Res* 12: 1262–1271, 1997.

44. Lau, E.M.C., Suriwongpaisal, P., Lee, J.K., Das De, S., Festin, M.R., Saw, S.M., Khir, A., Torralba, T., Sham, A., Sambrook, P. Risk factors for hip fracture in Asian men and women: the Asian Osteoporosis Study. *J Bone Miner Res* 16: 572–580, 2001.

45. Davis, J.W., Novotny, R., Wasnich, R.D., Ross, P.D. Ethnic, anthropometric, and lifestyle associations with regional variations in peak bone mass. *Calcif Tissue Int* 65: 100–105, 1999.

46. Prentice, A., Parsons, T.J., Cole, T.J. Uncritical use of bone mineral density in absorptiometry may lead to size-related artifacts in the identification of bone mineral determinants. *Am J Clin Nutr* 60: 837–842, 1994.

47. Ross, P.D., He, Y.-F., Yates, A.J., Coupland, C., Ravn, P., McClung, M., Thompson, D., Wasnich, R.D. Body size accounts for most differences in bone density between Asian and Caucasian women. *Calcif Tissue Int* 59: 339–343, 1996.

48. Cummings, S.R., Cauley, J.A., Palermo, L., Ross, P.D., Wasnich, R.D., Black, D., Faulkner, K.G. Racial differences in hip axis lengths might explain racial differences in rates of hip fracture. *Osteoporosis Int* 4: 226–229, 1994.

49. Nakamura, T., Turner, C.H., Yoshikawa, T., Slemenda, C.W., Peacock, M., Burr, D.B., Mizuno, Y., Orimo, H., Ouchi, Y., Johnston, C.C., Jr. Do variations in hip geometry explain differences in hip fracture risk between Japanese and white Americans? *J Bone Miner Res* 9: 1071–1076, 1994.

50. Alekel, D.L., Peterson, C.T., Werner, R.K., Mortillaro, E., Ahmed, N., Kukreja, S.C. Frame size, ethnicity, lifestyle, and biologic contributors to areal and volumetric lumbar spine bone mineral density in Indian/Pakistani and American Caucasian premenopausal women. *J Clin Densitometry* 5: 175–186, 2002.

51. Alekel, D.L., St. Germain, A., Peterson, C.T., Hanson, K.B., Stewart, J.W., Toda, T. Isoflavone-rich soy protein isolate attenuates bone loss in the lumbar spine of perimenopausal women. *Am J Clin Nutr* 72: 844–852, 2000.

52. Potter, S.M., Baum, J.A., Teng, H., Stillman, R.J., Shay, N.F., Erdman, J.W., Jr. Soy protein and isoflavones: their effects on blood lipids and bone density in postmenopausal women. *Am J Clin Nutr* 68: 1375S–1379S, 1998.

53. Chen, Z., Zheng, W., Custer, L.J., Dai, Q., Shu, X.-O., Jin, F., Franke, A.A. Usual dietary consumption of soy foods and its correlation with the excretion rate of isoflavonoids in overnight urine samples among Chinese women in Shanghai. *Nutr Cancer* 33: 82–87, 1999.

54. Kimira, M., Arai, Y., Shimoi, K., Watanabe, S. Japanese intake of flavonoids and isoflavonoids from foods. *J Epidemiol* 8: 168–175, 1998.

55. Maskarinec, G., Singh, S., Meng, L., Franke, A.A. Dietary soy intake and urinary isoflavone excretion among women from a multiethnic population. *Cancer Epidemiol Biomark Prev* 7: 613–619, 1998.

56. Ross, P.D., Fujiwara, S., Huang, C., Davis, J.W., Epstein, R.S., Wasnich, R.D., Kodama, K., Melton, J., III. Vertebral fracture prevalence in women in Hiroshima compared to Caucasians or Japanese in the U.S. *Int J Epidemiol* 24: 1171–1177, 1995.

57. Tsai, K., Twu, S., Chieng, P., Yang, R., Lee, T. Prevalence of vertebral fractures in Chinese men and women in urban Taiwanese communities. *Calcif Tissue Int* 59: 249–253, 1996.

58. Tsai, K., Huang, K., Chieng, P., Su, C. Bone mineral density of normal Chinese women in Taiwan. *Calcif Tissue Int* 48: 161–166, 1991.

59. Kin, K., Lee, E., Kushida, K., Sartoris, D.J., Ohmura, A., Clopton, P.L., Inque, T. Bone density and body composition on the Pacific Rim: a comparison between Japan-Born and U.S.-born Japanese American women. *J Bone Mineral Res* 8: 861–869, 1993.

60. Davis, J.W., Ross, P.D., Nevitt, M.C., Wasnich, R.D. Incidence rates of falls among Japanese men and women living in Hawaii. *J Clin Epidemiol* 50: 589–594, 1997.

61. Somekawa, Y., Chiguchi, M., Ishibashi, T., Aso, T. Soy intake related to menopausal symptoms, serum lipids, and bone mineral density in postmenopausal Japanese women. *Obstet Gynecol* 97: 109–115, 2001.

62. Tsuchida, K., Mizushima, S., Toba, M., Soda, K. Dietary soybeans intake and bone mineral density among 995 middle-aged women in Yokohama. *J Epidemiol* 9: 14–19, 1999.

63. Greendale, G.A., FitzGerald, G., Huang, M.-H., Sternfeld, B., Gold, E., Seeman, T., Sherman, S., Sowers, M.F. Dietary soy isoflavones and bone mineral density: results from the Study of Women's Health across the Nation. *Am J Epidemiol* 155: 746–754, 2002.

64. Kardinaal, A.F.M., Morton, M.S., Bruggemann-Rotgans, I.E.M., van Beresteijn, E.C.H. Phyto-oestrogen excretion and rate of bone loss in postmenopausal women. *Eur J Clin Nutr* 52: 850–855, 1998.

65. Thompson, L.U., Robb, P., Serraino, M., Cheung, F. Mammalian lignan production from various foods. *Nutr Cancer* 16: 43–52, 1991.

66. Zhang, X., Shu, X.-O., Li, H., Yang, G., Li, Q., Gao, Y.-T., Zheng, W. Prospective cohort study of soy food consumption and risk of bone fracture among postmenopausal women. *Arch Intern Med* 165: 1890–1895, 2005.

67. Riggs, B.L., Khosla, S., Melton, L.J., III. A unitary model for involutional osteoporosis: estrogen deficiency causes both type I and type II osteoporosis in postmenopausal women and contributes to bone loss in aging men. *J Bone Miner Res* 13: 763–773, 1998.

68. Komulainen, M., Kroger, H., Tuppurainen, M.T., Heikkinen, A.M., Alhava, E., Honkanen, R., Jurvelin, J., Saarikoski, S. Prevention of femoral and lumbar bone loss with hormone replacement therapy and vitamin D_3 in early postmenopausal women: a population-based 5-year randomized trial. *J Clin Endocrinol Metab* 84: 546–552, 1999.

69. Cauley, J.A., Seeley, D.G., Ensrud, K., Ettinger, B., Black, D., Cummings, S.R. Estrogen replacement therapy and fractures in older women. Study of Osteoporotic Fractures Research Group. *Ann Intern Med* 122: 9–16, 1995.

70. Manolagas, S.C., Jilka, R.L. Mechanisms of disease: bone marrow, cytokines, and bone remodeling: Emerging insights into the pathophysiology of osteoporosis. *N Engl J Med* 332: 305–311, 1995.

71. Scharbo-DeHaan, M. Hormone replacement therapy. *Nurs Pract* 21(12 Pt. 2): 1–13, 1996.

72. Beresford, S.A.A., Weiss, N.S., McKnight, B. Risk of endometrial cancer in relation to use of estrogen combined with cyclic progestagen therapy in postmenopausal women. *Lancet* 349: 458–461, 1997.

73. Writing Group for the Women's Health Initiative Investigators. Risks and benefits of estrogen plus progestin in healthy postmenopausal women. *JAMA* 288: 321–333, 2002.

74. McNagny, S.E. Prescribing hormone replacement therapy for menopausal symptoms. *Ann Intern Med* 131: 605–616, 1999.

75. Eastell, R. Treatment of postmenopausal osteoporosis. *N Engl J Med* 338: 736–746, 1998.

76. Kessel, B. Alternatives to estrogen for menopausal women. *Proc Soc Exp Biol Med* 217(1): 38–44, 1998.

77. Groeneveld, F.P., Bareman, F.P., Barentsen, R., Dokter, H.J., Drogendijk, A.C., Hoes, A.W. Duration of hormonal replacement therapy in general practice: a follow-up study. *Maturitas* 29: 125–131, 1998.

78. Schneider, D.L., Barrett-Connor, E.L., Morton, D.J. Timing of postmenopausal estrogen for optimal bone mineral density. The Rancho Bernardo Study. *JAMA* 277: 543–547, 1997.

79. U.S. Preventive Services Task Force. Postmenopausal hormone replacement therapy for primary prevention of chronic conditions: Recommendations and rationale. *Ann Intern Med* 137: 834–839, 2002.

80. Fleisch, H. Bisphosphonates in osteoporosis: an introduction. *Osteoporosis Int* 3: S3–S5, 1993.

81. Watts, N.B. Treatment of osteoporosis with bisphosphonates. *Rheum Dis Clin N Am* 27: 197–214, 2001.

82. Adachi, J.D., Bensen, W.G., Brown, J., Hanley, D., Hodsman, A., Josse, R., Kendler, D.L., Lentle, B., Olszynski, W., St. Marie, L.-G., Tenenhouse, A., Chines, A.A. Intermittent etidronate therapy to prevent corticosteroid-induced osteoporosis. *N Engl J Med* 337: 382–387, 1997.

83. Liberman, U.A., Weiss, S.R., Broll, J., Minne, H.W., Quan, H., Bell, N.H., Rodriguez-Portales, J., Downs, R.W., Jr., Dequeker, J., Favus, M. Effect of oral alendronate on bone mineral density and the incidence of fractures in postmenopausal osteoporosis. The Alendronate Phase III Osteoporosis Treatment Study Group. *N Engl J Med* 333(22): 1437–1443, 1995.

84. Karpf, D.B., Shapiro, D.R., Seeman, E., Ensrud, K.E., Johnston, C.C., Adami, S., Harris, S.T., Santora, A.C., II, Hirsch, L.J., Oppenheimer, L., Thompson, D. Prevention of Nonvertebral Fractures by alendronate: a meta-analysis. *JAMA* 277(14): 1159–1164, 1997.

85. Overgaard, K., Hansen, M.A., Jensen, S.B., Christiansen, C. Effect of calcitonin given intranasally on bone mass and fracture rates in established osteoporosis: a dose response study. *Br Med J* 305: 556–561, 1992.

86. Thamsborg, G. Effect of nasal salmon calcitonin on calcium and bone metabolism. *Dan Med Bull* 46: 118–126, 1999.

87. Silverman, S.L. Calcitonin. *Rheum Dis Clin N Am* 27: 187–196, 2001.

88. Ilich, J.Z., Kerstetter, J.E. Nutrition in bone health revisited: a story beyond calcium. *J Am Coll Nutr* 19: 715–737, 2000.

89. North American Menopause Society. The role of calcium in peri- and postmenopausal women: consensus opinion of the North American Menopause Society. *Menopause* 8: 84–95, 2001.

90. Morgan, S.L. Calcium and vitamin D in osteoporosis. *Rheum Dis Clin N Am* 27: 101–130, 2001.

91. Food and Nutrition Board, Institute of Medicine. *Dietary Reference Intakes for Calcium, Phosphorus, Magnesium, Vitamin D, and Fluoride*. Washington, D.C.: National Academy Press, 1997.

92. Heaney, R.P. Calcium, dairy products, and osteoporosis. *J Am Coll Nutr* 19: 83S–99S, 2000.

93. Nieves, J.W., Komar, L., Cosman, F., Lindsay, R. Calcium potentiates the effect of estrogen and calcitonin on bone mass: review and analysis. *Am J Clin Nutr* 67: 18–24, 1998.

94. Lips, P., Duong, T., Oleksik, A., Black, D., Cummings, S., Cox, D., Nickelsen, T. A global study of vitamin D status and parathyroid function in postmenopausal women with osteoporosis: baseline data from the multiple outcomes of raloxifene evaluation clinical trial. *J Clin Endocrinol Metab* 86: 1212–1221, 2001.

95. Kantorovich, V., Gacad, M.A., Seeger, L.L., Adams, J.S. Bone mineral density increases with vitamin D repletion in patients with coexistent vitamin D insufficiency and primary hyperparathyroidism. *J Clin Endocrinol Metab* 85: 3541–3543, 2000.

96. Adams, J.S., Kantorovich, V., Wu, C., Javanbakht, M., Hollis, B.W. Resolution of vitamin D insufficiency in osteopenic patients results in rapid recovery of bone mineral density. *J Clin Endocrinol Metab* 84: 2729–2730, 1999.

97. Bryant, H.U., Dere, W.H. Selective estrogen receptor modulators: an alternative to hormone replacement therapy. *Proc Soc Exp Biol Med* 217(1): 45–52, 1998.

98. Havsteen, B. Flavonoids, a class of natural products of high pharmacological potency. *Biochem Pharmacol* 32: 1141–1148, 1983.

99. Agnusdei, D., Zacchei, F., Bigazzi, S., Cepollaro, C., Nardi, P., Montagnani, M., Gennari, C. Metabolic and clinical effects of ipriflavone in established postmenopausal osteoporosis. *Drugs Exp Clin Res* 15: 97–104, 1989.

100. Yamazaki, I., Shino, A., Shimizu, Y., Tsukuda, R., Shirakawa, Y., Kinoshita, M. Effect of ipriflavone on glucocorticoid-induced osteoporosis in rats. *Life Sci* 38: 951–958, 1986.

101. Yamazaki, I., Shino, A., Tsukuda, R. Effect of ipriflavone on osteoporosis induced by ovariectomy in rats. *J Bone Min Metab* 3: 205–210, 1986.

102. Agnusdei, D., Gennari, C., Bufalino, L. Prevention of early postmenopausal bone loss using low doses of conjugated estrogens and the non-hormonal, bone-active drug ipriflavone. *Osteoporos Int* 5(6): 462–466, 1995.

103. Alexandersen, P., Toussaint, A., Christiansen, C., Devogelaer, J.-P., Roux, C., Fechtenbaum, J., Gennari, C., Reginster, J.Y., for the Ipriflavone Multicenter European Fracture Study: Ipriflavone in the treatment of postmenopausal osteoporosis. *JAMA* 285: 1482–1488, 2001.

104. Wright, C.D.P., Garrahan, N.J., Stanton, M., Gazet, J.-C., Mansell, R.E., Compston, J.E. Effect of long-term tamoxifen therapy on cancellous bone remodeling and structure in women with breast cancer. *J Bone Miner Res* 9: 153–159, 1994.

105. Love, R.R., Mazess, R.B., Barden, H.S., Epstein, S., Newcomb, P.A., Jordan, V.C., Carbone, P.P., DeMets, D.L. Effects of tamoxifen on bone mineral density in postmenopausal women with breast cancer. *N Engl J Med* 326: 852–856, 1992.

106. Fornander, T., Rutquist, L.E., Cedermark, B., Glas, U., Mattsson, A., Silfversward, C., Skoog, L., Somell, A., Theve, T., Wilking, N., Askergren, J., Hjalmar, M.-L. Adjuvant tamoxifen in early breast cancer: occurrence of new primary cancers. *Lancet* 1: 117–120, 1989.

107. Delmas, P.D., Bjarnason, N.H., Mitlak, B.H., Ravoux, A.-C., Shah, A.S., Huster, W.J., Draper, M., Christiansen, C. Effects of raloxifene on bone mineral density, serum cholesterol concentrations, and uterine endometrium in postmenopausal women. *N Engl J Med* 337: 1641–1647, 1997.

108. Heaney, R.P., Draper, M.W. Raloxifene and estrogen: Comparative bone-remodeling kinetics. *J Clin Endocrinol Metab* 82: 3425–3429, 1997.

109. Walsh, B.W., Kuller, L.H., Wild, R.A., Paul, S., Farmer, M., Lawrence, J.B., Shah, A.S., Anderson, P.W. Effects of raloxifene on serum lipids and coagulation factors in healthy postmenopausal women. *JAMA* 279(18): 1445–1451, 1998.

110. Gordon, S., Walsh, B.W., Ciaccia, A.V., Siddhanti, S., Rosen, A.S., Plouffe, L. Transition from estrogen-progestin to raloxifene in postmenopausal women: effect on vasomotor symptoms. *Obstet Gynecol* 103: 267–273, 2004.

111. St. Germain, A., Peterson, C.T., Robinson, J., Alekel, D.L. Isoflavone-rich or isoflavone-poor soy protein does not reduce menopausal symptoms during 24 weeks of treatment. *Menopause* 8(1): 17–26, 2001.

112. Arjmandi, B.H., Alekel, L., Hollis, B.W., Amin, D., Stacewicz-Sapuntzakis, M., Guo, P., Kukreja, S.C. Dietary soybean protein prevents bone loss in an ovariectomized rat model of osteoporosis. *J Nutr* 126: 161–167, 1996.

113. Arjmandi, B.H., Salih, M.A., Herbert, D.C., Sims, S.H., Kalu, D.N. Evidence for estrogen receptor-linked calcium transport in the intestine. *Bone Miner* 21: 63–74; 1993.

114. Spence, L.A., Lipscomb, E.R., Cadogan, J., Martin, B., Wastney, M.E., Peacock, M., Weaver, C.M. The effect of soy isoflavones on calcium metabolism in postmenopausal women: a randomized crossover study. *Am J Clin Nutr* 81: 916–922, 2005.

115. Pennington, J.A.T. *Bowes and Church's Food Values of Portions Commonly Used*, 17th ed. Harper and Row, New York, 1998.

116. Anderson, J.J.B., Thomsen, K., Christiansen, C. High protein meals, insular hormones and urinary calcium excretion in human subjects. In *Proceedings of the International Symposium on Osteoporosis*, Eds., C. Christiansen, J.S. Johansen, B.J. Riis. Nørhaven A/S, Viborg, Denmark, 1987.

117. Pie, J.-E., Paik, H.Y. The effect of meat protein and soy protein on calcium metabolism in young adult Korean women. *Korean J Nutr* 19: 32–40, 1986.

118. Sebastian, A. Low versus high meat diets: effects on calcium metabolism. *J Nutr* 133: 3237–3238, 2003.

119. Watkins, T.R., Pandya, K., Mickelsen, O. Urinary acid and calcium excretion: effect of soy versus meat in human diets. In *Nutritional Bioavailability of Calcium*, Ed., Kies, C. American Chemical Society, Washington, D.C., 1985.

120. Roughead, Z.K., Hunt, J.R., Johnson, L.K., Badger, T.M., Lykken, G.I. Controlled substitution of soy protein for meat protein: effects on calcium retention, bone, and cardiovascular health indices in postmenopausal women. *J Clin Endocrinol Metab* 90: 181–189, 2005.

121. Kerstetter, J.E., O'Brien, K., Insogna, K. Dietary protein and intestinal calcium absorption. *Am J Clin Nutr* 73: 990–992, 2001.

122. Pun, K.K., Chan, L.W.L., Chung, V., Wong, F.H.W. Calcium and other dietary constituents in Hong Kong Chinese in relation to age and osteoporosis. *J Appl Nutr* 43: 12–17, 1990.

123. Kung, A.W.C., Luk, K.D.K., Chu, L.W., Chiu, P.K.Y. Age-related osteoporosis in Chinese: an evaluation of the response of intestinal calcium absorption and calcitropic hormones to dietary calcium deprivation. *Am J Clin Nutr* 68: 1291–1297, 1998.

124. Heaney, R.P., Recker, R.R., Stegman, M.R., May, A.J. Calcium absorption in women: relationships to calcium intake, estrogen status, age. *J Bone Miner Res* 4: 469–475, 1989.

125. Weaver, C.M. Calcium requirements: the need to understand racial differences. Editorial. *Am J Clin Nutr* 68: 1153–1154, 1998.

126. Lau, E.M.C. Osteoporosis in Asians — the role of calcium and other nutrients. *Challenge Mod Med* 7: 45–54, 1995.

127. Kreijkamp-Kaspers, S., Kok, L., Grobbee, D.E., de Haan, E.H.F., Aleman, A., Lampe, J.W., van der Schouw, Y.T. Effect of soy protein containing isoflavones on cognitive function, bone mineral density, and plasma lipids in postmenopausal women. *JAMA* 292: 65–74, 2004.

128. Gallagher, J.C., Satpathy, R., Rafferty, K., Haynatzka, V. The effect of soy protein isolate on bone metabolism. *Menopause* 11: 290–298, 2004.

129. Dalais, F.S., Rice, G.E., Wahlqvist, M.L., Grehan, M., Murkies, A.L., Medley, G., Ayton, R., Strauss, B.J.G. Effects of dietary phytoestrogens in postmenopausal women. *Climacteric* 1: 124–129, 1998.

130. Lydeking-Olsen, E., Beck-Jensen, J.-E., Setchell, K.D.R., Holm-Jensen, T. Soymilk or progesterone for prevention of bone loss: a 2 year randomized, placebo-controlled trial. *Eur J Nutr* 43: 246–257, 2004.

131. Ho, S.C., Chan, S.G., Yi, Q., Wong, E., Leung, P.C. Soy intake and the maintenance of peak bone mass in Hong Kong Chinese women. *J Bone Miner Res* 16: 1363–1369, 2001.

132. Hsu, C.-S., Shen, W.W., Hsueh, Y.-M., Yeh, S.-L. Soy isoflavone supplementation in postmenopausal women: effects on plasma lipids, antioxidant enzyme activities, and bone density. *J Reprod Med* 46: 221–226, 2001.

133. Chen, Y.-M., Ho, S.C., Lam, S.S.H., Ho, S.S.S., Woo, J.L.F. Soy isoflavones have a favorable effect on bone loss in Chinese postmenopausal women with lower bone mass: A double-blind, randomized, controlled trial. *J Clin Endocrinol Metab* 88: 4740–4747, 2003.

134. Harkness, L.S., Fiedler, K., Sehgal, A.R., Oravec, D., Lerner, E. Decreased bone resorption with soy isoflavone supplementation in postmenopausal women. *J Womens Health* 13: 1000–1007, 2004.

135. Pines, A., Katchman, H., Villa, Y., Mijatovic, V., Dotan, I., Levo, Y., Ayalon, D. The effect of various hormonal preparations and calcium supplementation on bone mass in early menopause. Is there a predictive value for the initial bone density and body weight? *J Intern Med* 246: 357–61, 1999.

136. Heaney, R.P. The bone-remodeling transient: Implications for the interpretation of clinical studies of bone mass change. *J Bone Miner Res* 9: 1515–1523, 1994.

137. Souberbielle, J.C., Cormier, C., Kindermans, C. Bone markers in clinical practice. *Curr Opin Rheumatol* 11: 312–319, 1999.

138. Ross, P.D. Predicting bone loss and fracture risk with biochemical markers: a review. *J Clin Densitometry* 2: 285–294, 1999.

139. Garnero P. Markers of bone turnover for the prediction of fracture risk. *Osteoporos Int* 11(Suppl 6): S55–65, 2000.

140. Delmas, P.D., Eastell, R., Garnero, P., Seibel, M.J., Stepan, J. Committee of Scientific Advisors of the International Osteoporosis Foundation. The use of biochemical markers of bone turnover in osteoporosis. *Osteoporosis Int* 11(Suppl. 6): S2–17, 2000.

141. Murkies, A.L., Lombard, C., Strauss, B.J.G., Wilcox, G., Burger, H.G., Morton, M.S. Dietary flour supplementation decreases post-menopausal hot flushes: effect of soy and wheat. *Maturitas* 21: 189–195, 1995.

142. Washburn, S., Burke, G., Morgan, T., Anthony, M. Effect of soy protein supplementation on serum lipoproteins, blood pressure, and menopausal symptoms in perimenopausal women. *Menopause* 6: 7–11, 1999.

143. Arjmandi, B.H., Getlinger, M.J., Goyal, N.V., Alekel, L., Hasler, C.M., Juma, S., Drum, M.L., Hollis, B.W., Kukreja, S.C. The role of soy protein with normal or reduced isoflavone content in reversing bone loss induced by ovarian hormone deficiency in rats. *Am J Clin Nutr* 68(Suppl): 1358S–1363S, 1998.

144. Arjmandi, B.H., Lucas, E.A., Khalil, D.A., Devareddy, L., Smith, B.J., McDonald, A.B., Payton, M.E., Mason, C. One year soy protein supplementation has positive effects on bone formation markers but not bone density in postmenopausal women. *Nutr J* 4: 8–16, 2005.

145. Knight, D.C., Howes, J.B., Eden, J.A., Howes, L.G. Effects on menopausal symptoms and acceptability of isoflavone-containing soy powder dietary supplementation. *Climacteric* 4: 13–18, 2001.

146. Wangen, K.E., Duncan, A.M., Merz-Demlow, B.E., Xu, X., Marcus, R., Phipps, W.R., Kurzer, M.S. Effects of soy isoflavones on markers of bone turnover in premenopausal and postmenopausal women. *J Clin Endocrinol Metab* 85: 3043–3048, 2000.

147. Scheiber, M.D., Liu, J.H., Subbiah, M.T.R., Rebar, R.W., Setchell, K.D.R. Dietary inclusion of whole soy foods results in significant reductions in clinical risk factors for osteoporosis and cardiovascular disease in normal postmenopausal women. *Menopause* 8: 384–392, 2001.

148. Scambia, G., Mango, D., Signorile, P.G., Anselmi-Angeli, R.A., Palena, C., Gallo, D., Bombardelli, E., Morazzoni, P., Riva, A., Mancuso, S. Clinical effects of a standardized soy extract in postmenopausal women: a pilot study. *Menopause* 7(2): 105–111, 2000.

149. Upmalis, D.H., Lobo, R., Bradley, L., Warren, M., Cone, F.L., Lamia, C.A. Vasomotor symptom relief by soy isoflavone extract tablets in postmenopausal women: a multicenter, double-blind, randomized, placebo-controlled study. *Menopause* 7(4): 236–242, 2000.

150. Uesugi, T., Fukui, Y., Yamori, Y. Beneficial effects of soybean isoflavone supplementation on bone metabolism and serum lipids in postmenopausal Japanese women: a four-week study. *J Am Coll Nutr* 21: 97–102, 2002.

151. Zhang, Y., Wang, G.-J., Song, T.T., Murphy, P.A., Hendrich, S. Urinary disposition of the soybean isoflavones daidzein, genistein, and glycitein differs among humans with moderate fecal isoflavone degradation activity. *J Nutr* 129: 957–962, 1999.

152. Setchell, K.D.R., Brown, N.M., Desai, P., Zimmer-Nechemias, L., Wolfe, B.E., Brashear, W.T., Kirschner, A.S., Cassidy, A., Heubi, J.E. Bioavailability of pure isoflavones in healthy humans and analysis of commercial soy isoflavone supplements. *J Nutr* 131: 1362S–1375S, 2001.

153. Lampe, J.W., Skor, H.E., Li, S., Wahala, K., Howald, W.N., Chen, C. Wheat bran and soy protein feeding do not alter urinary excretion of the isoflavan equol in premenopausal women. *J Nutr* 131: 740–744, 2001.

154. Rowland, I.R., Wiseman, H., Sanders, T.A., Adlercreutz, H., Bowey, E.A. Interindividual variation in metabolism of soy isoflavones and lignans: Influence of habitual diet on equol production by the gut microflora. *Nutr Cancer* 36: 27–32, 2000.

155. Duncan, A.M., Merz-Demlow, B.E., Xu, X., Phipps, W.R., Kurzer, M.S. Premenopausal equol excretors show plasma hormone profiles associated with lowered risk of breast cancer. *Cancer Epidemiol Biomarkers Prev* 9: 581–586, 2000.

13 Applications of Herbs to Functional Foods

Susan S. Percival and R. Elaine Turner

CONTENTS

I. INTRODUCTION

Functional foods have been defined as foods and food components that provide a health benefit beyond basic nutrition.[1] Examples include conventional, fortified, enriched, or enhanced foods and dietary supplements. To date, however, no regulatory definition of *functional foods* or the similar terms *nutraceuticals* and *designer foods* has been proposed or approved by the Food and Drug Administration. Herbs or botanicals may have health benefits that are not derived from the plant's nutrient composition. When these herbs are provided in the form of a capsule, powder, softgel, gelcap, or other form that is not represented as a conventional food, these products are considered dietary supplements and are regulated quite differently from foods or food additives. Although the growing interest in herbal products has perhaps reached a plateau, an attitude toward health and wellness has not changed.[1] With an emphasis on quality and standardization, food manufacturers may find herbals to be a new source of functional ingredients. Herbal additives have begun to appear in conventional foods ranging from teas and juices to snack chips and energy bars. In the absence of a separate regulatory category for these and other functional foods, such products are regulated as conventional foods.

This chapter discusses botanicals as functional food ingredients, with the idea that the purported health benefits of the food are due to their botanical nature. Although other ingredients may also be beneficial, this chapter will describe benefits associated with the botanicals. Because botanically-enhanced functional foods are relatively new in the marketplace, little data exists regarding the efficacy of herbal compounds delivered in this way. Therefore, this chapter will review herbal compounds, their claims, and the evidence for their efficacy in dietary supplement form. In addition, we will describe some of the foods that contain herbal ingredients, and the challenges and uncertainties faced in this new functional food arena.

II. HERBAL MEDICINE

The use of herbal products became popular in the U.S. following the passage of the Dietary Supplements Health and Education Act of 1994 (DSHEA). This act amended the Federal Food, Drug, and Cosmetic Act to allow dietary supplements to be regulated differently from conventional foods or drugs. After the passage of this law, herbal and botanical supplements initially showed double-digit growth in sales; however, current rates of growth have slowed or even reversed that trend.[2]

Dietary supplements today are a far cry from the herbal medicine practiced in ancient China, Europe, or even by native Americans. Traditional herbalists used plant roots, leaves, bark, flowers, and seeds to prepare teas, broths, tinctures, poultices, etc. Today, highly purified extracts and powders are put into capsules and tablets. Modern herbal medicine (or phytotherapy) relies on standardization and demonstrated efficacy-constituent relationships.[3] Several comprehensive studies have been conducted to support or challenge the efficacy of modern herbal medicines; yet one of the greatest impediments today is the utilization of well-defined and standardized herbs. Different studies that use different preparations of the same herbal cannot be compared.

III. HERBS AS INGREDIENTS IN FUNCTIONAL FOODS

There is wide variation in the level of research available to support claims for many herbal supplements. Some, like *Ginkgo biloba*, have been studied extensively in Europe, and others, such as hawthorn leaves and berries, have only been tested in humans in a handful of studies.[4] Even less is known about herbals as food ingredients. When herbal compounds have been tested in clinical trials, it is usually as a standardized extract or specific supplement rather than as part of the food. From a scientific standpoint, a standardized extract or single compound is important in defining efficacy, but the results cannot necessarily be extrapolated to the whole herb as an ingredient to a food.

Numerous issues are raised when considering botanical ingredients as food additives, including regulatory requirements, safety, and identity, in addition to efficacy. One of the biggest questions is the stability of botanical ingredients in foods that must be processed by heat, air, or pressure.

A. REGULATORY STATUS

As mentioned previously, no separate regulatory category exists for functional foods. As such, regulations for conventional foods apply. To be used in a food, an herbal ingredient must be "generally recognized as safe" (GRAS) or approved as a food additive. This is one of the important distinctions between dietary supplements and foods. Notification of a new dietary ingredient (not in use prior to October 15, 1994) for a dietary supplement is given to the FDA 75 days before first marketing the supplement. The U.S. Food and Drug Administration (FDA) then evaluates the safety information provided and accepts or rejects the substance as a new dietary ingredient. For foods, however, if an herbal ingredient is not already GRAS, or has a reasonable chance of being affirmed as GRAS, a lengthy food-additive petition process is indicated.

The FDA has informally allowed companies to self-assert GRAS status provided notification is given to the FDA, and appropriate safety data are made available to the FDA upon request. However, no final rules have been published to guide this process, and there are no clear standards for judging the data provided by companies. As such, determining which herbs are considered GRAS is not a simple task. In 2001, the FDA issued a general letter to the industry suggesting that some herbal and botanical ingredients being added to foods may not be GRAS for their intended use. More specific warning letters were sent to several manufacturers questioning the basis for concluding that herbals such as echinacea, ginseng, and *Ginkgo biloba* were GRAS. Following this series of warning letters, many products with added herbal or botanical ingredients disappeared from the marketplace. Additional regulatory issues, such as label statements and claims, will be discussed later in this section.

B. Identity Dilemma

When considering botanicals as food ingredients, one of the fundamental issues is determining the correct identity of the plant compound. There are two issues with identity that have been documented in literature. The first case is the problem of harvesting the correct genus of plant. Two individuals were poisoned when the herbal preparation they consumed contained the *Digitalis lanata* plant rather than plantain, of the plantago genus.[5] Both individuals experienced cardiac symptoms as a result of elevated levels of digoxin. After tracing the product back through the manufacturer, supplier, and farmer, it was determined that the identity of the *D. lanata* had been confused with the plantain at harvest.

The other issue concerns identifying the correct species of plant. The efficacy of echinacea cannot be extended to all species: *E. purpurea, E. angustifolia,* and *E. pallida.* Studies can be flawed because although one species was studied, another species may have been reported. This confusion resulted in a denial by the German Commission E for approval of some of the echinacea preparations.[3] The Commission E has approved the oral use of *E. purpurea* herb, i.e., ground parts for colds, respiratory tract infections, urinary tract infections, and the topical use for poorly healing wounds. The *E. pallida* root (fresh or dried) has been approved for use in the treatment of influenza-like infections. The *E. angustifolia* root or herb and the *E. pallida* herb have not been approved due to the confusion in the identity of the actual plant that was studied.

C. Standardization Dilemma

Standardization of herbal ingredients is another relevant issue for both food manufacturers and consumers. Herbs are grown under different conditions, at different locations, and in different seasons of the year. These geographical and environmental differences result in variations in the levels of active compounds. The community of herbal growers, producers, etc., has called for standardization of herb products. But which compounds should be standardized? In some cases, the active compound is unknown. Even if the active ingredient is known, there are many different active compounds in herbs that may act additively or synergistically. Little is known about the optimum level of these compounds. Much research is needed to determine the appropriate standards for quantity, potency, and content uniformity.

D. Effect of Processing Dilemma

Clearly, we do not know many of the active compounds in the herbals that may be used in a functional food. More importantly, with the addition of those herbs to food and the processing that the food must undergo, even less is known about the effects of processing on the active compounds. Storage of *Echinacea purpurea* roots either at 24° or –18° resulted in significant losses in the alkamides, although drying and chopping had little effect.[6] Hyperforin, an ingredient in St. John's wort, has been shown to be very sensitive to oxidation, and storage conditions are critical to maintaining the levels found in the original harvested plant.[7] Thus, foods containing echinacea or St. John's wort that have been stored may lose efficacy. More research is needed on the stability of herbal active components. However, even if we were to determine that one compound is affected by processing, we would still need to determine whether the whole herb in a food product becomes ineffective.

E. Safety Dilemma

Another key question for herbal additives to food is the safety of the herb itself. Examples of herbs with known dangers include chaparral, ephedra, blue cohosh, and yohimbe, to name a few. Other safety concerns include potential interactions with other medicines (e.g., anticoagulants and *Ginkgo biloba*), and the possibility of contaminants, such as lead, in herbal preparations. This is discussed in more detail in the next section.

In many cases, the functional or active ingredients in an herb may have drug-like qualities. The suitability of providing such an herb in a food product for general consumption needs to be considered. Allergies to some herbal preparations exist; common allergens would need to be clearly identified in ingredient lists. Herbal preparations are, by definition, rather dilute. Adding the herb to a food may increase the dilution. However, when extracts are used, do the active compounds become more concentrated and thus potentially stronger? How much is effective? How much is too much? Concerns are raised regarding unintentional consumption and consumption by children. These are some of the many unanswered questions surrounding functional foods with herbal ingredients.

F. Interactions with Drugs Dilemma

Anecdotal incidences, case studies, and clinical trials have clearly shown an increase in the occurrence of complications between drugs and herbs. Interactions documented in the literature include herbs that increase the effects of anticoagulants, and those affecting brain neurotransmitters, immunity, or hormonal actions.[8–10] Some herbs act as hepatic enzyme inducers or inhibitors, thereby increasing or decreasing, respectively, plasma levels of prescribed drugs.[11] As these herbs can be added as ingredients to foods, it is important to pay attention to the levels that cause these drug interactions.

IV. LABEL STATEMENTS AND CLAIMS

When considering herbals in food products, the regulations for label statements or claims are different from herbal preparations that are sold as dietary supplements. As with all ingredients in a food, herbal compounds must be identified in the ingredient list by their common and usual name: "St. John's wort" instead of "*Hypericum perforatum*," for example. For foods with added herbal ingredients, these ingredients may be also identified in label statements such as "Contains kava kava" so long as such statements are truthful and not misleading. Comparison statements such as "Contains 50% more kava kava than brand X" must be accompanied by indications of the amounts of kava kava in each brand per serving. Other label terminology such as "High in ... " or "Good source of ... " is not applicable to herbal compounds because there are no daily values set for these ingredients like there are for essential nutrients.

One of the more controversial elements of DSHEA, and the resulting FDA regulations, relates to claims. Health claims are those FDA-approved statements that link a food or food component to reduced risk of a disease, e.g., calcium and osteoporosis, or fruits and vegetables and cardiovascular disease. To date, no health claims have been approved for herbal ingredients. Under current regulations, new health claims may be proposed at any time but must be supported by an authoritative statement from a recognized government entity (e.g., U.S. Department of Agriculture [USDA],

National Institutes of Health [NIH], and National Academy of Sciences [NAS]), have significant scientific agreement, or be a qualified claim. Further, the mention of a disease on a food label or in an advertisement in the absence of an approved health claim results in the product being considered an unapproved drug by FDA. Only approved drugs may claim to diagnose, cure, mitigate, treat, or prevent a disease. However, dietary supplement and food manufacturers may use what have come to be known as structure or function claims to promote the positive aspects of their products.

Structure or function claims are statements of an effect of an herb on a body function or structure (e.g., "Promotes urinary tract health"), or on general well being (e.g., "Gives energy and stamina"). Structure or function claims on a dietary supplement must be accompanied by the following disclaimer: *"This statement has not been evaluated by the FDA. This product is not intended to diagnose, cure, mitigate, treat, or prevent a disease."*

Structure or function claims have been used on food (e.g., "Calcium builds strong bones") but not extensively. As the regulations stand now, structure or function claims on foods must relate to the nutritive value of the food and not to another ingredient or property. For example, capsules of cranberry juice sold as a dietary supplement can carry the claim "Promotes urinary tract health," but bottles of cranberry juice (a conventional food) cannot because the beneficial effects of cranberry juice have not been linked to nutrient components. The current definition of nutritive value, "A value in sustaining human existence by such processes as promoting growth, replacing loss of essential nutrients, or providing energy," would seem to exclude herbal and botanical ingredients, as well as many other natural food components.[12] Further definition of structure or function claims on foods is needed to level the playing field with dietary supplements.

The remainder of this chapter will discuss individual herbs, their purported actions, active compounds, and clinical evidence that supports efficacy, if available. They are organized by the physiological system that they are reported to influence and summarized in Table 13.1. When known, food products containing these herbs are given; when examples do not exist, potential foods are suggested for the particular herb. Although we have reviewed and evaluated the current literature, it must be remembered that negative data may not be available because it was not published.

V. ACTIONS AND EVIDENCE OF HERBAL EFFICACY

A. NERVOUS SYSTEM

Touted as a memory booster, *Ginkgo biloba* has appeared in a variety of food products, generally beverages or energy bars. Products previously on the market had creative names to promote the idea of enhanced brain activity, e.g., Brain Broo, Think, BrainWash, and Wise Guy. According to *Nutraceuticals World, 2002*, ginkgo is the eighth best-selling herbal remedy by dollar sales in the U.S.[2] In Germany, ginkgo leaf extract was the most commonly prescribed single-ingredient phytomedicine in 1996.[3] Ginkgo is prescribed in Europe for the treatment of cerebral disturbances and circulatory disorders.

As sold in dietary supplement form, ginkgo is an extract of the leaves of *Ginkgo biloba*. This tree is native to China but seems to grow well in a range of climates. City-dwellers who may not know the name of the tree are probably quite familiar with the foul-smelling mature seeds it produces.

The active compounds in ginkgo are flavonoid glycosides and novel diterpene lactones, collectively known as ginkgolides. The ginkgolides are inhibitors of platelet-activating factor and thus may affect circulation, blood coagulation, and inflammation. The mechanism by which gingko has its effect is thought to be due to its ability to improve microvasculature insufficiency. An increase in blood flow to the brain may be the reason for the slowing of mental decline in dementia. This also has ramifications related to cardiovascular health and may be efficacious in treating tinnitis and vertigo.

Clinical trials have focused on cerebral insufficiency and peripheral arterial occlusive disease, and most of the research on *G. biloba* has been done in Europe. Published reviews indicate that

TABLE 13.1
Common Herbs, Active Ingredients, and Purported Function

Popular Name	Scientific Name	Active Compounds	Purported Function	Main Body System
Ginkgo biloba	*Ginkgo biloba*	Ginkolides: flavonoid glycosides, and diterpene lactones	Memory, cognition	Brain, circulatory system
St. John's wort	*Hypericum perforatum*	Hypericin, pseudohypericin, hyperforins, terpenes, catechin-type tannins, proanthocyanidins	Antidepressant for mild to moderate depression	Brain
Kava kava	*Piper methysticum*	Kavalactones	Antianxiety, relaxation	Brain
Valerian	*Valeriana officalis*	Valeptriates, valerenic acid, sesquiterpenes	Sleep inducement	Brain
Hawthorn berry	*Crataegus oxycantha*	Amygdalin, crategolic acid, oligomeric proanthocyanadins	Cardiac insufficiency	Circulatory system
Echinacea	*Echinacea purpurea* *E. pallida* *E. angustifolia*	Echinosides, caffeic, ferulic acids and cichoric acid, inulin and fructans	Immunomodulators	Innate immunity
Peppermint oil	*Mentha x piperita*	Menthol	Gastric intestinal distress	GI tract
Ginger	*Zingiber officinale*	Gingerols, gingerdiols	Antiemetic, nausea	GI tract
Licorice	*Glycyrrhiza glabra*	Glycyrrhetic acid, triterpene, saponins	Expectorant	Respiratory system
Saw palmetto berry	*Serenoa repens*	β-sitosterol, sterols, fatty acids	Alpha reductase inhibitor	Prostate gland
Feverfew	*Tancetum parthenuum*	Sesquiterpene lactones	Migraine prophylactic	Brain

most studies show clinically significant improvement.[13,14] Studies of patients with intermittent claudication show significant increases in pain-free walking distance for those treated with *G. biloba* extract.[14]

A standardized extract of ginkgo, called EGb 761, has been used in many clinical trials, making comparisons between studies easier and more valuable. Indeed, many studies have shown the ability of EGb 761 to improve or slow the dementia related to Alzheimer's disease.[15–17] A meta-analysis to determine the effects of ginkgo on cognitive function in patients with Alzheimer's disease located 50 trials. The authors determined that the majority of the studies did not provide clear diagnoses of dementia and Alzheimer's disease. Of the four studies that met all of the inclusion criteria for the analysis, there was a small but significant effect of ginkgo on cognitive function in Alzheimer's disease.[18] An examination of this meta-analysis suggests that an estimate of the quality of different types of studies on *G. biloba* is adequate to good and that methodological quality is good, resulting in the conclusion that ginkgo may be efficacious for preventing memory impairment, dementia, and tinnitus. Only for intermittent claudication (leg pain or leg pain while exercising) is the methodological quality considered very good for the beneficial effect of ginkgo.

The idea that ginkgo slows the rate of dementia in patients appears to have been extrapolated to suggest that consumption of this product will make the average healthy consumer smarter, better able to concentrate, and improve the ability to focus. No research has been able to support this notion. Because of the antioxidant compounds in ginkgo, its role in functional foods may be beneficial.

In clinical trials, mild side effects, including headaches, gastrointestinal disturbances, and skin allergies have been noted. Individuals who are already taking anticoagulant medication (e.g., warfarin or aspirin) or other dietary supplements with blood-thinning properties (e.g., vitamin E, garlic, ginger) should not take ginkgo without first consulting with their physician. Ginkgo did not influence the pharmacokinetics of warfarin on clotting status in healthy subjects[19] or bleeding time and platelet activity[20] at levels up to 240 mg/d. The safety of ginkgo for pregnant and lactating women or for infants and children has not been established.[14] As with most herbs, no studies have been conducted on *G. biloba*'s effectiveness when consumed as a food product.

St. John's wort, *Hypericum perforatum*, is a widely prescribed antidepressant in Europe and has become a top-selling dietary supplement in the U.S. Its common name (*wort* is Old English for *plant*) derives from the traditional belief that the plant blooms on the anniversary of the execution of St. John the Baptist. Although it has been suggested to have antiviral and anticancer properties, it is the antidepressive effects of St. John's wort that have garnered the attention of researchers and consumers.

Hypericum perforatum is a bushy plant with characteristic bright yellow flowers. The flowers and tops of the plant are considered the active parts. A number of compounds may contribute to the activity of St. John's wort, including naphthodianthroms, flavonoids, xanthose, and bioflavonoids,[21] although hypericin and pseudohypericin are the compounds that have been the subject of most investigations.[13]

The exact mechanism of action of St. John's wort has not been well defined. *In vitro* evidence initially suggested monoamine oxidase (MAO) inhibition, but this is unlikely, given the wide use in Europe without reported side effects usually associated with monoamine oxidase inhibitors (MAOI).[22] Other studies suggest effects on several neurotransmitters, including gamma-aminobutyric acid (GABA) affinity, activation of dopamine receptors, and inhibition of serotonin receptors. It is possible that small additive effects on several neurotransmitters combine to give the antidepressant effect.

Several large-scale clinical trials in the U.S. investigated the efficacy of St. John's wort with common prescription medications for depression and placebos in the treatment of mild to moderate depression.[23–25] Data are encouraging and suggest St. John's wort to be superior to fluoxetine.[23] Szegedi et al. concluded that hypericum extract WS 5570 was at least as effective as paroxetine.[24] Shelton et al., however, concluded St. John's wort was not effective; however, they studied people with major depression.[25] A meta-analysis compared outcomes of 23 randomized trials, determining a pooled estimate of the responder rate ratio (responder rate in treatment group or responder rate in control group) and found that hypericum extracts were superior to placebos, and equal to standard antidepressant drugs when standard depression scales were used.[26] In a review of many of the same studies, Volz came to the same conclusions regarding the efficacy of St. John's wort.[27] However, both reports cite a variety of shortcomings in the existing data, including variations in subject population, extract preparation, length of interventions, and dosages.

In dietary supplement form, most preparations are standardized extracts (0.3% hypericin), although random sampling of products indicated a wide variation in actual product contents. This may, in part, be due to the instability of some of the components of St. John's wort.[7] The dosage given in clinical trials is usually 300 mg three times per day. Side effects are minimal but have included photosensitivity, gastrointestinal upset, dizziness, sedation, restlessness, and constipation.[13] At least two studies have found an interaction with oral contraceptives that suggest the effectiveness of the contraceptive is less when St. John's wort is also consumed.[8,9] St. John's wort has also been shown to reduce blood levels of a common protease inhibitor used in the treatment of HIV and AIDS.[28,29] St. John's wort should not be taken in combination with other antidepressants, and its safety in pregnant and lactating women and in children is unknown. Like most herbal supplements, long-term safety has not been adequately evaluated, although the wide use of St. John's wort in Europe has not suggested any specific concerns.

One of the major concerns about St. John's wort is not related to its efficacy or safety, but rather to the wisdom of individuals choosing to self-medicate with a dietary supplement instead of seeking professional help for depression.[30] Clinical depression is a serious condition that should be evaluated by a health professional prior to treatment.

Tea, juice blends and other drinks, soups, and snack foods have been marketed with added St. John's wort, suggesting "calming" and "relaxing" effects of these products. No studies are available to lend weight to these implied claims, however, because St. John's wort has not been tested for efficacy when consumed as part of a food or when consumed by mentally healthy people.

Kava chips, kava chocolate, and kava juice are all used to relax and "mellow out" after a stressful day. After all, traditional ceremonies in Hawaii and other locations in the South Pacific used kava beverages as natural intoxicants. In addition to its relaxing effects, kava supplements are also promoted for antianxiety effects. Animal studies have also found anticonvulsive and antispasmodic effects.[3]

Traditional kava beverages are prepared from the root of the *Piper methysticum* plant. A group of at least six kavalactones are thought to be responsible for the sedative and intoxicating effects.[31] To date, the mechanism of action has not been defined. *In vitro* studies suggest that kavalactones affect benzodiazepine or GABA-binding sites, but results have been conflicting.

Meta-analyses of clinical trials using kava have found six well-controlled quality reports.[32,33] Both meta-analyses concluded that kava, particularly the standardized extract WS 1490 (standardized to 70% kavalactones), was effective. Volz and Kieser[34] described a 25-week placebo-controlled trial of kava with outpatients who had one of several nonpsychotic anxiety disorders. Outcomes on anxiety scales and self-reported impressions showed improvement in the kava group. Like other clinical trials to date, conclusions from this study are limited due to the heterogeneity of the subject group and the likelihood of depression as a comorbidity in several subjects.[13]

Adverse effects reported in clinical studies have been rare, mild, and reversible. Kava dermopathy (a temporary yellowish discoloration of the skin, hair, and nails) has been reported with higher doses, and heavy use is suggested to cause liver-related metabolic abnormalities, including increased liver enzymes.[35] Serious adverse events are, however, possible with kava ingestion, and liver damage is of the greatest concern.[35,36] In addition, because of its effects on the central nervous system, kava should not be used in conjunction with alcohol, barbituates, or psychopharmacological agents. Long-term safety is unknown.

Valerian root (species: *Valeriana officalis L.*) is well known in many cultures as a natural sleep aid. It is also promoted as having anxiolytic and antispasmodic activity. In Germany, it is approved as a mild sedative and sleep aid.[3] Animal studies support the benefits of valerian as a mild hypnotic agent but are inconsistent regarding effects relating to anticonvulsant or antidepressant activity. Several small human clinical trials have found valerian to be efficacious as a mild sedative, showing a significant decrease in sleep latency as compared to placebos.[13,21] A larger randomized placebo-controlled trial (n = 128) found that 400 mg of aqueous valerian extract before bedtime improved sleep quality and reduced sleep latency with no residual sedation upon awakening.[37] More recently, however, two trials did not show any reductions in sleep problems in affected individuals,[38,39] although one trial showed comparable efficacy to oxazepam but did not have a placebo-control group.[40]

The active ingredients in valerian are likely valepotriates and sesquiterpenes.[41] Both compounds are known to have sedative effects, and valepotriates are known to be cytotoxic. However, therapeutic preparations do not contain valepotriates as these are thermolabile and chemically unstable. Valerian has also been shown to be high in GABA.[13] The mechanism of action, however, is unknown. Extracts of valerian have affinity for GABA receptors, possibly due to the high GABA content, but this may have no sedating effect because GABA does not readily cross the blood–brain barrier. Other postulated mechanisms involve 5-hydroxy-tryptophan and adenosine receptors.

Reported dosages in literature vary widely from 500 mg to 12 g per day, given in single bedtime or divided doses.[41] A single case of overdose has been reported, but, otherwise, few adverse effects have been noted. There is no evidence that valerian is addictive. However, like most herbal remedies, there is insufficient evidence of safety in pregnant and lactating women. In addition, most sources recommend avoidance of alcohol and other CNS depressants when taking valerian.[13,21,22]

Valerian has been approved for use as a flavoring for foods and beverages and is considered GRAS. Few examples of products containing valerian have been found other than teas and beverages touted for relaxation. No studies have been done on valerian as a food ingredient.

B. HEART AND CIRCULATION

The hawthorn plant, *Crataegus oxycantha*, has been traditionally used for a number of cardiac complaints such as angina, hypertension, arrhythmia, and congestive heart failure. The medicinal parts of the hawthorn are the leaves, flowers, and berries, used singly or in combination. There is sufficient evidence in the literature for the Commission E to classify the hawthorn-leaf-with-flower combination as an approved herb for the treatment of mild cardiac insufficiency. Studies show that 160 to 1800 mg per day of an aqueous-alcoholic extract was effective for a period that lasted up to 56 d; however, no pharmacokinetics of the drug in humans are available. An improvement in subjective findings as well as an increase in work tolerance, ejection fraction, and a decrease in pressure and heart rate product was indicated.[4]

Animal studies in rats show that *in vitro* pretreatment of the isolated heart with dried hawthorn extract was protective against arrhythmia[42] and cell membrane damage[43] caused by no-flow ischemia. A tincture of hawthorn berries was effective in preventing lipid deposits in the liver and heart,[44] increasing LDL-receptor activity, and reducing cholesterol synthesis[45] in rats fed an atherogenic diet.

The active compounds of hawthorn are the flavones, flavanols, and oligomeric procyanidins (catechins and epicatechins). Other potential active compounds are the triterpene saponins, phenolics, and a few cardioactive amines. Like many other botanicals, the antioxidant and antithrombotic activities are likely to be responsible for improvement in cardiovascular symptoms.

Hawthorn has been previously added to beverages but, under current regulations, no claims could be made for management of vascular health. A precedent for a food with such a claim has been established — however, not with an herbal preparation. The HeartBar™ formulated by Cooke Pharmaceutical is the first nonprescription medical food on the market for dietary management of vascular disease. The active component of this bar is L-arginine, a precursor to nitric oxide. A functional food containing hawthorn has potential to be marketed for cardiovascular health as well. More human, controlled, randomized clinical trials are needed before this herb is found to be efficacious or accepted as a medical food.

C. IMMUNE SYSTEM

Herbs that are designed to stimulate the immune system include echinacea, astragalus, cat's claw, goldenseal, and pau d'arco (also known as lapacho). Each herb appears to influence different branches of the immune system. *Echinacea* is probably the best studied of the group.

The echinacea plant, also known as the purple coneflower, has been used for centuries. Although this is not an argument for efficacy, it does indicate some degree of safety. The herb is best known for its immuno-stimulating capabilities and is used for treating the common cold, flu, coughs, and bronchitis.[3]

Medicinally, three species of echinacea are important: *E. purpurea*, *E. angustifolia*, and *E. pallida*. Each has been alleged to have different medicinal properties, but little research has been done to compare them. The roots, the leaves, or the whole plant may be used in dietary supplement preparation. Standardized extracts may be aqueous extracts or ethanol extracts. The active components of echinacea are flavonoids, immuno-stimulating glycoproteins and polysaccharides, and caffeic acid and its derivatives.

A meta-analysis of randomized, placebo-controlled studies involving a total of 134 subjects was reported.[46] Two of the five studies showed an increase in phagocytic activity of peripheral blood neutrophils. Each of the five studies was done with different amounts of echinacea from different plant parts and in different preparation combinations. The inconsistent results underscore the importance of knowing the species of echinacea, the method of extraction, and the route of administration. A larger study by the same principal author looked at the ability of echinacea to prevent upper respiratory infection (URI).[47] "Time to event" was the primary outcome measure on 302 subjects who were healthy at the start of the study. Twelve weeks of oral ingestion of the herb preparations or a placebo did not prevent URI. Grimm and Muller completed a study with 109 healthy subjects using fresh juice of *Echinacea purpurea* or placebo juice. The number of subjects having URIs, the number of URIs per subject, and the duration of any colds was measured. There was no significant difference in these measures between the echinacea group and the placebo.[48] More recent studies have examined the efficacy of echinacea in virally-challenged subjects.[49,50] For those acquiring viruses naturally,[51–53] using *E. purpurea* or *E. angustifolia* show no significant effects on number of illnesses or duration or severity of symptoms.

Studies that examine echinacea's prophylactic ability to prevent illness show little to no significant benefit. Echinacea, because of its effect on the oxidative burst of phagocytic cells, would not be expected to prevent colds or flu; rather, it might be expected to enhance killing of the invading organisms. Thus, it has been thought more likely to be a therapeutic herb rather than a prophylactic herb. Recommendations for echinacea use suggest that it be consumed at the onset of symptoms.

A recent study in the *New England Journal of Medicine* evaluated three preparations of *E. angustifolia* roots in a viral challenge study.[51] *E. angustifolia* was given either 7 d prior to the challenge (prophylaxis) or at challenge (treatment). There were no significant effects of any of the echinacea extracts on rate of infection, severity of symptoms, or volume of nasal secretions. Neutrophil numbers and IL-8 concentration in nasal-lavage specimens were not significantly different among treatments. The echinacea preparations in this well-designed and controlled study showed neither a prophylactic nor a treatment against a common cold virus challenge.

If echinacea affects the phagocytes, long-term ingestion of echinacea may potentially do more harm than good. Increased reactivity of the phagocytic system may result in generation of more free radicals. Free radicals, in turn, may then cause damage to the host. Recommendations suggest that echinacea not be consumed for more than 6 to 8 weeks at a time.

In the U.S., echinacea was the top-selling product in natural food stores in 1997[3] and, while still in the top 20 supplements by dollar sales, echinacea saw a 23% drop in sales between 2001 and 2002.[2] Because of its popularity, several functional foods have been marketed with echinacea. Echinacea has been found in snack foods, beverages, and soups. More studies need to be done on the shelf life and heat stability of the active compounds, and also to identify the active compounds.

D. DIGESTIVE SYSTEM

Almost every herb listed in general reference books seems to have some influence on the digestive system. The alleged use of the botanical is to cleanse or purify the body. Cleansers and tonics are very difficult to study. Some of the herbs found to stimulate digestive juices include wormwood, dandelion, horseradish, chicory, and tarragon. Precautions should be noted for wormwood (daisy family) as this genus may contain thujone, a small molecule that has been responsible for convulsions, hallucinations, and kidney failure. Fennel is supposed to act as a carminative, a substance to relieve gas, cramps, and bloating. Aloe, when taken internally, acts as a laxative. Peppermint oil has been used in the relief of irritable bowel syndrome (IBS) and gastritis.

A meta-analysis of clinical trials done with peppermint oil (*Mentha x piperita*) described eight studies in which there was a global improvement in the symptoms associated with IBS.[54] The main active component in the oil is menthol. The authors of the meta-analysis noted several problems with existing studies, especially with the diagnosis of IBS. Only one out of eight trials properly diagnosed the condition. Three of the eight studies did not state their inclusion criteria. So although the global outcome suggested that peppermint oil is effective, the quality of the studies make the data circumspect. The authors of this meta-analysis note that, in early studies, peppermint oil acted as a calcium antagonist in human and animal studies. The consequence of calcium antagonism in the gut is relaxation of gastrointestinal smooth muscle, thus possibly promoting bowel rest. Peppermint oil has been successfully used as an antispasmodic agent.[55] The amount of peppermint oil needed to affect the gut is likely far too much to be palatable in food.

Another herb that has been suggested to promote gastrointestinal well-being is ginger (*Zingiber officinale*). Ginger is a common culinary spice, but levels that are recommended therapeutically (2 to 4 g of the rhizome daily) are far greater than what is incorporated into food as a seasoning. Clinical trials with ginger have focused on preventing postoperative nausea and motion sickness. One study found that ginger worked to prevent postoperative nausea as effectively as metoclopramide and better than placebos.[56] A ginger extract (200 mg) increased stomach motility,[57] but 1 g of the whole root did not alter gastric emptying.[58] Also, 1 g of the root did not prevent experimentally-induced motion sickness.[59] But in another study, 1 g of the root reduced the tendency to vomit on the high seas.[60] Available data is inconclusive on the antinausea mechanism of ginger, but it is generally believed to act differently than Dramamine. Benefits, if research bears it out, would be obtained with gram quantities of the root and therefore may not be palatable for a functional food. Teas, however, are currently used as a mode of administration, suggesting potential for ginger to be used in a beverage to prevent nausea.

E. RESPIRATORY SYSTEM

The coughs that accompany illness are sometimes treated with over-the-counter medicines designed to act as expectorants. The licorice root (*Glycyrrhiza glabra*) is claimed to act as an expectorant although, according to the *Physicians Desk Reference of Herbal Medicines*, this has only been researched in rabbits.[61] Licorice has been associated with hypertension,[62] and has been suggested to cause renal retention of sodium and a loss of body potassium. The mechanism by which it does this is unclear, but it may be through inhibiting 11 beta-hydroxy steroid dehydrogenase type 2.[62] The importance of replacing lost potassium should be stressed, and perhaps potassium could become a component of a functional food containing licorice root.

F. URINARY SYSTEM

There has been substantial interest in the benefits of cranberry (*Vaccinium macrocarpon*) for urinary tract health.[63] Cranberry appears to act as an antiseptic simultaneously preventing bacterial adherence to the epithelial cells of the urinary tract.[64] A Cochrane review concludes that cranberry juice decreases the number of symptomatic urinary tract infections in a 12-month period for women, but there is not enough evidence to conclude the same for children and the elderly.[65] Cranberry has been studied for a number of other conditions such as urinary stone formation,[66] neuropsychological effects,[67] and *Helicobacter pylori* infection.[68] Data is positive but not sufficient to draw conclusions. Other berries of the same family such as the blueberry (*V. angustifolium*) and bilberry (*V. myrtillus*) may also aid in urinary tract health. Bearberry (*Arctostaphylos uva-ursi*), a different family, is also indicated in urinary tract infections. The latter three have hardly been well studied in this respect.

Saw palmetto (*Serenoa repens*) is a very common palm plant indigenous to the southeastern U.S. The saw palmetto berry is used in the treatment of benign prostatic hyperplasia (BPH). Forty percent of men over the age of 70 have this condition. Frequent urination, nocturia, weak stream, incomplete emptying, and hesitancy, characterize BPH. The enlargement of the prostate is thought to occur via the action of dihydrotestosterone (DHT). DHT is derived from testosterone via an alpha reductase enzyme. The action of DHT is anabolic, hence the growth of the prostate. Treatment for this condition uses drugs designed to inhibit the alpha reductase enzyme. Saw palmetto berries contain compounds that inhibit the alpha reductase enzyme.

A meta-analysis of 18 randomized trials of the efficacy of saw palmetto berries for BPH symptoms was published in 1998.[69] Of a total of 2939 men that took part in these studies, 1118 of them were in studies that compared saw palmetto to placebos and 1821 compared saw palmetto to finasteride, a drug currently used in BPH treatment that acts as an alpha reductase inhibitor. The self-reported improvement from the men favored saw palmetto berries over placebos. Similarly, relief from nocturia and an increase in peak flow rates favored saw palmetto berries over placebo. When finasteride was compared to saw palmetto berries using the International Prostrate Symptoms Scale, no difference was observed between finasteride and saw palmetto, meaning that the saw palmetto was as effective as the drug. The authors noted two advantages of the berry over the drug: (1) saw palmetto berry is less expensive than finasteride and (2) erectile dysfunction was noted in 5% of the men on the drug, but there were no such side effects in the saw palmetto group.

Shortcomings of this meta-analysis included inconsistent reporting of outcomes, no attempts to assess the quality of blinding, only three trials using results from standardized, validated urological symptom scales, and the different doses and preparations of saw palmetto used in each study.

More recently, meta-analyses of a specific standardized lipid extract of *Serenoa repens* were published.[70,71] These reports concluded that there was significant (but small) improvement in peak flow rate, reductions in the International Prostate Symptoms scores, and nocturia compared to placebos.

Other botanicals that are becoming better known for the ability to reduce the symptoms associated with BPH include *Pygeum africanum* and *Urtica dioica*.[72,73] Less is known about these herbs, although *Pygeum* acts as an alpha reductase inhibitor.

For mild BPH, saw palmetto berries may be beneficial. Their actual benefit in a functional food rather than in capsule form is questionable, however. A quote from the 1696 diary of a young Quaker merchant, Jonathon Dickinson, said "We tasted them but not one amongst us could suffer them to stay in our mouths; for we could compare the taste of them to nothing else but rotten cheese steeped in tobacco."[74]

G. Musculoskeletal System

There are a number of herbal preparations designed to act as analgesics (relieve joint and muscle pain) and anti-inflammatory agents to reduce swelling and pain. The bark of the white willow is known to contain salicylates, the compound that is in aspirin. Feverfew (*Tancetum parthenuum*) is an herb resembling the daisy that has been reported as a prophylactic treatment for migraine headaches. The active components of feverfew are thought to be the sesquiterpene lactones.[75]

In 1985, subjects that were already taking feverfew preparations were studied.[76] Half of the group was given a placebo and the other half was given standardized capsules of feverfew. There was a significant increase in frequency and severity of attacks in those on the placebo, but those who took the feverfew-containing capsules had no change in their migraine attacks. In a crossover design study, patients who took feverfew experienced reduced and less severe attacks compared to the placebo group.[77] An *in vitro* study suggested that the mechanism by which feverfew worked was inhibition of 5-lipoxygenase and cyclo-oxygenase enzyme activities.[78] The five clinical trials that have been published suggest a beneficial effect of feverfew compared to placebos. However, the authors of the 1998 meta-analysis advise that the efficacy of feverfew has not been established beyond a reasonable doubt.[79] More recently, clinical trials with standardized extract (MIG-99) showed a significant reduction in the number and frequency of migraines.[80,81]

VI. SUMMARY AND CONCLUSION

Adding botanicals to foods to create functional products raises many issues including appropriate regulation, safety, stability, and efficacy. Individual food–herbal dynamics will create even more challenges, including ways to mask the unpleasant flavors of some herbs. Many gaps exist in our current knowledge, requiring caution on the part of both the manufacturer and consumer. However, as our knowledge base grows and confirms the suspected actions of many herbal compounds, our future food supply could be dramatically different than it is today.

REFERENCES

1. Functional Foods: Opportunities and Challenges, *IFT Expert Report* 1: 1–66, 2005.
2. Marra, J., The State of Dietary Supplements, November, http://www.nutraceuticalsworld.com/Nov022.htm 2002.
3. Blumenthal Med, *The Complete German Commission E Monographs, Therapeutic Guide to Herbal Medicines*, American Botanical Council, Austin, 1998.
4. Pittler, M.H., Schmidt, K., and Ernst, E., Hawthorn extract for treating chronic heart failure: meta-analysis of randomized trials, *Am. J. Med.* 114: 665–674, 2003.
5. Slifman, N.R., Obermeyer, W.R., Aloi, B.K., Musser, S.M., Correll, B.S., Cichowicz, B.S., Betz, J.M., and Love, L., Contamination of botanical dietary supplements by *Digitalis lanata*. *N. Engl. J. Med.* 339: 806–811, 1999.
6. Perry, N.B., van Klink, J.W., Burgess, E.J., and Parmenter, G.A., Alkamide levels in Echinacea purpurea: effects of processing, drying and storage, *Planta Med.* 66: 54–56, 2000.
7. Orth, H.C., Rentel, C., and Schmidt, P.C., Isolation, purity analysis and stability of hyperforin as a standard material from Hypericum perforatum L. *J. Pharm. Pharmacol.* 51: 193–200, 1999.
8. Hall, S.D., Wang, Z., Huang, S.M., Hamman, M.A., Vasavada, N., Adigun, A.Q., Hilligoss, J.K., Miller, M., and Gorski, J.C., The interaction between St John's wort and an oral contraceptive, *Clin. Pharmacol. Ther.* 74: 525–535, 2003.
9. Pfrunder, A., Schiesser, M., Gerber, S., Haschke, M., Bitzer, J., and Drewe, J., Interaction of St John's wort with low-dose oral contraceptive therapy: a randomized controlled trial, *Br. J. Clin. Pharmacol.* 56: 683–690, 2003.
10. Sparreboom, A., Cox, M.C., Acharya, M.R., and Figg, W.D., Herbal remedies in the United States: potential adverse interactions with anticancer agents, *J. Clin. Oncol.* 22: 2489–2503, 2004.
11. Gurley, B.J., Gardner, S.F., Hubbard, M.A., Williams, D.K., Gentry, W.B., Carrier, J., Khan, I.A., Edwards, D.J., and Shah, A., In vivo assessment of botanical supplementation on human cytochrome P450 phenotypes: citrus aurantium, Echinacea purpurea, milk thistle, and saw palmetto, *Clin. Pharmacol. Ther.* 76: 428–440, 2004.
12. Turner, R.E., Degnan, F.H., and Archer, D.L., Label claims for foods and supplements:a review of the regulations, *Nutr. Clin. Practice* 20: 21–32, 2005.
13. Wong, A.H.C., Smith, M., and Boon, H.S., Herbal remedies in psychiatric practice, *Gen. Psychiatry* 55: 1033–1044, 1998.
14. World Health Organization, *Folium Ginkgo, WHO Monographs on Selected Plants* 1: 154–167, 9 A.D.
15. Maurer, K., Ihl, R., Dierks, T., and Frolich, L., Clinical efficacy of Ginkgo biloba special extract EGb 761 in dementia of the Alzheimer type. *J. Psychiatr. Res.* 31: 645–655, 1997.
16. Le Bars, P.L., Katz, M.M., Berman, N., Itil, T.M., Freedman, A.M., and Schatzberg, A.F., A placebo-controlled, double-blind, randomized trial of an extract of Ginkgo biloba for dementia, North American EGb Study Group [see comments], *JAMA* 278: 1327–1332, 1997.
17. Kanowski, S., Herrmann, W.M., Stephan, K., Wierich, W., and Horr, R., Proof of efficacy of the ginkgo biloba special extract EGb 761 in outpatients suffering from mild to moderate primary degenerative dementia of the Alzheimer type or multi-infarct dementia, *Pharmacopsychiatry.* 29: 47–56, 1996.
18. Oken, B.S., Storzbach, D.M., and Kaye, J.A., The efficacy of *Ginkgo biloba* on cognitive function in Alzheimer disease, *Arch. Neurol.* 55: 1409–1415, 1998.
19. Jiang, X., Williams, K.M., Liauw, W.S., Ammit, A.J., Roufogalis, B.D., Duke, C.C., Day, R.O., and McLachlan, A.J., Effect of ginkgo and ginger on the pharmacokinetics and pharmacodynamics of warfarin in healthy subjects, *Br. J. Clin. Pharmacol.* 59: 425–432, 2005.
20. Kohler, S., Funk, P., and Kieser, M., Influence of a 7-day treatment with Ginkgo biloba special extract EGb 761 on bleeding time and coagulation: a randomized, placebo-controlled, double-blind study in healthy volunteers, *Blood Coagul. Fibrinolysis.* 15: 303–309, 2004.

21. Miller, L.G., Herbal medicinals: selected clinical considerations focusing on known or potential drug-herb interactions, *Arch. Intern. Med.* 158: 2200–2211, 1998.

22. O'Hara, M.A., Kiefer, D., Farrell, K., and Kemper, K., A review of 12 commonly used medicinal herbs, *Arch. Fam. Med.* 7: 523–526, 1998.

23. Fava, M., Alpert, J., Nierenberg, A.A., Mischoulon, D., Otto, M.W., Zajecka, J., Murck, H., and Rosenbaum, J.F., A Double-blind, randomized trial of St John's wort, fluoxetine, and placebo in major depressive disorder, *J. Clin. Psychopharmacol.* 25: 441–447, 2005.

24. Szegedi, A., Kohnen, R., Dienel, A., and Kieser, M., Acute treatment of moderate to severe depression with hypericum extract WS 5570 (St John's wort): randomised controlled double blind non-inferiority trial versus paroxetine, *Br. Med. J.* 330: 503, 2005.

25. Shelton, R.C., Keller, M.B., Gelenberg, A., Dunner, D.L., Hirschfeld, R., Thase, M.E., Russell, J., Lydiard, R.B., Crits-Cristoph, P., Gallop, R., Todd, L., Hellerstein, D., Goodnick, P., Keitner, G., Stahl, S.M., and Halbreich, U., Effectiveness of St John's wort in major depression: a randomized controlled trial, *JAMA* 285: 1978–1986, 2001.

26. Linde, K., Ramirez, G., Mulrow, C., Pauls, A., Weidenhammer, W., and Melchart, D., St. John's wort for depression — an overview and meta-analysis of randomized clinical trials, *Br. Med. J.* 313: 253–258, 1996.

27. Volz, H.-P., Controlled clinical trials of hypericum extracts in depressed patients: an overview, *Pharmacopsychiatry* 30: 72–76, 1997.

28. James, J.S., St. John's wort warning: do not combine with protease inhibitors, NNRTIs, *AIDS Treat. News.* 3–5, 2000.

29. Piscitelli, S.C., Burstein, A.H., Chaitt, D., Alfaro, R.M., and Falloon, J., Indinavir concentrations and St John's wort, *Lancet.* 355: 547–548, 2000.

30. Rey, J.M. and Wlater, G., Hypericum perforatum (St. John's wort) in depression: pest or blessing? *Med. J. Aust.* 169: 583–586, 1998.

31. Hu, L., Jhoo, J.W., Ang, C.Y., Dinovi, M., and Mattia, A., Determination of six kavalactones in dietary supplements and selected functional foods containing Piper methysticum by isocratic liquid chromatography with internal standard, *J. AOAC Int.* 88: 16–25, 2005.

32. Witte, S., Loew, D., and Gaus, W., Meta-analysis of the efficacy of the acetonic kava-kava extract WS1490 in patients with non-psychotic anxiety disorders, *Phytother. Res.* 19: 183–188, 2005.

33. Pittler, M.H. and Ernst, E., Kava extract for treating anxiety, *Cochrane. Database. Syst. Rev.* CD003383, 2003.

34. Volz, H.-P. and Kieser, M., Kava-kava extract WS1490 versus placebo in anxiety disorders — a randomized, placebo-controlled, 25-week outpatient trial, *Pharmacopsychiatry* 30: 1–5, 1997.

35. Stevinson, C., Huntley, A., and Ernst, E., A systematic review of the safety of kava extract in the treatment of anxiety, *Drug Saf.* 25: 251–261, 2002.

36. Clouatre, D.L., Kava kava: examining new reports of toxicity, *Toxicol. Lett.* 150: 85–96, 2004.

37. Leathwood, P.D., Chauffard, F., Heck, E., and Munoz-Box, R., Aqueous extract of valerian root improves sleep quality in man, *Pharmacol. Biochem. Behav.* 17: 65–71, 1982.

38. Diaper, A. and Hindmarch, I., A double-blind, placebo-controlled investigation of the effects of two doses of a valerian preparation on the sleep, cognitive and psychomotor function of sleep-disturbed older adults, *Phytother. Res.* 18: 831–836, 2004.

39. Gutierrez, S., Ang-Lee, M.K., Walker, D.J., and Zacny, J.P., Assessing subjective and psychomotor effects of the herbal medication valerian in healthy volunteers, *Pharmacol. Biochem. Behav.* 78: 57–64, 2004.

40. Ziegler, G., Ploch, M., Miettinen-Baumann, A., and Collet, W., Efficacy and tolerability of valerian extract LI 156 compared with oxazepam in the treatment of non-organic insomnia — a randomized, double-blind, comparative clinical study, *Eur. J. Med. Res.* 7: 480–486, 2002.

41. Heiligenstein, E. and Guenther, G., Over-the-counter psychotropics: a review of melatonin, St. John's wort, valerian, and kava-kava, *J. Am. Coll. Health* 46: 271–276, 1998.

42. al-Makdessi, S., Sweidan, H., Dietz, K., and Jacob, R., Protective effect of *Crataegus oxyacantha* against reperfusion arrhythmias after global no-flow ischemia in the rat heart, *Basic Res. Cardiol.* 94: 71–77, 1999.

43. al-Makdessi, S., Sweidan, H., Mullner, S., and Jacob, R., Myocardial protection by pretreatment with *Crataegus oxycantha*: an assessment by means of the release of lactate dehydrogenase by the ischemic and reperfused Langendorff heart, *Arzneimittelforschung* 46: 25–27, 1999.

44. Shanthi, S., Parasakthy, K., Deepalakshmi, P.D., and Devarag, S.J., Hypolipidemic activity of tincture of Crataegyus in rats. *Indian J. Biochem. Biophys.* 31: 143–146, 1994.

45. Rajendran, S., Deepalakshmi, P.D., Parasakthy, K., Devaraj, H., and Devaraj, S.N., Effect of tincture of *Crataegus* on the LDL-receptor activity of hepatic plasma membrane of rats fed an atherogenic diet. *Athersclerosis* 123: 235–241, 1996.

46. Melchart, D., Linde, K., Worku, F., Sarkady, L., Holzmann, M., Jurcic, K., and Wagner, H., Results of five randomized studies on the immunomodulatory activity of preparations of Echinacea, *J. Alt. Comp. Med* 1: 145–160, 1995.

47. Melchart, D., Walther, E., Linde, K., Brandmaier, R., and Lersch, C., Echinacea root extracts for the prevention of upper respiratory tract infections: a double-blind, placebo controlled randomized trial, *Arch. Fam. Med.* 7: 541–545, 1998.

48. Grimm, W. and Muller, H.-H., A randomized controlled trial of the effect of fluid extract of *Echinacea purpurea* on the incidence and severity of colds and respiratory infections, *Am. J. Med.* 106: 138–143, 1999.

49. Yale, S.H. and Liu, K., Echinacea purpurea therapy for the treatment of the common cold: a randomized, double-blind, placebo-controlled clinical trial, *Arch. Intern. Med.* 164: 1237–1241, 2004.

50. Sperber, S.J., Shah, L.P., Gilbert, R.D., Ritchey, T.W., and Monto, A.S., Echinacea purpurea for prevention of experimental rhinovirus colds, *Clin. Infect. Dis.* 38: 1367–1371, 2004.

51. Turner, R.B., Bauer, R., Woelkart, K., Hulsey, T.C., and Gangemi, J.D., An evaluation of Echinacea angustifolia in experimental rhinovirus infections, *N. Engl. J. Med.* 353: 341–348, 2005.

52. Taylor, J.A., Weber, W., Standish, L., Quinn, H., Goesling, J., McGann, M., and Calabrese, C., Efficacy and safety of echinacea in treating upper respiratory tract infections in children: a randomized controlled trial, *JAMA.* 290: 2824–2830, 2003.

53. Barrett, B.P., Brown, R.L., Locken, K., Maberry, R., Bobula, J.A., and D'Alessio, D., Treatment of the common cold with unrefined echinacea: a randomized, double-blind, placebo-controlled trial, *Ann. Intern. Med.* 137: 939–946, 2002.

54. Pittler, M.H. and Ernst, E., Peppermint oil for irritable bowel syndrome: a critical review and meta-analysis, *Am. J. Gastroenterol.* 93: 1131–1135, 1998.

55. Hiki, N., Kurosaka, H., Tatsutomi, Y., Shimoyama, S., Tsuji, E., Kojima, J., Shimizu, N., Ono, H., Hirooka, T., Noguchi, C., Mafune, K., and Kaminishi, M., Peppermint oil reduces gastric spasm during upper endoscopy: a randomized, double-blind, double-dummy controlled trial, *Gastrointest. Endosc.* 57: 475–482, 2003.

56. Phillips, S., Ruggier, R., and Hutchinson, S.E., Zingiber officinale (ginger) — an antiemetic for day case surgery [see comments], *Anaesthesia* 48: 715–717, 1993.

57. Micklefield, G.H., Redeker, Y., Meister, V., Jung, O., Greving, I., and May, B., Effects of ginger on gastroduodenal motility, *Int. J. Clin. Pharmacol. Ther.* 37: 341–346, 1999.

58. Phillips, S., Hutchinson, S., and Ruggier, R., Zingiber officinale does not affect gastric emptying rate: a randomized, placebo-controlled, crossover trial [see comments], *Anaesthesia* 48: 393–395, 1993.

59. Stewart, J.J., Wood, M.J., Wood, C.D., and Mims, M.E., Effects of ginger on motion sickness susceptibility and gastric function, *Pharmacology* 42: 111–120, 1991.

60. Grontved, A., Brask, T., Kambskard, J., and Hentzer, E., Ginger root against seasickness: a controlled trial on the open sea, *Acta Otolaryngol. (Stockh.)* 105: 45–49, 1988.

61. Gruenwald, J., Brendler, T., and Jaenicke, C.E., *PDR for Herbal Medicines*, Medical Economics Company, Montvale, NJ, 1998.

62. Serra, A., Uehlinger, D.E., Ferrari, P., Dick, B., Frey, B.M., Frey, F.J., and Vogt, B., Glycyrrhetinic acid decreases plasma potassium concentrations in patients with anuria, *J. Am. Soc. Nephrol.* 13: 191–196, 2002.

63. Fleet, J.C., New support for a folk remedy: cranberry juice reduces bacteriuria and pyuria in elderly women, *Nutr. Rev.* 52: 168–170, 1994.

64. Avorn, J., Monane, M., Gurwitz, J.H., Glynn, R.J., Choodnovskiy, I., and Lipsitz, L.A., Reduction of bacteriuria and pyuria after ingestion of cranberry juice [see comments], *JAMA* 271: 751–754, 1994.

65. Jepson, R.G., Mihaljevic, L., and Craig, J., Cranberries for preventing urinary tract infections, *Cochrane Database Syst. Rev.* CD001321, 2004.

66. Gettman, M.T., Ogan, K., Brinkley, L.J., Adams-Huet, B., Pak, C.Y., and Pearle, M.S., Effect of cranberry juice consumption on urinary stone risk factors, *J. Urol.* 174: 590–594, 2005.

67. Crews, W.D., Jr., Harrison, D.W., Griffin, M.L., Addison, K., Yount, A.M., Giovenco, M.A., and Hazell, J., A double-blinded, placebo-controlled, randomized trial of the neuropsychologic efficacy of cranberry juice in a sample of cognitively intact older adults: pilot study findings, *J. Altern. Complement Med.* 11: 305–309, 2005.

68. Zhang, L., Ma, J., Pan, K., Go, V.L., Chen, J., and You, W.C., Efficacy of cranberry juice on *Helicobacter pylori* infection: a double-blind, randomized placebo-controlled trial, *Helicobacter.* 10: 139–145, 2005.

69. Wilt, T.J., Ishani, A., Stark, G., MacDonald, R., Lau, J., and Mulrow, C., Saw palmetto extracts for treatment of benign prostatic hyperplasia, *JAMA* 280: 1604–1609, 1998.

70. Boyle, P., Robertson, C., Lowe, F., and Roehrborn, C., Updated meta-analysis of clinical trials of Serenoa repens extract in the treatment of symptomatic benign prostatic hyperplasia, *BJU. Int.* 93: 751–756, 2004.

71. Boyle, P., Robertson, C., Lowe, F., and Roehrborn, C., Meta-analysis of clinical trials of permixon in the treatment of symptomatic benign prostatic hyperplasia, *Urology.* 55: 533–539, 2000.

72. Chatelain, C., Autet, W., and Brackman, F., Comparison of once and twice daily dosage forms of Pygeum africanum extract in patients with benign prostatic hyperplasia: a randomized, double-blind study, with long-term open label extension, *Urology.* 54: 473–478, 1999.

73. Krzeski, T., Kazon, M., Borkowski, A., Witeska, A., and Kuczera, J., Combined extracts of Urtica dioica and Pygeum africanum in the treatment of benign prostatic hyperplasia: double-blind comparison of two doses, *Clin. Ther.* 15: 1011–1020, 1993.

74. Bennett, B.C. and Hicklin, J.R., Uses of saw palmetto (*Serenoa repens*, Arecaceae) in Florida, *Econ. Bot.* 52: 381–393, 1998.

75. Barsby, R.W., Salan, U., Knight, D.W., and Hoult, J.R., Feverfew and vascular smooth muscle: extracts from fresh and dried plants show opposing pharmacological profiles, dependent upon sesquiterpene lactone content, *Planta Med.* 59: 20–25, 1993.

76. Johnson, E.S., Kadam, N.P., Hylands, D.M., and Hylands, P.J., Efficacy of feverfew as prophylactic treatment of migraine, *Br. Med. J. (Clin. Res. Ed.)* 291: 569–573, 1985.

77. Murphy, J.J., Heptinstall, S., and Mitchell, J.R., Randomized double-blind placebo-controlled trial of feverfew in migraine prevention, *Lancet* 2: 189–192, 1988.

78. Sumner, H., Salan, U., Knight, D.W., and Hoult, J.R., Inhibition of 5-lipoxygenase and cyclo-oxygenase in leukocytes by feverfew, Involvement of sesquiterpene lactones and other components, *Biochem. Pharmacol.* 43: 2313–2320, 1992.

79. Vogler, B.K., Pittler, M.H., and Ernst, E., Feverfew as a preventive treatment for migraine: a systematic review, *Cephalalgia.* 18: 704–708, 1998.

80. Diener, H.C., Pfaffenrath, V., Schnitker, J., Friede, M., and Henneicke-von Zepelin, H.H., Efficacy and safety of 6.25 mg t.i.d. feverfew CO2-extract (MIG-99) in migraine prevention — a randomized, double-blind, multicentre, placebo-controlled study, *Cephalalgia.* 25: 1031–1041, 2005.

81. Pfaffenrath, V., Diener, H.C., Fischer, M., Friede, M., and Henneicke-von Zepelin, H.H., The efficacy and safety of Tanacetum parthenium (feverfew) in migraine prophylaxis — a double-blind, multicentre, randomized placebo-controlled dose-response study, *Cephalalgia.* 22: 523–532, 2002.

14 Conjugated Linoleic Acids: Biological Actions and Health

Yong Li and Bruce A. Watkins

CONTENTS

I. INTRODUCTION

Research on conjugated linoleic acid (CLA) continues to be of interest to nutritionists because of the potential biological actions of this group of dietary fatty acids. In our previous chapter, we comprehensively reviewed the numerous reported chemical, biochemical, molecular, and physiological properties of CLA.[1] Attention to the characterization of CLA isomers in food sources and investigations of their beneficial properties to reduce factors associated with cancer, cardiovascular diseases, and reducing body fat were of historical significance in the research on these fatty acids.[1,2] Although intriguing, the immediate focus of studies on CLA should be directed at demonstrating how specific isomers work on biological targets, their intrinsic value to human nutrition, and their impact on diet-related chronic diseases.[3,4]

As the relationship between dietary fat and human health continues to be explored as a chief research emphasis, to advance the understanding of nutrition for making recommendations to improve the human condition, CLA will be a part of this activity. In 2002, the report from the Institute of Medicine of the National Academies on Dietary Reference Intakes (DRIs) set forth new recommended levels for fat and individual fatty acids; however, no guidelines were provided for CLA. The DRIs establish an Adequate Intake (AI) of linoleic acid level at 17 g/d for young men and 12 g/d for young women in the U.S.[5,6] Though no DRIs are recommended for saturated fat and trans fatty acids because of their perceived adverse effects on health, the tolerable Upper Intake Levels (UL) were not set for these fatty acids because of practical issues. At this time, CLA isomers are a part of the fat component of a normal diet and are perceived as having a health benefit, but research has yet to associate a direct health benefit of these fatty acids.

CLA represents a family of fatty acids comprised of positional and geometric fatty acid isomers of octadecadienoic acid. The CLA isomers are reported to have antioxidant and anti-inflammatory properties. These chemical and biological actions have been investigated in various cell culture and animal models for cancer, atherosclerosis, bone metabolism, and fat metabolism. Some of the reported cellular effects include inducing apoptosis and cytotoxic activity, modulating fatty acid composition and prostanoid formation, and influencing the expression and action of cytokines and growth factors.[1] Though several actions of CLA have been reported, the most consistent findings include anticancer effects in rodents and cancer cells, and reducing body fat content in growing animals. In some cases, the biological responses observed from CLA isomers in animal models were influenced by the amounts of dietary n-6 and n-3 polyunsaturated fatty acids present (PUFA).[7–9] The purpose of this chapter is to present the recent published findings describing the actions of CLA in cell culture experiments and human studies.

II. ABSORPTION, METABOLISM, AND BODY WEIGHT

A. ABSORPTION

The level of CLA intake is closely associated with the concentrations in blood and certain tissues as found in animal and human studies.[1–4] Recently, Burdge et al. reported that the level of CLA intake for 8 weeks, followed by a 6-week washout period, is a major determinant of plasma and peripheral blood mononuclear cell (PBMC) concentrations.[10] The PBMC appear to incorporate both c9,t11 and t10,c12 CLA in healthy male subjects after consuming one, two, and four capsules containing about 600 mg of either c9,t11 or t10,c12 CLA per capsule.

Fernie et al. found that CLA administered in the triacylglycerol form in a study that evaluated triacylglycerols, free fatty acids, or fatty acid ethyl esters was the most suitable for incorporation into a food delivery system to optimize absorption and that the c9,t11 and t10,c12 isomers are absorbed similarly into chylomicrons in human subjects.[11] Even though the free acid form was absorbed into chylomicrons to the same extent as the triacylglycerol form, most subjects reported that the fatty acid formulation had poor taste characteristics.

Jewell et al. found that the overall transepithelial Ca transport as well as transcellular and paracellular Ca transport were significantly increased (P < 0.001) by exposure of Caco-2 cells to two isomers (18:2 c9,t11 or t10,c12) of CLA.[12] This effect appeared to be related to altered localization of zona occludens 1 (a tight junction protein).

B. LIPID METABOLISM

An important aspect of CLA actions is its potential effect on essential fatty acid desaturation leading to the long-chain PUFA which occurs to a great extent in liver tissue. Slomma et al. observed that the t10,c12 CLA isomer at 25 μM suppressed the $\Delta4$-desaturation process in HepG2 cells.[13] This step would result in potentially reduced long-chain production of essential fatty acids.

The effects of CLA on body fat and adipose tissue metabolism has been of great interest to nutritionists as the finding that these fatty acid isomers reduced fat content and altered body composition in growing animals. Granlund et al. reported that the t10,c12 CLA isomer inhibited lipid accumulation during adipocyte differentiation, and this effect was dependent on the stage of cell maturation and length of fatty acid treatment.[14] The inhibition of lipid accumulation by t10,c12 CLA treatment during adipocyte differentiation was associated with a tight regulatory cross-talk between early (PPARγ and C/EBPα) and late (LXRα, aP2 and CD36) adipogenic transcription factors and their marker genes.

The effect of CLA isomers on blood lipids has received some attention in an attempt to understand their role in controlling the development of atherosclerosis and body fat content. Pal et al. showed that apoB100 secretion was significantly decreased in HepG2 liver cells by treatment with 50 μM CLA (a blend of c9,t11 and t10,c12 isomers) treatment for 24 h.[15] A reduction in apoB100 production in the body would decrease the levels of VLDL and atherogenic LDL and thus reduce the risk of developing cardiovascular disease. Storkson et al. showed in HepG2 cells that the reduction of apoB secretion by a CLA mixture was a result of the unique structural features of the t10,c12 CLA isomer.[16] A trans double bond at the 10th position appeared to be a key feature in the molecular structure involved in the inhibition of apoB secretion.

Acting as a potential dietary factor in controlling body fat, the effect of CLA has also been investigated on insulin resistance. Chung et al. showed that CLA promoted insulin resistance through an NFκB-dependent pathway in human adipocytes; that is, the t10,c12 CLA isomer promoted NFκB activation and subsequent induction of IL-6, which are, at least in part, responsible for the t10,c12 CLA-mediated suppression of PPARγ target gene expression and insulin sensitivity in mature human adipocytes.[17]

Although many recent findings at the cellular and molecular levels suggest that CLA has a role in fat metabolism, it is important to demonstrate these effects *in vivo*. An appropriate response of fat loss in the human, or elucidation of the conditions for controlling body fat with CLA, is needed before application to food systems and dietary recommendations should be made.

C. Body Weight and Composition

The early literature on CLA described numerous experiments that showed a significant effect of dietary CLA mixtures on reducing body fat in growing animals.[1–4] In human studies where CLA supplements were given to adult subjects, the results were mixed, some with body weight loss and some body fat loss.[3,4]

After observing 81 middle aged, overweight healthy men and women consuming a daily dose of a drinkable dairy product containing up to 3 g of CLA isomers for 18 weeks, Malpuech-Brugere et al. concluded that there was no statistically significant effect on body composition in these subjects.[18] In another study, Desroches et al. reported that a 10-fold CLA enrichment of butter fat (4.22 g CLA/100 g butter fat) did not induce beneficial metabolic effects in overweight or obese men when compared to a control butter that was low in CLA (0.38 g CLA/100 g butter fat).[19] This study was conducted over a 4-week period utilizing a crossover design involving 16 men.

In contrast, Gaullier et al. found that long-term (1 yr) supplementation with CLA-FFA (CLA free fatty acid) or CLA-triacylglycerol reduced body fat mass in 180 healthy overweight adults in a double-blind, placebo-controlled study.[20] Riserus et al. reported that CLA (either a mix of isomers or t10,c12) might slightly decrease body fat in humans, particularly abdominal fat, but there was no effect on body weight or body mass index.[21] Gaullier et al. observed that CLA supplementation (a mixture of c9,t11 and t10,c12 at a ratio of 1:1, soft gel from Natural Lipids) for 24 months in healthy, overweight adults was well tolerated.[22] In this study, CLA decreased body fat mass in overweight humans (6 to 8% loss of body fat mass) compared to baseline values. A total of 134 subjects (24 men and 110 women) were enrolled in this study.

III. HEALTH ASPECTS

A. Blood Lipids

The effect of CLA isomeric mixtures on blood lipids continues to be an active area of discovery, but the research is not consistent in the human.[4] Thijssen et al. found that incorporation of both the c9,t11 and t10,c12 CLA isomers into plasma lipids reflects dietary intakes after giving healthy, overweight men and women a daily dose of 3 g of purified c9,t11 CLA or t10,c12 CLA in a drinkable dairy product for six weeks.[23] They also found that the Δ9 and Δ6 desaturation indices, based on product substrate ratios [18:1n-9/18:0 and (18:3n-6 + 20:3n-6)/18:2n-6] in plasma phospholipids, were decreased after consumption of c9,t11 or t10,c12 CLA, compared with oleic acid.

Tricon et al. observed divergent effects of c9,t11 CLA and t10,c12 CLA on blood lipid profiles in healthy male volunteers (aged 20 to 47 years).[24] The t10,c12 CLA isomer led to increased ratios of LDL cholesterol:HDL cholesterol and total cholesterol:HDL cholesterol, whereas the c9,t11 CLA isomer decreased both ratios. This study evaluated supplemented doses of highly enriched c9,t11 (0.59, 1.19, and 2.38 g/d) or t10,c12 (0.63, 1.26, and 2.52 g/d) CLA preparations administered for consecutive 8-week periods in a crossover design with a 6-week washout period in between.

Burdge et al. reported that selective assimilation of individual CLA isomers occurs in erythrocyte lipids and so does partial substitution for specific saturated and PUFA when healthy men (31 ± 8 years) consumed 1, 2, and 4 capsules containing approximately 80 g/100 g of either c9,t11 CLA or t10,c12 CLA for sequential 8-week periods.[25] The increase in the c9,t11 CLA concentration (0.31 g/100 g) was significantly greater than that of the t10,c12 CLA (0.19 g/100 g) in erythrocyte total lipids.

Herrera et al. found that CLA (450 mg/d), when given together with calcium (600 mg/d) to pregnant women who are at high risk for pregnancy-induced hypertension (PIH), decreased the incidence of PIH (8% in the study group vs. 42% in the placebo group, p = 0.1) and improved endothelial function in a randomized, double-blind, placebo-controlled trial.[26]

B. Cancer

As the first potential health benefit of CLA was an anticancer activity found in an animal model and extended to human cell cultures, the research continues to explain the extent of this outcome and exploit the application of CLA supplements to the human. Maggiora et al. commented in a review article that CLA may be regarded as a component of the diet that exerts antineoplastic activity, and its effect may be antiproliferative or proapoptotic.[27] The actions of CLA may be mediated, in part, through PPARs.

Kim et al. reported that treating mouse mammary tumor cell cultures with t10,c12 CLA reduced tumor cell growth, and the action of CLA may involve the suppression of the 5-lipoxygenase metabolite, 5-HETE, with subsequent effects on apoptosis and cell proliferation.[28] This effect was not observed with the c9,t11 CLA isomer or linoleic acid and may be specific to the different isomers of CLA. Yamasaki et al. also showed that the t10,c12 CLA isomer induced significant cytotoxic effects upon mitochondria-related apoptosis and lysosomal destabilization in rat hepatoma cells.[29]

Lim et al. showed that treating the HT-29 human colon carcinoma cell line with physiological concentrations of CLA (nondefined isomeric mixture, 0 to 20 μM) inhibited cancer cell growth of either the wild-type or mutant p53 and may have therapeutic benefits in vivo.[30] Lampen et al. reported that the c9,t11 CLA isomer had an antiproliferative effect at the cellular and molecular levels in human HT-29 and Caco-2 colon cells.[31] These results suggest that the anticancer effect of CLA in the development of colon cancer may be due to its downregulation of some target genes of the APC-beta-catenin-TCF-4 and PPARδ signaling pathways.

Albright et al. tested CLA isomers (c9,t11 and t10,c12) on human MCF-7 cells that were derived from a well-differentiated mammary adenocarcinoma and found that CLA (mixed isomers of c9, t11 and t10,c12) increased their sensitivity to oxidative stress and activation of p53 in these cell cultures, indicating a potential mechanism in the regulation of human breast cancer cell proliferation.[32] Other effects on cancer cell death include those reported by Bergamo et al.[33] This group found that CLA (from an organic butter containing 10.2 ± 0.5 mg c9,t11 CLA/100 g fat) increased apoptosis and IL-2 synthesis in human lymphoblastic Jurkat T-cells.

Ohtsu et al. used a mixture of CLA isomers (in free fatty acid form, containing 41% of c9,t11, 44% of t10,c12, 10% of c10,c12, and 5% of t9,t11 + t10,t12 + c9,c11 isomers) and found inhibition of cellular proliferation of androgen-independent PC3 prostate carcinoma cells in a dose-dependent manner.[34] The isomeric mixture also inhibited constitutive activation of NFκB and AP1 transcription factors in these cell cultures. Another study in prostate cancer cells conducted by Song et al. showed that CLA isomers (individual c9,t11 and t10,c12, and a 50:50 mixture of both) modulated the abundance of the PKC isoforms in LNCaP human prostate cancer cells, indicating a potential antitumor mechanism of action.[35]

Human breast cancer has also been a focus for the anticancer research on CLA isomers. Kim et al. reported that the t10,c12 CLA isomer reduced 5-hydroxyeicosatetraenoic acid (5-HETE) by competition with arachidonic acid and reduced the 5-lipoxygenase activating protein (FLAP) expression in MDA-MB-231 human breast tumor cells.[36] Liu and Sidell showed that the antiestrogenic activity of CLA (50% c9,t11; 40% t10,c12; 10% c10,c12) is caused by inducing the dephosphorylation of the estrogen receptor (ER) alpha through stimulation of protein phosphatase 2A (PP2A) activity in MCF-7 human breast cancer cells.[37] A study by Degner et al. showed that CLA (an isomeric mixture or selected isomers c9,t11 or t10,c12) attenuated cyclooxygenase-2 transcriptional activity via an anti-AP-1 mechanism in MCF-7 breast cancer cells.[38]

Yamasaki et al. evaluated the isomeric-specific cytotoxic effects of CLA on rat hepatoma dRLh-84 cells.[39] The researchers found a significant cytotoxic effect of the t10,c12 CLA isomer detected after only a 1.5-min incubation, and the most noticeable effect was seen after 3 h in culture at concentrations from 5 to 10 μM of this isomer.

Cimini et al. demonstrated that CLA and the PPARγ agonist GW347845X strongly inhibited cell growth and proliferation rate and induced apoptosis.[40] Both treatments (CLA and PPARγ agonist) also decreased cell migration and invasiveness. Lui et al. showed that CLA might exert its growth-inhibitory effects on murine myeloid leukemia WEHI-3B JCS cells by triggering their terminal differentiation, which is mediated, at least in part, by modulating cytokine gene expression of TNFα, IL-1 and IFNγ in leukemia cells.[41]

Larsson et al. reported that increased intakes of high-fat dairy foods that contain CLA may reduce the risk of colorectal cancer.[42] They examined long-term high-fat dairy food consumption and CLA intake on the incidence of colorectal cancer in a population consisting of 60,708 women aged 40 to 76 years who participated in the Swedish Mammography Cohort. They found in this study that each increment of two servings of high-fat dairy foods per day (whole milk, full-fat cultured milk, cheese, cream, sour cream, and butter) corresponded to a 13% reduction in the risk of colorectal cancer in the study population.

C. INFLAMMATION AND IMMUNE FUNCTION

The research on CLA has included some studies that examined the actions of these isomers on targets of inflammation including cytokines and prostanoids in immunocompetent cells, animal models, and human subjects.[1,4] Loscher et al. demonstrated that the c9,t11 CLA isomer enhanced transcription and production of the anti-inflammatory cytokine IL-10 while inhibiting the Th1-promoting cytokine IL-12, which may explain certain aspects of its immunosuppressive properties.[43] In contrast, Jaudszus et al. showed that the c9,t11 isomer exerted stronger anti-inflammatory effects in human bronchial epithelial cells and eosinophils compared to the t10,c12 CLA isomer and to linoleic acid.[44]

Ramakers et al. reported that daily consumption of 3 g of c9,t11 or t10,cl2 CLA isomers did not affect LPS-stimulated cytokine production by peripheral mononuclear cells and whole blood, and plasma C-reactive protein levels.[45] The inflammatory signatures in fasted, nonstimulated plasma as determined by an antibody array indicated enhanced immune function by both CLA isomers in these subjects. In another human study, Nugent et al. showed that CLA supplementation at 2 g/d had a minimal effect on the markers of human immune function.[46] Furthermore, supplementation with CLA had no immunological benefit compared with linoleic acid in a double-blind, randomized, placebo-controlled intervention trial involving a total of 55 healthy volunteers (20 male and 35 female subjects). Tricon et al. evaluated the effects of c9,t11 and t10,c12 CLA [3 doses of highly enriched c9,t11 CLA (0.59, 1.19, and 2.38 g/d) or t10,c12 CLA (0.63, 1.26, and 2.52 g/d)] isomers for 8 weeks on immune cell function in healthy human subjects following a randomized, double-blind, crossover design.[47] They found that CLA supplementation resulted in a dose-dependent reduction in the mitogen-induced activation of T lymphocytes. The effects of c9,t11 and t10,c12 CLA isomers were similar, and there was a negative correlation between mitogen-induced T lymphocyte activation and both the c9,t11 and t10,c12 CLA contents of mononuclear cells. In another CLA study with human subjects, Song et al. reported that supplementing CLA at 3 g (50:50 mixture of the 2 major isomers c9,t11 and t10,c12) per d for 12 weeks had a potentially beneficial effect on controlling immune function by decreasing the levels of the proinflammatory cytokines, TNFα and IL-1, while increasing the levels of the anti-inflammatory cytokine, IL-10, in young healthy volunteers in a double-blind, randomized, reference-controlled study.[48]

The research on many dietary factors that appear to modulate immune function is of importance for understanding mechanisms for controlling chronic inflammation related to disease. It will be critical to elucidate a clear mechanism of action for the various isomers of CLA on this process because it will have an impact on controlling diet-related chronic disease and aging.

D. BONE AND JOINT

Some research with CLA isomers has been conducted on bone metabolism and bone loss using rodents and cell cultures. In human chondrocytes, Shen et al. showed that CLA (39.1% c9,t11/t9,c11; 40.7% t10,c12; 1.8% c9,c11; 1.3% c10,c12; 1.9% t9,t11/t10,t12; 1.1% c9,c12; and 14.1% other isomers) alone or in combination with PUFA (AA, EPA, and linoleic acid) decreased prostaglandin E_2 and nitric oxide production in human osteoarthritic chondrocytes cultures.[49] These results might suggest that the 18:2 CLA isomers may have the potential to influence osteoarthritis pathogenesis by modulating inflammatory factors. Cusack et al. reported that CLA (either as pure c9,t11 and t10,c12 or a blend of these two isomers) did not show any cytotoxic effect on human osteoblast-like cell lines (SaOS2 and MG63), and this could suggest a potential action that may be beneficial to bone formation.[50]

Doyle et al. reported that daily supplementation with CLA [3.0 g CLA isomeric blend (50:50% c9,t11: t10,c12 isomers as a triacylglycerol)] or placebo (a palm or bean oil blend) for 8 weeks had no significant effect on markers of bone formation (serum osteocalcin and bone-specific alkaline phosphatase), bone resorption (serum C-telopeptide-related fraction of type 1 collagen degradation products, urinary N-telopeptide-related fraction of type 1 collagen degradation products, urinary pyridinoline and deoxypyridinoline), or on serum or urinary calcium levels in a double-blind, placebo-controlled trial with 60 healthy adult males (aged 39 to 64 years).[51] However, Brownbill et al. showed that dietary CLA was positively correlated with Ward's triangle bone mineral density (P = 0.04) in a multiple regression model in a cross-sectional analysis of 136 Caucasian, healthy, postmenopausal women, with a mean age of 68.6 years.[52]

E. DIABETES

Eyjolfson et al. reported that giving a common dosage of a commercially available CLA supplement (4 g/d of a mixed CLA isomeric blend containing 35.5% c9,t11 and 36.8% t10,c12) improved insulin sensitivity index in 16 young, sedentary individuals (12 females and 4 males) after 8 weeks, compared to the placebo control group.[53] However, Riserus et al. found that supplementing 3.4 g of the t10,c12 CLA isomer to nondiabetic abdominally obese men for 12 weeks induced hyper-proinsulinaemia that is related to impaired insulin sensitivity, independent of changes in insulin concentrations.[54] These results are of clinical interest, as hyperproinsulinaemia predicts diabetes and cardiovascular disease in this randomized double-blind study. Moloney et al. observed that supplementing CLA (3.0 g/d; 50:50 blend of c9,t11 and t10,c12 CLA) to subjects with stable, diet-controlled type 2 diabetes for 8 weeks significantly increased fasting glucose concentrations (6.3%; $P < 0.05$) and reduced insulin sensitivity as measured by a homeostasis model assessment, oral glucose insulin sensitivity, and the insulin sensitivity index (composite) ($P = 0.05$).[55] This investigation followed a randomized, double-blind, placebo-controlled design. Although some data appear promising for CLA in diabetes, the results of a few trials are inconclusive and may be specific to the physiological state and the age of the subjects studied.

F. CLA Adverse Effects

Several questions have been raised regarding the safety of CLA preparations for use as supplements that are derived from chemical isomerized vegetable oils. Other issues have evolved from studies that utilized large amounts of specific isomers of CLA. For example, Riserus et al. reported that CLA supplementation to humans did not provide improvement in lipid or glucose metabolism.[54] Rather, the t10,c12 CLA isomer caused significant impairment of peripheral insulin sensitivity as well as blood glucose and serum lipid concentrations. At the same time, CLA significantly elevated lipid peroxidation. In another study, Riserus et al. evaluated a CLA preparation containing the purified c9,t11 CLA isomer and reported increased insulin resistance and lipid peroxidation in subjects compared with the placebo group in 25 abdominally obese men that received 3 g of c9,t11 CLA/d or placebo (olive oil).[56] Compared with the placebo, the c9,t11 CLA decreased insulin sensitivity by 15% ($P < 0.05$) and increased 8-iso-prostaglandin $F_{2\alpha}$ and 15-keto-dihydroprostaglandin $F_{2\alpha}$ excretion by 50% ($P < 0.01$) and 15% ($P < 0.05$), respectively.

Taylor et al. reported that a CLA isomeric mixture had at most modest effects on adiposity and worsened endothelial function as brachial artery flow-mediated dilatation declined (-1.3%, $P = 0.013$) and plasma F_2-isoprostanes increased ($+91$ pg/mL, $P = 0.042$) significantly in a 12-week double-blind study involving 40 healthy volunteers with BMI > 27 kg/m.[57] On the basis of these results, the authors do not recommend the use of the isomeric mixtures of CLA as an aid to weight loss.

Smedman et al. reported that 4.2 g/d of the isomers c9,t11 CLA and t10,c12 CLA increased levels of C-reactive protein ($P = 0.003$), compared with the control group.[58] This investigation included 53 human subjects (27 men and 26 women, aged 23 to 63 years) that were supplemented with either the CLA treatment or a control oil for 3 months in a double-blind, placebo-controlled study.

In a study with mice, Poirier et al. reported that supplementation with an isomeric mixture of CLA (47% c9,t10 and 48% t10,c12; Tonalin CLA 90%; Natural Lipids, Hovdebygda, Norway) at 1% of the diet for 28 days induced a profound reduction of leptinemia and adiponectinemia, followed by hyperinsulinemia.[59] It was concluded that CLA caused an increased secretory capacity of pancreatic islets, leading, in turn, to liver steatosis in C57BL/6J female mice.

G. Safety

In a study, Whigham et al. evaluated the safety of one CLA product (Clarinol™) over a one-year period in obese healthy humans (35 females and 15 males with BMI from 27 and 35 kg/m²) and found that CLA as Clarinol™ was safe for use in obese humans for at least 1 year as laboratory tests showed no adverse effects of CLA, and subject complaints related to the study were less in the CLA group compared to placebo.[60] Although body composition was not different between groups, the use of this commercial supplement did not result in any adverse actions over a one year period.

IV. CONCLUSIONS

A significant body of evidence indicates that CLA isomers demonstrate effects on blood lipids, tissue metabolism, cell functions, and transcription factors that potentially could improve health status. However, at the same time, studies with dietary supplements of various CLA isomers alone or in combination have resulted in undesirable effects on human nutrition and health. The next few years of research on CLA should focus on distinguishing the positive and negative actions of specific isomers and their impact on nutrition and health for different age groups and conditions in the human population where a justification of use is warranted. Care must be given to conduct research in appropriate animal and cell culture models for elucidating mechanisms of action and safety of the CLA isomers.

REFERENCES

1. Watkins, B.A. and Li, Y., Conjugated linoleic acid: the present state of knowledge, in *Handbook of Nutraceuticals and Functional Foods*, CRC Press, Boca Raton, FL, 2001.
2. Watkins, B.A. and Li, Y., Conjugated linoleic acids, in *Nutrition and Biology, Food Lipids*, Marcel Dekker, New York, 2001.
3. Watkins, B.A. and Li, Y., Conjugated linoleic acids (CLAs): food, nutrition, and health, in *Nutraceutical and Speciality Lipids and Their Co-Products*, CRC Press, Boca Raton, FL, 2006.
4. Li, Y. and Watkins, B.A., CLA in human nutrition and health: human studies, in *Handbook of Functional Lipids*, CRC Press, Boca Raton, FL, 2006.
5. Dietary fats: total fat and fatty acids, in *Dietary Reference Intakes — Energy, Carbohydrate, Fiber, Fat, Fatty Acids, Cholesterol, Protein, and Amino Acids*, (8): 8-1–8–97, Washington, D.C., The National Academies Press, 2002.
6. Dietary fats: total fat and fatty acids, in *Dietary Reference Intakes — Energy, Carbohydrate, Fiber, Fat, Fatty Acids, Cholesterol, Protein, and Amino Acids*, (11): 11-1–11-87, Washington, D.C., The National Academies Press, 2002.
7. Turek, J.J., Li, Y., Schoenlein, I.A., Allen, K.G.D., and Watkins, B.A., Modulation of macrophage cytokine production by conjugated linoleic acids is influenced by the dietary n-6:n-3 fatty acid ratio, *J. Nutr. Biochem.*, 9(5): 258–266, 1998.
8. Li, Y. and Watkins, B.A., Conjugated linoleic acids alter bone fatty acid composition and reduce ex vivo prostaglandin E2 biosynthesis in rats fed n-6 or n-3 fatty acids, *Lipids*, 33(4): 417–425, 1998.
9. Li, Y., Seifert, M.F., Ney, D.M., Grahn, M., Grant, A.L., Allen, K.G., and Watkins, B.A., Dietary conjugated linoleic acids alter serum IGF-I and IGF binding protein concentrations and reduce bone formation in rats fed (n-6) or (n-3) fatty acids, *J. Bone Miner. Res.*, 14(7): 1153–1162, 1999.
10. Burdge, G.C., Lupoli, B., Russell, J.J., Tricon, S., Kew, S., Banerjee, T., Shingfield, K.J., Beever, D.E., Grimble, R.F., Williams, C.M., Yaqoob, P., and Calder, P.C., Incorporation of cis-9,trans-11 or trans-10,cis-12 conjugated linoleic acid into plasma and cellular lipids in healthy men, *J. Lipid Res.*, 45(4): 736–741, 2004.
11. Fernie, C.E., Dupont, I.E., Scruel, O., Carpentier, Y.A., Sebedio, J.L., and Scrimgeour, C.M., Relative absorption of conjugated linoleic acid as triacylglycerol, free fatty acid and ethyl ester in a functional food matrix, *Eur. J. Lipid Sci. Technol.*, 106(6): 347–354, 2004.
12. Jewell, C., Cusack, S., and Cashman, K.D.., The effect of conjugated linoleic acid on transepithelial calcium transport and mediators of paracellular permeability in human intestinal-like Caco-2 cells, *Prostaglandins Leukot Essent Fatty Acids*, 72(3): 163–171, 2005.
13. Slomma, N., Becker, K., and Eder K., The effects of cis-9, trans-11 and trans-10, cis-12 conjugated linoleic acids on Delta 4-desaturation in HepG2 cells, *Int. J. Vitam. Nutr. Res.*, 74(4): 243–246, 2004.
14. Granlund, L., Pedersen, J.I., and Nebb, H.I., Impaired lipid accumulation by trans 10, cis 12 CLA during adipocyte differentiation is dependent on timing and length of treatment, *Biochim. Biophy. Acta Mol. Cell Biol. Lipids*, 1687(1–3): 11–22, 2005.
15. Pal, S., Takechi, R., and Ho, S.S., Conjugated linoleic acid suppresses the secretion of atherogenic lipoproteins from human HepG2 liver cells, *Clin. Chem. Lab. Med.*, 43(3): 269–274, 2005.
16. Storkson, J.M., Park, Y., Cook, M.E., Pariza, M.W., Effects of trans-10,cis-12 conjugated linoleic acid and cognates on apolipoprotein B secretion in HepG2 cells, *Nutr. Res.*, 25(4): 387–399, 2005.
17. Chung, S.K., Brown, J.M., Provo, J.N., Hopkins, R., and McIntosh, M.K.., Conjugated linoleic acid promotes human adipocyte insulin resistance through NF kappa B-dependent cytokine production, *J. Biol. Chem.*, 280(46): 38445–38456, 2005.

18. Malpuech-Brugere, C., Verboeket-van de Venne, W.P.H.G., Mensink, R.P., Arnal, M.A., Morio, B., Brandolini, M., Saebo, A., Lassel, T.S., Chardigny, J.M., Sebedio, J.L., and Beaufrere, B., Effects of two conjugated linoleic acid isomers on body fat mass in overweight humans, *Obes. Res.*, 12(4): 591–598, 2004.

19. Desroches, S., Chouinard, P.Y., Galibois, I., Corneau, L., Delisle, J., Lamarche, B., Couture, P., and Bergeron, N., Lack of effect of dietary conjugated linoleic acids naturally incorporated into butter on the lipid profile and body composition of overweight and obese men, *Am. J. Clin. Nutr.*, 82(2): 309–319, 2005.

20. Gaullier, J.M., Halse, J., Hoye, K., Kristiansen, K., Fagertun, H., Vik, H., and Gudmundsen, O., Conjugated linoleic acid supplementation for 1 y reduces body fat mass in healthy overweight humans, *Am. J. Clin. Nutr.*, 79(6): 1118–1125, 2004.

21. Riserus, U., Smedman, A., Basu, S., and Vessby, B., Metabolic effects of conjugated linoleic acid in humans: the Swedish experience, *Am. J. Clin. Nutr.*, 79(6 Suppl. S): 1146S–1148S, 2004.

22. Gaullier, J.M., Halse, J., Hoye, K., Kristiansen, K., Fagertun, H., Vik, H., and Gudmundsen, O., Supplementation with conjugated linoleic acid for 24 months is well tolerated by and reduces body fat mass in healthy, overweight humans, *J. Nutr.*, 135(4): 778–784, 2005.

23. Thijssen, M.A.M.A., Malpuech-Brugere, C., Gregoire, S., Chardigny, J.M., Sebedio, J.L., and Mensink, RP., Effects of specific CLA isomers on plasma fatty acid profile and expression of desaturases in humans, *Lipids*, 40(2): 137–145, 2005.

24. Tricon, S., Burdge, G.C., Kew, S., Banerjee, T., Russell, J.J., Jones, E.L., Grimble, R.F., Williams, C.M., Yaqoob, P., and Calder, P.C., Opposing effects of cis-9,trans-11 and trans-10,cis-12 conjugated linoleic acid on blood lipids in healthy humans, *Am. J. Clin. Nutr.*, 80(3): 614–620, 2004.

25. Burdge, G.C., Derrick, P.R., Russell, J.J., Tricon, S., Kew, S., Banerjee, T., Grimble, R.F., Williams, C.M., Yaqoob, P., and Calder, P.C., Incorporation of cis-9, trans-11 or trans-10, cis-12 conjugated linoleic acid into human erythrocytes in vivo, *Nutr. Res.*, 25(1): 13–19, 2005.

26. Herrera, J.A., Shahabuddin, A.K.M., Ersheng, G., Wei, Y., Garcia, R.G., and Lopez-Jaramillo, P., Calcium plus linoleic acid therapy for pregnancy-induced hypertension, *Int. J. Gynecol. Obstet.*, 91(3): 221–227, 2005.

27. Maggiora, M., Bologna, M., Ceru, M.P., Possati, L., Angelucci, A., Cimini, A., Miglietta, A., Bozzo, F., Margiotta, C., Muzio, G., and Canuto, R.A., An overview of the effect of linoleic and conjugated-linoleic acids on the growth of several human tumor cell lines, *Int. J. Cancer*, 112(6): 909–919, 2004.

28. Kim, J.H., Hubbard, N.E., Ziboh, V., and Erickson, K.L., Conjugated linoleic acid reduction of murine mammary tumor cell growth through 5-hydroxyeicosatetraenoic acid, *Biochim. Biophys. Acta Mol. Cell Biol. Lipids*, 1687(1–3): 103–109, 2005.

29. Yamasaki, M., Miyamoto, Y., Chujo, H., Nishiyama, K., Tachibana, H., and Yamada, K., Trans 10, cis12-conjugated linoleic acid induces mitochondria-related apoptosis and lysosomal destabilization in rat hepatoma cells, *Biochim. Biophys. Acta Mol. Cell Biol. Lipids*, 1735(3): 176–184, 2005.

30. Lim, D.Y., Tyner, A.L., Park, J.B., Lee, J.Y., Choi, Y.H., and Park, J.H.Y., Inhibition of colon cancer cell proliferation by the dietary compound conjugated linoleic acid is mediated by the CDK inhibitor p21(CIP1/WAF1), *J. Cell. Physiol.*, 205(1): 107–113, 2005.

31. Lampen, A., Leifheit, M., Voss, J., and Nau, H., Molecular and cellular effects of cis-9, trans-11-conjugated linoleic acid in enterocytes: Effects on proliferation, differentiation, and gene expression, *Biochim. Biophys. Acta Mol. Cell Biol. Lipids*, 1735(1): 30–40, 2005.

32. Albright, C.D., Klem, E., Shah, A.A., and Gallagher, P., Breast cancer cell-targeted oxidative stress: Enhancement of cancer cell uptake of conjugated linoleic acid, activation of p53, and inhibition of proliferation, *Exp. Mol. Pathol.*, 79(2): 118–125, 2005.

33. Bergamo, P., Luongo, D., Maurano, F., and Rossi, M., Butterfat fatty acids differentially regulate growth and differentiation in Jurkat T-cells, *J. Cell. Biochem.*, 96(2): 349–360, 2005.

34. Ohtsu, H., Ho, E., Huang, Y.S., Chuang, L.T., and Bray, T.M., Congulated linoleic acid decreases cellular proliferation and inhibits nuclear factor-kappa B and activator protein 1 activation in PC3 cancerous prostate epithelial cells, *Nutr. Res.*, 25(7): 655–662, 2005.

35. Song, H.J., Sneddon, A.A., Barker, P.A., Bestwick, C., Choe, S.N., McClinton, S., Grant, I., Rotondo, D., Heys, S.D., and Wahle, K.W.J., Conjugated linoleic acid inhibits proliferation and modulates protein kinase C isoforms in human prostate cancer cells, *Nutr. Cancer Int. J.*, 49(1): 100–108, 2004.

36. Kim, J.H., Hubbard, N.E., Ziboh, V., and Erickson, K.L., Attenuation of breast tumor cell growth by conjugated linoleic acid via inhibition of 5-lipoxygenase activating protein, *Biochim. Biophys. Acta Mol. Cell Biol. Lipids*, 1736(3): 244–250, 2005.

37. Liu, J.B. and Sidell, N., Anti-estrogenic effects of conjugated linoleic acid through modulation of estrogen receptor phosphorylation, *Breast Cancer Res. Treat.*, 94(2): 161–169, 2005.

38. Degner, S.C., Kemp, M.Q., Bowden, G.T., and Romagnolo, D.F., Conjugated linoleic acid attenuates cyclooxygenase-2 transcriptional activity via an anti-AP-1 mechanism in MCF-7 breast cancer cells, *J. Nutr.*, 136(2): 421–427, 2006.

39. Yamasaki, M., Nishida, E., Nou, S., Tachibana, H., and Yamada, K., Cytotoxity of the trans10,cis12 isomer of conjugated linoleic acid on rat hepatoma and its modulation by other fatty acids, tocopherol, and tocotrienol, *In Vitro Cell. Dev. Biol. Anim.*, 41(7): 239–244, 2005.

40. Cimini, A.M., Cristiano, L., Colafarina, S., Benedetti, E., Di Loreto, S., Festuccia, C., Amicarelli, F., Canuto, R.A., and Ceru, M.P., PPAR gamma-dependent effects of conjugated linoleic acid on the human glioblastoma cell line (ADF), *Int. J. Cancer*, 117(6): 923–933, 2005.

41. Lui, O.L., Mak, N.K., and Leung, K.N., Conjugated linoleic acid induces monocytic differentiation of murine myeloid leukemia cells, *Int. J. Oncol.*, 27(6): 1737–1743, 2005.

42. Larsson, S.C., Bergkvist, L., and Wolk, A., High-fat dairy food and conjugated linoleic acid intakes in relation to colorectal cancer incidence in the Swedish Mammography Cohort, *Am. J. Clin. Nutr.*, 82(4): 894–900, 2005.

43. Loscher, C.E., Draper, E., Leavy, O., Kelleher, D., Mills, K.H.G., and Roche, H.M., Conjugated linoleic acid suppresses NF-kappa B activation and IL-12 production in dendritic cells through ERK-mediated IL-10 induction, *J. Immunol.*, 175(8): 4990–4998, 2005.

44. Jaudszus, A., Foerster, M., Kroegel, C., Wolf, I., and Jahreis, G., Cis-9,Trans-11-CLA exerts anti-inflammatory effects in human bronchial epithelial cells and eosinophils: comparison to Trans-10,Cis-12-CLA and to linoleic acid, *Biochim. Biophys. Acta Mol. Cell Biol. Lipids*, 1737(2–3): 111–118, 2005.

45. Ramakers, J.D., Plat, J., Sebedio, J.L., and Mensink, R.P., Effects of the individual isomers cis-9, trans-11 vs. trans-10,cis-12 of conjugated linoleic acid (CLA) on inflammation parameters in moderately overweight subjects with LDL-phenotype B, *Lipids*, 40(9): 909–918, 2005.

46. Nugent, A.P., Roche, H.M., Noone, E.J., Long, A., Kelleher, D.K., and Gibney, M.J., The effects of conjugated linoleic acid supplementation on immune function in healthy volunteers, *Eur. J. Clin. Nutr.*, 59(6): 742–750, 2005.

47. Tricon, S., Burdge, G.C., Kew, S., Banerjee, T., Russell, J.J., Grimble, R.F., Williams, C.M., Calder, P.C., and Yaqoob, P., Effects of cis-9,trans-11 and trans-1 0,cis-12 conjugated linoleic acid on immune cell function in healthy humans, *Am. J. Clin. Nutr.*, 80(6): 1626–1633, 2004.

48. Song, H.J., Grant, I., Rotondo, D., Mohede, I., Sattar, N., Heys, S.D., and Wahle, K.W.J., Effect of CLA supplementation on immune function in young healthy volunteers, *Eur. J. Clin. Nutr.*, 59(4): 508–517, 2005.

49. Shen, C.L., Dunn, D.M., Henry, J.H., Li, Y., and Watkins, B.A., Decreased production of inflammatory mediators in human osteoarthritic chondrocytes by conjugated linoleic acids, *Lipids*, 39(2): 161–166, 2004.

50. Cusack, S., Jewell, C., and Cashman, K.D., The effect of conjugated linoleic acid on the viability and metabolism of human osteoblast-like cells, *Prostaglandins Leukot Essent Fatty Acids*, 72(1): 29–39, 2005.

51. Doyle, L., Jewell, C., Mullen, A., Nugent, A.P., Roche, H.M., and Cashman, K.D., Effect of dietary supplementation with conjugated linoleic acid on markers of calcium and bone metabolism in healthy adult men, *Eur. J. Clin. Nutr.*, 59(3): 432–440, 2005.

52. Brownbill, R.A., Petrosian, M., and Ilich, J.Z., Association between dietary conjugated linoleic acid and bone mineral density in postmenopausal women, *J. Am. Coll. Nutr.*, 24(3): 177–181, 2005.

53. Eyjolfson, V., Spriet, L.L., and Dyck, D.J., Conjugated linoleic acid improves insulin sensitivity in young, sedentary humans, *Med. Sci. Sports Exercise*, 36(5): 814–820, 2004.

54. Riserus, U., Vessby, B., Arner, P., and Zethelius, B., Supplementation with trans10cis12-conjugated linoleic acid induces hyperproinsulinaemia in obese men: close association with impaired insulin sensitivity, *Diabetologia*, 47(6): 1016–1019, 2004.

55. Moloney, F., Yeow, T.P., Mullen, A., Nolan, J.J., and Roche, H.M., Conjugated linoleic acid supplementation, insulin sensitivity, and lipoprotein metabolism in patients with type 2 diabetes mellitus, *Am. J. Clin. Nutr.*, 80(4): 887–895, 2004.

56. Riserus, U., Vessby, B., Arnlov, J., and Basu, S., Effects of cis-9,trans-11 conjugated linoleic acid supplementation on insulin sensitivity, lipid peroxidation, and proinflammatory markers in obese men, *Am. J. Clin. Nutr.*, 80(2): 279–283, 2004.

57. Taylor, J.S.W., Williams, S.R.P., Rhys, R., James, P., and Frenneaux, M.P., Conjugated linoleic acid impairs endothelial function, *Arterioscl. Throm. Vasc. Biol.*, 26(2): 307–312, 2006.

58. Smedman, A., Basu, S., Jovinge, S., Fredrikson, G.N., and Vessby, B., Conjugated linoleic acid increased C-reactive protein in human subjects, *Br. J. Nutr.*, 94(5): 791–795, 2005.

59. Poirier, H., Rouault, C., Clement, L., Niot, I., Monnot, M.C., Guerre-Millo, M., and Besnard, P., Hyperinsulinaemia triggered by dietary conjugated linoleic acid is associated with a decrease in leptin and adiponectin plasma levels and pancreatic beta cell hyperplasia in the mouse, *Diabetologia*, 48(6): 1059–1065, 2005.

60. Whigham, L.D., O'Shea, M., Mohede, I.C.M., Walaski, H.P., and Atkinson, R.L., Safety profile of conjugated linoleic acid in a 12-month trial in obese humans, *Food Chem. Toxicol.*, 42(10): 1701–1709, 2004.

15 Olive Oil and Health Benefits

Denis M. Medeiros and Meghan Hampton

CONTENTS

I. INTRODUCTION

The olive is a common name for a plant family and its representative genus, and for the fruit of the olive tree. There are approximately 900 species of olives in 24 genera. Most of us are familiar with the olive that is cultivated for its fruit, which are sometimes referred to as drupes. Olives for eating are harvested or picked when they are either unripe or ripe. The unripe olives are green and remain so during pickling. Ripe olives are dark bluish when fresh and turn blackish during pickling.

Olives have been associated with Mediterranean cultures for some time. The cultivated olive is originally native to the eastern Mediterranean region but is cultivated throughout that area and in other parts of the world that have climates similar to the Mediterranean area. The genus and species of the cultivated olive is *Olea europea*, which is grown between the 30th and 45th parallels. Spain, Italy, and Greece are the major producers of olives, with Spain being the biggest producer, followed by Italy and then Greece. Other producers in the area include Portugal, Turkey, Morocco, Tunisia, and France. More countries and regions of the world (U.S., Canada, Japan, Chile, Argentina, New Zealand, and Australia) are cultivating olives because of interest in the health benefits of the Mediterranean diet. In the U.S. most of the production is in California due to its more Mediterranean-like climate. Olive trees normally thrive in regions where there are mild winters and hot summers. The trees cannot normally tolerate temperatures below 10°C, but they can withstand hot temperatures and are drought-resistant.

TABLE 15.1
Selected Nutrient Compositions of Olives

Nutrient	1 large olive (4.4 g)
Macronutrients	
Water	3.52 g
Energy	5.05 Kcal
Protein	0.037 g
Total lipid	0.47 g
Carbohydrate	0.28 g
Total dietary fiber	0.14 g
Ash	0.10 g
Lipids	
Palmitic (16:0)	0.05 g
Stearic (18:0)	0.01 g
Oleic (18:1)	0.34 g
Linoleic (18:2)	0.04 g
Linolenic (18:3)	0.003 g

Source: From USDA Nutrient Database for Standard Reference, Release 12. U.S. Department of Agriculture, Agriculture Research Service, Nutrient Data Laboratory Home Page, http://www.nal.usda.gov/fnic/foodcomp, 1998.

II. NUTRITIONAL COMPONENTS OF OLIVES

Harvesting of olives may influence their nutrient composition. A point worth noting is to not let them over-ripen as the acidity level will increase too much. If the harvest is too early, there is limited oil in the olive. When the olives turn green it is a good time to pick them. The acidity and oil content will continue to increase as they turn purple and black. For the most part, the nutrient composition of olives shown in Table 15.1 is fairly representative. One large olive will supply 5.1 Kcal. Most of the caloric value is supplied by fat, followed by carbohydrate and protein, respectively. Olive oil is derived from the fresh, ripe fruit and comprises about 20% of the olive by weight. One of the most studied aspect of olives is the fatty acid content, with the oil being a good source of the monounsaturated fatty acid oleate. Oleate may range from 56 to 84% of the fatty acid content.[1] Olive oil also contains the saturated fatty acids palmitoleate and stearate in small amounts, the polyunsaturated fatty acids linoleate, and to a small degree, linolenate.[2] Linoleate may comprise 3 to 21% of the fatty acid content.[1]

III. OLIVE OIL

The best quality olive oil is termed *virgin* oil or *extra virgin* olive oil (EVO). This is the oil that is first expressed under light pressure during processing and not further refined. This process is a very significant part of olive oil production. On the other hand, the fact that it has less polyunsaturated fatty acids than other oils gives it a better shelf life. Furthermore, it has a mixture of tocopherols, including vitamin E, which can give a protective effect.[4]

Figure 15.1 illustrates the method commonly used in production of extra virgin olive oil. The olives can be hand-picked from the olive tree or the trees may be beaten with poles to loosen the olives. Some machines collect the olives into nets as a tractor shakes the branches of the olive trees. Most olive oil on the market is expressed under heavy pressure and undergoes further refinement. Olives should be processed within 24 h of picking, especially if the weather is hot.

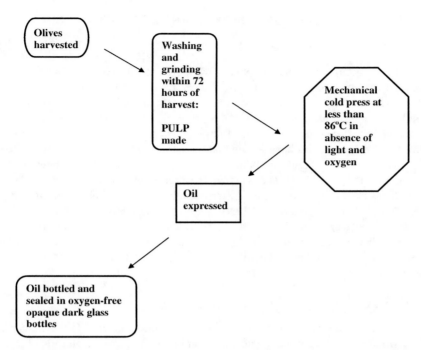

FIGURE 15.1 Scheme on the production of extra virgin olive oil. After olives are harvested and cleaned, within 72 h they must be crushed and made into a pulp. After that point, the pulp is cold pressed in the absence of light and oxygen and the oil expelled and bottled in opaque glass bottles.

They should be processed regardless within 72 h of picking. Typically, olive oil may oxidize easily and produce a strong flavor. Thus, protection from light and heat will increase its shelf life considerably.[3] It is important that during processing no heat or chemicals are used to produce extra virgin olive oil. After the olives are harvested, they are washed and then ground up with the pits into a pulp in a mill made from stainless steel. Before industrialization granite rocks were used to grind the olives. All of the oil is pressed from the pulp and then collected. If the process occurs above 86°C, it is no longer considered "cold press," which is one of the characteristics of extra virgin olive oil. Using this method 90% of the oil is extracted from the olives. To obtain the remaining 10% requires heat and/or a chemical process, producing an oil that would not be considered extra virgin olive oil. The three basic grades of olive oils that consumers have access to are: (1) extra virgin, (2) virgin, and (3) olive oils.

The interest in the health benefits of olive oil is due to the low incidence of coronary heart disease and even cancer, particularly breast cancer, in cultures that consume a "Mediterranean diet." This diet is rather high in fruits, vegetables, grains, and legumes, but low in meat. Much of the evidence that links the Mediterranean diet to a lower incidence of coronary heart disease has centered around the relatively high oleate, but low saturated, fat content. In fact, this diet is associated with a lower incidence of several chronic diseases.[5,6] Diets in the Mediterranean area are characterized by a high content of oleic acid compared to diets in other Northern European cultures and North America. It is well known that monounsaturated fatty acids may lower blood cholesterol levels and may increase HDL cholesterol levels, which could be a link between olive consumption and the lower incidence of coronary heart disease. With respect to olive oil intake and cancer rate, the mechanism for such observations are less clear.

This review will focus on two health conditions as affected by olive consumption: coronary heart disease (CHD) and cancer — but will also consider generalized health aspects. The components of olives, in addition to fatty acids, will be evaluated as will other compounds such as polyphenols.

IV. CORONARY HEART DISEASE

A. FATTY ACIDS IN THE MEDITERRANEAN DIET

Prescription of a Mediterranean diet to patients who have had a myocardial infarct decreases the risk of a second cardiovascular accident,[7] which may be due to several factors. It is commonly accepted that saturated fatty acids are twice as effective at raising blood cholesterol as are polyunsaturated and monounsaturated fatty acids at lowering blood cholesterol. The general consensus appears to be that mono- and polyunsaturated fatty acids are similar in terms of their cholesterol-lowering abilities. Several studies have shown that monounsaturated fatty acids decrease total blood cholesterol, LDL cholesterol, apolipoprotein B and triglycerides, with no changes in HDL cholesterol and Apo-I plasma levels.[8] Elder and Kirchgessner[9] reported that rats fed linseed oil, as opposed to olive oil, had lower concentrations of cholesterol, triglycerides, and phospholipids in plasma and lipoproteins, but a higher susceptibility of LDL to lipid peroxidation. This latter factor, the susceptibility of low-density lipoprotein (LDL) cholesterol to oxidation, yields a more potent atherogenic compound and may be more significant. Also, although polyunsaturated fatty acids may lower blood lipids,[10,11] they elevate the oxidative susceptibility of LDL, in contrast to fats that contain elevated saturated and monounsaturated fatty acids.[12, 13]

B. OTHER OLIVE CONSTITUENTS AND THEIR EFFECTS

It is not always clear if the resistance to oxidation resulting from the Mediterranean diet is due only to oleic acid or to other nontriglyceride components present in oleic acid-rich oils. The minor constituents of virgin olive oil are nonglycerides such as hydrocarbons, monoglyceride esters, tocopherols, alkanols, flavenoids, anthocyanins, hydroxy and dihydroxyterpenic acids, sterols, polyphenols, and phosopholipids.[1,14,15] The Mediterranean diet is high in polyphenolic compounds, and olives have a high amount of these substances. The level of these compounds is variable, with 50 to 800 mg/kg olive oil reported, and is dependent upon several agronomic factors, including soil, degree of olive ripeness, and cultivar or olive variety.[1] There are a number of phenolic compounds in extra virgin oil (Table 15.2). The simple phenolic compounds are hydroxytyrosol (3,4-dihydroxyphenylethanol), tyrosol, and phenolic acids such as vanillic and caffeic acids. The complex phenolic compounds are tyrosol, hydroxytyrosol esters, oleuropein, and its aglycone. Oleuropein is the phenol that contributes primarily to the bitter taste of olives,[1, 15] but other phenolic compounds may contribute some bitterness as well. In addition to the phenolic compounds described, newer information has revealed the presence of the lignan class of phenolics such as (+)-1-acetoxypinoresinol, (+)-pinoresinol and (+)-1-hydroxypinoriesinol.[4] For extra virgin olive oil, the levels of these lignans can be as high as 100 mg/kg in the oils, but variation does exist.[4]

TABLE 15.2
Phenolic Compounds in Extra Virgin Olive Oil

Hydroxytyrosol
Tyrosol
Oleuropein
Vanillic acid
Caffeic acid
Lignans:
    (+)-1-acetoxypinoresinol
    (+)-pinoresinol
    (+)-1-hydroxypinoriesinol

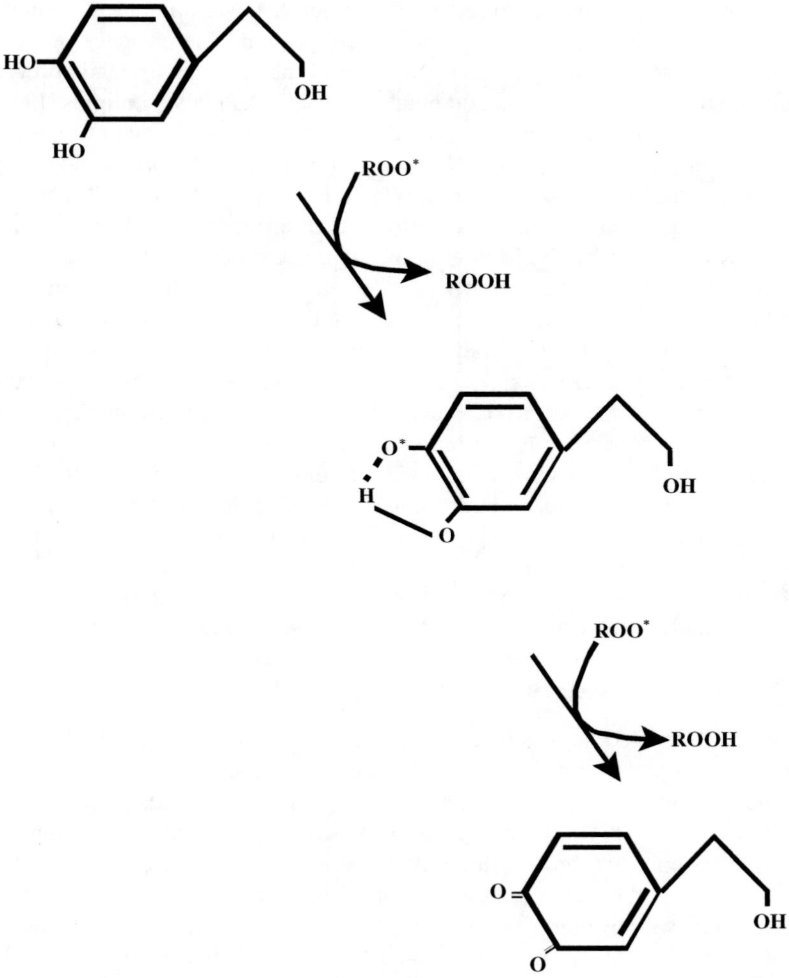

FIGURE 15.2 Hydroxytyrosol's antioxidant mechanism. Hydrogen is donated from the hydroxyl groups of the phenol ring structure to free radicals to generate stable compounds. Two hydrogen atoms per compound can react, resulting in a carbonyl structure on the phenol ring of the hydroxytyrosol.

C. OLIVES AS SOURCES OF ANTIOXIDANTS

Phenols are very good antioxidants. The greater the phenol content in virgin olive oil, the better the oxidative stability. Hydroxytyrosol can donate a hydrogen to free radicals, thereby neutralizing their potential harmful effects as demonstrated in Figure 15.2. Another factor is that hydroxytyrosol is able to chelate metal ions, which are themselves prooxidant agents. However, it is important that metal ions be removed during processing as their presence can lead to partial degradation of the phenolic compounds in the oil.[16]

With respect to the ability of the various phenolic compounds to protect against LDL cholesterol oxidation, both hydroxytyrosol and oleuropein inhibit $CuSO_4$-induced oxidation of LDL, and the effect appears to be dose dependent. Luteolin and lutean aglycon are both effective in protecting against LDL oxidation.[17,18] Visioli and Galli[1] reported that oleuropein and hydroxytyrosol are equally or more effective than other antioxidants such as butylated hydroxytoluene (BHT), vitamin C, and vitamin E. Incubation of LDL with olive oil phenolics (oleuropein or hydroxytyrosol) reduced the fall in vitamin E levels. Normally, virtually all of the vitamin E would have disappeared in 30 min, but 80% remained in the presence of phenols. A lower amount of compounds such as isoprostanes, malonaldehyde, and lipid peroxides were present. The presence of these substances is relatively indicative of free-radical activity. Also, both phenolic compounds prevented the oxidation of linoleic and docosahexaenoic compounds in the LDL phosopholipids. Phenols can also inhibit platelet aggregation. Reduced TXB_2 and LTB_4 production by activated leukocytes is a known effect of olive phenolics.[1,15] In one study, Nicolaiew et al.[14] used 10 normolipidemic subjects in a crossover design in which they received virgin olive oil or sunflower oil for 3 weeks each. Plasma levels of LDL cholesterol did not change in both diets in either the fasting or postprandial states. LDL oxidation, as measured by the formation of conjugated dienes, decreased after the olive oil diet. The results were mixed, in that there was a decrease in the level of conjugated dienes at the beginning and at the end of the oxidation reaction, but the total diene production (maximal-diene at time zero) in the presence of $CuSO_4$ did not differ.

Many studies on olive oil are linked to studies on the Mediterranean diet where other dietary factors could play a role in the findings. However, recent studies have demonstrated that antioxidant capacity is enhanced by adherence to the Mediterranean diet.[19] The Attica area of Greece studied 3042 male and female adult subjects without evidence of cardiovascular disease. Total antioxidant capacity of the serum samples were obtained. This approach involves determining the extent to which the addition of exogenous hydrogen peroxide reacts with antioxidants already in the serum. Total antioxidant capacity was positively correlated with fruits, vegetables, and olive oil intake as found in a Mediterranean diet, but inversely correlated with consumption of red meat. Furthermore, low oxidized LDL cholesterol levels were reported for those with greater total antioxidant capacity.

D. Olive Oil and Inflammation

Another theory has emerged suggesting olive oil and its phenolic compounds are mediators of inflammation. Miles et al.[20] conducted a systematic study of the different components of olive oil such as vanillic, p-coumaric, syringic, homovanillic and caffeic acids, kaempferol, oleuropein glycoside, and tyrosol to determine the degree to which they were able to inhibit the proinflammatory effects of lipopolysaccharide using diluted human blood cultures. They studied a number of cytokines, and the results suggested that the phenolic compounds all had differing degrees of inhibiting the cytokines at different concentrations. For instance, oleuropein glycoside and caffeic acid decreased the concentration of interleukin-1β. However, oleuropein at a concentration of 10^{-4} M inhibited interleukin-1β production by 80%, but caffeic acid only reduced it by 40% at the same concentration. Kaemferol decreased prostaglandin E_2 by 95% at a concentration of 10^{-4} M. These phenolics did not appear to affect interleukin-6 or tumor necrosis in this *in vitro* study. Moreover, a study on human subjects who consumed the Mediterranean diet reported that serum levels of tumor-necrosis factor-α and vascular cell adhesion molecule (VCAM)-1 were markedly decreased.[21] Further, the authors were able to separate out the effects of olive oil vs. other components of the diet and found that both gave similar results. Ruano et al.[22] studied endothelial function in hypercholesterolemic men as a result of an acute response to a meal high in virgin olive oil. Five men and 16 women from Cordoba, Spain, with cholesterol between 200 and 350 mg/100 ml were also studied. In a crossover design, subjects received two fat meals consisting of 60 g of white bread and 40 ml of virgin olive oil with either low or high phenolic acid content. Venous blood was sampled for periods of time after ingestion up to 240 min after consumption. Ischemic reactive hyperemia was measured with a Laser-Doppler probe. Subjects on the high phenolic acid olive oil diet had significantly greater increases in ischemic reactive hyperemia starting 120 min after meal ingestion than those on the low phenolic acid diet. This suggested improved endothelial function among these subjects. Further analysis revealed a reduction in oxidative stress and an increase in nitric oxide metabolites.

Hydroxytyrosol, present in olives, is a diphenolic compound common in extra virgin olive oil and may be a potent antioxidant. The superoxide radical (O_2^-) and nitric oxide (NO^-) react rapidly to form peroxynitrite (ONOO⁻), which is a chemical that is very reactive and can cause tissue damage. Nitric oxide may contribute to inflammatory diseases and cardiovascular disease. Hydroxytyrosol has been shown to be highly protective against the peroxynitrite-dependent nitration of tyrosine and DNA damage by peroxynitrite *in vitro*.[23] On the other hand, oleuropein can increase nitric oxide release by cultured macrophages after endotoxin challenge by increasing nitric oxide-synthase expression. This may be beneficial in the sense that NO may guard against infectious agents and parasites.[24]

E. HYPERTENSION AND OLIVE OIL CONSUMPTION

There is some evidence that olive oil may lower blood pressure. One study reported that a diet enriched with olive oil reduced the mean blood pressure in adult men and women.[25] For those with hypertension, a crossover study in women revealed that olive oil, as opposed to high oleic-acid sunflower oil, significantly reduced both systolic and diastolic blood pressure.[26] This suggests that constituents of olive oil other than fatty acids may be contributing to these findings. A recent study by Alonso and Martinez-Gonzalez[27] in Spain of 6863 adults in the Seguimiento Universidad de Navarra (SUN) study revealed lower blood pressure among men who consumed more olive oil in their diets, but no such relationship was observed among women. Furthermore, Fito et al.[28] reported that extra virgin olive oil, as compared to refined olive oil, lowered systolic blood pressure in hypertensive patients. However, diastolic blood pressure, blood glucose, lipids, and even oxidized LDL cholesterol did not differ between the refined olive oil group and the extra virgin olive oil group.

V. CANCER

A. BREAST CANCER AND OLIVE OIL

In modern cultures, a switch from a low fat diet that contains a high proportion of monounsaturated fatty acids to a high fat diet containing a high proportion of saturated fatty acids may be contributing to the increased incidence of cancer, including breast cancer. There is geographic variation in the incidence of breast cancer, and this variation is coincident with the consumption of a high oleic acid intake derived from olive oil, typical of the Mediterranean diet.[29] Case control studies have yielded evidence of a protective association between oleic acid or olive oil consumption and breast cancer. Animal experiments indicate that oleic acid may be protective when ingested in a vehicle both very high in oleic acid and very low in linoleic acid, which is typical of olive oil. Consumption of olive oil has been shown to reduce mammary tumor incidence even when compared with safflower oil which contains similar amounts of oleic acid but higher levels of linoleic acid.[30,31] Moreover, experiments with feeding rats a 15% olive oil diet significantly reduced tumor incidence caused by the carcinogenic compound, 9, 10-dimethyl-1,2-benzanthracene.[32]

Simsonsen et al.[33] hypothesized that an olive oil diet could reduce susceptibility of tissue structures to damage by free radicals, and thus the incidence of breast cancer. This research group used gluteal fat aspirates and measured the fatty-acid profiles of subjects from various European cultures. The study included 291 postmenopausal incident breast cancer patients and 351 control subjects. Oleic acid showed a strong inverse relationship with breast cancer in Spanish cultures, but not among subjects from Berlin, Northern Ireland, the Netherlands, and Switzerland, or non-Spanish residents. One reason for the failure of this study to show any relationship of oleic acid levels to breast cancer in the non-Spanish population could be because olive oil contains other compounds such as the phenols and flavenoids which are good antioxidants. Moreover, the Spanish residents obtained their oleic acid from olive oil whereas the other residents obtained theirs from other sources, which possibly explains these results.

Epidemiological studies have yielded consistent results on the association of monounsaturated fatty acids or olive oil consumption and the incidence of breast cancer. Omega-6 fatty acids enhance carcinogenesis promotion[34,35] but omega-3 fatty acids from fish inhibit this phase.[36,37] The impact of omega-6 fatty acid-rich diets is thought to be related to eicosanoid products, such as prostaglandins E_2 and $F_{2\alpha}$, and thromboxane B_2, which are elevated in N-nitrosomethylurea-induced rat mammary cancer.[38] On the other hand, there have been epidemiology studies reporting a higher risk from increased polyunsaturated fat consumption for breast cancer. Landa et al.[39] studied 100 breast cancer subjects and 100 controls using a food-frequency instrument. Those with breast cancer reported lower intakes of fish, fruits, and vegetables compared to controls. Those with breast cancer also had lower intakes of vitamin C and monounsaturated fatty acids. Martin-Moreno et al.[40] used a case-control study in Spain and examined specific nutrient intakes using a food-frequency questionnaire in 762 newly diagnosed breast cancer women and compared this to 988 randomly selected control females. Both total fat and type of fat intake were not associated with breast cancer in either pre- or postmenopausal women, after adjustment for energy intake. However, a lower risk of breast cancer was reported in those who consumed higher amounts of olive oil. Trichopoulou et al.[41] used a semi-quantitative food-frequency instrument administered to 820 women with breast cancer and 1548 control women from Greece to estimate the intakes of olive oil, margarine, and other food items. After adjustment for some other potential confounding factors, increased olive oil consumption was associated with a significantly reduced risk for breast cancer. Margarine consumption was associated with a greater risk of breast cancer. They also reported that fruit and vegetable consumption was inversely related to breast cancer in the same study. In a much larger study in Italy, 2,564 women hospitalized with breast cancer were compared to 2,588 women admitted to the same hospital for other health conditions not related to breast cancer, hormone problems, or gastric disorders[42]. Using a food-frequency questionnaire, this study demonstrated an inverse relationship with olive oil and other vegetable oil consumption and the incidence of breast cancer. No relationship for butter or margarine were reported.

B. Prostate Cancer and Olive Oil

Olive oil may protect against prostate cancer. Southern European populations of Greece, Italy, Portugal, and Spain have lower rates of prostate cancer and perhaps the Mediterranean diet that is high in olive oil may be a factor.[43,44] Studies have suggested that diets high in olive oil may afford protection against prostate cancer. Hodge et al.[45] reported in a case-controlled study of 858 men below 70 years of age with prostate cancer, compared to 905 age-frequency-matched men in Australia, that diets with high levels of olive oil, tomatoes, and allium containing vegetables reduce the risk of prostate cancer. However, the association with olive oil in that study was weak. It was also unclear whether the fatty acids or the antioxidants in olive oil were the responsible factor. Many studies on prostate cancer have reported inconsistent results for the effect of fatty acid intake on prostate cancer.[46,47] However, margarine consumption was related to an increased risk of prostate cancer. A New Zealand study revealed that diet patterns high in monounsaturated fatty acid-rich vegetable oils reduced the risk of prostate cancer in 317 prostate cancer cases compared to 480 controls.[48] However, the association was with the foods high in monounsaturated fatty acids and not the fatty acids *per se*. This suggested that other components in these foods (eg., phenolic compounds) could be contributing factors.

C. Other Cancers and Olive Oil

In addition to the role of olive oil in lowering the incidence of breast tumors, later studies have suggested that other cancer types may benefit from a diet high in olive oil. Franceschi et al.[49] examined cases of 512 men and 86 women from Northeastern Italy who had cancer of the oral cavity and pharynx and compared them to 1008 men and 483 women controls who had been admitted to area hospitals for ailments other than neoplastic conditions. Subjects were administered a dietary questionnaire to evaluate fat intake and other lifestyle aspects. Risk for these cancers was reduced by at least 50% in subjects with the highest intakes of several food items, including poultry, fish, raw and cooked vegetables, citrus fruits, and olive oil.

D. SUMMARY AND FUTURE NEED FOR CANCER RESEARCH AND OLIVE OIL

While much of the work on olive oil intake and cancer has focused upon the monounsaturated fatty acid content, the antioxidant compounds present may play an important role in its benefits as it apparently does for heart disease, as reviewed in earlier text. Furthermore, the studies examining the antioxidant effects of olive oil on various cancers are surprisingly limited and thus afford more opportunity for investigation.

VI. OTHER DISEASE CONDITIONS AND OLIVE OIL

Heart disease and cancer are the two diseases that show a reduction in risk with increased olive oil intake as found in the Mediterranean diet. Recently it has been suggested that metabolic syndrome can be prevented by adherence to the Mediterranean diet.[50] Metabolic syndrome consists of a combination of conditions, including hypertension, abdominal obesity, increased fibrinogen, insulin resistance, increased blood viscosity, and uric acid levels.[51] These conditions predispose the individuals to be at high risk for cardiovascular disease. Esposito et al.[52] conducted a randomized clinical trial among 90 men and women with metabolic syndrome. The intervention group followed a Mediterranean diet and the control group followed the prudent diet where carbohydrates provided 50 to 60%; protein, 15 to 20%; and total fat was less than 30%. Two years later, serum C-reactive protein levels, whose elevation indicates metabolic syndrome, were significantly reduced. Furthermore, insulin resistance, interleukin-6, and improved endothelial function were found in those on the Mediterranean diet.

Interestingly, some recent studies have suggested that a combination of fish oil with olive oil may prove beneficial in treatments of inflammation-related conditions. The omega-3 fatty acids present in fish oils have a well-known impact upon attenuating the inflammatory response. Berbert et al.[53] reported that treatment of rheumatoid arthritis patients with fish oil plus olive oil resulted in superior relief of clinical arthritic symptoms as opposed to those supplemented with fish oil only. The control group received soy oil. Subjects consuming both supplements of fish and olive oils were better able to withstand pain on handgrip tests, had reduced duration of morning stiffness, and increased time before fatigue became apparent. Camuesco et al.[54] reported that fish oil and olive oil were superior in reducing inflammation in the colons of rats that were induced to develop colitis with dextran sodium sulfate (DSS). Tumor necrosis factor-α and LTB_4 levels were reduced in rats treated with both fish and olive oils.

VII. SUMMARY OF A CONSENSUS REPORT

A recent international conference developed a consensus report on the health benefits of virgin olive oil. In addition to the influence of extra virgin olive oil (EVO) upon cardiovascular disease and cancer, the report goes further to suggest that EVO may be protective against age-related cognitive decline and Alzheimer's disease. They further recommended that olive oil intake is especially important during the first decades of life and particularly that EVO intake should begin before puberty and continued throughout life.[55]

VIII. SUMMARY

Clearly the monounsaturated content of the Mediterranean diet, with respect to the intake of olive oil, plays a significant role in the lower incidence of both coronary heart disease and cancer, particularly breast cancer. The anti-oxidant compounds present in extra virgin olive oil allow for the protection against LDL cholesterol oxidation and thus spare other antioxidant nutrients. The role of these same antioxidants in protecting against various cancers should be pursued. Therefore, further examination of olive oil intake and other cancer types may also yield beneficial information.

The health benefits of olive oil due to its active compounds should focus more on those agronomic factors that optimize their content. Additionally, further knowledge on the genetic regulation of the production of antioxidant phenolic compounds would be worthwhile. Increasing the content of these valuable nutrients to protect against both coronary heart disease and cancers is a good example of functional food for health. Furthermore, extraction of these compounds from olives and concentrating them for clinical trials, both animal and human, may provide better insights into their utility as nutraceuticals for the future.

REFERENCES

1. Visioli, F. and Galli, C. The effect of minor constituents of olive oil on cardiovascular disease: new findings. *Nutr. Rev.* 56: 142–147, 1998.
2. USDA Nutrient Database for Standard Reference, Release 12. U.S. Department of Agriculture, Agriculture Research Service, Nutrient Data Laboratory Home Page, http://www.nal.usda.gov/fnic/foodcomp, 1998.
3. Freeland-Graves, J.M. and Peckham, G.C., *Foundations of Food Preparation*. 5th ed. MacMillan, New York, 1987.
4. Owen, R.W., Mier, W., Giacosa, A., Hull, W.E., Spiegelhalder, B., and Bartsch, H. Identification of lignans as major compounds in the phenolic fraction of olive oil. *Clin. Chem.* 46: 976–988, 2000.
5. World Health Organization Study Group. Diet, Nutrition, and the Prevention of Chronic Diseases. World Health Organization Tech. Rep. Ser. 16, 2003.
6. Ganji, V. and Kafai, M.R. Demographic, health, lifestyle and blood vitamin determinants of serum total homocysteine concentrations in the third National Health and Nutrition Examination Survey, 1988–1994. *Am. J. Clin. Nutr.* 77: 826–833, 2003.
7. Renaud, S., DeLorgeril, M., Delaye, J., Guidollet, J., Jacquard, F., Mamelle, N., Martin, J.L., Monjaud, I., Salen, P., and Toubol, P. Cretan Mediterranean diet for prevention of coronary heart disease. *Am. J. Clin. Nutr.* 61: 1360–1367, 1995.
8. Baggio, G., Pagnan, A., Muraca, M., Martini, S., Opportuno, A., Bonanome, A., Ambrosio, G.B., Ferrari, S., and Crepaldi, G. Olive oil-enriched diet: effect on serum lipoprotein levels and biliary cholesterol saturation. *Am. J. Clin. Nutr.* 47: 960–964, 1998.
9. Elder, K. and Kirchgessner, M. Concentrations of lipids in plasma and lipoproteins and oxidative susceptibility of low-density lipoproteins in zinc-deficient rats fed linseed oil or olive oil. *J. Nutr. Biochem.* 8: 461–468, 1997.
10. Stangl, G.I., Kirchgessner, M., Reichlmayr-Lais, A.M., and Eder, K. Serum lipids and lipoproteins from rats fed different dietary oils. *J. Anim. Physiol. Anim. Nutr.* 71: 87–97, 1994.
11. Balasubramaniam, S., Simons, L.A., Chang, S., and Hickie, J.B. Reduction in plasma cholesterol and increase in biliary cholesterol by a diet rich in n-3 fatty acids in the rat. *J. Lipid Res.* 26: 684–689, 1985.
12. Scaccini, C., Nardini, M., D'Aquino, M., Gentili, V., Di Felice, M., and Tomassi, G. Effect of dietary oils on lipid peroxidation and on antioxidant parameters of rat plasma and lipoprotein fractions. *J. Lipid Res.* 33: 627–633, 1992.
13. Parthasarthy, S., Khoo, J.C., Miller, E., Barnett, J., Witztum, J.L., and Steinberg, D. Low density lipoprotein rich in oleic acid is protective against oxidative modification: implication for dietary prevention of atherosclerosis. *Proc. Natl. Acad. Sci. USA.* 87: 3894–3898, 1990.
14. Nicolaiew, N., Lemort, N., Adorni, L., Berra, B., Montorfano, G., Rapelli, S., Cortesi, N., and Jacotot, B. Comparison between extra virgin olive oil and oleic acid rich sunflower oil: effect on postprandial lipemia and LDL susceptibility to oxidation. *Ann. Nutr. Metab.* 42: 251–260, 1998.
15. Visioli, F. and Galli, C. Olive oil phenols and their potential effects on human health. *J. Agric. Food Chem.* 46: 4292–4296, 1998.

16. Angerosa, F. and DiGiacinto, L. Oxidation des huiles d'olive vierges par le métaux manganese et nickel, Note 1 (Metal-induced oxidation of virgin olive oils: manganese and nickel. Note 1), *Rev. Fr. Corps Gras*. 40: 41–44, 1993.

17. Visioli, F., Bellomo, G., Montedoro, G.F., and Galli, C. Low-density lipoprotein oxidation is inhibited in vitro by olive oil constituents. *Atherosclerosis* 117: 25–42, 1995.

18. Visioli, F. and Galli, C. Oleuropein protects low-density lipoprotein from oxidation. *Life Sci*. 55: 1965–1971, 1994.

19. Pitsavos, C., Panagiotakos, B.B., Tzima, N., Chrysohoou, C., Economou, M., Zampelas, A., and Stefanadis, C. Adherence to the Mediterranean diet is associated with total anti-oxidant capacity in healthy adults: the ATTICA study. *Am. J. Clin. Nutr*. 82: 694–699, 2005.

20. Miles, E.A., Znoubouli, P., and Calder, P.C. Differential anti-inflammatory effects of phenolic compounds from extra virgin olive oil identified in human whole blood cultures. *Nutrition* 21: 389–394, 2005.

21. Serrano-Martinez, M., Palacios, M., Martinez-Losa, E., Lezaun, R., Maravi, C., Prado, M., Martinez, J.A., and Martinez-Gonzalez, M.A. A Mediterranean dietary style influences TNF-alpha and VCAM-1 coronary blood levels in unstable angina patients. *Eur. J. Nutr*. 44: 349–354, 2005.

22. Ruano, J., Lopez-Miranda, J., Fuentes, F., Morena, J.A., Bellido, C., Perez-Martinez, P., Lozano, A., Jiménez, Y., and Jiménez, F.P. Phenolic content of virgin olive oil improves ischemic reactive hyperemia in hypercholesterolemic patients. *J. Am. Coll. Cardiol*. 46: 1864–1868, 2005.

23. Deiana, M., Aruoma, O.I., Bianchi, M.L.P., Spencer, J.P.E., Kaur, H., Halliwell, B., Aeschbach, R., Banni, S., Dessi, M.A. and Corongiu, F.P. Inhibition of peroxynitrite dependent DNA base modification and tyrosine nitration by the extra virgin olive oil-derived antioxidant hydroxytyrosol. *Free Radic. Biol. Med*. 26: 762–769, 1999.

24. Visioli, F., Bellosta, S., and Galli, C. Oleuropein, the bitter principles in olives, enhances nitric oxide production by murine macrophages. *Life Sci*. 62: 541–546, 1998.

25. Lahoz, C., Alonso, R., Porres, A., and Mata, P. Las Dietas Enriquecidas en Ácidos Gracos Monoinsaturadoes y Ácidos Gracos Poliinsaturado Omega 3 Disminuyen la Presion Artersial, sin Modificar la Concentración de Insulina Plasmática en Sujetos Sanos. *Med. Clin. (Barc)*. 112: 133–137, 1999.

26. Ruiz-Gutierres, V., Muriana, F.J., Guerrero, A., Cert, A.M., and Villar, J. Plasma lipids, erythrocyte membrane lipids and blood pressure of hypertensive women after ingestion of dietary oleic acid from two different sources. *J. Hypertens*. 14: 1483–1490, 1996.

27. Alonso, A. and Martinez-González, M.Á. Olive oil consumption and reduced incidence of hypertension: the SUN study. *Lipids*. 39: 1233–1238, 2004.

28. Fito, M., Cladellas, M., de la Torre, R., Marti, J., Alcántara, M., Pujadas-Bastardes, M., Marrugat, J., Bruguera, J., López-Sabater, M.C., Vila, J., and Covas, M.I. Antioxidant effect of virgin olive oil in patients with stable coronary heart disease: a randomized, crossover, controlled, clinical trial. *Atherosclerosis* 181: 149–158, 2005.

29. Berrino, F. and Muti, P. Mediterranean diet and cancer. *Eur. J. Clin. Nutr*. 43: 49–55, 1989.

30. Cohen, L.A., Thompson, D.O., Maeura, Y., Choi, K., Blank, M.E., and Rose, D.P. Dietary fat and mammary cancer. I. Promoting effects of different dietary fats on N-nitrosomethylurea-induced rat mammary tumorigenesis. *J. Natl. Cancer Inst*. 77: 33–42, 1986.

31. Lasekan, J.B., Clayton, M.K., Gendron-Fitzpatrick, A., and Ney, D.M. Dietary olive and safflower oil in promotion of DMBA-induced mammary tumorigenesis in rats. *Nutr. Cancer*. 13: 153–163, 1990.

32. Zusman, I. Comparative anticancer effects of vaccination and dietary factors on experimentally-induced cancers. *In vivo* 12: 675–689, 1998.

33. Simsonsen, N.R., Navajas, J.F.C., Martin-Moreno, J.M., Strain, J.J., Huttnen, J.K., Martin, B.C., Thamm, M., Kardinaal, A.F.M., van't Veer, P., Kok, F.J., and Kohlmeier, L. Tissue stores of individual monounsaturated fatty acids and breast cancer: the EURAMIC study. *Am. J. Clin. Nutr*. 68: 134–141, 1998.

34. Carrol, K.K. Experimental evidence of dietary factors and hormone-dependent cancers. *Cancer Res*. 35: 3374–3383, 1975.

35. Cohen, L.A., Thompson, D.O., Maeura, Y., Choi, K., Blank, M.E., and Rose, D.P. Dietary fat and mammary cancer. I. Promoting effects of different dietary fats on N-nitrosomethylurea-induced rat mammary tumorigenesis. *J. Natl. Cancer Inst*. 77: 33–42, 1986.

36. Jurkowski, J.J. and Cave, W.T., Jr. Dietary effects of menhaden oil on the growth and membrane lipid composition of rat mammary tumors. *J. Natl. Cancer. Inst.* 74: 1145–1150, 1985.

37. Cohen, L.A., Chen-Backlund, J.Y., Sepkovic, D.W., and Sugie, S. Effect of varying proportions of dietary menhaden corn oil on experimental rat tumor promotion. *Lipids* 28: 449–456, 1993.

38. Karmali, R.A., Thaler, H.T., and Cohen, L.A. Prostaglandin concentrations and prostaglandin synthase activity in N-nitrosomethylurea-induced rat mammary adenocarcinoma. *Eur. J. Clin. Oncol.* 19: 817–823, 1983.

39. Landa, M.C, Frago, N., and Tres, A. Diet and the risk of breast cancer in Spain. *Eur. J. Cancer Prev.* 3: 313–320, 1994.

40. Martin-Moreno, J.M., Willett, W.C., Gorgojo, L., Banegas, J.R., Rodriguez-Artalejo F., Fernandez-Rodrigues J.C., Maisonneuve, P., and Boyle, P. Dietary fat, olive oil intake and breast cancer risk. *Int. J. Cancer.* 58: 774–780, 1994.

41. Trichopoulou, A., Katsouyanni, K., Stuver, S., Tzala, L., Gnardellis, C., Rimm, E., Trichopoulos, D. Consumption of olive oil and specific food groups in relation to breast cancer in Greece. *J. Natl. Cancer. Inst.* 87: 110–116, 1995.

42. La Vecchia, C., Negri, E., Franceschi, S., Decarli, A., Giacosa, A., and Lipworth, L. Olive oil, other dietary fats, and the risk of breast cancer (Italy). *Cancer Causes Control.* 6: 545–550, 1995.

43. Helsing, E. Traditional diets and disease patterns of the Mediterranean, circa 1960. *Am. J. Clin. Nutr.* 61 (Suppl.): 1329S–1337S, 1995.

44. Mezzanotte, G., Cislagni, C., Decarli, A., and LaVecchia, C. Cancer mortality in broad Italian geographic areas, 1975–1977. *Tumori* 72: 145–152, 1986.

45. Hodge, A.M., English, D.R., McCredie, M.R.E., Severi, G., Boyle, P., Hopper, J.L. and Giles, G.G. Foods, nutrients and prostate cancer. *Cancer Causes Control.* 15: 11–20, 2004.

46. Clinton, S.K. and Giovannucci, E. Diet, nutrition, and prostate cancer. *Annu. Rev. Nutr.* 18: 413–440, 1998.

47. Kolonel, L.N. Fat, meat and prostate cancer. *Epidemiol. Rev.* 23: 72–81, 2001.

48. Norrish, A.E., Jackson, R.T., Sharpe, S.J., and Skeaff, C.M. Men who consume vegetable oils rich in monounsaturated fat: their dietary patterns and risk of prostate cancer (New Zealand). *Cancer Causes Control.* 11: 609–615, 2000.

49. Franceschi, S., Favero, A., Conti, E., Talamini, R., Volpe, R., Negri, E., Barzan, L., and La Vecchia, C. Food groups, oils and butter, and cancer of the oral cavity and pharynx. *Br. J. Cancer.* 80: 614–620, 1999.

50. Panagiotakos, D., and Polychronopoulos, E. The role of Mediterranean diet in the epidemiology of metabolic syndrome: converting epidemiology to clinical practice. *Lipids Health Dis.* 4: 7, 2005 http://www/lipiworld.com/content/4/1/7.

51. Hansen, B.C. The metabolic syndrome X. *Ann. N. Y. Acad Sci.* 892: 1–24, 1999.

52. Esposito, K., Marfella, R., Ciotola, M., DiPalo, C., Giugliano, F., Giuliano, G., D'Armiento, M., D'Andrea, F., and Gingliano, D. Effect of a Mediterranean-style diet on endothelial dysfunction and markers of vascular inflammation in the metabolic syndrome: a randomized trial. *JAMA* 292: 1440–1446, 2004.

53. Berbert, A.A., Kondo, C.R.M., Almendra, C.L., Matsuo, T., and Dichi, I. Supplementation of fish oil and olive oil in patients with rheumatoid arthritis. *Nutrition* 21: 131–136, 2005.

54. Camuesco, D., Galvez, J., Nieto, A., Comalada, M., Rodrigues-Cabezas, M.E., Concha, A., Xaus, J., and Zarzuelo, A. Dietary olive oil supplemented with fish oil, rich in EPA and DHA (n-3) polyunsaturated fatty acids, attenuates colonic inflammation in rats with DDS-induced colitis. *J. Nutr.* 135: 687–694, 2005.

55. Perez-Jimenez, F. International conference on the health effect of virgin olive oil. *Eur. J. Clin. Invest.* 35: 421–424, 2005.

16 The Role of α- and γ-Tocopherols in Health

Richard S. Bruno

CONTENTS

I. INTRODUCTION

The term vitamin E is used to describe eight lipophilic, naturally occurring compounds, which include four tocopherols and four tocotrienols (Figure 16.1).[1] Tocopherols have a saturated phytyl tail whereas the tocotrienols have an unsaturated tail. Within each class, four forms exist as α-, β-, γ-, and δ- that differ according to the number and position of methyl groups present on the chromanol head. For example, when the chromanol head is fully methylated and the phytyl tail is saturated,

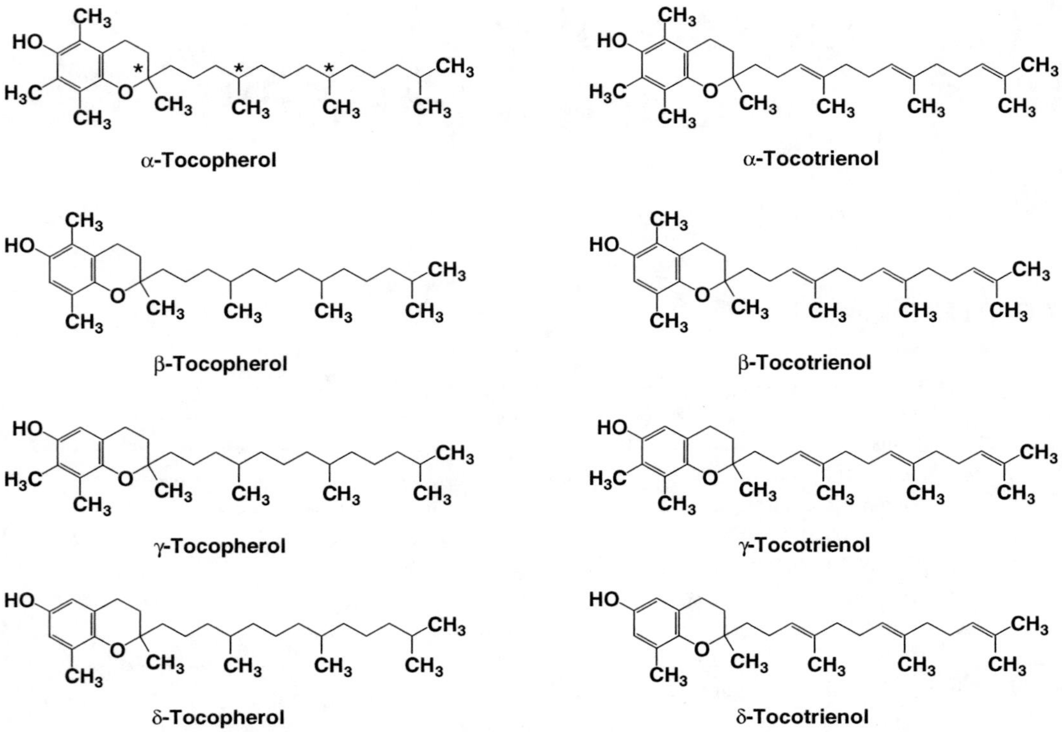

FIGURE 16.1 Vitamin E structures: tocopherols and tocotrienols. Vitamin E consists of four tocopherols and four tocotrienols. α-Tocopherol, either naturally occurring or in synthetic preparations, is widely consumed in supplement form. Synthetic preparations of α-tocopherol result in the formation of 8 stereoisomers (2R forms: *RRR*, *RSR*, *RRS*, *RSS*; 2S forms: *SRR*, *SSR*, *SRS*, *SSS*) as three chiral centers (denoted by asterisks) are present along the phytyl tail, whereas naturally occurring α-tocopherol occurs only in the *RRR* configuration.

then this vitamer is identified as α-tocopherol (2,5,7,8-tetramethyl-2R-(4′R,8′R,12 trimethyltride-cyl)-6-chromanol). α- and γ-Tocopherol are the most abundant forms of vitamin E found biologically and in the diet.[2] Structurally, they are quite similar and differ only in that γ-tocopherol has an unsubstituted position on the chromanol head (Figure 16.1). Thus, due to the dietary and biological abundance of these vitamin E forms, a considerable body of knowledge has accumulated since their discovery. Therefore, this chapter will be limited only to these vitamin E forms.

II. HISTORY

Vitamin E was discovered in 1922 as a compound necessary to sustain reproductive ability in rodents.[3] Evans and Bishop determined that rodents fed diets containing rancid fat (i.e., vitamin E-deficient) produced offspring that were mostly sterile in the first generation and completely sterile in the second generation. From their work, they concluded that fetal resorption occurred despite the presence of normal ovarian structure and function. About this time, the same conclusion was formed by Barnett Sure who performed similar dietary experiments, but he coined the term *vitamin E* since vitamins A, B, C, and D were already identified.[4]

Further work led to the isolation of α-tocopherol from wheat germ that had the biological activity of vitamin E.[5] In the subsequent year, β- and γ-tocopherols were isolated from vegetable oils, but it was determined that these vitamin E homologues had lower biological activity than α-tocopherol.[6] Although these non-α-tocopherol forms of vitamin E have been reported to possess vitamin E biological activity, the purity of these compounds as well as the analytical methods used have been recently questioned. Currently, the purity of commercially available γ-tocopherol is identified as ~97% pure with much of the "contamination" attributed to α-tocopherol. Therefore, some of the early research regarding vitamin E biological activity may need to be repeated.

Historically, the fetal resorption assay has been used to define vitamin E biological activity despite the fact that the assay is very tedious and time consuming.[7] However, the assay does provide useful information as it determines vitamin E biological activity and quantifies the amount of vitamin E necessary to maintain the maximal number of live fetuses. Whereas vitamin E deficiency can be induced in laboratory animals, it is quite difficult to do so in humans. Horwitt and others[8–10] studied the effects of chronically low vitamin E intakes among hospitalized volunteers. After nearly 2 years of the 6-year-long investigation, plasma vitamin E dropped into the deficient range, but anemia did not develop despite increased sensitivity of erythrocytes to hydrogen peroxide-induced hemolysis.

Despite efforts to produce chronic dietary vitamin E restriction in humans, symptoms of vitamin E deficiency such as peripheral neuropathy, spinocerebellar ataxia, skeletal myopathy, and pigmented retinopathy have not been observed in the laboratory. In addition, free living humans usually become vitamin E-deficient secondary only to other pathologies including fat maldigestion disorders,[11] dysfunctional lipid metabolism,[12] and severe protein-energy malnutrition.[13] However, the discoveries of the α-tocopherol transfer protein and its rarely occurring mutation have led to the identification of vitamin E deficiency independently of other pathologies in humans,[14] which has also been confirmed with the use of α-tocopherol transfer protein knock-out mice.[15]

III. FUNCTIONS

A. ANTIOXIDANT

The most well known biological function of vitamin E is as a chain-breaking antioxidant (Figure 16.2) that prevents the propagation of lipid peroxidation.[16] In this role, vitamin E acts as a peroxyl radical scavenger and is able to protect PUFAs from lipid peroxidation.[17] Vitamin E has been found to "outcompete" the propagation reactions so that a single vitamin E molecule is able to protect ~1000 lipid molecules from the chain-reaction propagation step.[18] This phenomenon is attributed to the higher rate constant between vitamin E and peroxyl radicals compared to the rate constant between PUFAs and peroxyl radicals. When vitamin E scavenges peroxyl radicals, it loses an electron, and becomes oxidized to form a tocopheroxyl radical (Figure 16.2). The tocopheroxyl radical then has one of several biological fates: (1) it can lose a second electron, becoming further oxidized to form a tocopherol quinone,[19] (2) it can react with another radical to yield a nonreactive product, (3) it can be recycled (i.e., reduced to tocopherol) by other antioxidants such as vitamin C,[20] or (4) it could potentially reinitiate lipid peroxidation through a process termed *tocopherol-mediated peroxidation* due to its relatively long half-life.[21]

Of all the tocopherols, α-tocopherol is the most potent biological form based on methodology that quantifies the inhibited auto-oxidation of styrene (e.g., peroxyl radical generation).[22] The potencies of the tocopherols occur in the following order: $\alpha > \gamma > \beta > \delta$ with respective rate coefficients of 320, 140, 130, and 44 × 10[4] (M^{-1} sec^{-1}). It seems that α-tocopherol is the superior tocopherol form because it contains three methyl groups (Figure 16.1) on the chromanol head that function to stabilize phenoxyl radicals, whereas the other tocopherols lack one or more methyl groups.

Despite vitamin E's known *in vitro* antioxidant activity, it is often argued whether vitamin E functions as an antioxidant in humans. Although there are eight forms of vitamin E, only α- and γ-tocopherols are generally detected in tissues and plasma of unsupplemented individuals (discussed further under *Bioavailability* section). In fact, plasma α-tocopherol concentrations (~20 to 40 μmol/L) are significantly higher than those of γ-tocopherol (~1 to 5 nmol/L) whereas the other six vitamin E forms are generally low (<500 μmol/L) or undetectable in human plasma. Thus, these more abundant forms represent the logical possibilities for having an *in vivo* antioxidant function.

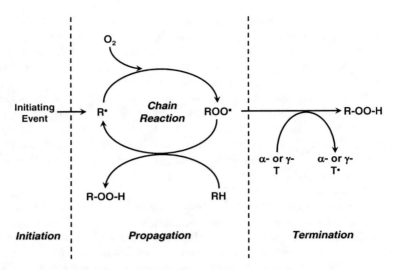

FIGURE 16.2 Chain-breaking antioxidant ability of α- and γ-tocopherol. Oxidative stress may result in the formation of carbon-centered radicals that can react with oxygen to form peroxyl radicals. In the absence of α- or γ-tocopherol, lipid peroxidation is continually propagated through the regeneration of a carbon-centered radical. In the presence of α- or γ-tocopherol, peroxyl radicals are scavenged, which ends the chain reaction of lipid peroxidation. Abbreviations: R,[•] carbon-centered radical; ROO,[•] peroxyl radical; R-OO-H, lipid hydroperoxide; RH, polyunsaturated fatty acid; α- or γ-T, α- or γ-tocopherol; α- or γ-T[•], α- or γ-tocopheroxyl radical. (Adapted from Burton, G.W. and Traber, M.G., Vitamin E: antioxidant activity, biokinetics, and bioavailability, *Annu Rev Nutr*, 10: 357–82, 1990.)

Oxidative stress results in the imbalance between free radicals and antioxidant defenses in favor of the former.[23] Therefore, excess free radicals can damage various biomolecules including proteins, DNA, and lipids. Similarly, antioxidants such as α- and γ-tocopherol should be oxidized by free radicals, which consequently would result in their increased disappearance from biological systems. This phenomenon has been clearly demonstrated *in vitro* showing that vitamin E can be oxidized by oxidant-rich cigarette smoke[24–26] or chemically by peroxynitrite.[27] However, considerably less is known regarding the effects of oxidative stress on vitamin E in humans. This is partly due to the availability of few experimental human models to evaluate the extent to which oxidative stress alters vitamin E concentrations.

To circumvent the limited human models, investigators have evaluated alterations in vitamin E utilization in aerobically exercising individuals and cigarette smokers. Although these activities are on opposite ends of the health spectrum, they serve their purpose well because each of them is well characterized as having increased oxidative stress, which is seen by the measurement of various oxidative-damage markers. The large difference between them is due to the fact that smokers represent a model of chronic oxidative stress resulting not only from the direct effects attributed to cigarette smoke itself, but also from the activated inflammatory processes that smoke induces.[20,25] Alternatively, aerobic exercise increases the magnitude of oxidative stress due to increased mitochondrial oxygen consumption and electron-transport flux.[28] Nonetheless, smoking and exercise increase oxidative damage markers[20,29] including F_2-isoprostanes, which are considered to be the "gold standard" measurement of oxidative damage.[30]

To evaluate the effects of oxidative stress attributed to cigarette smoke, smokers and non-smokers orally ingested 150 mg of deuterium-labeled α-tocopherols for 6 d.[20] After the supplementation period, smokers and nonsmokers had similar plasma concentrations of labeled α-tocopherols. However, during the post supplementation period, the smokers' plasma α-tocopherol-disappearance rates were ~13% significantly faster than those of the nonsmokers and they had plasma α-tocopherol half-lives that were significantly shorter by ~10 h. Moreover, at the end of the study, smokers had significantly lower plasma-labeled α-tocopherols than those of nonsmokers. Interestingly, the smokers' α-tocopherol-disappearance rates were inversely correlated with their plasma vitamin C concentrations (further discussion follows later under Section IX). Thus, smokers with the lowest vitamin C had the fastest rates of α-tocopherol disappearance. Therefore, the investigators conducted a follow-up trial in which they supplemented smokers and nonsmokers with vitamin C or placebo for 2 weeks prior to the ingestion of a single dose of deuterium-labeled α- and γ-tocopherols.[31] As observed in the previous study, during the placebo phase smokers had faster plasma α- and γ-tocopherol-disappearance rates. However, vitamin C supplementation completely restored smokers' α- and γ-tocopherol disappearance rates to levels similarly observed in the nonsmokers. Thus, they concluded that vitamin C recycled α- and γ-tocopheroxyl radicals to their reduced tocopherol forms, which enabled smokers to have increased α- and γ-tocopherol plasma half-lives. Such studies in smokers and nonsmokers have improved our understanding that α- and γ-tocopherol function as antioxidants *in vivo* and that they act along with vitamin C as members of an antioxidant network.[18]

Similarly, aerobic exercise also increased α-tocopherol disappearance.[29] Ultramarathon runners completed two trials in which they ingested deuterium-labeled α-tocopherols prior to a 50 km race (trial 1) or during a sedentary period (trial 2) that occurred 1 month after the race. From the plasma samples they measured labeled α-tocopherols during both trials and determined that extreme aerobic exercise resulted in ~22% faster plasma α-tocopherol disappearance compared to the sedentary phase. Importantly, exercise nearly doubled plasma isoprostanes from pre-race to post-race samples whereas the sedentary trial resulted in no changes in plasma isoprostanes. Thus, exercise-induced oxidative stress resulted in increased lipid peroxidation concomitant with increased α-tocopherol disappearance.

B. NONANTIOXIDANT

1. α-Tocopherol

In addition to α-tocopherol's antioxidant ability, α-tocopherol may have a contributory role in cell signaling. In particular, protein kinase C, a protein involved in cell proliferation and differentiation, may be inhibited by α-tocopherol in smooth muscle cells,[32,33] monocytes,[34] and platelets.[35] Other proteins that were altered by α-tocopherol include VCAM-1 and ICAM-1,[36] which are important factors in cardiovascular disease risk since they cause adhesion of certain blood cell components to the vascular endothelium. In addition, vitamin E upregulates the expression of both COX-1[37] and phospholipase A_2.[38] Further studies suggested that α-tocopherol dose dependently increased the production of vasodilator prostanoids (prostaglandin I_2 and prostaglandin E_2) in human aortic endothelial cells.[39] In this investigation, however, α-tocopherol inhibited COX activity, but did not change the expression of COX-1 or COX-2. Additionally, α-tocopherol supplementation decreased C-reactive protein and monocyte interleukin-6 concentrations in both healthy volunteers, as well as type 2 diabetics.[40] Also, α-tocopherol decreased TNF-α from activated human monocytes and also NF-κB binding activity by 5-lipoxygenase inhibition.[41] NF-κB, a redox-sensitive transcription factor, was inhibited by α-tocopherol succinate.[42] However, this effect was not observed for α-tocopherol or α-tocopheryl acetate. In contrast, it was reported in an animal investigation of phenobarbital-induced oxidative stress that α-tocopherol acetate in dietary doses of 50 and 250 mg/kg decreased liver NF-κB activation without affecting other endogenous antioxidant systems.[43]

2. γ-Tocopherol

γ-Tocopherol, as well as its physiological metabolite, γ-CEHC (γ-carboxy-ethyl-hydroxy-chroman; Figure 16.3), may possess anti-inflammatory activity.[44,45] γ-Tocopherol and γ-CEHC inhibited COX activity in lipopolysaccharide-stimulated macrophages and interleukin-1β-stimulated epithelial cells.[44] However, it should be noted that the γ-CEHC concentrations (10 to 50 μmol/L) used in

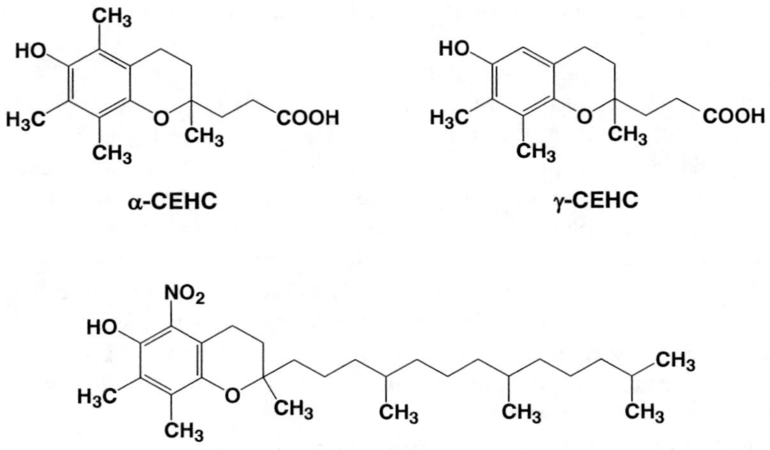

FIGURE 16.3 Structures of vitamin E metabolites and 5-nitro-γ-tocopherol. Vitamin E metabolites, α- and γ-CEHC (carboxyethyl-hydroxychromanol) are formed via P450-mediated metabolism of α- and β-tocopherol, respectively. 5-nitro-γ-Tocopherol, a nitration product of γ-tocopherol, is formed through reactions with reactive nitrogen oxides such as peroxynitrite.

these experiments exceeded physiological concentrations. Further investigations demonstrated that γ-tocopherol treatment reduced the synthesis of prostaglandin E_2 and leukotriene B_4 at the site of inflammation in a rodent model of arthritis.[45] Moreover, γ-tocopherol supplementation, but not α-tocopherol supplementation, inhibited protein nitration and spared vitamin C in rats subjected to zymosan-induced inflammation.[46]

In humans, animals, and *in vitro* models of inflammation and nitrosative stress, γ-tocopherol can be nitrated by reactive nitrogen species to yield 5-NO_2-γ-tocopherol (Figure 16.3). γ-Tocopherol, but not α-tocopherol, can be nitrated due to the subtle structural differences between the two molecules (Figure 16.1). As γ-tocopherol has an unsubstituted position on the chromanol head, it can scavenge reactive nitrogen oxides.[47] In fact, 5-NO_2-γ-tocopherol is the major product formed from the reaction between γ-tocopherol and peroxynitrite.[48] Thus, 5-NO_2-γ-tocopherol may serve as a biomarker of nitrosative stress and γ-tocopherol may also protect other biomolecules, such as tyrosine, from nitration.[25] In patients with coronary artery disease, 5-NO_2-γ-tocopherol was elevated in the plasma, as well as in the carotid-artery atherosclerotic plaque.[49] Evidence from postmortem brains of Alzheimer's patients also indicated that 5-NO_2-γ-tocopherol was elevated.[50] Cigarette smoke, in addition to its extremely high levels of reactive oxygen species, also contains 500 to 1000 ppm nitric oxide.[51] Thus, following the analysis of plasma from smokers and nonsmokers, it was determined that smokers had plasma 5-NO_2-γ-tocopherol concentrations that doubled those of nonsmokers despite no differences between the groups for plasma α- or γ-tocopherol concentrations.[25]

IV. DIETARY SOURCES

A. FOOD

Humans and animals lack the ability to synthesize vitamin E and must therefore obtain it from plants that synthesize it. The predominate forms of vitamin E found in foods are α- and γ-tocopherol.[52] Figure 16.4 illustrates the amounts of α- and γ-tocopherol in some commonly consumed foods. Notably, α-tocopherol is found in copious amounts in almonds, safflower oil, sun-

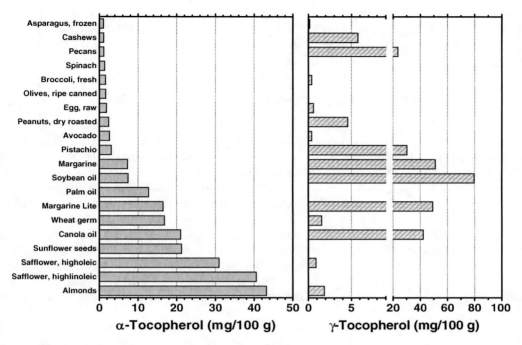

FIGURE 16.4 α- and γ-Tocopherol content of select foods.

flower seeds, and canola oil, whereas abundant sources of γ-tocopherol include certain vegetable oils (soybean and canola) and nuts (walnuts, peanuts, pecans). Interestingly, due to the high consumption of γ-tocopherol-rich foods in the typical American diet, it is estimated that γ-tocopherol represents nearly 70% of the total vitamin E content consumed.[53] Probably, this is the result of the increased consumption of fats and oils which are derived from soybean oil.[54]

B. SUPPLEMENTS

The majority of dietary vitamin E supplements contain α-tocopherol although γ-tocopherol supplements have recently emerged in the marketplace. The latter, however, generally contains a mixed tocopherol/tocotrienol formulary with γ-tocopherol as the predominant form. With regard to α-tocopherol, most dietary supplements and fortified foods contain synthetic α-tocopherol (*all rac-α*-tocopherol or commonly labeled as *dl-α*-tocopherol), rather than naturally occurring α-tocopherol (*RRR-α*-tocopherol or labeled as *d-α*-tocopherol). Although natural and synthetic compounds are often similar for most dietary supplements, this is not the case with α-tocopherol. α-Tocopherol has three chiral centers (carbon positions 2, 4′, and 8′; Figure 16.1), which can yield up to 8 stereoisomers (2R forms: *RRR, RSR, RRS, RSS*; 2S forms: *SRR, SSR, SRS, SSS*). In fact, synthetic preparations contain equal proportions of each stereoisomer whereas naturally occurring α-tocopherol only contains the *RRR* stereoisomer.[55] There are no differences in the intestinal absorption or chylomicron secretion (Figure 16.5) of synthetic and natural α-tocopherol forms.[56] However, the biopotency of *all rac-α*-tocopherol is lower than that of *RRR-α*-tocopherol so that the liver, via the α-tocopherol transfer protein, preferentially secretes *RRR-α*-tocopherol into very low-density lipoproteins, whereas *all rac-α*-tocopherol seems to be preferentially metabolized to α-CEHC. Further illustrating this point were studies conducted in healthy human participants who were simultaneously supplemented with equal amounts of deuterium-labeled natural (d_3-*RRR-α*-tocopheryl acetate) and synthetic (d_6-*all rac-α*-tocopheryl acetate) tocopherols orally.[20,57,58] In these studies, plasma concentrations of naturally occurring α-tocopherol (d_3-α-tocopherol) were approximately 2 times higher than those of synthetic α-tocopherol (d_6-α-tocopherol). Moreover, plasma d_6-α-CEHC[59] and urinary d_6-α-CEHC[20] were significantly higher (1.7 to 4.7 times) than that of d_3-α-CEHC, which suggested a greater metabolic conversion of synthetic α-tocopherol to α-CEHC (synthesis of CEHC discussed further under Subsection VI.C. Hepatic Metabolism).

V. HUMAN REQUIREMENTS AND DIETARY INTAKE

Currently, vitamin E dietary recommendations only exist for α-tocopherol because the other seven forms of vitamin E are poorly recognized by the α-tocopherol transfer protein and they are not interconverted to α-tocopherol.[60] Based on the available data, the Recommended Dietary Allowance (RDA) for men and women was established at 15 mg/d for α-tocopherol. By extrapolation it was determined that this quantity would achieve a plasma α-tocopherol concentration that would be sufficient to prevent hydrogen peroxide-induced erythrocyte lysis. In an effort to make dietary recommendations as accurate as possible, the stereochemistry of α-tocopherol was also considered when these recommendations were developed.[60] Whereas naturally occurring α-tocopherol exists only as *RRR*-α-tocopherol, synthetic preparations result in a *racemic* mixture of eight stereoisomers because the α-tocopherol phytyl tail contains three chiral centers. As 2*S*-stereoisomers of α-tocopherol are not maintained in the plasma or tissues, they were not included in the definition of active components of vitamin E, and the dietary recommendations were limited to the 2*R*-stereoisomers only.

As vitamin E is a lipophilic, chain-breaking antioxidant, it would be expected that diets rich in PUFAs could potentially increase the requirements for vitamin E.[61] Human studies are limited, but in animal studies in which the degree of lipid unsaturation ingested was increased, the result was a reduction in the time required to develop symptoms of vitamin E deficiency. Thus, it has been suggested that at least 0.6 mg of α-tocopherol equivalents per gram of PUFA should be ingested. Continued studies in humans are clearly warranted to further understand this relationship.

In comparison to the current dietary recommendations, it appears that Americans are not consuming diets adequate in α-tocopherol.[60] Recently, it was suggested that >90% of American men and women do not consume diets that meet the Estimated Average Requirement (EAR; 12 mg/d) for α-tocopherol.[62] In further support of this were data from the Third National Heath and Nutrition Examination Survey, which indicated that median α-tocopherol intakes from food alone for men and women (19 to 30 years) were only 9.4 and 6.4 mg, respectively.[60] However, it is possible that these values might be underestimated due to several sources of measurement error, which include the underreporting of total energy[63] and fat intake,[64] the amounts of fats and oils used in food preparation, the uncertainty of the specific oils consumed, and inaccuracies in the food composition databases.[60] Nonetheless, the collective data suggested that Americans are most likely not meeting the dietary recommendations for α-tocopherol intake and the available data regarding dietary intakes of α-tocopherol are probably misleading and inaccurate.

VI. BIOAVAILABILITY

A. DIGESTION AND ABSORPTION

Since vitamin E is lipophilic, its absorption from the intestinal lumen is highly dependent on the same processes that enable fat digestion and uptake into the enterocytes (Figure 16.5). In addition to pancreatic esterases that are required to cleave fatty acids from triglycerides, bile acid secretion is equally important, as both are necessary for the formation of mixed micelles that makes vitamin E absorption possible.[65] In fact, the absence of either of these components results in poor vitamin E absorption, which is why vitamin E deficiency can be observed in patients with biliary obstruction, cholestatic liver disease, pancreatitis, or cystic fibrosis.[66] Upon enterocyte uptake of vitamin E,

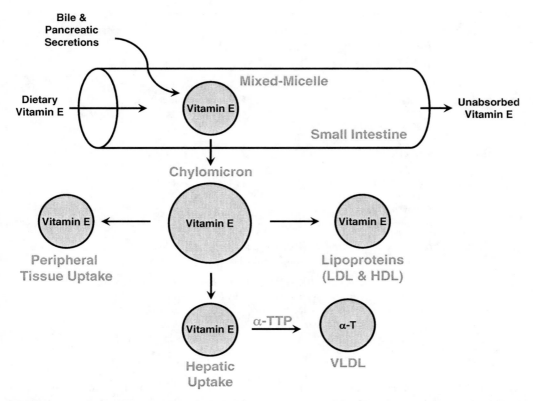

FIGURE 16.5 Vitamin E intestinal absorption. All ingested vitamin E forms are equally incorporated into micelles, absorbed in the small intestine, and packaged into chylomicrons prior to secretion into the lymph. Chylomicrons containing newly absorbed vitamin E can be catabolized by lipoprotein lipase to facilitate the transfer of vitamin E to peripheral tissues or lipoproteins (HDL or LDL). However, chylomicron remnants containing newly absorbed vitamin E are taken up by the liver by a receptor mediated process. The liver then secretes VLDL containing mostly α-tocopherol (α-T) into the plasma through a process that is mediated by the α-tocopherol transfer protein (α-TTP).

absorption into the lymphatic system is then dependent on chylomicron synthesis and secretion (Figure 16.5). In the enterocytes, chylomicrons containing triglycerides, cholesterol, phospholipids, and apolipoprotein are synthesized.[67] During that process, lipophilic compounds such as vitamin E and carotenoids are incorporated into chylomicrons and then secreted into the lymph (Figure 16.5). In healthy individuals, the absorption of vitamin E was estimated to range between 15 to 45% of the ingested dose when using radioactive α-tocopherol.[68] However, in thoracic duct-cannulated rats, the absorption of vitamin E became less efficient as the amount of α-tocopherol ingested increased.[69] The bioavailability of α-tocopherol was recently examined in healthy human participants who consumed three test meals of varying lipid amounts (0 to 11 g fat) along with deuterium-labeled *RRR*-α-tocopherol (22 mg) that was impregnated into apple pieces.[70] From blood sampling obtained up to 72 h following breakfast and deuterium-labeled *RRR*-α-tocopherol inges-tion, they determined that the bioavailability was increased up to 3-fold when 11 g of fat was co-ingested with the labeled α-tocopherol. They further calculated that at least 33% of the dose had to be absorbed during the 11 g fat trial. Moreover, it was estimated that 0.33 mg of α-tocopherol was absorbed for each gram of fat consumed, which confirmed the necessity of fat in the diet for adequate vitamin E absorption. Further studies are needed to determine the lower limit of fat ingestion necessary for optimal vitamin E absorption.

TABLE 16.1
Binding Affinity of the α-Tocopherol Transfer Protein with Tocopherols

Vitamin E Form	α-Tocopherol Transfer Protein Binding Affinity (% of *RRR*-α-Tocopherol)
RRR-α-Tocopherol	100
β-Tocopherol	38
γ-Tocopherol	9
δ-Tocopherol	2
α-Tocopherol acetate	2
α-Tocopherol quinone	2
SRR-α-Tocopherol	11
α-Tocotrienol	12

Note: The α-tocopherol transfer protein has the highest-binding affinity for naturally occurring stereoisomer of α-tocopherol (*RRR*-α-tocopherol).

Source: Data adapted from Hosomi, A., Arita, M., Sato, Y., Kiyose, C., Ueda, T., Igarashi, O., Arai, H., and Inoue, K., Affinity for alpha-tocopherol transfer protein as a determinant of the biological activities of vitamin E analogs, *FEBS Lett*, 409(1): 105–108, 1997.

B. Hepatic Secretion

Differences in plasma concentrations of the various forms of vitamin E were initially attributed to differences in intestinal absorption.[65] However, investigations using deuterated tocopherols have demonstrated that the absorptive discrimination between vitamin E forms was not due to enterocyte uptake or chylomicron secretion.[56,71] In fact, the liver is responsible for the preferential secretion of α-tocopherol into the plasma.[72] Furthermore, VLDL containing newly absorbed vitamin E (containing mostly α-tocopherol) is secreted by the liver into the plasma.[73]

The likely cause for hepatic discrimination of vitamin E is probably attributed to the α-tocopherol transfer protein.[60] This protein was first identified by Catignani and Bieri,[74] purified and characterized from liver cytosol,[75,76] and was recently crystallized.[77] The α-tocopherol transfer protein is expressed mainly in the liver[78] and purportedly functions to preferentially transfer/secrete α-tocopherol from the liver (Figure 16.5) to the plasma[79] by an incompletely understood mechanism. In comparison to α-tocopherol, other vitamin E forms bind with significantly less affinity to this protein (Table 16.1),[80] thus providing a suitable explanation for hepatic discrimination of the various vitamin E forms. In the absence of the α-tocopherol transfer protein, such as in α-tocopherol transfer protein knock-out mice[81] or humans with a genetic defect for this protein,[82] the result is vitamin E deficiency.

C. Hepatic Metabolism

Excretion of α- and γ-tocopherol occurs via two predominant pathways. It can either be excreted intact, or in its oxidized form, into bile. Alternatively, tocopherols can be metabolized by a cytochrome P450-dependent mechanism to yield a final urinary excretory product, CEHC (α- or γ-carboxyethyl-hydroxychroman; Figure 16.3). Tocopherol metabolism occurs predominately in the liver. The specific P450 enzyme responsible for initiating the metabolism of tocopherols has been a subject of debate,[83–87] but much evidence has accumulated for a cytochrome P450 of the 3A type (CYP3A). Tocopherol metabolism is initiated by ω-hydroxylation (P450 specific) of the phytyl tail, followed by subsequent cycles of β-oxidation that each remove 2 carbon units from the phytyl tail until the final product, CEHC, is produced. CEHC is then glucuronidated or sulfated prior to urinary excretion.

α- and γ-Tocopherols are metabolized at different rates. This is exemplified by a trial in which equal amounts of deuterium-labeled α- and γ-tocopherol were orally ingested by healthy participants.[88] Following the single dose of tocopherols, plasma γ-tocopherol disappeared 3 times faster than α-tocopherol. Furthermore, deuterium-labeled plasma α-CEHC was undetectable, but plasma deuterium-labeled γ-CEHC was readily detectable. Importantly, similar rates of disappearance for γ-CEHC and γ-tocopherol were observed, which suggested that γ-tocopherol disappearance was largely attributed to P450-mediated metabolism.

As noted earlier in this chapter, the diet contains mostly γ-tocopherol, but human plasma contains significantly more α-tocopherol than γ-tocopherol. This is partly explained by the higher binding affinity of the α-tocopherol transfer protein to α-tocopherol compared to γ-tocopherol (Table 16.1). As γ-tocopherol is not well recognized by the α-tocopherol transfer protein, it seems that it is more actively metabolized to γ-CEHC than α-tocopherol is metabolized to α-CEHC.[88] In fact, plasma γ-CEHC concentrations are generally in the range of 50 to 150 nmol/L whereas α-CEHC concentrations are either low (<5 nmol/L) or undetectable in unsupplemented individuals.[59] However, with α-tocopherol supplementation, a concomitant increase in α-CEHC is observed.[89] Interestingly, because CEHC is a truncation of the tocopherol's phytyl tail, CEHC retains antioxidant activity due to the intactness of the chromal head (Figure 16.3).[90] However, the extent to which that provides any antioxidant activity in humans has yet to be determined. Although it seems logical that metabolism of tocopherols would prevent vitamin E toxicity in humans, its purpose still remains unclear.

VII. DEFICIENCY

Dietary intakes of α-tocopherol are rarely low enough in the American diet to induce vitamin E deficiency symptoms (no level of deficiency has yet to be determined for γ-tocopherol). The first reports of vitamin E deficiency were characterizations of children with fat malabsorption syndromes such as abetalipoproteinemia, cholestasis, and cystic fibrosis.[73] More recently, in persons without any apparent lipid absorption or lipoprotein metabolism dysfunction, vitamin E deficiency was observed.[91] In these patients it was determined that they had a defect in the gene that encoded for the α-tocopherol transfer protein. Thus, vitamin E could be absorbed, packaged into chylomicrons, and taken up by the liver (Figure 16.5), but in the absence of the hepatic α-tocopherol transfer protein, vitamin E could not be secreted into the plasma. Understanding the role of the α-tocopherol transfer protein in human health is an area under extensive investigation. In α-tocopherol transfer-protein knockout mice, mice become vitamin E deficient and have difficulties with reproduction.[15] Additionally, these mice are more susceptible to developing atherosclerosis. Little is known about the regulation of the α-tocopherol transfer protein. Oxidative stress, induced by hyperoxia exposure for 48 h, resulted in decreased α-tocopherol transfer protein mRNA, but no apparent changes in protein levels.[92] Zinc deficiency in rats induced dramatic reductions in α-tocopherol absorption and reduced plasma α-tocopherol concentrations.[93] However, it is unclear if zinc is necessary for α-tocopherol transfer-protein expression. Importantly, dietary protein intakes are integral for maintaining vitamin E concentrations. In rats fed a low protein diet, α-tocopherol concentrations decreased and α-tocopherol transfer protein mRNA and protein levels were significantly decreased.[94]

VIII. TOXICITY

The Institute of Medicine's Food and Nutrition Board adopted a tolerable upper limit (UL) of consumption for vitamin E as 1000 mg/d.[60] This amount is considered to pose no adverse risk on health in nearly all individuals of the general population.[95] However, it should be noted that no important adverse effects have been attributed to vitamin E intakes up to 3200 IU/d.[96] Recently, a meta-analysis was conducted using data from 19 clinical trials that investigated the potential health benefits of α-tocopherol supplementation in a variety of populations (i.e., patients with cardiovascular disease, renal failure, and Alzheimer's).[97] From the analysis, it was suggested that adults ingesting >400 IU/d of α-tocopherol were 6% more likely to die prematurely. However, further analysis according to dose ingested and controlling for other nutrient intakes indicated that a significant relationship was only found among participants ingesting 2000 IU/d, which is well above the UL of 1000 mg/d. Thus, the data suggested that persons supplementing with α-tocopherol up to the UL should attract little or no risk. This is further supported by additional meta-analyses[98–100] that did not observe an adverse relationship between α-tocopherol supplementation up to 800 IU/d on the incidence of cardiovascular disease mortality or all-cause mortality.

IX. α- AND γ-TOCOPHEROL INTERACTIONS WITH VITAMIN C

Various *in vitro* investigations have indicated that the antioxidants vitamin C and vitamin E interact. Such investigations, conducted under varying conditions of oxidative stress, have suggested the ability of ascorbic acid to either spare α-tocopherol from oxidation[26,101,102] or to enable α-tocopherol regeneration from its oxidized form (α-tocopheroxyl radical) via a recycling mechanism.[103] From these investigations, α-tocopheroxyl radicals formed within micellar and bilayer membrane systems were effectively "recycled" back to α-tocopherol by ascorbic acid found within the aqueous phase. Thus, the hydrophobic α-tocopheroxyl radical likely interacts with the hydrophilic ascorbic acid at the lipid membrane interface.[18]

Limited evidence exists to support an interactive relationship between vitamin E and C in animals or humans. In fact, no interaction was observed between vitamins C and E in guinea pigs fed two concentrations of deuterium-labeled α-tocopherol and three varying concentrations of ascorbic acid.[104] However, the guinea pigs were not subjected to any form of oxidative stress, which may have limited this investigation. Alternatively, in humans this relationship has been supported in recent years. In the ASAP trial,[105,106] co-supplementation with vitamin C and α-tocopherol, but not individual nutrient supplementation, for 3 years, significantly reduced carotid artery intima-media thickness among hypercholesterolemic male smokers. This interaction between nutrients was further supported from a human trial in which smokers and nonsmokers were supplemented with ascorbic acid for 2 weeks prior to the ingestion of a single dose of deuterium-labeled α- and γ-tocopherols.[31] Among the smokers, but not the nonsmokers, vitamin C supplementation significantly attenuated plasma α- and γ-tocopherol disappearance by 25% and 45%, respectively. These dramatic decreases in tocopherol disappearance from the smokers were observed despite no reductions in the magnitude of oxidative stress as measured by plasma $F_{2\alpha}$-isoprostanes. Thus, this suggested that oxidative stress from cigarette smoking resulted in the oxidation of tocopherols and that enhanced plasma concentrations of ascorbic acid reduced (i.e., recycled) α- and γ-tocopheroxyl radicals to their respective tocopherol forms in order to attenuate vitamin E disappearance in humans.

X. ROLE IN CHRONIC DISEASE PREVENTION

Oxidative stress as it relates to aerobic organisms is often defined as an imbalance between antioxidant defenses and the production of free radicals.[23] An imbalance in favor of free radicals is often an exacerbating factor for a variety of chronic diseases.[107] This disturbance may arise from diminished antioxidants, increased production of reactive oxygen species/reactive nitrogen species or, in many cases, from a combination of these two factors. Because of vitamin E's antioxidant function, numerous investigations have been conducted to assess if vitamin E can ameliorate the risk of developing chronic diseases, particularly heart disease, certain cancers, and Alzheimer's disease.

A. CARDIOVASCULAR DISEASE

Heart disease is the leading cause of death in the U.S. accounting for nearly 700,000 deaths annually.[108] It is well accepted that oxidative stress, characterized by lipid and protein oxidation in the vascular wall, is implicated in the pathogenesis of atherosclerosis.[109] The major underlying mechanism suggests that LDL oxidation precipitates atherosclerosis. LDL that becomes trapped in the subendothelial space may become oxidized, which could lead to the stimulation of chemotaxis for monocytes and ultimately result in the formation of foam cells. Consequently, foam cells become necrotic, which leads to endothelial dysfunction and injury.

Epidemiological data suggested that low levels of α-tocopherol were inversely related to cardiovascular disease risk and that higher α-tocopherol intakes may be protective.[110,111] Moreover, individuals with coronary risk factors such as hypertriglyceridemia and low HDL levels had low serum α-tocopherol concentrations.[112] The protective role of α-tocopherol in cardiovascular disease has been supported by numerous *in vitro* studies. For example, LDL isolated from patients ingesting α-tocopherol supplements is more resistant to oxidation.[113,114] Furthermore, beyond α-tocopherol's antioxidant function, it inhibits smooth muscle cell proliferation, platelet adhesion and aggregation, and endothelial monocyte adhesion.[115] In humans, α-tocopherol's role in cardiovascular health was supported by data indicating that α-tocopherol supplementation decreased lipid peroxidation, reduced platelet aggregation, and functioned as an anti-inflammatory agent.

Prospective clinical trials using α-tocopherol alone or simultaneously with other nutrients have failed to provide convincing or consistent evidence that it decreased cardiovascular risk. Although limited in number, several clinical trials have observed positive results for α-tocopherol supplementation in the risk reduction of cardiovascular disease. Such trials include the CHAOS trial,[116] the SPACE trial,[117] the Transplant Associated Arteriosclerosis Study,[118] and the ASAP study.[105] The CHAOS and SPACE trials evaluated the effects of α-tocopherol alone whereas the ASAP and Transplant Associated Arteriosclerosis studies evaluated α-tocopherol in combination with ascorbic acid supplementation. In the CHAOS study, a 47% reduction in coronary artery disease (CAD) associated death and nonfatal myocardial infarction was observed with α-tocopherol supplementation whereas in the SPACE trial, a 39% nonsignificant reduction in CAD mortality was observed. However, in this same trial, a 70% significant reduction in myocardial infarction rate was also observed. The Transplant Associated Arteriosclerosis Study evaluated co-supplementation of α-tocopherol and ascorbic acid in patients within 2 years of cardiac transplantation. Interestingly, after a 1-year follow-up, patients randomized to the antioxidant cocktail had significantly reduced plaque area and maximal intimal thickness. Similar findings were found in the ASAP study, although this study evaluated these nutrients for a 3-year period in hypercholesterolemic patients. Interestingly, no significant reductions in the rates of intima media thickness were observed with individual nutrient supplementation, but co-supplementation with α-tocopherol and ascorbic acid significantly decreased these rates. Moreover, these effects were most pronounced in men who smoked compared to those who were nonsmokers. Most recently, results from the Women's Health Study were reported.[119] In this study, it was evaluated whether α-tocopherol supplementation among women decreased the risks of developing cardiovascular disease and cancer. During the >10-year follow-up period, 482 cardiovascular events were observed in the α-tocopherol group compared with 517 in the placebo group (7% risk reduction; nonsignificant p > 0.05). The overall conclusion of this trial was that α-tocopherol supplementation offered no cardioprotective benefit. However, subgroup analyses of women aged >65 years old indicated that this population accounted for 10% of the study population but contributed to 31% of the endpoints. Furthermore, women supplemented from this older group had a significant 26% reduction in major cardiovascular events due to a 34% reduction in myocardial infarction and 49% reduction in cardiovascular death rates.

Although the clinical trials that observed "positive" findings, with respect to α-tocopherol supplementation, on cardiovascular risk are highlighted in this chapter, caution should be applied as most clinical trials to date have provided neutral effects. Accordingly, continued studies are certainly warranted to understand the mechanisms responsible for these positive effects and to determine the limiting factors in the neutral trials that prevented a positive outcome. In addition, no clinical trials to date have evaluated the role of γ-tocopherol in cardiovascular disease risk.

B. ALZHEIMER'S DISEASE

There has been a great amount of interest to assess the extent to which α-tocopherol supplementation can prevent or slow the development of Alzheimer's disease. Like most chronic diseases, increased oxidative stress has also been implicated in the pathogenesis of Alzheimer's disease. Thus, it would be expected that improvements in antioxidant concentrations, such as vitamin E, would attenuate the risk of developing Alzheimer's disease.

Alzheimer's disease is believed to occur as a result of excessive β-amyloid formation and/or aggregation due to alterations in the processing of the amyloid precursor protein.[120] Consequently, β-amyloid toxicity induces oxidative stress. The rationale for the potential role of vitamin E as a preventative strategy for Alzheimer's disease is that the central nervous system contains a large proportion of polyunsaturated fatty acids, which are highly susceptible to lipid peroxidation. Supporting this rationale are the observations that Alzheimer's disease patients have elevated concentrations of malondialdehyde, an oxidative damage marker of lipid peroxidation.[121]

Various in vitro studies have supported the use of α-tocopherol as a strategy to attenuate the risk of Alzheimer's disease. Specifically, α-tocopherol can prevent hydrogen peroxide mediated cytotoxicity.[122] Also, α-tocopherol inhibited amyloid β-protein-induced cell death.[123] Furthermore, it can protect cells against oxidative cell death mediated by amyloid β-protein, hydroperoxide, and glutamate as it also induces the activity of the NF-κB.[124] Various studies in animals have indicated that α-tocopherol supplementation increased brain concentrations of α-tocopherol.[125,126] Moreover, cognitive performance of aged rats improved with α-tocopherol supplementation such that they had greater memory retention.[127] Likewise, α-tocopherol treatment protected against an oxidative stress-inducing neurotoxin that normally causes impaired water maze performance.[128] Lastly, α-tocopherol prevented brain lipofuscin accumulation in rats[129] and protected against ischemic neural damage in the hippocampus of gerbils.[130]

In humans, vitamin E-supplement users were less likely to develop Alzheimer's disease.[131] Somewhat conflicting data from a prospective study claimed an inverse relationship between dietary vitamin E intake from foods only and the incidence of Alzheimer's disease.[132] Therefore, it has been suggested that supplements alone (containing only α-tocopherol) were not effective because of the fact that vitamin E is comprised of 8 closely related molecules. In a follow-up study by the Chicago Health and Aging Project, it was determined that the various vitamin E forms, rather than α-tocopherol alone, were collectively protective against Alzheimer's disease.[133] Although a relationship was observed for α-tocopherol equivalents, it appeared that the strongest relationships occurred for α- and γ-tocopherols whereas lesser relationships were observed for β- and δ-tocopherols.

Importantly, peroxynitrite, the reaction product between superoxide and nitric oxide,[134] is a highly reactive molecule that initiates protein nitration to yield the formation of nitro-tyrosine. Increased neuron nitro-tyrosine concentrations have been observed and implicated in the pathogenesis of Alzheimer's disease.[135,136] γ-Tocopherol, but not α-tocopherol, is highly effective in scavenging reactive nitrogen species, which leads to the formation of 5-NO$_2$-γ-tocopherol (Figure 16.3). Recent evidence suggested that γ-tocopherol may be an important nutrient in attenuating the risk of developing Alzheimer's disease.[50] In postmortem brains of Alzheimer's disease patients, 5-NO$_2$-γ-tocopherol was increased 2 to 3-fold. Additionally, γ-tocopherol, but not α-tocopherol, attenuated SIN-1 mediated mitochondrial damage. Thus, γ-tocopherol may have unique health benefits beyond those of α-tocopherol.

C. CANCER

The role of dietary antioxidants has garnered a great deal of attention from our increased understanding that the consumption of fruits and vegetables is inversely related to the incidence of cancer.[137] Such studies have prompted investigators to search for bioactive or antioxidant components that may thwart the development and progression of cancer as oxidative stress is highly implicated in cancer pathogenesis. Specifically, oxidative stress disrupts apoptotic processes and damages various cellular components, including DNA, which suggests that antioxidants like vitamin E may inhibit carcinogenesis.[138] With respect to vitamin E and cancer, much of the attention has been focused on the protective role of α-tocopherol on cancer incidence although γ-tocopherol is now being recognized as a potentially important form of vitamin E.[139]

1. Lung Cancer

The large incidence of lung cancer and the lack of implementation of risk-lowering lifestyle strategies (i.e., smoking cessation) has spawned a great deal of scientific interest into the potential use of antioxidants in the chemoprevention of this disease.[140] The ATBC study tested the potential benefits of α-tocopherol and β-carotene supplementation, individually and in combination, in >29,000 male smokers.[141] Unfortunately, this trial was halted prematurely because it was determined that β-carotene increased lung cancer incidence despite the prior epidemiological data that suggested an inverse correlation between β-carotene and lung cancer incidence. Nonetheless, the analysis indicated that α-tocopherol's effects on lung cancer were neutral. Recently, several human trials were conducted to evaluate potential differences in vitamin E utilization between smokers and nonsmokers. Consistent with γ-tocopherol's reactive nitrogen species-scavenging ability it was determined that smokers' plasma 5-nitro-γ-tocopherol concentrations were double those of non-smokers'. This suggested that γ-tocopherol utilization increased due to increased reactive nitrogen species attributed to smoking and that γ-tocopherol might be potentially protecting other biomolecules from nitration.[25] Additionally, cigarette smoking resulted in faster plasma α- and γ-tocopherol disappearance compared to that in nonsmokers, suggesting that smokers need additional tocopherols to offset the deleterious effects of cigarette smoke.[20,31] Collectively, these findings could potentially indicate an increased risk for smokers to develop lung cancer if it is determined that α- and γ-tocopherols play a significant role in the pathogenesis of this disease. Certainly this is an area for continued investigation.

2. Prostate Cancer

In the U.S., prostate cancer has a relatively high incidence, prevalence, and mortality rate.[142] The ATBC study suggested a protective role for α-tocopherol in prostate health.[142] Among the participants receiving α-tocopherol in this study there was a significant, 32% reduction in prostate cancer incidence, as well as a 41% decreased mortality rate. However, the study was halted prematurely due to increased cancer incidence attributed to β-carotene. Nonetheless, a more recent follow-up analysis of the ATBC study participants was conducted.[143] Interestingly, the relative risk of prostate cancer incidence and mortality increased among those who were previously receiving α-tocopherol supplements, which suggested that the positive effects of α-tocopherol were diminished over time after supplementation ceased. The CARET trial provided further support of α-tocopherol in prostate health although in this trial vitamin E was not administered.[144] However, serum vitamin E analysis indicated that those with the lowest α-tocopherol concentrations had the highest risk for developing prostate cancer, whereas no interrelationship was observed for γ-tocopherol. The SELECT trial is currently under way to investigate α-tocopherol and selenium, alone and in combination, on prostate cancer incidence.[145] However, data from this trial are not expected to be available until 2013.[146]

The mechanisms by which α- and γ-tocopherol may influence the development of prostate cancer are under intense investigation. Participants with increased prostate-specific antigen (PSA) and/or abnormal digital rectal examination on initial evaluation were randomized to receive 400 IU α-tocopherol or placebo.[147] α-Tocopherol supplementation had no effect on serum androgens, IGF-1, or PSA levels, which suggested that if α-tocopherol was to have a beneficial effect, it would be mediated through a mechanism that is nonhormonally related and independent of IGF-1. In cell culture, treatment with α-tocopheryl succinate, a derivative of α-tocopherol, resulted in G1 cell-cycle arrest by attenuating various cell-cycle regulatory proteins.[148] However, as with most vitamin E esters such as α-tocopheryl succinate or acetate, the esters are cleaved in the gut prior to enterocyte uptake of free α-tocopherol. The growth of prostate cells was inhibited *in vitro* by α-tocopherol.[149] Additionally, α-tocopherol may protect prostate cells by reducing cellular androgen hormone concentrations.[150] Interestingly, γ-tocopherol more effectively inhibited prostate tumor cell growth *in vitro* to a larger extent than α-tocopherol.[151] Furthermore, γ-tocopherol induced apoptosis in androgen-responsive prostate cancer cells through caspase-dependent and γ-independent mechanisms.[152] Additionally, γ-tocopherol (alone or with other vitamin E forms) also disrupted the sphingolipid pathway and induced cell death in prostate cancer cells. Interestingly, both γ-tocopherol and γ-CEHC were the most effective inhibitors of prostate cancer cell proliferation compared to α-tocopherol, γ-CEHC, and trolox (a vitamin E metabolite analogue).[153] Given the possible benefits of α- and γ-tocopherol in prostate health, it can be expected that additional studies will be conducted to understand the mechanisms involved.

3. Colon Cancer

Colon cancer is the second leading cause of cancer-related deaths in the U.S.[154] The gastrointestinal (GI) tract is believed to be a major site where antioxidants could exert protective effects.[155] Oxidative stress and dysregulation of apoptotic processes appear to contribute to GI cancer pathogenesis. Consequently, this has led investigators to search our complex diet for bioactive components that may attenuate our risk for developing GI cancers. It has been suggested that vitamin E may prevent colon cancer by decreasing the production of mutagens that arise from the free radical-mediated oxidation of fecal lipids or by other nonoxidative stress-related mechanisms.

In vitro studies suggested that the protection of free radical-mediated damage to DNA is dependent upon the ability of tocopherols to be incorporated into cells.[154] γ-Tocopherol, compared to α-tocopherol, was preferentially increased threefold in endothelial cells after a 4-h incubation[156] although other similar studies indicated that these effects may be similar between the two vitamin E forms, or slightly higher for γ-tocopherol.[44] In human colon cancer cells, both α- and γ-tocopherol increased mRNA expression of PPAR-γ, but γ-tocopherol was more effective.[154] However, α-tocopherol was more effective than γ-tocopherol in regulating PPAR-γ protein levels. This is of interest because PPAR-γ activation induces growth inhibition in colonocytes by G1 cell-cycle arrest and by induction of apoptosis. Additionally, γ-tocopherol was more effective than α-tocopherol in preventing cell proliferation, cell cycle progression, and DNA synthesis.[157] In rats supplemented with α- or γ-tocopherol, those supplemented with γ-tocopherol had lower levels of fecal lipid hydroperoxides and ras-P21 protein levels (colon cancer biomarker) compared to those supplemented with α-tocopherol.[158]

Largely, epidemiological studies regarding vitamin E and colon cancer have produced inconsistent results, although it is often observed that patients with colon cancer tend to have lower serum vitamin E concentrations.[154,159] One of the most well-known studies, the ATBC trial, suggested a decreased incidence of colon and prostate cancer, despite the negative findings observed in this study with respect to lung cancer incidence.[141] Nonetheless, it is speculated that these inconsistencies between large trials may be attributed to differences in dietary vitamin E forms or supplementation forms of α-tocopherol (ie., natural vs. synthetic α-tocopherol). Specifically, most trials have only provided data on α-tocopherol and have used synthetic α-tocopherol supplements as a therapeutic strategy. Continued studies with other vitamin E forms may improve our understanding of vitamin E in the chemoprevention of colon cancer.

XI. CONCLUSIONS

The goal of this chapter was to provide an overview of the potential health benefits of α- and γ-tocopherols. As illustrated throughout the chapter much of the scientific data accumulated to date has mainly been in reference to α-tocopherol. With our increased understanding of the physiological and molecular actions of γ-tocopherol, it can only be expected that additional data will be forthcoming in the near future.

With that in mind, even though γ-tocopherol appears to exert beneficial effects beyond its traditional antioxidant function, it is probably premature to recommend that the general population obtain γ-tocopherol from supplements but, rather, from some of the dietary sources listed in Figure 16.4. As for α-tocopherol, supplementation in moderate doses may exert some health benefits, but until some of the inconsistencies in data from large prospective trials can be clarified, it is probably best to obtain α-tocopherol from dietary sources as well. Given the recent data demonstrating that Americans in general have low intakes of α-tocopherol, individuals should strive to make additional efforts to improve their α-tocopherol intakes. For example, the daily inclusion of a small serving of nuts or seeds such as almonds or sunflower seeds (Figure 16.4) would probably bridge the gap in most individual's diets. In addition to improving α-tocopherol intake, one would potentially benefit from all the purported cardioprotective benefits associated with the consumption of nuts.

Lastly, continued investigations into elucidating the molecular mechanisms associated with α- and γ-tocopherols' antioxidant and nonantioxidant functions are clearly warranted. Such investigations will further our understanding of why γ-tocopherol is preferentially metabolized and not well maintained in plasma or tissues peripheral to the liver. Additionally, it is hopeful that these investigations will provide a clear biological basis for γ-tocopherol in human health.

ABBREVIATIONS

ASAP	Antioxidant Supplementation in Atherosclerosis Prevention Study
CARET	β-Carotene and Retinol Efficacy Trial
CHAOS	Cambridge Heart Antioxidant Study
COX	Cyclooxygenase
HDL	High-density lipoprotein
ICAM-1	Intracellular adhesion molecule-1
LDL	Low-density lipoprotein
NF-κB	Nuclear factor kappa B
PPAR-γ	Peroxisome proliferator activated receptor-γ
PUFA	Polyunsaturated fatty acid
SELECT	Selenium and Vitamin E Cancer Prevention Trial
SPACE	Secondary Prevention with Antioxidants of Cardiovascular Disease in Endstage Renal Disease
VCAM-1	Vascular cell adhesion molecule-1
VLDL	Very low-density lipoprotein

REFERENCES

1. Traber, M.G. and Arai, H., Molecular mechanisms of vitamin E transport, *Annu Rev Nutr*, 19: 343–55, 1999.
2. Bruno, R.S. and Traber, M.G., Cigarette smoke alters human vitamin E requirements, *J Nutr*, 135(4): 671–4, 2005.
3. Evans, H.M. and Bishop, K.S., On the existence of a hitherto unrecognized dietary factor essential for reproduction, *Science*, 56: 650–651, 1922.
4. Sure, B., Dietary requirements for reproduction. II. The existence of a specific vitamin for reproduction, *J Biol Chem*, 58(1): 693–709, 1924.

5. Evans, H.M., Emerson, O.H., and Emerson, G.A., The isolation from wheat germ oil of an alcohol, alpha-tocopherol, having the properties of vitamin E., *J. Biol. Chem.*, 113: 319–332, 1936.

6. Emerson, O.H., Emerson, G.A., Mohammad, A., and Evans, H.M., The chemistry of vitamin E tocopherols from various sources, *J. Biol. Chem.*, 122(1): 99–107, 1937.

7. Machlin, L.J., *Handbook of Vitamins.* 2nd, rev. and expand ed. 1991, New York: Marcel Dekker, p. 595.

8. Horwitt, M.K., Century, B., and Zeman, A.A., Erythrocyte survival time and reticulocyte levels after tocopherol depletion in man, *Am J Clin Nutr*, 12: 99–106, 1963.

9. Horwitt, M.K., Harvey, C.C., Duncan, G.D., and Wilson, W.C., Effects of limited tocopherol intake in man with relationships to erythrocyte hemolysis and lipid oxidations, *Am J Clin Nutr*, 4: 408–419, 1956.

10. Horwitt, M.K., Vitamin E and lipid metabolism in man, *Am J Clin Nutr*, 8: 451–461, 1960.

11. Sokol, R.J., Heubi, J.E., Iannaccone, S.T., Bove, K.E., and Balistreri, W.F., Vitamin E deficiency with normal serum vitamin E concentrations in children with chronic cholestasis, *N Engl J Med*, 310(19): 1209–1212, 1984.

12. Rader, D.J. and Brewer, H.B., Jr., Abetalipoproteinemia. New insights into lipoprotein assembly and vitamin E metabolism from a rare genetic disease, *JAMA*, 270(7): 865–869, 1993.

13. Kalra, V., Grover, J., Ahuja, G.K., Rathi, S., and Khurana, D.S., Vitamin E deficiency and associated neurological deficits in children with protein-energy malnutrition, *J Trop Pediatr*, 44(5): 291–295, 1998.

14. Cavalier, L., Ouahchi, K., Kayden, H.J., Di Donato, S., Reutenauer, L., Mandel, J.L., and Koenig, M., Ataxia with isolated vitamin E deficiency: heterogeneity of mutations and phenotypic variability in a large number of families, *Am J Hum Genet*, 62(2): 301–310, 1998.

15. Terasawa, Y., Ladha, Z., Leonard, S.W., Morrow, J.D., Newland, D., Sanan, D., Packer, L., Traber, M.G., and Farese, R.V., Jr., Increased atherosclerosis in hyperlipidemic mice deficient in alpha-tocopherol transfer protein and vitamin E, *Proc Natl Acad Sci USA*, 97(25): 13830–13834, 2000.

16. Burton, G.W. and Ingold, K.U., Vitamin E as an in vitro and in vivo antioxidant, *Ann NY Acad Sci*, 570: 7–22, 1989.

17. Burton, G.W., Joyce, A., and Ingold, K.U., Is vitamin E the only lipid-soluble, chain-breaking antioxidant in human blood plasma and erythrocyte membranes? *Arch Biochem Biophys*, 221(1): 281–290, 1983.

18. Buettner, G.R., The pecking order of free radicals and antioxidants: lipid peroxidation, alpha-tocopherol, and ascorbate, *Arch Biochem Biophys*, 300(2): 535–543, 1993.

19. Terentis, A.C., Thomas, S.R., Burr, J.A., Liebler, D.C., and Stocker, R., Vitamin E oxidation in human atherosclerotic lesions, *Circ Res*, 90(3): 333–339, 2002.

20. Bruno, R.S., Ramakrishnan, R., Montine, T.J., Bray, T.M., and Traber, M.G., {alpha}-Tocopherol disappearance is faster in cigarette smokers and is inversely related to their ascorbic acid status, *Am J Clin Nutr*, 81(1): 95–103, 2005.

21. Upston, J.M., Terentis, A.C., and Stocker, R., Tocopherol-mediated peroxidation of lipoproteins: implications for vitamin E as a potential antiatherogenic supplement, *FASEB J*, 13(9): 977–994, 1999.

22. Burton, G.W., Doba, T., Gabe, E.J., Hughes, L., Lee, F.L., Prasad, L., and Ingold, K.U., Autoxidation of Biological Molecules. 4. Maximizing the Antioxidant Activity of Phenols, *J Am Chem Soc*, 107(24): 7053–7065, 1985.

23. Halliwell, B. and Gutteridge, J.M.C., *Free Radicals in Biology and Medicine*, 3rd ed., 1999, New York: Oxford University Press, 936 pp.

24. Handelman, G.J., Packer, L., and Cross, C.E., Destruction of tocopherols, carotenoids, and retinol in human plasma by cigarette smoke, *Am J Clin Nutr*, 63(4): 559–565, 1996.

25. Leonard, S.W., Bruno, R.S., Paterson, E., Schock, B.C., Atkinson, J., Bray, T.M., Cross, C.E., and Traber, M.G., 5-nitro-gamma-tocopherol increases in human plasma exposed to cigarette smoke in vitro and in vivo, *Free Radic Biol Med*, 35(12): 1560–1567, 2003.

26. Frei, B., England, L., and Ames, B.N., Ascorbate is an outstanding antioxidant in human blood plasma, *Proc Natl Acad Sci USA*, 86(16): 6377–6381, 1989.

27. Botti, H., Batthyany, C., Trostchansky, A., Radi, R., Freeman, B.A., and Rubbo, H., Peroxynitrite-mediated alpha-tocopherol oxidation in low-density lipoprotein: a mechanistic approach, *Free Radic Biol Med*, 36(2): 152–162, 2004.

28. Sacheck, J.M. and Blumberg, J.B., Role of vitamin E and oxidative stress in exercise, *Nutrition*, 17(10): 809–814, 2001.

29. Mastaloudis, A., Leonard, S.W., and Traber, M.G., Oxidative stress in athletes during extreme endurance exercise, *Free Radic Biol Med*, 31(7): 911–922, 2001.

30. Basu, S. and Helmersson, J., Factors regulating isoprostane formation in vivo, *Antioxid Redox Signal*, 7(1–2): 221–235, 2005.

31. Bruno, R.S., Leonard, S.W., Atkinson, J., Montine, T.J., Bray, T.M., and Traber, M.G., Vitamin C supplementation normalizes smokers' faster plasma vitamin E disappearance, *Free Radic Biol Med*, 40(4): 689–697, 2006.

32. Boscoboinik, D., Szewczyk, A., and Azzi, A., Alpha-tocopherol (vitamin E) regulates vascular smooth muscle cell proliferation and protein kinase C activity, *Arch Biochem Biophys*, 286(1): 264–269, 1991.

33. Chatelain, E., Boscoboinik, D.O., Bartoli, G.M., Kagan, V.E., Gey, F.K., Packer, L., and Azzi, A., Inhibition of smooth muscle cell proliferation and protein kinase C activity by tocopherols and tocotrienols, *Biochim Biophys Acta*, 1176(1–2): 83–89, 1993.

34. Devaraj, S., Li, D., and Jialal, I., The effects of alpha tocopherol supplementation on monocyte function. Decreased lipid oxidation, interleukin 1 beta secretion, and monocyte adhesion to endothelium, *J Clin Invest*, 98(3): 756–763, 1996.

35. Freedman, J.E., Farhat, J.H., Loscalzo, J., and Keaney, J.F.J., Alpha-tocopherol inhibits aggregation of human platelets by a protein kinase C-dependent mechanism, *Circulation*, 94(10): 2434–2440, 1996.

36. Cominacini, L., Garbin, U., Pasini, A.F., Davoli, A., Campagnola, M., Contessi, G.B., Pastorino, A.M., and Lo Cascio, V., Antioxidants inhibit the expression of intercellular cell adhesion molecule-1 and vascular cell adhesion molecule-1 induced by oxidized LDL on human umbilical vein endothelial cells, *Free Radic Biol Med*, 22(1–2): 117–127, 1997.

37. Chan, A.C., Wagner, M., Kennedy, C., Mroske, C., Proulx, P., Laneuville, O., Tran, K., and Choy, P.C., Vitamin E up-regulates phospholipase A2, arachidonic acid release and cyclooxygenase in endothelial cells., *Akt. Ernahr-Med.*, 23: 1–8, 1998.

38. Chan, A.C., Wagner, M., Kennedy, C., Chen, E., Lanuville, O., Mezl, V.A., Tran, K., and Choy, P.C., Vitamin E up-regulates arachidonic acid release and phospholipase A2 in megakaryocytes., *Mol Cell Biochem*, 189: 153–159, 1998.

39. Wu, D., Liu, L., Meydani, M., and Meydani, S.N., Vitamin E increases production of vasodilator prostanoids in human aortic endothelial cells through opposing effects on cyclooxygenase-2 and phospholipase A2, *J Nutr*, 135(8): 1847–1853, 2005.

40. Devaraj, S. and Jialal, I., Alpha tocopherol supplementation decreases serum C-reactive protein and monocyte interleukin-6 levels in normal volunteers and type 2 diabetic patients, *Free Radic Biol Med*, 29: 790–792, 2000.

41. Devaraj, S. and Jialal, I., Alpha-tocopherol decreases tumor necrosis factor-alpha mRNA and protein from activated human monocytes by inhibition of 5-lipoxygenase, *Free Radic Biol Med*, 38(9): 1212–1220, 2005.

42. Suzuki, Y.J. and Packer, L., Inhibition of NF-kappa B DNA binding activity by alpha-tocopheryl succinate, *Biochem Mol Biol Int*, 31(4): 693–700, 1993.

43. Calfee-Mason, K.G., Spear, B.T., and Glauert, H.P., Vitamin E inhibits hepatic NF-kappaB activation in rats administered the hepatic tumor promoter, phenobarbital, *J Nutr*, 132(10): 3178–3185, 2002.

44. Jiang, Q., Elson-Schwab, I., Courtemanche, C., and Ames, B.N., Gamma-tocopherol and its major metabolite, in contrast to alpha-tocopherol, inhibit cyclooxygenase activity in macrophages and epithelial cells, *Proc Natl Acad Sci U S A*, 97(21): 11494–11499, 2000.

45. Jiang, Q. and Ames, B.N., Gamma-tocopherol, but not alpha-tocopherol, decreases proinflammatory eicosanoids and inflammation damage in rats, *FASEB J*, 17(8): 816–822, 2003.

46. Jiang, Q., Lykkesfeldt, J., Shigenaga, M.K., Shigeno, E.T., Christen, S., and Ames, B.N., Gamma-tocopherol supplementation inhibits protein nitration and ascorbate oxidation in rats with inflammation, *Free Radic Biol Med*, 33(11): 1534–1542, 2002.

47. Christen, S., Woodall, A.A., Shigenaga, M.K., Southwell-Keely, P.T., Duncan, M.W., and Ames, B.N., Gamma-tocopherol traps mutagenic electrophiles such as NO(X) and complements alpha-tocopherol: physiological implications, *Proc Natl Acad Sci U S A*, 94(7): 3217–3222, 1997.

48. Hoglen, N.C., Waller, S.C., Sipes, I.G., and Liebler, D.C., Reactions of peroxynitrite with gamma-tocopherol, *Chem Res Toxicol*, 10(4): 401–407, 1997.

49. Morton, L.W., Ward, N.C., Croft, K.D., and Puddey, I.B., Evidence for the nitration of gamma-tocopherol in vivo: 5-nitro-gamma-tocopherol is elevated in the plasma of subjects with coronary heart disease, *Biochem J*, 364(Pt. 3): 625–628, 2002.

50. Williamson, K.S., Gabbita, S.P., Mou, S., West, M., Pye, Q.N., Markesbery, W.R., Cooney, R.V., Grammas, P., Reimann-Philipp, U., Floyd, R.A., and Hensley, K., The nitration product 5-nitro-gamma-tocopherol is increased in the Alzheimer brain, *Nitric Oxide*, 6(2): 221–227, 2002.

51. Church, D.F. and Pryor, W.A., Free-radical chemistry of cigarette smoke and its toxicological implications, *Environ Health Perspect*, 64: 111–126, 1985.

52. Dial, S. and Eitenmiller, R.R., Tocopherols and tocotrienols in key foods in the U.S. diet, in *Nutrition, Lipids, Health, and Disease*, A.S.H. Ong, E. Niki, and L. Packer, Eds., 1995, AOCS Press: Champaign, IL, pp. 327–342.

53. McLaughlin, P.J. and Weihrauch, J.L., Vitamin E content of foods, *J Am Diet Assoc*, 75: 647–665, 1979.

54. Bieri, J.G. and Evarts, R.P., Gamma tocopherol: metabolism, biological activity and significance in human vitamin E nutrition, *Am J Clin Nutr*, 27(9): 980–986, 1974.

55. Muller, P.Y., Netscher, T., Frank, J., Stoecklin, E., Rimbach, G., and Barella, L., Comparative quantification of pharmacodynamic parameters of chiral compounds (RRR- vs. all-rac-alpha tocopherol) by global gene expression profiling, *J Plant Physiol*, 162(7): 811–817, 2005.

56. Traber, M.G., Burton, G.W., Ingold, K.U., and Kayden, H.J., RRR- and SRR-alpha-tocopherols are secreted without discrimination in human chylomicrons, but RRR-alpha-tocopherol is preferentially secreted in very low-density lipoproteins, *J Lipid Res*, 31(4): 675–685, 1990.

57. Burton, G.W., Traber, M.G., Acuff, R.V., Walters, D.N., Kayden, H., Hughes, L., and Ingold, K.U., Human plasma and tissue alpha-tocopherol concentrations in response to supplementation with deuterated natural and synthetic vitamin E, *Am J Clin Nutr*, 67(4): 669–684, 1998.

58. Traber, M.G., Rader, D., Acuff, R.V., Brewer, H.B., Jr., and Kayden, H.J., Discrimination between RRR- and all-racemic-alpha-tocopherols labeled with deuterium by patients with abetalipoproteinemia, *Atherosclerosis*, 108(1): 27–37, 1994.

59. Bruno, R.S., Leonard, S.W., Li, J., Bray, T.M., and Traber, M.G., Lower plasma alpha-carboxyethylhydroxychroman after deuterium-labeled alpha-tocopherol supplementation suggests decreased vitamin E metabolism in smokers, *Am J Clin Nutr*, 81(5): 1052–1059, 2005.

60. Institute of Medicine (U.S.). Panel on Dietary Antioxidants and Related Compounds., Dietary Reference Intakes for Vitamin C, Vitamin E, Selenium, and Carotenoids: A Report of the Panel on Dietary Antioxidants and Related Compounds, Subcommittees on Upper Reference Levels of Nutrients and of Interpretation and Use of Dietary Reference Intakes, and the Standing Committee on the Scientific Evaluation of Dietary Reference Intakes, Food and Nutrition Board, Institute of Medicine. 2000, Washington, D.C.: National Academy Press. p. 506.

61. Valk, E.E. and Hornstra, G., Relationship between vitamin E requirement and polyunsaturated fatty acid intake in man: a review, *Int J Vitam Nutr Res*, 70(2): 31–42, 2000.

62. Maras, J.E., Bermudez, O.I., Qiao, N., Bakun, P.J., Boody-Alter, E.L., and Tucker, K.L., Intake of alpha-tocopherol is limited among U.S. adults, *J Am Diet Assoc*, 104(4): 567–575, 2004.

63. Mertz, W., Tsui, J.C., Judd, J.T., Reiser, S., Hallfrisch, J., Morris, E.R., Steele, P.D., and Lashley, E., What are people really eating? The relation between energy intake derived from estimated diet records and intake determined to maintain body weight, *Am J Clin Nutr*, 54(2): 291–295, 1991.

64. Briefel, R.R., Sempos, C.T., McDowell, M.A., Chien, S., and Alaimo, K., Dietary methods research in the third National Health and Nutrition Examination Survey: underreporting of energy intake, *Am J Clin Nutr*, 65(4 Suppl.): 1203S–1209S, 1997.

65. Traber, M.G., *Vitamin E*, in *Modern Nutrition in Health and Disease*, Shils, M.E. et al., Eds., 1999, Williams and Wilkins: Baltimore, MD, pp. 347–362.

66. Sokol, R.J., *Vitamin E Deficiency and Neurological Disorders*, in *Vitamin E in Health and Disease*, Packer, L. and Fuchs, J., Eds., 1993, Marcel Dekker: New York, pp. 815–849.

67. Cohn, J.S., McNamara, J.R., Cohn, S.D., Ordovas, J.M., and Schaefer, E.J., Plasma apolipoprotein changes in the triglyceride-rich lipoprotein fraction of human subjects fed a fat-rich meal, *J Lipid Res*, 29(7): 925–936, 1988.

68. Blomstrand, R. and Forsgren, L., Labelled tocopherols in man. Intestinal absorption and thoracic-duct lymph transport of dl-alpha-tocopheryl-3,4-14C2 acetate dl-alpha-tocopheramine-3,4-14C2 dl-alpha-tocopherol-(5-methyl-3H) and N-(methyl-3H)-dl-gamma-tocopheramine, *Int Z Vitaminforsch*, 38(3): 328–344, 1968.

69. Traber, M.G., Kayden, H.J., Green, J.B., and Green, M.H., Absorption of water-miscible forms of vitamin E in a patient with cholestasis and in thoracic duct-cannulated rats, *Am J Clin Nutr*, 44(6): 914–923, 1986.

70. Bruno, R.S., Leonard, S.W., Park, S.I., Zhao, Y., and Traber, M.G., Human vitamin E requirements assessed using apples fortified with deuterium-labeled alpha-tocopheryl acetate, *Am J Clin Nutr*, submitted, 2005.

71. Traber, M.G., Burton, G.W., Hughes, L., Ingold, K.U., Hidaka, H., Malloy, M., Kane, J., Hyams, J., and Kayden, H.J., Discrimination between forms of vitamin E by humans with and without genetic abnormalities of lipoprotein metabolism, *J Lipid Res*, 33(8): 1171–1182, 1992.

72. Traber, M.G., Rudel, L.L., Burton, G.W., Hughes, L., Ingold, K.U., and Kayden, H.J., Nascent VLDL from liver perfusions of cynomolgus monkeys are preferentially enriched in RRR- compared with SRR-alpha-tocopherol: studies using deuterated tocopherols, *J Lipid Res*, 31(4): 687–694, 1990.

73. Kayden, H.J. and Traber, M.G., Absorption, lipoprotein transport, and regulation of plasma concentrations of vitamin E in humans, *J Lipid Res*, 34(3): 343–358, 1993.

74. Catignani, G.L. and Bieri, J.G., Rat liver alpha-tocopherol binding protein, *Biochim Biophys Acta*, 497(2): 349–357, 1977.

75. Sato, Y., Hagiwara, K., Arai, H., and Inoue, K., Purification and characterization of the alpha-tocopherol transfer protein from rat liver, *FEBS Lett*, 288(1–2): 41–45, 1991.

76. Yoshida, H., Yusin, M., Ren, I., Kuhlenkamp, J., Hirano, T., Stolz, A., and Kaplowitz, N., Identification, purification, and immunochemical characterization of a tocopherol-binding protein in rat liver cytosol, *J Lipid Res*, 33(3): 343–350, 1992.

77. Min, K.C., Kovall, R.A., and Hendrickson, W.A., Crystal structure of human {alpha}-tocopherol transfer protein bound to its ligand: Implications for ataxia with vitamin E deficiency, *Proc Natl Acad Sci U S A*, 100(25): 14713–14718, 2003.

78. Arita, M., Sato, Y., Miyata, A., Tanabe, T., Takahashi, E., Kayden, H.J., Arai, H., and Inoue, K., Human alpha-tocopherol transfer protein: cDNA cloning, expression and chromosomal localization, *Biochem J*, 306 (Pt. 2): 437–443, 1995.

79. Traber, M.G., Vitamin E, nuclear receptors and xenobiotic metabolism, *Arch Biochem Biophys*, 423(1): 6–11, 2004.

80. Hosomi, A., Arita, M., Sato, Y., Kiyose, C., Ueda, T., Igarashi, O., Arai, H., and Inoue, K., Affinity for alpha-tocopherol transfer protein as a determinant of the biological activities of vitamin E analogs, *FEBS Lett*, 409(1): 105–108, 1997.

81. Schock, B.C., Van Der Vliet, A., Corbacho, A.M., Leonard, S.W., Finkelstein, E., Valacchi, G., Obermueller-Jevic, U., Cross, C.E., and Traber, M.G., Enhanced inflammatory responses in alpha-tocopherol transfer protein null mice, *Arch Biochem Biophys*, 423(1): 162–169, 2004.

82. Cellini, E., Piacentini, S., Nacmias, B., Forleo, P., Tedde, A., Bagnoli, S., Ciantelli, M., and Sorbi, S., A family with spinocerebellar ataxia type 8 expansion and vitamin E deficiency ataxia, *Arch Neurol*, 59(12): 1952–1953, 2002.

83. Birringer, M., Drogan, D., and Brigelius-Flohe, R., Tocopherols are metabolized in HepG2 cells by side chain omega-oxidation and consecutive beta-oxidation, *Free Radic Biol Med*, 31(2): 226–232, 2001.

84. Parker, R.S., Sontag, T.J., and Swanson, J.E., Cytochrome P4503A-dependent metabolism of tocopherols and inhibition by sesamin, *Biochem Biophys Res Commun*, 277(3): 531–534, 2000.

85. Sontag, T.J. and Parker, R.S., Cytochrome P450 omega-hydroxylase pathway of tocopherol catabolism. Novel mechanism of regulation of vitamin E status, *J Biol Chem*, 277(28): 25290–25296, 2002.

86. Kluth, D., Landes, N., Pfluger, P., Muller-Schmehl, K., Weiss, K., Bumke-Vogt, C., Ristow, M., and Brigelius-Flohe, R., Modulation of Cyp3a11 mRNA expression by alpha-tocopherol but not gamma-tocotrienol in mice, *Free Radic Biol Med*, 38(4): 507–514, 2005.

87. Traber, M.G., Siddens, L.K., Leonard, S.W., Schock, B., Gohil, K., Krueger, S.K., Cross, C.E., and Williams, D.E., Alpha-tocopherol modulates Cyp3a expression, increases gamma-CEHC production, and limits tissue gamma-tocopherol accumulation in mice fed high gamma-tocopherol diets, *Free Radic Biol Med*, 38(6): 773–785, 2005.

88. Leonard, S.W., Paterson, E., Atkinson, J.K., Ramakrishnan, R., Cross, C.E., and Traber, M.G., Studies in humans using deuterium-labeled alpha- and gamma-tocopherols demonstrate faster plasma gamma-tocopherol disappearance and greater gamma-metabolite production, *Free Radic Biol Med*, 38(7): 857–866, 2005.

89. Schultz, M., Leist, M., Petrzika, M., Gassmann, B., and Brigelius-Flohe, R., Novel urinary metabolite of alpha-tocopherol, 2,5,7,8-tetramethyl-2(2-carboxyethyl)-6-hydroxychroman, as an indicator of an adequate vitamin E supply? *Am J Clin Nutr*, 62(6 Suppl.): 1527S–1534S, 1995.

90. Betancor-Fernandez, A., Sies, H., Stahl, W., and Polidori, M.C., In vitro antioxidant activity of 2,5,7,8-tetramethyl-2-(2-carboxyethyl)-6-hydroxychroman (alpha-CEHC), a vitamin E metabolite, *Free Radic Res*, 36(8): 915–921, 2002.

91. Ouahchi, K., Arita, M., Kayden, H., Hentati, F., Ben Hamida, M., Sokol, R., Arai, H., Inoue, K., Mandel, J.L., and Koenig, M., Ataxia with isolated vitamin E deficiency is caused by mutations in the alpha-tocopherol transfer protein, *Nat Genet*, 9(2): 141–145, 1995.

92. Ban, R., Takitani, K., Kim, H.S., Murata, T., Morinobu, T., Ogihara, T., and Tamai, H., alpha-Tocopherol transfer protein expression in rat liver exposed to hyperoxia, *Free Radic Res*, 36(9): 933–938, 2002.

93. Kim, E.S., Noh, S.K., and Koo, S.I., Marginal zinc deficiency lowers the lymphatic absorption of alpha-tocopherol in rats, *J Nutr*, 128(2): 265–270, 1998.

94. Shaw, H.M. and Huang, C., Liver alpha-tocopherol transfer protein and its mRNA are differentially altered by dietary vitamin E deficiency and protein insufficiency in rats, *J Nutr*, 128(12): 2348–2354, 1998.

95. Hathcock, J.N., Azzi, A., Blumberg, J., Bray, T., Dickinson, A., Frei, B., Jialal, I., Johnston, C.S., Kelly, F.J., Kraemer, K., Packer, L., Parthasarathy, S., Sies, H., and Traber, M.G., Vitamins E and C are safe across a broad range of intakes, *Am J Clin Nutr*, 81(4): 736–745, 2005.

96. Kappus, H. and Diplock, A.T., Tolerance and safety of vitamin E: a toxicological position report, *Free Radic Biol Med*, 13(1): 55–74, 1992.

97. Miller, E.R., III, Pastor-Barriuso, R., Dalal, D., Riemersma, R.A., Appel, L.J., and Guallar, E., Meta-analysis: high-dosage vitamin E supplementation may increase all-cause mortality, *Ann Intern Med*, 142(1): 37–46, 2005.

98. Eidelman, R.S., Hollar, D., Hebert, P.R., Lamas, G.A., and Hennekens, C.H., Randomized trials of vitamin E in the treatment and prevention of cardiovascular disease, *Arch Intern Med*, 164(14): 1552–1556, 2004.

99. Shekelle, P.G., Morton, S.C., Jungvig, L.K., Udani, J., Spar, M., Tu, W., Suttorp, M.J., Coulter, I., Newberry, S.J., and Hardy, M., Effect of supplemental vitamin E for the prevention and treatment of cardiovascular disease, *J Gen Intern Med*, 19(4): 380–389, 2004.

100. Vivekananthan, D.P., Penn, M.S., Sapp, S.K., Hsu, A., and Topol, E.J., Use of antioxidant vitamins for the prevention of cardiovascular disease: meta-analysis of randomised trials, *Lancet*, 361(9374): 2017–2023, 2003.

101. Huang, J. and May, J.M., Ascorbic acid spares alpha-tocopherol and prevents lipid peroxidation in cultured H4IIE liver cells, *Mol Cell Biochem*, 247(1–2): 171–176, 2003.

102. May, J.M., Qu, Z.C., and Mendiratta, S., Protection and recycling of alpha-tocopherol in human erythrocytes by intracellular ascorbic acid, *Arch Biochem Biophys*, 349(2): 281–289, 1998.

103. Bisby, R.H. and Parker, A.W., Reaction of ascorbate with the alpha-tocopheroxyl radical in micellar and bilayer membrane systems, *Arch Biochem Biophys*, 317(1): 170–178, 1995.

104. Burton, G.W., Wronska, U., Stone, L., Foster, D.O., and Ingold, K.U., Biokinetics of dietary RRR-alpha-tocopherol in the male guinea pig at three dietary levels of vitamin C and two levels of vitamin E. Evidence that vitamin C does not "spare" vitamin E in vivo, *Lipids*, 25(4): 199–210, 1990.

105. Salonen, J.T., Nyyssonen, K., Salonen, R., Lakka, H.M., Kaikkonen, J., Porkkala-Sarataho, E., Voutilainen, S., Lakka, T.A., Rissanen, T., Leskinen, L., Tuomainen, T.P., Valkonen, V.P., Ristonmaa, U., and Poulsen, H.E., Antioxidant Supplementation in Atherosclerosis Prevention (ASAP) study: a randomized trial of the effect of vitamins E and C on 3-year progression of carotid atherosclerosis, *J Intern Med*, 248(5): 377–386, 2000.

106. Salonen, R.M., Nyyssonen, K., Kaikkonen, J., Porkkala-Sarataho, E., Voutilainen, S., Rissanen, T.H., Tuomainen, T.P., Valkonen, V.P., Ristonmaa, U., Lakka, H.M., Vanharanta, M., Salonen, J.T., and Poulsen, H.E., Six-year effect of combined vitamin C and E supplementation on atherosclerotic progression: the Antioxidant Supplementation in Atherosclerosis Prevention (ASAP) Study, *Circulation*, 107(7): 947–953, 2003.

107. Betteridge, D.J., What is oxidative stress? *Metabolism*, 49(2 Suppl. 1): 3–8., 2000.

108. Anderson, R.N. and Smith, B.L., Deaths: leading causes for 2002, *Natl Vital Stat Rep*, 53(17): 1–89, 2005.

109. Stocker, R. and Keaney, J.F., Jr., Role of oxidative modifications in atherosclerosis, *Physiol Rev*, 84(4): 1381–1478, 2004.

110. Harris, A., Devaraj, S., and Jialal, I., Oxidative stress, alpha-tocopherol therapy, and atherosclerosis, *Curr Atheroscler Rep*, 4(5): 373–380, 2002.

111. Jialal, I. and Devaraj, S., Scientific evidence to support a vitamin E and heart disease health claim: research needs, *J Nutr*, 135(2): 348–353, 2005.

112. Miwa, K., Okinaga, S., and Fujita, M., Low serum alpha-tocopherol concentrations in subjects with various coronary risk factors, *Circ J*, 68(6): 542–546, 2004.

113. Fuller, C.J., Chandalia, M., Garg, A., Grundy, S.M., and Jialal, I., RRR-alpha-tocopheryl acetate supplementation at pharmacologic doses decreases low-density-lipoprotein oxidative susceptibility but not protein glycation in patients with diabetes mellitus., *Am J Clin Nutr*, 63(5): 753–759, 1996.

114. Devaraj, S., Adams-Huet, B., Fuller, C.J., and Jialal, I., Dose-response comparison of RRR-alpha-tocopherol and all-racemic alpha-tocopherol on LDL oxidation., *Arterioscler Thromb Vasc Biol*, 17(10): 2273–2279, 1997.

115. Devaraj, S. and Jialal, I., The effects of alpha-tocopherol on critical cells in atherogenesis, *Curr Opin Lipidol*, 9(1): 11–15, 1998.

116. Stephens, N.G., Parsons, A., Schofield, P.M., Kelly, F., Cheeseman, K., and Mitchinson, M.J., Randomized controlled trial of vitamin E in patients with coronary disease: Cambridge Heart Antioxidant Study (CHAOS), *Lancet*, 347(9004): 781–786, 1996.

117. Boaz, M., Smetana, S., Weinstein, T., Matas, Z., Gafter, U., Iaina, A., Knecht, A., Weissgarten, Y., Brunner, D., Fainaru, M., and Green, M.S., Secondary prevention with antioxidants of cardiovascular disease in end stage renal disease (SPACE): randomized placebo-controlled trial, *Lancet*, 356: 1213–1218, 2000.

118. Fang, J.C., Kinlay, S., Beltrame, J., Hikiti, H., Wainstein, M., Behrendt, D., Suh, J., Frei, B., Mudge, G.H., Selwyn, A.P., and Ganz, P., Effect of vitamins C and E on progression of transplant-associated arteriosclerosis: a randomized trial, *Lancet*, 359(9312): 1108–1113, 2002.

119. Lee, I.M., Cook, N.R., Gaziano, J.M., Gordon, D., Ridker, P.M., Manson, J.E., Hennekens, C.H., and Buring, J.E., Vitamin E in the primary prevention of cardiovascular disease and cancer: the Women's Health Study: a randomized controlled trial, *JAMA*, 294(1): 56–65, 2005.

120. Grundman, M., Vitamin E and Alzheimer disease: the basis for additional clinical trials, *Am J Clin Nutr*, 71(2): 630S–636S, 2000.

121. Palmer, A.M. and Burns, M.A., Selective increase in lipid peroxidation in the inferior temporal cortex in Alzheimer's disease, *Brain Res*, 645(1–2): 338–342, 1994.

122. Behl, C., Davis, J.B., Lesley, R., and Schubert, D., Hydrogen peroxide mediates amyloid beta protein toxicity, *Cell*, 77(6): 817–827, 1994.

123. Behl, C., Davis, J., Cole, G.M., and Schubert, D., Vitamin E protects nerve cells from amyloid beta protein toxicity, *Biochem Biophys Res Commun*, 186(2): 944–950, 1992.

124. Behl, C., Vitamin E protects neurons against oxidative cell death in vitro more effectively than 17-beta estradiol and induces the activity of the transcription factor NF-kappaB, *J Neural Transm*, 107(4): 393–407, 2000.

125. Leonard, S.W., Terasawa, Y., Farese, R.V., Jr., and Traber, M.G., Incorporation of deuterated RRR-or all-rac-alpha-tocopherol in plasma and tissues of alpha-tocopherol transfer protein — null mice, *Am J Clin Nutr*, 75(3): 555–560, 2002.

126. Pillai, S.R., Traber, M.G., Steiss, J.E., Kayden, H.J., and Cox, N.R., Alpha-tocopherol concentrations of the nervous system and selected tissues of adult dogs fed three levels of vitamin E, *Lipids*, 28(12): 1101–1105, 1993.

127. Socci, D.J., Crandall, B.M., and Arendash, G.W., Chronic antioxidant treatment improves the cognitive performance of aged rats, *Brain Res*, 693(1–2): 88–94, 1995.

128. Wortwein, G., Stackman, R.W., and Walsh, T.J., Vitamin E prevents the place learning deficit and the cholinergic hypofunction induced by AF64A, *Exp Neurol*, 125(1): 15–21, 1994.

129. Monji, A., Morimoto, N., Okuyama, I., Yamashita, N., and Tashiro, N., Effect of dietary vitamin E on lipofuscin accumulation with age in the rat brain, *Brain Res*, 634(1): 62–68, 1994.

130. Hara, H., Kato, H., and Kogure, K., Protective effect of alpha-tocopherol on ischemic neuronal damage in the gerbil hippocampus, *Brain Res*, 510(2): 335–338, 1990.

131. Morris, M.C., Beckett, L.A., Scherr, P.A., Hebert, L.E., Bennett, D.A., Field, T.S., and Evans, D.A., Vitamin E and vitamin C supplement use and risk of incident Alzheimer disease., *Alzheimer Dis Assoc Disord*, 12: 121–126, 1998.

132. Morris, M.C., Evans, D.A., Bienias, J.L., Tangney, C.C., Bennett, D.A., Aggarwal, N., Wilson, R.S., and Scherr, P.A., Dietary intake of antioxidant nutrients and the risk of incident Alzheimer disease in a biracial community study, *JAMA*, 287(24): 3230–3237, 2002.

133. Morris, M.C., Evans, D.A., Tangney, C.C., Bienias, J.L., Wilson, R.S., Aggarwal, N.T., and Scherr, P.A., Relation of the tocopherol forms to incident Alzheimer disease and to cognitive change, *Am J Clin Nutr*, 81(2): 508–514, 2005.

134. Beckman, J.S., Beckman, T.W., Chen, J., Marshall, P.A., and Freeman, B.A., Apparent hydroxyl radical production by peroxynitrite: implications for endothelial injury from nitric oxide and super-oxide, *Proc Natl Acad Sci USA*, 87(4): 1620–1624, 1990.

135. Smith, M.A., Richey Harris, P.L., Sayre, L.M., Beckman, J.S., and Perry, G., Widespread peroxynitrite-mediated damage in Alzheimer's disease, *J Neurosci*, 17(8): 2653–2657, 1997.

136. Good, P.F., Werner, P., Hsu, A., Olanow, C.W., and Perl, D.P., Evidence of neuronal oxidative damage in Alzheimer's disease, *Am J Pathol*, 149(1): 21–28, 1996.

137. Block, G., Patterson, B., and Subar, A., Fruit, vegetables, and cancer prevention: a review of the epidemiological evidence, *Nutr Cancer*, 18(1): 1–29, 1992.

138. Bjelakovic, G., Nikolova, D., Simonetti, R.G., and Gluud, C., Antioxidant supplements for preventing gastrointestinal cancers, *Cochrane Database Syst Rev* (4): CD004183, 2004.

139. Wagner, K.H., Kamal-Eldin, A., and Elmadfa, I., Gamma-tocopherol — an underestimated vitamin? *Ann Nutr Metab*, 48(3): 169–188, 2004.

140. Hirsch, F.R. and Lippman, S.M., Advances in the biology of lung cancer chemoprevention, *J Clin Oncol*, 23(14): 3186–3197, 2005.

141. Albanes, D., Heinonen, O.P., Huttunen, J.K., Taylor, P.R., Virtamo, J., Edwards, B.K., Haapakoski, J., Rautalahti, M., Hartman, A.M., Palmgren, J. et al., Effects of alpha-tocopherol and beta-carotene supplements on cancer incidence in the alpha-tocopherol beta-carotene cancer prevention study., *Am J Clin Nutr*, 62(6 Suppl.): 1427S–1430S, 1995.

142. Klein, E.A., Chemoprevention of prostate cancer, *Crit Rev Oncol Hematol*, 54(1): 1–10, 2005.

143. Virtamo, J., Pietinen, P., Huttunen, J.K., Korhonen, P., Malila, N., Virtanen, M.J., Albanes, D., Taylor, P.R., and Albert, P., Incidence of cancer and mortality following alpha-tocopherol and beta-carotene supplementation: a postintervention follow-up, *JAMA*, 290(4): 476–485, 2003.

144. Goodman, G.E., Schaffer, S., Omenn, G.S., Chen, C., and King, I., The association between lung and prostate cancer risk, and serum micronutrients: results and lessons learned from beta-carotene and retinol efficacy trial, *Cancer Epidemiol Biomarkers Prev*, 12(6): 518–526, 2003.

145. Klein, E.A., Thompson, I.M., Lippman, S.M., Goodman, P.J., Albanes, D., Taylor, P.R., and Coltman, C., SELECT: the selenium and vitamin E cancer prevention trial, *Urol Oncol*, 21(1): 59–65, 2003.

146. Klein, E.A., Selenium and vitamin E cancer prevention trial, *Ann N Y Acad Sci*, 1031: 234–241, 2004.

147. Hernandez, J., Syed, S., Weiss, G., Fernandes, G., von Merveldt, D., Troyer, D.A., Basler, J.W., and Thompson, I.M., Jr., The modulation of prostate cancer risk with alpha-tocopherol: a pilot randomized, controlled clinical trial, *J Urol*, 174(2): 519–522, 2005.

148. Ni, J., Chen, M., Zhang, Y., Li, R., Huang, J., and Yeh, S., Vitamin E succinate inhibits human prostate cancer cell growth via modulating cell cycle regulatory machinery, *Biochem Biophys Res Commun*, 300(2): 357–363, 2003.

149. Sigounas, G., Anagnostou, A., and Steiner, M., dl-alpha-tocopherol induces apoptosis in erythroleukemia, prostate, and breast cancer cells, *Nutr Cancer*, 28(1): 30–35, 1997.

150. Hartman, T.J., Dorgan, J.F., Virtamo, J., Tangrea, J.A., Taylor, P.R., and Albanes, D., Association between serum alpha-tocopherol and serum androgens and estrogens in older men, *Nutr Cancer*, 35(1): 10–15, 1999.

151. Moyad, M.A., Brumfield, S.K., and Pienta, K.J., Vitamin E, alpha- and gamma-tocopherol, and prostate cancer, *Semin Urol Oncol*, 17(2): 85–90, 1999.

152. Jiang, Q., Wong, J., and Ames, B.N., Gamma-tocopherol induces apoptosis in androgen-responsive LNCaP prostate cancer cells via caspase-dependent and independent mechanisms, *Ann N Y Acad Sci*, 1031: 399–400, 2004.

153. Galli, F., Stabile, A.M., Betti, M., Conte, C., Pistilli, A., Rende, M., Floridi, A., and Azzi, A., The effect of alpha- and gamma-tocopherol and their carboxyethyl hydroxychroman metabolites on prostate cancer cell proliferation, *Arch Biochem Biophys*, 423(1): 97–102, 2004.

154. Stone, W.L., Krishnan, K., Campbell, S.E., Qui, M., Whaley, S.G., and Yang, H., Tocopherols and the treatment of colon cancer, *Ann N Y Acad Sci*, 1031: 223–233, 2004.

155. Bjelakovic, G., Nikolova, D., Simonetti, R.G., and Gluud, C., Antioxidant supplements for prevention of gastrointestinal cancers: a systematic review and meta-analysis, *Lancet*, 364(9441): 1219–1228, 2004.

156. Tran, K. and Chan, A.C., Comparative uptake of alpha- and gamma-tocopherol by human endothelial cells, *Lipids*, 27(1): 38–41, 1992.

157. Gysin, R., Azzi, A., and Visarius, T., Gamma-tocopherol inhibits human cancer cell cycle progression and cell proliferation by down-regulation of cyclins, *FASEB J*, 16(14): 1952–1954, 2002.

158. Stone, W.L., Papas, A.M., LeClair, I.O., Qui, M., and Ponder, T., The influence of dietary iron and tocopherols on oxidative stress and ras-p21 levels in the colon, *Cancer Detect Prev*, 26(1): 78–84, 2002.

159. Campbell, S., Stone, W., Whaley, S., and Krishnan, K., Development of gamma (gamma)-tocopherol as a colorectal cancer chemopreventive agent, *Crit Rev Oncol Hematol*, 47(3): 249–59, 2003.

160. Burton, G.W. and Traber, M.G., Vitamin E: antioxidant activity, biokinetics, and bioavailability, *Annu Rev Nutr*, 10: 357–82, 1990.

17 Probiotics and Prebiotics

Edward R. Farnworth

CONTENTS

I. PROBIOTICS

Within the definition of functional foods, there is a subset of foods believed to be good for health that are produced by or that contain live microorganisms. These foods are called *probiotics*. The earliest definition of a probiotic was very narrow and applied specifically to animals (see Table 17.1). As the metabolism of bacteria became better defined, more studies pointed out the role that microorganisms play in human health and disease resistance, and more microorganisms were identified that may be included in probiotic products, a need to expand the definition of a probiotic became obvious. The recent WHO definition of probiotics includes the word *administered* to acknowledge that routes of administration other than oral can be used for probiotics. It should be noted that discussions of probiotics are usually limited to bacteria; the use and importance of yeasts in probiotic foods have not received much attention.

A. CRITERIA FOR PROBIOTICS

As researchers and food manufacturers started to appreciate the potential for including microorganisms in probiotic foods, various criteria were suggested to screen candidate microorganisms that would at the same time satisfy regulatory bodies and ensure consumer acceptance (see Table 17.2). The first three criteria address practical aspects of selection of appropriate microorganisms for inclusion in

TABLE 17.1
Evolving Definitions of Probiotics

Definition

"Animal feed supplements that have a beneficial effect on the host animal by affecting its gut microflora"

"A live microbial feed supplement which beneficially affects the host animal by improving its intestinal microbial balance"

"A viable mono- or mixed culture of microorganisms which, when applied to animals or man, beneficially affects the host by improving the properties of the indigenous microbiota"

"A microbial preparation which contains live and/or dead cells, including their metabolites, which is intended to improve the microbial or enzymatic balance at mucosal surfaces or to stimulate immune mechanisms"

"Live microorganisms which, when administered in adequate amounts, confer a health benefit on the host"

Source: Parker, R.B., Probiotics, the other half of the antibiotics story, *Anim. Nutr. Health*, 29: 4–8, 1974; Fuller, R., Probiotics in man and animals, *J. Appl. Bacteriol.*, 66: 365–378, 1989; Havenaar, R. and Huis in't Veld, J.H.J., Probiotics: a general view, in *The Lactic Acid Bacteria in Health and Disease*, Vol. 1, Wood, B.J.B., Ed., Elsevier Applied Science, London, 1992; Reuter, G., Present and future probiotics in Germany and in Central Europe, *Biosci. Microflora*, 16: 43–51, 1997; Report of a Joint FAO/WHO Working Group, Guidelines for the Evaluation of Probiotics in Food, London, Ont. Canada, 2002.

probiotic foods, and the latter two may be more important from a consumer-acceptance and regulatory point of view. The ideal probiotic bacteria would possess all of the criteria. However, the list of bacteria that meet several of the criteria and, in particular, those that have sound scientific evidence of efficacy and that have been incorporated into foods, is not long. Debate over what is truly a microorganism of human origin has prompted many to downplay the importance of this criterion.

Several of the criteria listed in Table 17.2 are obviously related. To be effective, the probiotic bacteria must arrive at the site of action in large enough numbers to exert their effect. This may most easily be achieved by using resistant bacteria or by providing large numbers of live bacteria at the time of consumption to compensate for losses during passage through the upper gastrointestinal (GI) tract. Some manufacturers are also using enteric coated capsules that do not dissolve in the low pH environment of the stomach to protect the bacteria.

TABLE 17.2
Proposed Criteria for Microorganisms to Be Included in Probiotic Foods and Drinks

1. Microorganism of human origin
2. Resistance to acid conditions of stomach, bile, and digestive enzymes normally found in the human GI tract
3. Ability to colonize human intestine
4. Safe for human consumption
5. Scientifically proven efficacy

Source: Lee, Y.-K. and Salminen, S., The coming of age of probiotics, *Trends Food Sci. Technol.*, 6: 241–244, 1995; Huis in't Veld, J.H.J. and Havenaar, R., Probiotics and health in man and animal, *J. Chem. Tech. Biotechnol.*, 51: 562–567, 1991; Huis in't Veld, J.H.J. and Havenaar, R., Selection criteria and application of probiotic microorganisms in man and animal, *Microbiol. Ther.*, 26: 43–57, 1997; O'Sullivan, M.G., Thornton, G., O'Sullivan, G.C., and Collins, J.K., Probiotic bacteria: myth or reality, *Trends Food Sci. Technol.*, 3: 309–314, 1992; Rambaud, J.-C., Bouhnik, Y., Marteau, P., and Pochart, P., Manipulation of the human gut microflora, *Proc. Nutr. Soc.*, 52: 357–366, 1993.

Knowledgeable consumers are now looking for products that contain live bacteria. Meanwhile, manufacturers are becoming more aware of the need to provide accurate information about the levels and types of bacteria in their products.[4] The setting of a minimum number of viable microorganisms in a food to ensure probiotic effects is an important decision. The Fermented Milks and Lactic Acid Bacteria Beverages Association in Japan has set a minimum of 10^7 bifidobacteria/g or ml.[11] Others have suggested a lower level (10^5).[5] However, experimental evidence in which various levels of bacteria were fed and viable numbers counted after passage through the stomach would indicate that probiotic products may have to deliver even higher ($>10^{10}$ to 10^{11}) levels of microorganisms to survive the conditions of the GI tract.[12] This conclusion is supported by *in vitro* tests done on a variety of potential probiotic bacteria using simulated digestive systems.[13,14] This wide diversity of opinion may only reflect the differences in the ability of different bacteria to survive passage through the stomach. To set one level for all bacteria may not be possible because the numbers of bacteria required to produce a certain metabolic change will vary depending on the effect to be achieved.

Only bacteria that can survive passage through the stomach and can colonize the intestines will exert any effect on the host. This was most clearly shown by Pedrosa and colleagues.[15] In healthy elderly persons fed yogurt containing *Lactobacillus bulgaricus* and *Streptococcus thermophilus*, these two organisms could not be found in intestinal contents after feeding, and there were no changes in three bacterial enzyme activities. When healthy subjects were fed live *Lb. gasseri* (*Lb. acidophilus* strain MS 02), a human strain capable of adhering to intestinal cells, the organism was found in all subjects and the activities of β-glucuronidase, nitroreductase, and azoreductase were all significantly reduced. This study emphasizes the need to measure both the fate of the ingested bacteria and metabolic effects to ensure proper interpretation of results.

Various reports have included lists of bacteria that can be considered as candidates for inclusion in probiotic products (Table 17.3). The whole premise of a functional food is that certain commonly eaten foods contain active ingredients that can fight or prevent disease and infection. With advances in analytical techniques, the identification of new active ingredients occurs every day. For probiotics, however, the identity of the active ingredient may not be as straightforward because there is always more than one possibility. The active agent could be one or more of the live microorganisms in the food, or it could be a metabolite produced by one of the microorganisms themselves, or it could be a fermentation product that has been formed due to the action of the microorganism(s) on the original product. Indeed, depending on the probiotic in question, each of the above arguments has been used to explain the beneficial effects of the probiotic.

B. PROBIOTIC PRODUCTS ON THE MARKET

In Japan, there is a long tradition of believing that health is dependent on food and that the maintenance of a population of beneficial intestinal bacteria is important to overall health. In 1981, the Japanese established the Japan Bifidus Foundation to encourage research on bifidobacteria which, in part, may explain why 53 probiotic products containing bifidobacteria were for sale in Japan by 1993.[11] Japan is often lauded as an example of how cooperation between industry and government health agencies can lead to a system of approval and labeling of foods that are good for health. The "foods for specific health uses" (FOSHU) system provides consumers with products with a distinctive logo indicating that the product (or product ingredients) have been judged as being good for health. There are 11 categories of functional components that qualify under the FOSHU system. Three of these categories, namely, dietary fiber, oligosaccharides, and lactic acid bacteria, refer specifically to intestinal function and control. Recent listings show 43 probiotic products that have been given FOSHU status.[16]

Reuter[4] pointed out that in both Germany and Switzerland, there is wide consumer interest in probiotic products. He lists 21 products (produced in seven European countries) for sale in Germany of either a yogurt-type or a yogurt drink format in 1997. Regulatory concerns have slowed the

TABLE 17.3
Possible Probiotic Microorganisms

Lactobacillus Bacteria

Lb. acidophilus
   Lb. acidophilus LC1
   Lb. acidophilus NCFB 1748
Lb. plantarum
Lb. casei
   Lb. casei Shirota
Lb. rhamnosus (strain GG)
Lb. brevis
Lb. delbrueckii subsp. *bulgaricus*
Lb. fermentum
Lb. helveticus

Bifidobacterium Bacteria

B. bifidum
B. longum
B. infantis
B. breve
B. adolescentis

Other Bacteria

Streptococcus salvarius subsp. *thermophilus*
Lactococcus lactis subsp. *lactis*
Lac. lactis subsp. *cremoris*
Enterococcus faecium
Leuconostoc mesenteroides subsp. *dextranicum*
Propionibacterium freudenreichii
Pediococcus acidilactici
Escherichia coli

Yeasts

Saccharomyces boulardii

Note: The identification and classification of bacteria and yeasts change as more sophisticated methods are used. The nomenclature used throughout this chapter is that found in the references cited to avoid confusion.

Source: Lee, Y.-K. and Salminen, S., The coming of age of probiotics, *Trends Food Sci. Technol.*, 6: 241–244, 1995; Huis in't Veld, J.H.J. and Havenaar, R., Probiotics and health in man and animal, *J. Chem. Tech. Biotechnol.*, 51: 562–567, 1991; Huis in't Veld, J.H.J. and Havenaar, R., Selection criteria and application of probiotic microorganisms in man and animal, *Microbiol. Ther.*, 26: 43–57, 1997.

introduction of such products in North America. As of 2004, no probiotic products sold in North America carry a government-approved health claim.

II. PREBIOTICS

The concept of a prebiotic arose from two observations: (1) bacteria, like any other living organism, have (sometimes specific) nutrient requirements[17] and (2) some nutrients, particularly complex carbohydrates, pass undigested into the colon where they are utilized by resident bacteria.[18] In

---

TABLE 17.4
Some Proposed Prebiotics

Neosugars
(GFn n = 1–4)
Inulin-like fructans (fructooligosaccharides of chain length up to 60 units)
Soy oligosaccharides
Galacto-oligosaccharides
Isomalto-oligosaccharides
Gentio-oligosaccharides
Xylo-oligosaccharides
Lactulose (fructose-galactose disaccharide)
Raffinose
Stachyose
Sorbitol
Xylitol
Palatinose
Lactosucrose

Source: Tannock, G.W., Exploring the intestinal ecosystem using molecular methods, in *Probiotics and Health, The Intestinal Microflora,* Roy, E. Ed., Edisem Publ. Co., Saint-Hyacinthe, Canada, pp. 14–26; Macfarlane, G.T. and Macfarlane, S., Human colonic microbiota: ecology, physiology and metabolic potential of intestinal bacteria, *Scand. J. Gastroenterol.,* 32 (Suppl. 222): 3–9, 1997.

1995, Gibson and Roberfroid[19] defined a prebiotic as "nondigestible food ingredient that beneficially affects the host by selectively stimulating the growth or activity of a limited number of bacteria in the colon." Rather than supplying an exogenous source of beneficial bacteria, the concept of a prebiotic proposes to increase the number of certain target bacteria already in the colon. Attention has centered mainly on the increase of *Lactobacillus* and *Bifidobacterium* as the two main groups of "friendly bacteria" to increase.[20–23] Variation in individual response is often high and, as cautioned by Roberfroid,[24] the prebiotic effect may depend on the initial level of target bacteria. Some carbohydrates of interest as prebiotics are listed in Table 17.4.

The goal of increasing selected bacteria by feeding prebiotics has often been the production of various short-chain fatty acids (SCFAs) because of their impact on the lower gut environment, metabolism, and disease prevention.[25–26] The SCFAs are quickly absorbed and can serve as an energy source for the host, especially between meals. They contribute to fecal pH and thereby influence colonic function and perhaps the risk of cancer.[27] The effects of feeding a prebiotic such as galacto-oligosaccharide on constipation are not conclusive,[28,29] although gut-transit time can be shortened by feeding particular bacterial strains.[30,31]

The combination of live bacteria in a food and the inclusion of nutrients (usually sugars) that can be used by those bacteria as the two traverse the GI tract has resulted in what have been termed symbiotic foods.[24] The most popular combination to date appears to be *Bifidobacterium* and fructooligosaccharides, but other combinations are possible, if not practical.[23,32]

III. MICROBIOLOGY OF THE GASTROINTESTINAL TRACT

The human microbiota is complex, difficult to study, and is influenced by many factors. Study of the microorganisms that populate human GI tracts is hampered by the fact that sampling opportunities are limited, variation between individuals is great, there is no totally relevant animal model, such research is time-consuming and expensive, and advances in this area of research are obviously

---

TABLE 17.5
Bacterial Genera Found in Human Intestinal and Fecal Samples

Bacteroidaceae	*Eubacteria*	*Staphylococci*
Peptococcaceae	*Bifidobacteria*	*Leuconostoc*
Streptococci	*Enterobacteria*	*Fusobacteria*
Lactobacilli	*Vellonella*	*Magasphaera*
Clostridia	*Lactococci*	

Source: Conly, J.M., Stein, K., Worobetz, L., and Rutledge-Harding, S., The contribution of vitamin K2 (menaquinones) produced by the intestinal microflora to human nutritional requirements for vitamin K, *Am. J. Gastroenterol.*, 89: 915–923, 1994; Mitsuoka, T., Intestinal flora and aging, *Nutr. Rev.*, 50: 438–446, 1992; Gorbach, S.L., Perturbation of intestinal microflora, *Vet. Hum. Toxicol.*, 35 (Suppl. 1): 15–23, 1993.

---

dependent on advances in microbiology. The recent use of molecular biology techniques has allowed the study of the human GI tract microbiota using non-media dependent methods. Fluorescent *in situ* hybridization (FISH), and polymer chain reaction (PCR) together with denaturing gradient gel electrophoresis (DGGE) are now being used for definitive and comparative bacterial population studies.[33,34]

Even the simplest questions, such as how many and what kind of bacteria are important in the human GI tract, are not easy to answer or to find a consensus in the literature. Indeed, at least one author has stated that due to difficulties in obtaining proper samples, the crudeness of the methods used to count the various types of bacteria, and the short duration of most diet intervention studies, very little is really known about the human microbiota and factors that affect it.[35] To date, most of our understanding of the human microflora comes from analyses of fecal contents, which may severely limit our understanding of events further up the GI tract.

There is agreement about the changes, in general terms, in the bacterial population that occur during the passage from newborn to infant to adult. Vaginally delivered babies have nearly sterile GI tracts, which soon become colonized, either with large numbers of *Bifidobacterium* and *Lactobacillus* in the case of breast-fed babies or *Bacteroides sp.* and *Eschericha coli* in the case of bottle-fed babies.[36] *Bifidobacterium* are considered as desirable, and so attempts have been made to add prebiotics to infant formula to encourage the growth of bifidobacteria.[37] By adulthood, over 400 different species may be present (see Table 17.5) but only the most abundant bacteria have been well identified, because of limitations in methodology. Resident bacteria can be found starting with the mouth and working down the GI tract. The stomach and the upper small intestine may have as many as 10^5 colony-forming units (CFU/ml), the ileum 10^7, and the colon 10^{11} to 10^{12}.[38] Anaerobic bacteria outnumber aerobic by a factor of 1000 to 1.[39]

The bacteria that reside in the human intestinal tract have both beneficial and harmful effects on the host. The production of vitamins, SCFAs, some proteins, the role played in digestion and absorption of nutrients, the production of protective bacteriocins, and the stimulation of the immune system are all positive effects of the intestinal microflora.[40,41] At the same time, intestinal bacteria produce carcinogens and mutagens directly during their metabolism and also enzymes that convert digesta contents into carcinogens and mutagens. Products of fermentation such as ammonia, amines, and phenols may be harmful and some bacteria are pathogenic. Mitsuoka[42] and Gorbach[43] list the many enzymatic reactions of intestinal bacteria and their impact on health, disease, and infection.

Because of the difficulties in identifying and enumerating various microorganisms that inhabit the GI tract, several authors have suggested that a more sensitive and perhaps more relevant approach

---

TABLE 17.6
Microflora-Associated Characteristics Indicative of Intestinal Microflora Changes

1. Cellular fatty acid profiles of washed bacteria pellet of fecal or cecal contents
2. Primary to secondary bile acid ratio
3. Ratio of primary to secondary sterols
4. Molar ratio of SCFAs in intestinal material

Source: Carman, R.J., Van Tassall, R.L., and Wilkins, T.D., The normal intestinal microflora: ecology, variability and stability, *Vet. Hum. Toxicol.*, 35(Suppl. 1): 11–14, 1993. With permission.

---

is to measure effects on the metabolic activities of the bacterial flora because of their potential impact on metabolism and disease. Carman and colleagues[44] used the term microflora-associated characteristics (MACs) and argued that changes in MACs brought about by dietary (probiotic or not) interventions were true indicators of changes in the intestinal flora, and a more useful way of establishing the consequences of such changes. Goldin and Gorbach[45] used much the same reasoning when they measured bacterial enzymes associated with the production of carcinogens in the intestine. Table 17.6 lists the MACs suggested by Carman and colleagues.[44] Other characteristics could be added that also reflect changes to the intestinal tract.

IV. PROBIOTIC PRODUCTS

A. Yogurt

Yogurt is defined as a fermented milk obtained by specific lactic acid fermentation, brought about by *Lb. bulgaricus* and *S. thermophilus*. Other bacteria may be added to enhance organoleptic properties or, more recently, to increase the probiotic properties. Yogurt can now be found on the market that contains *Lactobacillus*, *Streptococcus*, *Leuconostoc*, and *Bifidobacterium* bacteria. Yogurt and yogurt-like products can be found in many countries.[46]

The amount of research on yogurt far surpasses any other probiotic product. Yogurt has been studied to determine its effects on lactase deficiency, cholesterol metabolism, immunity, infantile diarrhea, and certain cancers with varying levels of success.

1. Lactase Deficiency

Yogurt has been shown to be a dairy product that may be tolerated by people with a lactase (β-galactosidase) deficiency. It is more accurate to refer to a lactase deficiency as opposed to a lactose intolerance. Lactase is the digestive enzyme found in the intestinal brush border responsible for the hydrolysis of the milk sugar lactose into glucose and galactose. A lactase deficiency results in the buildup of unabsorbed lactose which acts osmotically to retain water. The deficiency is characterized by diarrhea, excessive flatulence, bloating, and abdominal pain after the ingestion of milk or milk products. Measurement of the enzyme activity, the concentration of lactose or glucose or galactose in digesta, or the measurement of breath hydrogen are ways of evaluating dietary treatment effects on lactase activity.

In 1984, two groups, Kolars and colleagues[47] and Savaiano and colleagues,[48] demonstrated that yogurt reduced the symptoms of lactase deficiency and speculated that this was due to the live bacteria in yogurt. Yogurt was said to be able to autodigest lactose, resulting in 20 to 30% lower lactose levels in yogurt compared to unfermented milk when consumed. Yogurt, but not heat-treated yogurt, improves lactose digestion, indicating that the live bacteria in yogurt are responsible, and long-term ingestion (8 d) does not seem to change this.[49,50] The bacteria in yogurt survive passage through the stomach due to the enhanced protective (buffering) properties of the yogurt compared with milk. However, the buffering capacity of yogurt may also slow hydrolysis until the digesta passes to a point in the intestinal tract where the pH favors β-galactosidase activity.[49] The β-galactosidase activity in commercial yogurts has been found to vary depending on the manufacturer, whether fruit is added, the addition of additional bacteria, and whether the yogurt is frozen or not. Frozen yogurt that is pasteurized before freezing has no β-galactosidase activity. To overcome this, some manufacturers add starter culture to the pasteurized yogurt before freezing, but this does not necessarily increase enzyme activity.[51]

In addition to the *in vivo* bacterial hydrolysis, there also appears to be a slower rate of stomach emptying after a yogurt load compared to milk due to differences in physical properties. This effect may contribute to the enhanced digestion of the lactose in yogurt.[52,53]

The beneficial effects of yogurt on healthy individuals may not be as obvious as for those who have a defined medical problem. Guerin-Danan et al.[54] saw few changes in the fecal bacteria and the bacterial enzyme activity of healthy infants (10 to 18 months old) over a 1-month supplementation trial. Branch-chain and long-chain fatty acid levels were significantly reduced during yogurt consumption, however.

2. Cholesterol Metabolism

The research into the effects of yogurt consumption on blood cholesterol has been difficult to understand because of the contradictory results that have been reported over the years. It is now clear that, in many cases, results and conclusions from one experiment cannot be compared with those of others because of differences in experimental protocol. The sex, age, general health status, initial cholesterol level, and level of physical activity of subjects all influence cholesterol metabolism. The diet before and during the experiment can also influence results, as can the time of day the yogurt is consumed, whether it is consumed with other food or not, and the position in the meal (beginning or end of meal). One of the most important details of many yogurt–blood cholesterol experiments, namely, the type of yogurt fed (including details of the levels and an unambiguous identification of bacteria in the test yogurt or fermented milk), are often not well described. This, together with the fact that proper controls for such feeding trials were often not included, reduces the scientific validity of many studies.[55,56]

The observation that even though the Masai of Africa ate a diet rich in saturated fats and fermented milk, they had low blood cholesterol levels (compared with Western standards) and were free of signs of coronary heart disease, prompted Mann and Spoerry[57] to carry out their much reported study involving fermented milk. Yogurt trials carried out since that time use this as a starting point, despite of the fact that Mann[58] later emphasized that he believed that it was a milk factor responsible for the hypocholesterolemic effect, which was enhanced by fermentation to yogurt. Taylor and Williams[55] list 12 publications (13 trials) in which yogurt has been fed in an attempt to lower blood cholesterol. As they point out, many of the study protocols can be criticized — too few subjects, too short a feeding trial, no or improper control diets, and unrealistic feeding levels. Of the 13 trials, 8 reported reduced blood total cholesterol levels, 1 reported an increase, and 4 reported no difference from control. Two studies, one showing "no difference from control"[59] and one showing nonsignificant positive effects on serum cholesterol levels have been published.[60] Adding oligofructose and two probiotic bacteria to traditional yogurt (3.5% fat) did not change total serum cholesterol, but did significantly lower the LDL/HDL ratio in women after consumption for 6 months.[61] Feeding healthy residents in a gerontology institute bioyogurt — yogurt made with *Lb. acidophilus*, *B. bifidum*, and *Strep. salivarius* subsp. *thermophilus* — significantly reduced serum cholesterol levels.[62]

Various suggestions have been made regarding the possible active ingredient(s) or the mode of action of yogurt, which might affect cholesterol metabolism.[63] *In vivo* cholesterol synthesis may be related to, and controlled by, the availability of certain short chain fatty acids (SCFAs) produced by bacteria in the gut; interest has centered on acetate and propionate.[64,65] Several bacteria have been shown to be capable of hydrolyzing bile acids, which would prevent reabsorption in the intestine and facilitate elimination from the body. Bile acids are formed from cholesterol in the liver and, therefore, any increase in elimination of bile acids from the body would increase the rate of conversion of cholesterol to bile acids. It has also been hypothesized that a reduced pH in the gut as a result of lactic acid produced by some bacteria can cause cholesterol and deconjugated bile salts to coprecipitate, facilitating elimination of cholesterol from the body.

Until a mechanism is clearly demonstrated, the claim that yogurt or fermented milk reduces serum cholesterol remains in doubt.

3. Immune Function

The organs of the immune system (spleen, appendix, lymph nodes, Peyer's patches, etc.) are varied, but the intestine is generally considered the most important component of the immune system. A wide variety of parameters, including levels of specific immunoglobulins, numbers of different cell types, and measurement of specific metabolite concentrations, are used to measure immune function. To date, several hypotheses have been put forward regarding how yogurt might improve the immune system. Interaction of the yogurt bacteria with intestinal bacteria could produce indirect effects, or the gut-associated or systemic immune system might be affected by metabolites of the bacteria themselves or fermentation products in the yogurt.[66]

Perdigon's group[67–69] has published several studies using animals that show that yogurt consumption does improve immune function. Consuming yogurt has also been reported to modulate some components of the immune system (lymphocytes and CD56 cells) in stressed individuals.[70] However, Wheeler and colleagues[71] measured a wide variety of cellular, humoral, phagocytic, and mucosal immunity parameters in patients with preexisting atopic disease and found no significant differences in any parameters whether the patients were consuming yogurt or milk. Spanhaak and colleagues[72] similarly reported no changes in immunity parameters in healthy subjects who had been fed milk fermented with *Lb. casei* strain Shirota, even though fecal bacteria patterns were changed and fecal enzyme activities were significantly decreased. Gill's[73] review of the literature emphasized the difficulties in comparing the results from different studies but concluded that there is enough evidence to suggest that certain lactic acid bacteria, given at adequate levels of intake, can influence immune function in humans. Additional published data showing positive effects would strengthen this conclusion.

4. Diarrhea

Diarrhea, particularly in young children, can be problematic because of the need to rehydrate the patient as quickly as possible combined with the problems associated with decreased nutrient intake. The detrimental consequences of complete withdrawal of food from infants as a treatment have been defined, but withholding food during early stages of diarrhea is still widespread.[74] Fermented milk or yogurt can supply liquid and simultaneously may supply natural antibiotics produced by the lactic acid bacteria to prevent or reduce the severity of infantile diarrhea. Gonzalez and colleagues[75] showed that milk fermented with *Lb. casei* and *Lb. acidophilus* could be used to prevent the incidence of diarrhea (17% vs. 59% for controls receiving unfermented milk) in infants 5 to 29 months old, and that the protective effect of the fermented milk appeared to be correlated to the level of fecal lactic acid bacteria. Isolauri and coworkers[76] used milk fermented with the human strain *Lb. casei* sp. strain GG to reduce the duration of acute diarrhea in children. This same strain of bacteria was shown to be effective in the prevention of antibiotic (erythromycin) associated diarrhea, partly due to its ability to colonize the intestinal tract.[77] Yogurt containing *Lb. bulgaricus* and *S. thermophilus* and the probiotic strain *Lb. casei* DN-114 001 has been shown in several large trials with children to significantly reduce the duration of diarrhea.[78,79] However, positive results only appear to be applicable in infants who are otherwise well nourished.[80] A nonsignificant reduction in the incidence of diarrhea in healthy adults consuming yogurt containing *Lb. casei* has recently been reported.[81]

5. Cancer

The beneficial effect of yogurt consumption on reduced cancer incidence is not well established. The article published by Van't Veer and colleagues[82] is often quoted as proof of a link between yogurt consumption and a low incidence of breast cancer. Based on a daily food-consumption questionnaire of newly diagnosed breast cancer patients or a group of healthy women (control), they concluded that eating fermented milk products (yogurt, buttermilk, Gouda cheese) may have a protective effect against breast cancer. Two more recent dietary survey studies came to different conclusions about the effect of yogurt (fermented milk products) on colorectal cancer.[83,84]

The work of Goldin and Gorbach[45] and Goldin and colleagues[85] supports the idea that the *Lb. acidophilus* found in yogurt may impact on marker enzymes related to cancer. They found two to 6-fold reductions in the activities of β-glucuronidase, nitroreductase, and azoreductase enzyme activities after 4-week supplementation with 10^9 to 10^{10} viable *Lb. acidophilus*. These bacterial enzymes produce carcinogens from procarcinogens in the lower intestine. This work, together with positive *in vitro* and experimental animal results, suggests that the bacteria in yogurt may act directly or indirectly to prevent cancer.[86–89] Recent data using mice fed yogurt has indicated that the immune system may be involved in inhibiting the promotion and progression of colorectal cancer.[90] Other work on the cancer-fighting properties of yogurt has centered on the isolation and identification of bioactive peptides. Caseins found in milk are themselves antimutagenic; totally hydrolyzed caseins are not. A wide variety of peptides of various lengths are formed from milk during fermentation or in the stomach during the digestion of yogurt.[91–93] Low-molecular-weight peptides have a wide variety of activities *in vitro* and *in vivo*, including antimutagenic and antitumor properties that may be responsible for the beneficial effects of yogurt on cancer initiation and progression.

6. A Vehicle for Other Nutrients

The popularity of yogurt has prompted several studies that have investigated the feasibility of using yogurt as a vehicle for other important nutrients that normally would not be found in yogurt. Fernandez-Garcia and colleagues[94] have recently shown that oat fiber can be added to plain yogurt and still maintain commercially acceptable sensory qualities. Plant sterols have been added to yogurt producing a product that significantly lowers serum cholesterol after only three weeks of consumption.[95]

In spite of the potential problems of off-flavor and encouragement of growth of contaminating bacteria, Hekmat and McMahon[96] were able to produce a yogurt with up to 40 mg/kg of added iron that was acceptable particularly to untrained consumers. In addition, it has been shown that yogurt consumption can increase zinc bioavailability in humans eating a diet high in plant-based phytates without affecting iron bioavailability.[97]

B. Kefir

Kefir is a fermented milk drink that is believed to have its origins in the Caucasus Mountains of the former U.S.S.R. Traditionally, it was made from goat or cow milk that was stored in animal skin bags. Over time, a mass of bacteria, yeasts, proteins, and carbohydrates precipitated out from the drink and was used to inoculate new milk. This mass is called *kefir grains*, and it is the grains that give kefir its texture, taste, and possible health benefits. Kefir has a long oral tradition for its health-promoting properties in Eastern Europe and has only recently been produced in North America on a commercial scale.[98] A product of the fermentation process is CO_2 gas, which continues to be produced after packaging and results in a thick drink with a "sparkling" mouth-feel when consumed.

TABLE 17.7
Microorganisms Reported to Be Found in Kefir and Kefir Grains

Bacteria

Lactobacillus Bacteria	*Lactococcus* Bacteria
Lb. acidophilus	L. lactis subsp. lactis
Lb. johnsonii	L. lactis subsp. cremoris
Lb. kefirgranum	L. lactis subsp. lactis biovar diacetylactis
Lb. helveticus	
Lb. delbrueckii subsp. bulgaricus	**Leuconostoc Bacteria**
Lb. kefiranofaciens	Ln. lactis
Lb. casei	Ln. mesenteroides subsp. mesenteroides
Lb. zeae	Ln. mesenteroides subsp. cremoris
Lb. rhamnosus	Ln. mesenteroides subsp. dextranicum
Lb. plantarum	
Lb. brevis	**Other Bacteria**
Lb. buchneri	Streptococcus thermophilus
Lb. fermentum	
Lb. kefir	
Lb. parakefir	

Yeasts

Saccharomyces Yeasts	*Kluyveromyces* Yeasts
S. cerevisiae	K. marxianus var. marxianus
S. unisporus	K. marxianus var. lactis
S. turicersis	

Other Yeasts

Candida kefyr
Torulaspora delbrueckii
Geotrichum candidum Link

Source: Mainville, I., Robert, N., Lee, B., and Farnworth, E.R., Polyphasic characterization of the lactic acid bacteria in kefir. *Syst. Appl. Microbiol.*, 29, 59–68, 2006; Vayssier, Y., Le kéfir: etude et mise au point d'un levain pour la préparation d'une boisson, *Rev. Lait Fr.*, 362: 131–134, 1978; Zourari, A. and Anifantakis, E.M., Le kéfir caractères physico-chimiques, microbiologiques et nutritionnels. Technologie et production. Une revue, *Lait*, 68: 373–392, 1988

Unlike yogurt, which requires only two well-defined bacteria for production, the microbiology of kefir is much more complex (Table 17.7) and has been shown to vary from country to country, thus making a comparison of its properties difficult. The use of molecular biological techniques has shown that many bacteria have been misidentified in the past, and the list of bacteria and yeasts in kefir may not be as long as once believed.[99] Changes that occur during fermentation promote the growth of certain microorganisms, while reducing the growth of others. Therefore, reports of the composition and properties of the grains may not be totally applicable to the finished product.

1. Fabrication

Three different types of kefir drink are produced — traditional kefir, Russian-type kefir, and industrial kefir — depending on whether the grains or a mother culture from the grains is used to inoculate the pasteurized milk.[103,104] No studies have been published that compare the properties (health benefits or otherwise) of kefir produced by different processes. Incubation is carried out at 20 to 22°C for 18 to 20 h until a specific pH is reached and then packaged, or a maturation period can be introduced. The grains themselves have a strong yeasty taste and, therefore, using a mother culture or sieving out the grains may be ways of making a product closer to buttermilk in taste.[104,105] A double-fermentation process was proposed by Marshall and Cole[105] as a way of making the taste of traditional kefir more acceptable to the consumer.[106] Today, commercial kefir is only produced from cow milk, but other milks, including soymilk, can be fermented with kefir grains.[107,108]

Studies of the microflora of kefir grains led to the formulation of less complex starter cultures that could replace kefir grains. A method using as few as four bacteria and one yeast type has been reported as being used to produce "kefir."[109] However, apart from very gross characteristics, there is little reason to believe that the two beverages (produced from traditional grains or simpler starter cultures) are the same. Today, lyophilized kefir starter culture mixtures are used by some manufactures instead of kefir grains.

2. Health Benefits

The (Western) scientific literature to support the beneficial health claims of kefir is not extensive and few human feeding trials using kefir have been performed. The Russian literature lists peptic ulcers, biliary tract diseases, chronic enteritis, bronchitis, and pneumonia as all being treated with kefir.[98] Kefir is included as a regular part of hospital diets, is a recommended food for nursing mothers, and is often used as an initial weaning food for babies in Russia. Both kefir grains and the drink itself have been shown to have antitumoral, antibacterial, and antifungal properties that may explain the diverse list of diseases and infections it is used to treat. In the tests carried out by Cevikbas and colleagues,[110] the kefir grains were more effective than the drink. Osada and coworkers[111] reported the isolation of a sphingomyelin from kefir grains, which they showed enhanced interferon-β production in a human cancer cell line that had been challenged with a chemical inducer. They concluded that this sphingomyelin could be important in treating viral diseases.

Several Japanese studies using experimental animals have indicated anticancer properties of kefir for a variety of cancers.[111–117] These studies have used kefir grains, kefir-grain polysaccharides, or both to prevent the onset of cancer if given before a cancer challenge or to slow the growth and spread of cancer if given after the cancer challenge. However, to date, such experiments have not been carried out on humans.

Vujicic and colleagues[118] incubated milk samples with kefir grains from six different sources and showed that after 24 h, between 22 and 63% of the cholesterol originally in the milk was assimilated. They concluded that the grains possessed a cholesterol-degrading enzyme system. In a study in which hypercholesterolemic men were given 500 ml of kefir daily for 1 month, no changes (compared with values obtained after 1 month of milk feeding) were measured in serum cholesterol levels or cholesterol metabolism, despite the fact that a reference organism (*Lb. brevis*) could be found in fecal samples and changes in fecal volatile fatty acids were found.[119]

V. FERMENTED VEGETABLES AND OTHER FOODS

The most well-known and popular probiotic foods in industrialized countries are milk based. Yakult®, a milk product containing the probiotics bacteria *L. casei* Shirota, is believed to be the largest-selling probiotic product in the world. However, fermented foods are produced and consumed around the world based on vegetables, fruits, cereals, grains, root crops, fish, and meat. Some of these foods may have health-promoting properties.[120]

Fermentation is often considered an effective method to preserve vegetables, without regard to any health benefits. Reddy and colleagues[121] list 23 legume-based fermented foods, the majority of which are soybean products. Only *natto*, a popular fermented soybean product from Japan, is mentioned as encouraging the growth of Bifidobacterium in animals.[122] Most reports of fermented vegetables have centered on the organism(s) used to produce the fermentation and on any increases in the protein, amino acid, and vitamin concentrations of the final product, not any possible probiotic effects.[123–125]

Various other foods have been tested as possible vectors to carry probiotic bacteria. Verification of the efficacy of these products has not been given much attention to date, but, rather, investigation of whether the bacteria will survive in the food matrix and during processing and storage. Cheddar cheese containing *Enterococcus faecium*,[126] *B. longum* in frozen yogurt,[127] and *B. longum, B. infantis, B. brevis*,[32] *L. acidophilus*, and *B. bifidum*[125] in ice cream are examples.[128]

Lee and Salminen[6] predicted that probiotic infant formulae, baby food, fermented fruit juices, fermented soy products, cereal-based products, as well as disease-specific products, are possible products of the future.

VI. THE FUTURE FOR PROBIOTICS AND PREBIOTICS

The market for probiotic and prebiotic products will continue to grow as our knowledge of the intestinal microflora and its role in the maintenance of health and disease resistance advances. Food manufacturers will have to be able to commercialize products that maintain viable bacteria up until the time of consumption, and in many cases, will also have to provide encapsulation or other protective mechanisms for the live microorganisms in their products to be able to deliver bacteria to the correct site of action in the GI tract.

REFERENCES

1. Parker, R.B., Probiotics, the other half of the antibiotics story, *Anim. Nutr. Health*, 29: 4–8, 1974.
2. Fuller, R., Probiotics in man and animals, *J. Appl. Bacteriol.*, 66: 365–378, 1989.
3. Havenaar, R. and Huis in't Veld, J.H.J., Probiotics: a general view, in *The Lactic Acid Bacteria in Health and Disease*, Vol. 1, Wood, B.J.B., Ed., Elsevier Applied Science, London, 1992.
4. Reuter, G., Present and future probiotics in Germany and in Central Europe, *Biosci. Microflora*, 16: 43–51, 1997.
5. Report of a Joint FAO/WHO Working Group, Guidelines for the Evaluation of Probiotics in Food, London, Ont. Canada, 2002.
6. Lee, Y.-K. and Salminen, S., The coming of age of probiotics, *Trends Food Sci. Technol.*, 6: 241–244, 1995.
7. Huis in't Veld, J.H.J. and Havenaar, R., Probiotics and health in man and animal, *J. Chem. Tech. Biotechnol.*, 51: 562–567, 1991.
8. Huis in't Veld, J.H.J. and Havenaar, R., Selection criteria and application of probiotic microorganisms in man and animal, *Microbiol. Ther.*, 26: 43–57, 1997.
9. O'Sullivan, M.G., Thornton, G., O'Sullivan, G.C., and Collins, J.K., Probiotic bacteria: myth or reality, *Trends Food Sci. Technol.*, 3: 309–314, 1992.
10. Rambaud, J.-C., Bouhnik, Y., Marteau, P., and Pochart, P., Manipulation of the human gut microflora, *Proc. Nutr. Soc.*, 52: 357–366, 1993.
11. Ishibashi, N. and Shimamura, S., Bifidobacteria: research and development in Japan, *Food. Technol.*, 126, 129–130, 132–135, 1993.
12. Saxelin, M., Elo, S., Salminen, S., and Vapaatalo, H., Dose response colonization of faeces after oral administration of *Lactobacillus casei* strain GG, *Microb. Ecol. Health Dis.*, 4: 209–214, 1991.
13. Molly, K., Vande Woestyne, M., and Verstraete, W., Development of a 5-step multi-chamber reactor as a simulation of the human intestinal microbial ecosystem, *Appl. Microbiol. Biotechnol.*, 39: 254–258, 1993.
14. Alander, M., De Smet, I., Nollet, L., Verstraete, W., von Wright, A., and Mattila-Sandholm, T., The effect of probiotic strains on the microbiota of the simulator of the human intestinal microbial ecosystem (SHIME), *Int. J. Food. Microbiol.*, 46: 71–79, 1999.

15. Pedrosa, M.C., Golner, B.B., Goldin, B.R., Barakat, S., Dallal, G.E., and Russel, R.M., Survival of yogurt-containing organisms and *Lactobacillus gasseri* (ADH) and their effect on bacterial enzyme activity in the gastrointestinal tract of healthy and hypochlorhydric elderly subjects, *Am. J. Clin. Nutr.*, 61: 353–358, 1995.

16. http://www.jhnfa.org/index.htm (in Japanese).

17. Yazawa, K. and Tamura, Z., Search for sugar sources for selective increase of Bifidobacteria, *Bifidobact. Microflora*, 1: 39–44, 1982.

18. Mitsuoka, T., Hidaka, H., and Eida, T., Effect of fructo-oligosaccharides on intestinal microflora, *Nahrung*, 31: 5–6, 427–436, 1987.

19. Gibson, G.R. and Roberfroid, M.B., Dietary modulation of the human colonic microbiota: introducing the concept of prebiotics, *J. Nutr.*, 125: 1401–1412, 1995.

20. Hidaka, H., Eida, T., Takizawa, T., Tokunaga, T., and Tashiro, Y., Effects of fructooligosaccharides on intestinal flora and human health, *Bifidobact. Microflora*, 5: 37–50, 1986.

21. Koo, M. and Rao, A.V., Long-term effect of Bifidobacteria and neosugar on precursor lesions of colonic cancer in CF1 mice, *Nutr. Cancer*, 16: 249–257, 1991.

22. Grill, J.P., Manginot-Durr, C., Schneider, F., and Ballongue, J., Bifidobacteria and probiotic effects: action of Bifidobacterium species on conjugated bile salts, *Curr. Microbiol.*, 31: 23–27, 1995.

23. Schaafsma, G., Meuling, W.J.A., van Dokkum, W., and Bouley, C., Effects of a milk product, fermented by *Lactobacillus acidophilus* and with fructo-oligosaccharides added, on blood lipids in male volunteers, *Eur. J. Clin. Nutr.*, 52: 436–440, 1998.

24. Roberfroid, M.B., Prebiotics and symbiotics: concepts and nutritional properties, *Br. J. Nutr.*, 80: (Suppl. 2): S197–S202, 1998.

25. Jenkins, D.J.A., Kendall, C.W.C., and Vuksan, V., Inulin, oligosaccharides and intestinal function, *J. Nutr.*, 129: 1432S–1433S, 1999.

26. Elsen, R.J. and Bistrain, B.R., Recent developments in short-chain fatty acid metabolism, *Nutrition*, 7: 7–10, 1991.

27. Fleming, S.E. and Arce, D.S., Volatile fatty acids: their production, absorption, utilization and roles in human health, *Clin. Gastroenterol.*, 15: 787–814, 1986.

28. Teuri, U. and Korpela, R., Galacto-oligosaccharides relieve constipation in elderly people, *Ann. Nutr. Metab.*, 42: 319–327, 1998.

29. Ito, M., Deguchi, Y., Miyamori, A., Matsumoto, K., Kikuchi, H., Matsumoto, K., Kobayashi, Y., Yajima, T., and Kan, T. Effects of administration of galactoologosaccharides on the human faecal microflora, stool weight and abdominal sensation. *Microb. Ecol. Health Dis.* 3: 285–292, 1990.

30. Meance, S., Cayuela, C., Turchet, P., Raimondi, A., Lucas, C., and Antoine, J.M., A fermented milk with *Bifidobacterium* probiotic strain DN-173 010 shortened oro-fecal gut transit time in elderly, *Microb. Ecol. Health Dis.* 13: 217–222, 2001.

31. Marteau, P., Cuillerier, E., and Meance, S. Gerhard, M.F., Myara, A., Bouvier, M., Bouley, C., Tondu, F., Bommelaer, G., and Grimaud, J.C., *Bifidobacterium animalis* strain DN-173 010 shortens the colonic transit time in healthy women: a double blind, randomized, controlled study, *Aliment Pharmacol. Ther.* 16: 587–593, 2002.

32. Modler, H.W., McKellar, R.C., Goff, H.D., and Mackie, D.A., Using ice cream as a mechanism to incorporate bifidobacteria and fructooligosaccharides into the human diet, *Cult. Dairy Prod. J.*, 25: 4–6, 7, 1990.

33. Farnworth, E.R., The future for fermented foods, in *Handbook of Fermented Functional Foods*, Farnworth, E.R. Ed., CRC Press, Boca Raton, FL, pp. 361–378.

34. Tannock, G.W., Exploring the intestinal ecosystem using molecular methods, in *Probiotics and Health, The Intestinal Microflora*, Roy, D. Ed., Edisem Publ. Co., Saint-Hyacinthe, Canada, pp. 14–26.

35. Hill, M.J., Diet and the human intestinal bacterial flora, *Cancer Res.*, 41: 3778–3780, 1981.

36. Benno, Y., Sawada, K., and Mitsuoka, T., The intestinal microflora of infants: composition of fecal flora in breast-fed and bottle-fed infants, *Microbiol. Immunol.*, 28: 975–986, 1984.

37. Rubaltelli, F.F., Biadaioli, R., Pecile, P., and Nicoletti, P., Intestinal flora in breast- and bottle-fed infants, *J. Perinat. Med.*, 26: 186–191, 1998.

38. Evaldson, G., Heimdahl, A., Kager, L., and Nord, C.E., The normal human anaerobic microflora, *Scand. J. Infect. Dis.*, 35(Suppl.): 9–15, 1982.

39. Gorbach, S.L. and Goldin, B.R., Nutrition and the gastrointestinal microflora, *Nutr. Rev.*, 50: 378–381, 1992.

40. Macfarlane, G.T. and Macfarlane, S., Human colonic microbiota: ecology, physiology and metabolic potential of intestinal bacteria, *Scand. J. Gastroenterol.*, 32 (Suppl. 222): 3–9, 1997.

41. Conly, J.M., Stein, K., Worobetz, L., and Rutledge-Harding, S., The contribution of vitamin K2 (menaquinones) produced by the intestinal microflora to human nutritional requirements for vitamin K, *Am. J. Gastroenterol.*, 89: 915–923, 1994.

42. Mitsuoka, T., Intestinal flora and aging, *Nutr. Rev.*, 50: 438–446, 1992.

43. Gorbach, S.L., Perturbation of intestinal microflora, *Vet. Hum. Toxicol.*, 35 (Suppl. 1): 15–23, 1993.

44. Carman, R.J., Van Tassall, R.L., and Wilkins, T.D., The normal intestinal microflora: ecology, variability and stability, *Vet. Hum. Toxicol.*, 35(Suppl. 1): 11–14, 1993.

45. Goldin, B.R. and Gorbach, S.L., The effect of milk and lactobacillus feeding on human intestinal bacterial enzyme activity, *Am. J. Clin. Nutr.*, 39: 756–761, 1984.

46. Farnworth, E.R., The beneficial health effects of fermented foods — potential probiotics around the world, *J. Nutraceuticals Funct. Med. Food*. 4: 93–117, 2004.

47. Kolars, J.C., Levitt, M.D., Aouji, M., and Savaiano, D.A., Yogurt — an autodigesting source of lactose, *N. Engl. J. Med.*, 310: 1–3, 1984.

48. Savaiano, D.A., AbouElAnouar, A., Smith, D.E., and Levitt, M.D., Lactose malabsorption from yogurt, pasteurized yogurt, sweet acidophilus milk, and cultured milk in lactase-deficient individuals, *Am. J. Clin. Nutr.*, 40: 1219–1223, 1984.

49. Pochart, P., Dewit, O., Desjeux, J.-F., and Bourlioux, P., Viable starter culture, b-galactosidase activity, and lactose in duodenum after yogurt ingestion in lactase-deficient humans, *Am. J. Clin. Nutr.*, 49: 828–831, 1989.

50. Lerebours, E., N'Djitoyap Ndam, C., Lavoine, A., Hellot, M.F., Antoine, J.M., and Colin, R., Yogurt and fermented-then-pasteurized milk: effects of short-term and long-term ingestion on lactose absorption and mucosal lactase activity in lactase-deficient subjects, *Am. J. Clin. Nutr.*, 49: 823–827, 1989.

51. Martini, M.C., Smith, D.E., and Savaiano, D.A., Lactose digestion from flavored and frozen yogurts, ice milk, and ice cream by lactase-deficient persons, *Am. J. Clin. Nutr.*, 46: 636–640, 1987.

52. Arrigoni, E., Marteau, P., Briet, F., Pochart, P., Rambaud, J.-C., and Messing, B., Tolerance and absorption of lactose from milk and yogurt during short-bowel syndrome in humans, *Am. J. Clin. Nutr.*, 60: 926–929, 1994.

53. Vesa, T.H., Marteau, P., Zidi, S., Briet, F., Pochart, P., and Rambaud, J.C., Digestion and tolerance of lactose from yogurt and different semi-solid fermented dairy products containing *Lactobacillus acidophilus* and bifidobacteria in lactose maldigesters — is bacterial lactase important? *Eur. J. Clin. Nutr.* 50: 730–733, 1996.

54. Guerin-Danan, C., Chabanet, C., Pedone, C., Popot, F., Vaissade, P., Bouley, C., Szylit, O., and Andrieux, C., Milk fermented with yogurt cultures and *Lactobacillus casei* compared with yogurt and gelled milk: influence on intestinal microflora in healthy infants, *Am. J. Clin. Nutr.*, 67: 111–117, 1998.

55. Taylor, G.R.J. and Williams, C.M., Effects of probiotics and prebiotics on blood lipids, *Br. J. Nutr.*, 80 (Suppl. 2): S225–S230, 1998.

56. Farnworth, E.R., Designing a proper control for testing the efficacy of a probiotic product. *J. Nutraceuticals Funct. Med. Food* 2: 55–63, 2000.

57. Mann, G.V. and Spoerry, A., Studies of a surfactant and cholesteremia in the Masai, *Am. J. Clin. Nutr.*, 27: 464–469, 1974.

58. Mann, G.V., The Masai, milk and the yogurt factor: an alternative explanation, *Atherosclerosis*, 29: 265, 1978.

59. de Roos, N.M., Schoouten, G., and Katan, M.B., Yoghurt enriched with *Lactobacillus acidophilus* does not lower blood lipids in healthy men and women with normal to borderline high serum cholesterol levels, *Eur. J. Clin. Nutr.*, 53: 277–280, 1999.

60. Xiao, J.Z., Kondo, S., Takahashi, N., Miyaji, K., Oshida, K., Hiramatsu, A., Iwatsuki, K., Kokubo, S., and Hosono, A., Effects of milk products fermented by *Bifidobacterium longum* on blood lipids in rats and healthy adult male mice, *J. Dairy Sci.* 86: 2452–2461, 2003.

61. Kiebling, G., Schneider, J., and Jahreis, G., Long-term consumption of fermented dairy products over 6 months increases HDL cholesterol, *Eur. J. Clin. Nutr.* 56: 843–849, 2002.

62. Chagarovskii, V.P., and Zholkevskaya, I.G. Biotechnology for producing bioyogurts and biokefir: study of their effect on human health. *Mikrobiol. Z.* 65: 67–73, 2003 (translated from Russian).

63. St-Onge, M.-P., Farnworth, E.R., and Jones, P.J.H., Fermented and non-fermented dairy product consumption: effects on cholesterol levels and metabolism, *Am J. Clin. Nutr.*, 71: 674–681, 2000.

64. Wolever, T.M.S., Spadafora, P., and Eshuis, H., Interaction between colonic acetate and propionate in humans, *Am. J. Clin. Nutr.*, 53: 681–687, 1991.

65. Wolever, T.M.S., Spadafora, P.J., Cunnane, S.C., and Pencharz, P.B., Propionate inhibits incorporation of colonic (1,2–13C) acetate into plasma lipids in humans, *Am. J. Clin. Nutr.*, 61: 1241–1247, 1995.

66. Farnworth, E.R., Kefir: a complex probiotic, *Food. Sci. Technol. Bull.* 2: 1–17, 2005.

67. Perdigon, G., Alvarez, S., Rachid, M., Aguero, G., and Gobbato, N., Symposium: probiotic bacteria for humans: clinical systems for evaluation of effectiveness, *J. Dairy Sci.*, 78: 1597–1606, 1995.

68. Perdigon, G., Valdez, J.C., and Rachid, M., Antitumour activity of yogurt: study of possible immune mechanisms, *J. Dairy Res.*, 65: 129–138, 1998.

69. Cano, P.G., Aguero, G., and Perdigon, G., Immunological effects of yogurt addition to a re-nutrition diet in a malnutrition experimental model, *J Dairy Res.* 69: 303–316, 2002.

70. Marcos, A., Warnberg, J., Nova, E., Gomez, S., Alvarez, A., Alvarez, R., Mateos, J.A., and Cobo, J.M., The effect of milk fermented by yogurt cultures plus *Lactobacillus casei* DN-114001 on the immune response of subjects under academic examination stress, *Eur J Nutr.* 43: 381–389, 2004.

71. Wheeler, J.G., Bogle, M.L., Shema, S.J., Shirrell, M.A., Stine, K.C., Pittler, A.J., Burks, A.W., and Helm, R.M., Impact of dietary yogurt on immune function, *Am. J. Med. Sci.*, 313: 120–123, 1997.

72. Spanhaak, S., Havenaar, R., and Schaafsma, G., The effect of consumption of milk fermented by *Lactobacillus casei* strain Shirota on the intestinal microflora and immune parameters in humans, *Eur. J. Clin. Nutr.*, 52: 899–907, 1998.

73. Gill, H.S., Stimulation of the immune system by lactic cultures, *Int. Dairy J.*, 8: 535–544, 1998.

74. Sullivan, P.B., Nutritional management of acute diarrhea, *Nutrition*, 14: 758–762, 1998.

75. Gonzalez, S., Albarracin, G., Locascio de Ruiz Pesce, M., Male, M., Apella, M.C., Pesce de Ruiz Holgado, A., and Oliver, G., Prevention of infantile diarrhoea by fermented milk, *Microbiol. Aliments Nutr.*, 8: 349–354, 1990.

76. Isolauri, E., Juntunen, M., Rautanen, T., Sillanaukee, P., and Koivula, T., A human Lactobacillus strain (Lactobacillus casei sp. strain GG) promotes recovery from acute diarrhea in children, *Pediatrics*, 88: 90–97, 1991.

77. Siitonen, S., Vapaatalo, H., Salminen, S., Gordin, A., Saxelin, M., Wikberg, R., and Kirkkola, A.-L., Effect of Lactobacillus GG yoghurt in prevention of antibiotic associated diarrhoea, *Ann. Med.*, 22: 57–59, 1990.

78. Pedone, C.A., Bernabeu, A.O., Postaire, E.R., Bouley, C.F., and Reinert, P., The effect of supplementation with milk fermented by *Lactobacillus casei* (strain DN-114 001) on acute diarrhea in children attending day care centers, *Int. J. Clin. Pract.* 53: 179, 181–184, 1999.

79. Pedone, C.A., Arnaud, C.C., Postaire, E.R., Bouley, C.F., and Reinert, P., Multicentric study of the effect of milk fermented by *Lactobacillus casei* on the incidence of diarrhea, *Int. J. Clin. Pract.* 54: 568–571, 2000.

80. Bhatnagar, S., Singh, K.D., Sazawal, S., Saxena, S. K., and Bhan, M.K., Efficacy of milk versus yogurt offered as part of a mixed diet in acute noncholera diarrhea among malnourished children, *J. Pediatr.*, 132: 999–1003, 1998.

81. Pereg, D., Kimhi, O., Tirosh, A., Orr, N., Kayouf, R., and Lishner, M., The effect of fermented yogurt on the prevention of diarrhea in a healthy adult population, *Am. J. Infect. Control* 33: 122–125, 2005.

82. Van't Veer, P., Dekker, J.M., Lamers, J.W.J., Kok, F.J., Schouten, E.G., Brants, H.A.M., Sturmans, F., and Hermus, R.J.J., Consumption of fermented milk products and breast cancer: a case–control study in the Netherlands, *Cancer Res.*, 49: 4020–4023, 1989.

83. Kampman, E., Goldbohm, R.A., van den Brandt, P.A., and van't Veer, P., Fermented dairy products, calcium, and colorectal cancer in the Netherlands cohort study, *Cancer Res.*, 54: 3186–3190, 1994.

84. Boutron, M.-C., Faivre, J., Marteau, P., Couillault, C., Senesse, P., and Quipourt, V., Calcium, phosphorus, vitamin D, dairy products and colorectal carcinogenesis: a French case-control study, *Br. J. Cancer*, 74: 145–151, 1996.

85. Goldin, B.R., Swenson, L., Dwyer, J., Sexton, M., and Gorbach, S.L., Effect of diet and Lactobacillus acidophilus supplements on human fecal bacterial enzymes, *J. Natl. Cancer Inst.*, 64: 255–261, 1980.

86. Tsuru, S., Shinomiya, N., Taniguchi, M., Shimazaki, H., Tanigawa, K., and Nomoto, K., Inhibition of tumor growth by dairy products, *J. Clin. Lab. Immunol.*, 25: 177–183, 1988.

87. Renner, H.W. and Münzner, R., The possible role of probiotics as dietary antimutagens, *Mutat. Res.*, 262: 239–245, 1991.

88. Rice, L.J., Chai, Y.-J., Conti, C.J., Willis, R.A., and Locniskar, M.F., The effect of dietary fermented milk products and lactic acid bacteria on the initiation and promotion stages of mammary carcinogenesis, *Nutr. Cancer*, 24: 99–109, 1995.

89. Bakalinsky, A.T., Nadathur, S.R., Carney, J.R., and Gould, S.J., Antimutagenicity of yogurt, *Mutat. Res.*, 350: 199–200, 1996.

90. De Moreno de LeBlanc, A., and Perdigon, G., Yogurt feeding inhibits promotion and progression of experimental colorectal cancer, *Med. Sci. Monit.* 10: BR96–104, 2004.

91. Matar, C., Amiot, J., Savoie, L., and Goulet, J., The effect of milk fermentation by *Lactobacillus helveticus* on the release of peptides during in vitro digestion, *J. Dairy Sci.*, 79: 971–979, 1996.

92. Matar, C., Nadathur, S.S., Bakalinsky, A.T., and Goulet, J., Antimutagenic effects of milk fermented by Lactobacillus helveticus L89 and a protease-deficient derivative, *J. Dairy Sci.*, 80: 1965–1970, 1997.

93. Chabance, B., Marteau, P., Rambaud, J.C., Migliore-Samour, D., Boynard, M., Perrotin, P., Guillet, R., Jollès, P., and Fiat, A.M., Casein peptide release and passage to the blood in humans during digestion of milk or yogurt, *Biochimie*, 80: 155–165, 1998.

94. Fernandez-Garcia, E., McGregor, J.U., and Traylor, S., The addition of oat fiber and natural alternative sweeteners in the manufacture of plain yogurt, *J. Dairy Sci.*, 81: 655–663, 1998.

95. Clifton, P.M., Noakes, M., Sullivan, D., Erichsen, N., Ross, D., Annison, G., Fassoulakis, A., Cehun, M., and Nestel, P., Cholesterol-lowering effects of plant sterol esters differ in milk, yogurt, bread and cereal, *Eur. J. Clin. Nutr.* 58: 503–509, 2004.

96. Hekmat, S. and McMahon, D.J., Manufacture and quality of iron-fortified yogurt, *J. Dairy Sci.*, 80: 3114–3122, 1997.

97. Rosado, J.L., Diaz, M., Gonzalez, K., Griffin, I., and Abrams, S.A., The addition of milk or yogurt to a plant-based diet increases zinc bioavailability but does not affect iron bioavailability in women, *J. Nutr.* 135: 465–468, 2005.

98. Farnworth, E.R., Kefir: from folklore to regulatory approval, *J. Nutraceuticals Funct. Med. Food*, 1: 57–68, 1999.

99. Mainville, I., Robert, N., Lee, B., and Farnworth, E.R., Polyphasic characterization of the lactic acid bacteria in kefir. *Syst. Appl. Microbiol.*, 29, 59–68, 2006.

100. Hallé, C., Leroi, F., Dousset, X., and Pidoux, M., Les Kéfirs des associations bactéries lactiques — levures, in Bactéries *Lactiques: Aspects Fondamentaux et Technologiques*, Vol. 2, de Roissart, H. and Luquet, F.M., Eds., Uriage, France, 1994, pp. 169–181.

101. Vayssier, Y., Le kéfir: etude et mise au point d'un levain pour la préparation d'une boisson, *Rev. Lait Fr.*, 362: 131–134, 1978.

102. Zourari, A. and Anifantakis, E.M., Le kéfir caractères physico-chimiques, microbiologiques et nutritionnels. Technologie et production. Une revue, *Lait*, 68: 373–392, 1988.

103. Duitschaever, C.L., Kemp, N., and Emmons, D., Pure culture formulation and procedure for the production of kefir, *Milchwissenschaft*, 42: 80–82, 1987.

104. Kroger, M., Kefir, *Cult. Dairy Prod.*, 28: 26, 28, 29, 1993.

105. Marshall, V.M. and Cole, W.M., Methods for making kefir and fermented milks based on kefir, *J. Dairy Res.*, 52: 451–456, 1985.

106. Duitschaever, C.L., Toop, D.H., and Buteau, C., Consumer acceptance of sweetened and flavored kefir, *Milchwissenschaft*, 46: 227–229, 1991.

107. Kneifel, W. and Mayer, H.K., Vitamin profiles of kefirs made from milks of different species, *Int. J. Food Sci. Technol.*, 26: 423–428, 1991.

108. Liu, J.R., Chen, M-J., and Lin, C-W., Characterization of polysaccharides and volatile compounds produced by kefir grains grown in soymilk, *J. Food. Sci.*, 67: 104–108, 2002.

109. Duitschaever, C.L., Kemp, N., and Emmons, D., Comparative evaluation of five procedures for making kefir, *Milchwissenschaft*, 43: 343–345, 1988.

110. Cevikbas, A., Yemni, E., Ezzedenn, F.W., Yardimici, T., Cevikbas, U., and Stohs, S.J., Antitumoral antibacterial and antifungal activities of kefir and kefir grain, *Phytother. Res.*, 8: 78–82, 1994.

111. Osada, K., Nagira, K., Teruya, K., Tachibana, H., Shirahata, S., and Murakami, H., Enhancement of interferon-b production with sphingomyelin from fermented milk, *Biotherapy*, 7: 115–123, 1994.

112. Shiomi, M., Sasaki, K., Murofushi, M., and Aibara, K., Antitumor activity in mice of orally administered polysaccharide from kefir grain, *Jpn. J. Med. Sci. Biol.*, 35: 75–80, 1982.

113. Murofushi, M., Shiomi, M., and Aibara, K., Effect of orally administered polysaccharide from kefir grain on delayed type-hypersensitivity and tumor growth in mice, *Jpn. J. Med. Sci. Biol.*, 36: 49–53, 1983.

114. Murofushi, M., Mizuguchi, J., Aibara, K., and Matuhasi, T., Immunopotentiative effect of polysaccharide from kefir grain, KGF-C, administered orally in mice, *Immunopharmacology*, 12: 29–35, 1986.

115. Furukawa, N., Matsuoka, A., and Yamanaka, Y., Effects of orally administered yogurt and kefir on tumor growth in mice, *J. Jpn. Soc. Nutr. Food Sci.*, 43: 450–453, 1990 (in Japanese, abstract only).

116. Furukawa, N., Matsuoka, A., Takahashi, T., and Yamanaka, Y., Effects of fermented milk on the delayed-type hypersensitivity response and survival day in mice bearing Meth-A, *Anim. Sci. Technol.*, 62: 579–585, 1991 (in Japanese).

117. Kubo, M., Odani, T., Nakamura, S., Tokumaru, S., and Matsuda, H., Pharmacological study of kefir — a fermented milk product in Caucasus. I. On antitumor activity (1), *Yakugaku Zasshi*, 112: 489–495, 1992 (in Japanese, abstract only).

118. Vujicic, I.F., Vulic, M., and Konyves, T., Assimilation of cholesterol in milk by kefir cultures, *Biotechnol. Lett.*, 14: 847–850, 1992.

119. St-Onge, M-P., Farnworth, E.R., Savard, T., Chabot, D., Mafu, A., and Jones, P.J.H., Kefir consumption does not alter plasma lipid levels or cholesterol fractional synthesis rates relative to milk in hyperlipidemic men, *BMC Compl. Altern. Med. J.*, 2002. http://www.biomedcentral.com/1472-6882/2/1/.

120. Farnworth, E.R., The beneficial health effects of fermented foods — potential probiotics around the world, *J. Nutraceuticals Funct. Med. Food* 4: 93–117.

121. Reddy, N.R., Pierson, M.D., and Salunkhe, D.K., Introduction, in *Legume-Based Fermented Foods*, Reddy, N.R., Pierson, M.D., and Salunkhe, D.K., Eds., CRC Press, Boca Raton, FL, 1986.

122. Ohta, T., Natto, in *Legume-Based Fermented Foods*, Reddy, N.R., Pierson, M.D., and Salunkhe, D.K., Eds., CRC Press, Boca Raton, FL, 1986.

123. Cheigh, H.-S. and Park, K.-Y., Biochemical, microbiological, and nutritional aspects of Kimchi (Korean fermented vegetable products), *Crit. Rev. Food Sci. Nutr.*, 34: 175–203, 1994.

124. Steinkraus, K.H., Classification of fermented foods: worldwide review of household fermentation techniques, *Food Control*, 8: 311–317, 1997.

125. Harris, L.J., The microbiology of vegetable fermentations, in *Microbiology of Fermented Foods*, Wood, B.J.B., Ed., Blackie Academic and Professional, Tomson Science, London, 1998, pp. 45–72.

126. Gardiner, G., Stanton, C., Lynch, P.B., Collins, J.K., Fitzgerald, G., and Ross, R.P., Evaluation of cheddar cheese as a carrier for delivery of a probiotic strain to the gastrointestinal tract, *J. Dairy Sci.*, 82: 1379–1387, 1999.

127. Modler, H.W. and Villa-Garcia, L., The growth of *Bifidobacterium longum* in a whey-based medium and viability of this organism in frozen yogurt with low and high levels of developed acidity, *Cult. Dairy Prod. J.*, 28: 4–8, 1993.

128. Hekmat, S. and McMahon, D.J., Survival of *Lactobacillus acidophilus* and *Bifidobacterium bifidum* in ice cream for use as a probiotic food, *J. Dairy Sci.*, 75: 1415–1422, 1992.

18 Exopolysaccharides from Lactic Acid Bacteria: Food Uses, Production, Chemical Structures, and Health Effects

Edward R. Farnworth, Claude P. Champagne,
and Marie-Rose Van Calsteren

CONTENTS

I. INTRODUCTION

Exopolysaccharides (EPSs) are metabolites of some bacteria and yeasts. EPSs can have simple or complex compositions and structures and are produced by the cell for a variety of reasons (see Table 18.1). The composition and structure of EPSs give them physical and chemical properties that were initially used to modify food texture characteristics. As the structures of EPSs were identified, their similarities to dietary fiber were noted and research was undertaken to show how EPSs affected digestion, metabolism, and immune function. The development of functional foods

TABLE 18.1
The Roles of Exopolysaccharides Produced by Bacteria

Protection of the Cell Against:
Desiccation
Phagocytosis
Phage attack
Antibiotics
Osmotic stress
Metal ions
Bacteriocins

Other Functions:
Contribute to cell recognition
Facilitate adhesion to surfaces
Form biofilms
Sequestering of essential cations

Source: From Looijesteijn, P.J., Trapet, L., de Vries, E., Abee, T., and Hugenholtz, J., Physiological function of exopolysaccharides produced by *Lactococcus lactis*, *Int. J. Food Microbiol.*, 64: 71–80, 2001; Ruas-Madiedo, P., Hugenholtz, J., and Zoon, P., An overview of the functionality of exopolysaccharides produced by lactic acid bacteria, *Int. Dairy J.*, 12: 163–171, 2002; De Vuyst, L., De Vin, F., Vaningelgem, F., and Degeest, B., Recent developments in the biosynthesis and applications of heteropolysaccharides from lactic acid bacteria, *Int. Dairy J.*, 11: 687–707, 2001.

containing EPSs has been the result of collaborations between microbiologists, chemists, food scientists, and biochemists.

Several microorganisms produce polysaccharides: some are storage polysaccharides localized in the cytoplasm; others are components of the cell wall of both gram-positive and gram-negative bacteria or of the outer membrane of gram-negative bacteria; others still are excreted outside the cell, hence the term *exopolysaccharides*. These EPSs can either be tightly bound to the cells to form a capsule, in which case they are called *capsular polysaccharides* (CPSs), or be secreted into the environment as slime. Microbial EPSs are divided into two classes according to their biosynthesis mechanism: homopolysaccharides and heteropolysaccharides. Homopolysaccharides are made up of only one type of monosaccharide, whereas heteropolysaccharides contain different types of sugar monomers and sometimes substituents arranged in repeating units.

II. EXOPOLYSACCHARIDES IN FOODS

A. INTRODUCTION

The two most important polysaccharides produced by bacteria that are found in foods as ingredients are xanthan gum and gellan. With the exception of dextran and levan, EPSs produced by lactic acid bacteria (LAB) are not currently marketed.[3] Dextran and levan are used in filtration and medical applications. EPSs of LAB origin are presently found in foods that are fermented by the LAB, but are not found in nutraceutical products.

There are many fermented foods: milk (yogurt, cheese), vegetables (sauerkraut), meats (dry sausages), fruits (wine), and cereals (bread, beer). However, only a few benefit from the production of EPS from LAB (Table 18.2). In many countries, the addition of stabilizers is not allowed in fermented milks[8] and the use of EPS-producing strains becomes imperative. The most common

TABLE 18.2
Some Technological Consequences of EPS Production in Foods and Beverages

Type	Food	Effect	Reference
Desirable	Yogurt	Improved water retention/less syneresis	4, 5
	Yogurt	Increased viscosity	6, 7
	Kefir	Grain structure	8
	Kefir	Increased viscosity	8
	Low-fat mozzarella	Higher water content	9–11
	Low-fat mozzarella	Better melt properties	9–11
	Ogi	Increased viscosity	12
	Cheesemaking	Potential protection against bacteriophages	13–16
	Ice cream	Better survival in freezing and storage	17
	Fermented oats	Improved texture	18
	Bread	Replace hydrocolloids currently used as texturizing or antistaling agents	19
Undesirable	Cheese whey	Higher viscosity during membrane processing	9
	Yoghurt	Slower fermentation	20
	Beer	Defect in texture; filtration problems	21

fermented milks with EPSs include yogurt, cheese, ropy milks (Swedish "Langmjulk," Finnish ropy milk) and kefir.[8] Many milk products are fermented by LAB and could benefit from EPS production, such as cultured buttermilk, dahi, cultured cream, Nordic (Sweden, Norway, Denmark, Finland) traditional fermented milks, and various probiotic-containing fermented milks.[3] A study was conducted to ascertain the level of EPS production in bacterial strains used in commercial European food products. Of the 26 strains isolated, EPS production in milk varied between 20 to 100 mg/L.[22] In yogurt, kefir, and other fermented milks, there are two important benefits: improved viscosity and less syneresis (Table 18.2). In cheesemaking, EPS-producing strains only appear to be used in mozzarella manufacture, partially because the resulting whey is more difficult to process (Table 18.2).

In fermented milks, viscosity does not always correlate with EPS production;[23–26] this is partially because viscosity and firmness in yogurt is linked to both protein coagulation and EPS production.[6,27] Good reviews of this aspect have been published.[3,28] Some strains produce many EPSs with variable molecular weight or chemical structures,[2,22,25,29–31] and ratios of high and low MW affect texturing more than their total concentration.[32] Drying of EPS may result in a reduction in molecular mass.[1]

EPS produced by LAB have no taste, but they can enhance the taste of the product because the increased viscosity they bring to products can increase residence time in the mouth.[33]

Studies with *Lb. sanfranciscensis* have shown that as the sucrose levels were increased from 2 to 15%, not only was EPS production increased, but there was also a proportional increase of the oligosaccharide kestose.[34] Thus, a process aimed at producing high levels of EPS might generate a valuable by-product in the form of a prebiotic oligosaccharide. This adds to the potential role of the EPS as a prebiotic for bifidobacteria.[3] The extent to which oligosaccharides are produced in addition to the EPS is largely unknown.

LAB-produced EPSs appear to be as good a technological tool as the current bacterial stabilizers on the market. For example, carboxymethylation of kefiran has increased its viscosity 14-fold.[8] At 1%, a *Lb. sake* EPS had a better viscosifying property than xanthan gum.[35]

The determination of EPS production has mostly been carried out following extraction with ethanol, but methods based on ultrafiltration cells,[36] ultracentrifugation with anion-exchange chromatography,[37] and near infrared spectroscopy[38] have been proposed. The values will obviously vary as a function of the method used.[36,37]

B. FACTORS INFLUENCING THE PRODUCTION OF EXOPOLYSACCHARIDES BY LACTIC ACID BACTERIA

The ability of bacteria to produce viscous compounds is notoriously variable,[25,39–41] but a certain number of parameters have been shown to affect EPS production by LAB.[42] Fermentations that are carried out with pH continuously maintained at a set point generally result in higher yields (Table 18.3). However, because all the foods that are currently available with LAB-derived EPSs are fermented without pH control, factors that affect EPS synthesis under these conditions have been examined.

1. Fermentation Conditions

a. Bacterial Growth and Exopolysaccharide Production

Most studies have found a link between the biomass (or bacterial population) reached in the fermentation and the quantity of EPS produced.[23,53,58–60] Generally, EPS is growth-associated[56] — the greater the number of cells in the product or the system, the more EPS is produced. However, fermentation conditions can also have significant effects on EPS yields.

EPS production can be important in the stationary growth phase (SGP).[32,48,59] However, in most of these cases, the fermentations are carried out without pH control,[60] with pH being the limiting growth factor, not the carbohydrate source. Generally, when fermentations are carried out with pH control, growth often stops when the carbohydrates have been consumed, which would theoretically prevent any extensive EPS production during the SGP. Thus, in instances where EPS production occurs in the SGP during pH-controlled fermentations, there are excess carbohydrates in the medium[48,55] and lactate becomes the element inhibiting growth rather than low pH.[55] To prevent the inhibitory effect of lactate accumulation on growth, lactate-consuming yeast can be added, as has been done very effectively with the organisms used in kefir manufacture.[49]

b. Temperature, pH, and Stirring during Fermentation

Exceptions do exist,[51,56] but with mesophilic lactococci,[26,55,56] *Sc. thermophilus*,[61,62] and *Lb. rhamnosus*,[63,64] suboptima incubation temperatures result in higher EPS production. Over-optimal temperatures tend to decrease the specific EPS production ability.[47,65,66] However, with most lactobacilli, a correlation between the optimum growth temperature and that for obtaining maximum EPS production is observed.[51,61,67] When EPS is mostly produced in the SGP, much higher levels are obtained if the culture is grown at its optimum growth temperature and then cooled to 10°C during the SGP.[52,59]

With LAB, pH control generally enables higher cell counts and thus higher EPS levels.[68,69] For most cultures, pHs between 5.5 and 6.2 give best EPS yields,[47,52,56,64,66,70] and only *Lb. helveticus* seems to prefer lower optimum pH values. Not only does pH affect yields, it also affects the soluble:insoluble ratios and EPS degradation during storage.[48,52,71]

Stirring can improve EPS production,[23] but it also increases oxygen dissolution in the medium. With *Sc. thermophilus*, higher oxygen levels promoted growth and subsequently higher EPS levels.[56] However, the effect of oxygen on EPS production can be the opposite.[55,56]

2. Effect of Growth Media on Exopolysaccharide Production

There have been several defined media for growth and EPS production of lactobacilli, some media containing over 50 ingredients.[62,72]

Numerous studies demonstrate the effect of carbon source on EPS yields.[32,44,47,59,63,71,73] Without pH control, the initial carbohydrate level is not as important.[32] Obviously, the quantity of carbohydrates in the medium affects EPS yields[74] and high initial carbohydrate levels tend to enhance final EPS levels.[33,49,56]

TABLE 18.3
Exopolysaccharide Yields from Lactic Acid Bacteria in Fermentation Processes

Species	Medium	Fermentation Technology		Yield (mg/L)	References
		Type	pH Control		
Lactobacillus casei	Whey + sucrose + AA[a]	Single batch — free cells	No	195	43
	BMM (synthetic)	Single batch — free cells	No	160	44
Lactobacillus delbrueckii ssp. *bulgaricus*	Protein-hydrolyzed whey	Single batch—free cells	Yes at 5.0	330	45
	Defined	Chemostat — free cells	Yes at 6.5	2310 [110 at D = 0.055 h^{-1}][b]	46
	Defined	Chemostat — free cells	Yes at 6.0	85	47
	Defined	Chemostat — free cells	Yes at 6.0	200	38
Lactobacillus kefranofaciens	Modified MRS	Single batch — free cells	Yes at 5.5	2000	48
	MRS + yeast	Single batch — free cells	Yes at 5.5	3400	49
	MRS + yeast	Fed batch — free cells	Yes at 5.5	5400	49
Lactobacillus helveticus	Milk	Single batch — free cells	No	399	23
	Milk	Single batch — free cells	Yes 4.5–6.2	549	50
Lactobacillus rhamnosus	BMM (synthetic)	Single batch — free cells	Yes at 6.0	1275	51
	MRS	Single batch — free cells	Yes 5.2–7.2	150	52
	Whey + YE[a] + minerals	Single batch — free cells	Yes at 6.0	2350	53
	Whey + YE + minerals	Chemostat — ICT (30%)[c]	Yes at 6.0	1250–1802 [540–2240 at D = 0.3 h^{-1}][b]	54
	Whey + YE + minerals	Multiple batch — ICT (25%)	Yes at 6.0	1750	53
Lactococcus lactis	Milk	Single batch — free cells	No	600	43
	Defined medium	Single batch — free cells	Yes at 5.8	590	55
	Defined medium	Chemostat — free cells	Yes at 5.8	180	55
Streptococcus thermophilus	Milk	Single batch — free cells	No	277–3640	24, 25
	Milk + lactose + YE + peptone	Single batch — free cells	Yes pH 6.2	546	56
	MRS + lactose + YE + peptone	Single batch — free cells	Yes pH 6.2	1142	57

[a] Supplements: AA = amino acids, YE = yeast extracts, ICT = immobilized cell technology.
[b] Data in brackets, [], represent productivity expressed as mg/l/h.
[c] Represents the % of the fermentor volume occupied by the immobilized cell carriers.

The LAB require many amino acids for growth,[72] and media rich in peptones or yeast extracts tend to promote high biomass levels, which often translates into high EPS levels.[41,45,57,64,67,70,75,76] However, excess nitrogen-based supplements can sometimes reduce EPS production.[57,77] Interestingly, when the same strains were cultured in milk, amino-acid-supplement whey, or laboratory media for equal cell counts, EPS production was generally higher in milk.[25,45]

Other supplements that enhance growth, such as minerals or vitamins, will tend to increase bacterial populations, and thus EPS production.[78–82]

3. Interactions between Strains

Most studies on EPS production have been carried out with pure cultures, and very little data are available with respect to interactions between strains. Cocultures do affect productivity,[83,84] and the most fruitful combination seems to be between kefir cultures *Lb. kefiranofaciens* and *Saccharomyces cerevisiae*.[48,49,85] In this coculture, carried out under pH control, the yeast consumes the lactic acid, thus reducing the product inhibition and direct contact of the lactobacilli with the yeast results in higher kefiran production.[86] The *Lb. kefiranofaciens* and *S. cerevisiae* coculture gave the highest reported EPS yield for LAB (Table 18.3). However, this EPS yield may be influenced by yeast-based polymers,[87] which can interfere with EPS analyses.[53]

4. Effect of Fermentation Technology

Food fermentations are typically done in batch processes, and LAB EPS-containing foods currently on the market are produced by this method. However, highest yields in EPSs are attained with fed-batch or continuous fermentation techniques (Table 18.3). A carbon-based fed-batch process would not seem appropriate for EPS production because of unfavorable carbon-to-nitrogen ratios.[42,55,57,77] However, a fed-batch process was successful using a coculture of *Lb. kefiranofaciens* and *S. cerevisiae*. This seems to be associated with the fact that a high carbohydrate level was initially added in the medium.[49]

If pure cultures are to be used for EPS production, immobilized cell technology (ICT) may give higher yields in the future. EPS production is much more rapid once the biomass is reached.[53] Furthermore, ICT also enables multiple batch fermentations, which reduce the fermentation time from 32 to 7 h.[53]

III. CHEMICAL STRUCTURE OF EXOPOLYSACCHARIDES

The diversity of heteropolysaccharides comes from the following characteristics: the number of sugar residues in the repeating unit; their identity, hexoses, or their deoxy, amino, or uronic derivatives, pentoses, polyols, etc.; the absolute configuration of each sugar residue, D or L; its anomeric configuration, α or β; its cyclic conformation, pyranose or furanose; the sequence of glycosidic linkages between residues, including branching; and, if present, the nature and linkage position of substituents, organic or inorganic. The molar mass of EPSs range from 4×10^4 to 6×10^6 Da.[87] The large diversity in the primary structure results in a large number of possible conformations that could be adopted by these EPSs, and therefore the study of structure–properties relationships is still in its infancy.

A. Methods of Structural Characterization

High-resolution nuclear magnetic resonance (NMR) spectroscopy is the most powerful technique for structure determination. ^1H, ^{13}C, and sometimes ^{31}P are the most common nuclei observed. One-dimensional as well as homonuclear and heteronuclear two-dimensional NMR techniques provide information on the number and identity of sugar residues, their anomeric configuration and cyclic conformation, the proximity or linkages between residues, and the nature and position of substituents.

Chemical and chromatographic methods are used to substantiate NMR findings. High-performance liquid chromatography (HPLC) is mostly used for sugar and substituent analysis after hydrolysis of the EPS. Gas chromatography (GC), coupled or not with mass spectrometry (MS), is also used after the sugar monomers have been rendered volatile by derivatization. The sugar monomers can be tagged by methylation prior to hydrolysis in order to determine the linkage and substitution positions of each sugar.

The only information not obtainable by NMR is the absolute configuration of the sugars, which has to be determined independently, either by polarimetry or by derivatizing the sugars with a chiral alcohol to form one of two possible diastereoisomers that can be separated by GC.

The usefulness of elemental analysis lies mainly in detecting the presence of amino sugars and inorganic substituents. In some instances, it is interesting to chemically or enzymatically modify a polysaccharide in order to produce oligosaccharides, representative of the repeating unit but with a lower molecular mass, that are possible to analyze directly by mass spectrometry and give narrower lines on NMR spectra. Enzymes are highly specific, but few have proven useful for that purpose because of the diversity of linkages in EPSs. Some chemical reactions, such as periodate oxidation and diazotization, have a high degree of specificity and yield products easier to purify than those produced by partial hydrolysis unless a particularly weak linkage is present in the structure. Molecular masses are determined by gel-permeation chromatography or light scattering. Finally, molecular modeling is useful to predict the conformations and three-dimensional structure adopted by EPSs and possibly, when more structures become available in the future, to understand their structure–properties relationships.

IV. HEALTH BENEFITS OF EXOPOLYSACCHARIDES

EPSs were originally added to various food formulations as gelling agents and stabilizers and were popular in the food industry long before their effects on digestion, metabolism, and human health were identified. Early human feeding trials confirmed that EPSs were safe to consume at concentrations higher than those added to alter food texture.[100,101]

A. DIGESTION OF EPSs

The high viscosity of EPSs in solutions makes them act as fecal bulking agents that can alter transit time, fecal weight, and fecal water content. In rats, structural differences in the surface structures of the ileum and cecum have been observed after eating diets containing the homopolymer curdlan →3)-β-D-Glcp-(1→ or the heteropolymer gellan gum (Figure 18.1, structure 1).[88] The structure and chemical bonding within EPSs leads to their resistance to normal carbohydrate digestive enzymes. Most EPSs remain intact until they reach the lower GI tract, where they act like other nondigestible fibers (see Table 18.4).

Using fecal slurry, Ruijssenaars et al.[103] compared the degradation of six EPSs produced from lactic acid bacteria and the EPS produced by *Xanthomonas campestris* (xanthan gum). They found that only the EPSs produced by *Streptococcus thermophilus* SFi39 (Figure 18.1, structure 2), SFi12 (Figure 18.1, structure 3), and *Xanthomonas campestris* (Figure 18.1, structure 4) were degraded after a 5-d incubation period. The repeating units of the two EPSs that were degraded have only a β-galactosyl residue as a side chain, and xanthan gum has a cellulose backbone.

EPSs are digested in the colon, if they are digested at all. For example, the total recovery of EPS from *Lactococcus lactis* subsp. *cremoris* B40 (Figure 18.1, structure 5) was 96% when fed to rats.[1] EPSs fermented by colonic bacteria produce short-chain fatty acids (SCFAs), which are sources of energy to the host and are believed to protect against colorectal cancer.[104]

Few digestion-related enzymes were found to act on EPSs from LAB, no enzymes with *endo* activity. However, EPSs from *Lactobacillus helveticus* TY1-2 (Figure 18.1, structure 6)[93] and TN-4 (Figure 18.1, structure 7),[94] *Lactococcus lactis* subsp. *cremoris* B39 (Figure 18.1, structure 8),[95] as

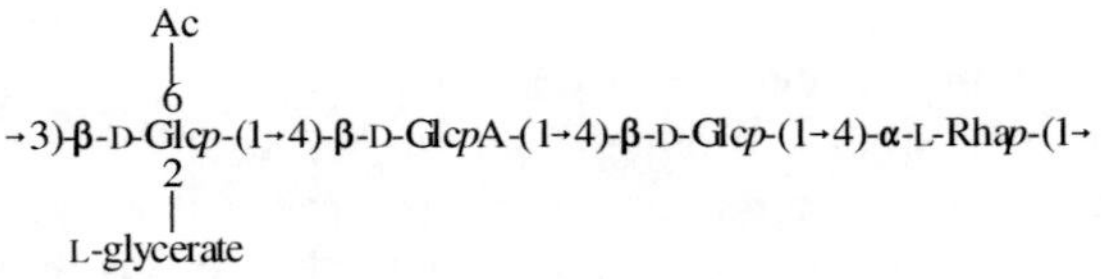

$$Ac$$
$$\downarrow$$
$$6$$
$$\rightarrow3)\text{-}\beta\text{-}D\text{-}Glcp\text{-}(1\rightarrow4)\text{-}\beta\text{-}D\text{-}GlcpA\text{-}(1\rightarrow4)\text{-}\beta\text{-}D\text{-}Glcp\text{-}(1\rightarrow4)\text{-}\alpha\text{-}L\text{-}Rhap\text{-}(1\rightarrow$$
$$2$$
$$\downarrow$$
$$L\text{-glycerate}$$

Structure 1: native gellan gum[88]

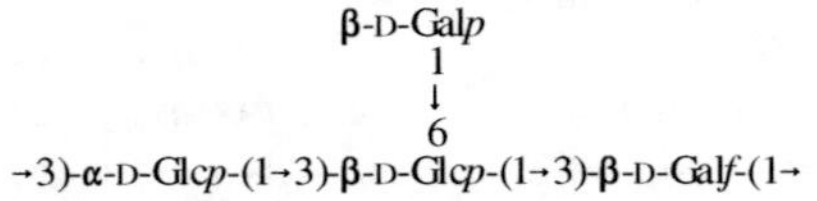

$$\beta\text{-}D\text{-}Galp$$
$$1$$
$$\downarrow$$
$$6$$
$$\rightarrow3)\text{-}\alpha\text{-}D\text{-}Glcp\text{-}(1\rightarrow3)\text{-}\beta\text{-}D\text{-}Glcp\text{-}(1\rightarrow3)\text{-}\beta\text{-}D\text{-}Galf\text{-}(1\rightarrow$$

Structure 2: EPS from *Streptococcus thermophilus* SFi39[89]

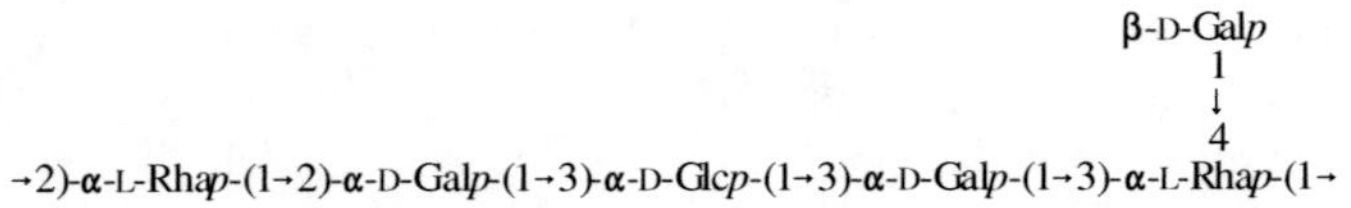

$$\beta\text{-}D\text{-}Galp$$
$$1$$
$$\downarrow$$
$$4$$
$$\rightarrow2)\text{-}\alpha\text{-}L\text{-}Rhap\text{-}(1\rightarrow2)\text{-}\alpha\text{-}D\text{-}Galp\text{-}(1\rightarrow3)\text{-}\alpha\text{-}D\text{-}Glcp\text{-}(1\rightarrow3)\text{-}\alpha\text{-}D\text{-}Galp\text{-}(1\rightarrow3)\text{-}\alpha\text{-}L\text{-}Rhap\text{-}(1\rightarrow$$

Structure 3: EPS from *Streptococcus thermophilus* Sfi12[89]

FIGURE 18.1 Structures 1 through 3.

TABLE 18.4
Effects of Nondigestible Fiber on the Gastrointestinal Tract and Its Function

1. Increase viscosity of digesta
2. Increase transit time
3. Alter pH
4. Change to digestive enzyme activity
5. Decrease absorption of nutrients
6. Enlarge digestive organs
7. Change to intestinal surface layer

Source: From Ikegami, S., Tsuchihashi, F., Harada, H., Tsuchihashi, N., Nishide, E., and Innami, S., Effect of viscous indigestible polysaccharides on pancreatic-biliary secretion and digestive organs in rats, *J. Nutr.*, 120: 353–360, 1990.

---

well as the O-deacetylated polysaccharide from *Lactococcus lactis* subsp. *cremoris* B891 (Figure 18.1, structure 9),[96] having the disaccharide fragment lactose β-D-Galp-(1→4)-β-D-Glcp-(1→ in their side chains, were susceptible to enzyme preparations having *exo* β-galactosidase activity.

The EPS produced by *Lb. sanfranciscensis* is a fructan that is not degraded in the stomach or small intestine. Human strains of bifidobacteria that reside in the large intestine are able to metabolize this EPS, which would make the *Lb. sanfranciscensis* EPS a potential prebiotic.[105]

Curdlan, an EPS produced by *Alcaligenes faecalis* var. *myxogenes,* is easily digested and fermented by intestinal bacteria, whereas gellan gum, produced by *Pseudomonus elodea,* is more resistant to intestinal breakdown. In rats, both EPSs increased colon plus rectum weights, lowered fecal pH, increased % fecal moisture content, lowered fecal dry weight, and both decreased cecum ammonia concentration compared to rats consuming a diet containing cellulose. However, rats eating gellan gum had lower amounts of SCFAs per g cecal contents and lower total cecal SCFAs compared to rats eating the diet containing cellulose. The diet containing curdlan had the opposite effect on cecal SCFAs; the beneficial effects of the high levels of butyric, propionic, and lactic acids in cecal

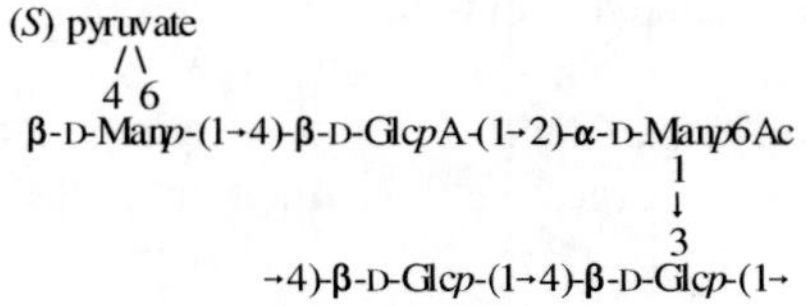

(S) pyruvate
/\
4 6
β-D-Man*p*-(1→4)-β-D-Glc*p*A-(1→2)-α-D-Man*p*6Ac
|
↓
3
→4)-β-D-Glc*p*-(1→4)-β-D-Glc*p*-(1→

Structure 4: xanthan gum from *Xanthomonas campestris* [90]

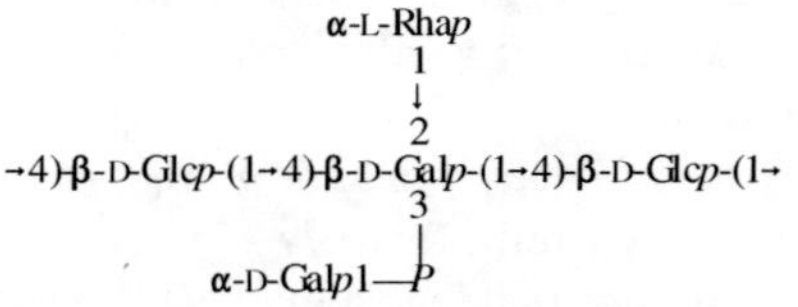

α-L-Rha*p*
1
↓
2
→4)-β-D-Glc*p*-(1→4)-β-D-Gal*p*-(1→4)-β-D-Glc*p*-(1→
3
|
α-D-Gal*p*1—P

Structure 5: EPS from *Lactococcus lactis* subsp. *cremoris* B40 [91] **and viilian from *Lactococcus lactis* subsp. *cremoris* SBT 0495** [92]

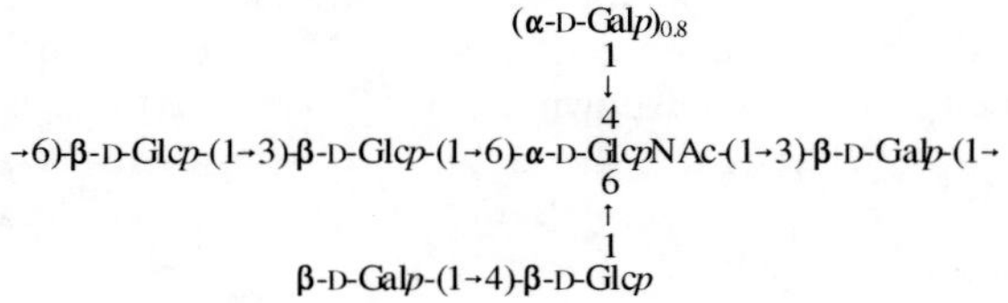

(α-D-Gal*p*)$_{0.8}$
1
↓
4
→6)-β-D-Glc*p*-(1→3)-β-D-Glc*p*-(1→6)-α-D-Glc*p*NAc-(1→3)-β-D-Gal*p*-(1→
6
↑
1
β-D-Gal*p*-(1→4)-β-D-Glc*p*

Structure 6: EPS from *Lactobacillus helveticus* TY1-2 [93]

FIGURE 18.1 Structures 4 through 6.

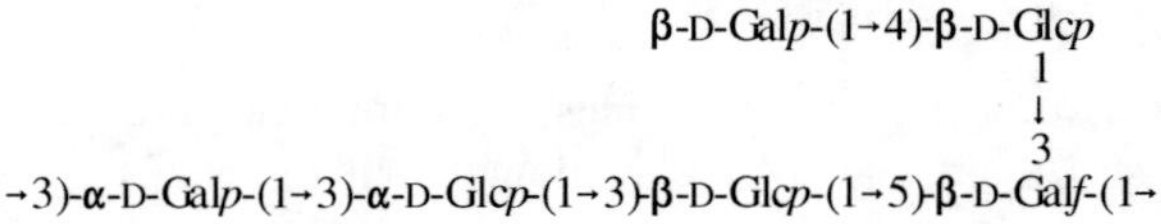

β-D-Gal*p*-(1→4)-β-D-Glc*p*
1
↓
3
→3)-α-D-Gal*p*-(1→3)-α-D-Glc*p*-(1→3)-β-D-Glc*p*-(1→5)-β-D-Gal*f*-(1→

Structure 7: EPS from *Lactobacillus helveticus* TN-4 [94]

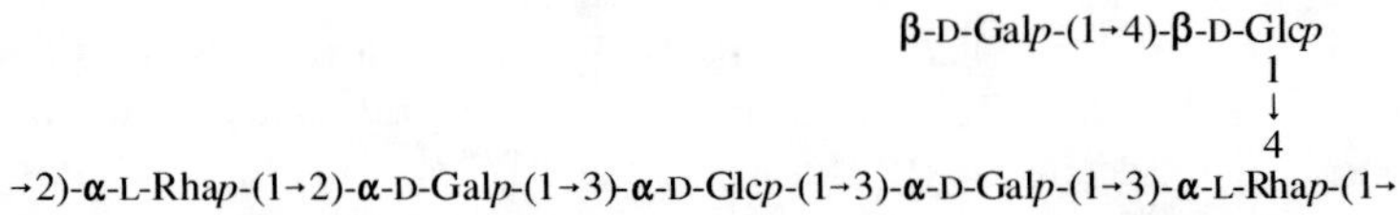

β-D-Gal*p*-(1→4)-β-D-Glc*p*
1
↓
4
→2)-α-L-Rha*p*-(1→2)-α-D-Gal*p*-(1→3)-α-D-Glc*p*-(1→3)-α-D-Gal*p*-(1→3)-α-L-Rha*p*-(1→

Structure 8: EPS from *Lactococcus lactis* subsp. *cremoris* B39 [95]

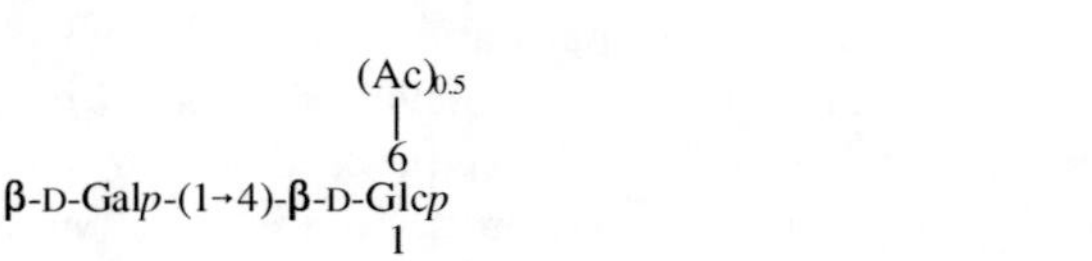

(Ac)$_{0.5}$
|
6
β-D-Gal*p*-(1→4)-β-D-Glc*p*
1
↓
6
→4)-α-D-Glc*p*-(1→4)-β-D-Gal*p*-(1→4)-β-D-Glc*p*-(1→

Structure 9: EPS from *Lactococcus lactis* subsp. *cremoris* B891 [96]

FIGURE 18.1 Structures 7 through 9.

contents were noted.[106] Rats eating the diet containing the curdlan had ceca that were twice as heavy as rats eating other sources of fiber. Similar results have been published earlier.[88] The ease of fermentation and the production of SCFAs from EPSs may impact on fecal water content and fecal output, which may ultimately affect digestive tract function and diseases.[107]

B. ANTITUMOR EFFECTS

Some bacteria have been shown to have antimutagenic properties. The production of EPS and its ability to bind mutagens may partly explain this phenomenon. For example, the EPS produced by *Bifidobacterium longum* can bind to heterocyclic amines.[108] In other cases, the effect may be mediated through the immune system.

EPS (Figure 18.1, structure 10) isolated from kefir grain — a mass of bacteria, yeasts, and milk protein used to produce the fermented milk kefir[109] — has been shown to inhibit the growth of Ehrlich carcinoma (up to 64% inhibition) and sarcoma 180 (up to 90% inhibition) in mice.[110] The tumor growth was inhibited when the EPS was administered orally or intraperitoneally. Tests of delayed-type hypersensitivity in mice given tumors and kefir EPS prompted this same group to conclude that a cell-mediated response was occurring and that the EPS exerted inhibitory effects when it was given before or after tumor inoculation.[111] Using radio-labeled EPS, the group then showed that some of the EPS or its breakdown products were able to reach the spleen and thymus, which would support the hypothesis that the antitumor effects were the result of a delayed-type hypersensitivity.[112] An EPS formed by *Lb. helveticus* var. *jugurii* was shown to prolong the life of mice injected with sarcoma 180 cells.[113]

More recently, another Japanese group has shown that kefir grain EPS stimulates *in vitro* Peyer's patch cells in tumor-bearing mice, which causes the secretion of water-soluble factors that stimulate the mitogenic response in T and B lymphocytes in normal mice.[114] They then showed that the same EPS protects mice against pulmonary metastasis, again either when the EPS was given before or after the tumor.[115]

C. IMMUNE FUNCTION EFFECTS

Some EPSs, like other polysaccharides, have immune-stimulating properties that depend on their stereochemistry, molecular size, or the number and kinds of sugar residues making up the EPS. Most interest has centered on the stimulation of Th1 response that is responsible for resistance to infectious agents and allergens. Kitazawa and coworkers were able to show that the EPS produced by *Lactococcus lactis* ssp. *cremoris* KVS20, one of the starter cultures from the Scandinavian ropy sour milk viili, was able to stimulate the mitogenic response in murine spleen cells of C57BL/6 mice, particularly in a fraction enriched in B cells, and also in spleen cells from athymic *nu/nu* mice.[116] They then showed that the EPS was not a lipopolysaccharide and that its mode of action was different from a lipopolysaccharide.[117] This particular EPS appears to be a phosphopolysaccharide, and its composition suggests it could have the same structure as viilian from strain SBT 0495 (Figure 18.1, structure 5), although this was not confirmed.[118] It may be a biological response modifier that is able to stimulate the production of IFN-γ and IL-1α in antigen presenting macrophages (Mφ).[118]

As early as 1987, there was speculation that the slime material produced by *Streptococcus cremoris* in the production of the Scandinavian fermented milk drink called viili was capable of stimulating the immune system.[119] Nakajima et al.[120] showed that the ESP[92] in viili was able to increase serum DNP-specific antibody production in mice, indicating its adjuvant properties. Stimulated lymphocytes and enhanced macrophage activity were suggested as possible mechanisms. The EPS produced by *Lb. rhamnosus* RW-9595M (Figure 18.1, structure 11) stimulated the production of TNF, IL-6, and IL-12 in human and mouse cells and IFN-γ in mouse splenocytes.[121]

The EPS structure is important to its immunostimulating effect, but the phosphate group in some EPSs is also critical. Thus, the EPS produced by *Lactobacillus delbrueckii* ssp. *bulgaricus*

OLL 1073R-1 can enhance macrophage phagocytosis *in vivo* and *in vitro,* but only when the phosphate is in place.[122] The mode of action of the phosphate-containing EPS is different from lipopolysaccharide (LPS). Nitric oxide (NO) production is not induced but mRNA expression of cytokines in microphages does occur.[123] The importance of the phosphate group was also underlined in the mitogenic activation of lymphocytes by the EPS of *Lactobacillus delbrueckii* ssp. *bulgaricus,* and Kitazawa et al.[124] stated that the magnitude of EPS mitogenic activity may be directly related to the phosphate content of an EPS.

D. CHOLESTEROL DIGESTION AND METABOLISM EFFECTS

EPSs probably act as typical dietary fibers in terms of how they decrease serum cholesterol levels. The increased viscosity associated with EPSs may coat the unstirred layer of the intestinal mucosus, thereby cutting down on cholesterol absorption. Also, there may be direct chemical binding depending on the chemical structure of the EPS and conditions (such as pH) in the gut. Such binding would increase excretion, induce bile acid synthesis in the liver, and reduce cholesterol via oxidation. It is also possible that EPSs are being fermented in the colon, producing SCFAs, especially propionate, which can impact on cholesterol-synthesis pathways.

Direct binding of cholesterol has been shown by *in vitro* tests for both xanthan gum and, to a lesser extent, gellan gum.[125] Binding of EPS to free bile acids has also been reported *in vitro.*[126] EPSs produced by two strains of *Lb. delbrueckii* had the greatest ability to bind free cholic acid (up to 15% of a 1.5 mM solution), and coincidentally were also the highest producers of EPS. None of the EPSs from the *Lb. delbrueckii* or *Sc. thermophilus* strains tested were able to bind free glycocholic acid.

Nakajima et al. fed a milk fermented with *Lactococcus lactis* subsp. *cremoris* SBT 0495 to rats fed a high-cholesterol diet and found significant reductions in total serum cholesterol and a significant increase in the HDL/total cholesterol ratio compared to controls.[127] The action of the bacteria gives the milk a ropy texture due to the production of the EPS viilian.[127] The cholesterol-lowering effect was attributed to "dietary fiber action."

Consumption of a diet with as little as 1% xanthan gum significantly reduced plasma and liver cholesterol levels in rats[128] that was linked to significant decreases in apparent cholesterol absorption and digestibility. Rats eating the diets containing xanthan gum also had significantly reduced serum and liver triglyceride levels. A mixture of xanthan gum (1%) and guar gum (2%) had a hypocholesterolemic effect on plasma and liver of diabetic rats and on plasma of nondiabetic rats, and a hypotriacylglycerolemic effect on the liver of both diabetic and nondiabetic rats.[129]

Feeding humans the EPS gellan gum (175 and 200 mg/kg body weight) for 30 d decreased serum cholesterol in both the females (−13%) and the males (−11%).[101] Kefiran, the EPS obtained from by kefir-producing bacteria, has also been reported to lower serum and liver cholesterol levels and to lower blood pressure in hypertensive rats.[130]

E. EFFECTS ON DIABETES

Food viscosity influences the speed at which food exits the stomach. One strategy for slowing the glycemic response has been to slow gastric emptying using the EPS xanthan gum, which in turn delays intestinal digestion and absorption. Xanthan is more viscous than guar gum or methylcellulose on a per weight basis measured *in vitro*, but all three have equal ability to lower the blood glucose response curve in rats fed a carbohydrate challenge.[131] Feeding humans xanthan gum (12 g/d) in muffins significantly lowered fasting serum glucose levels and blood glucose concentrations 1 h after a glucose challenge in borderline type II diabetics.[132] After 6 weeks of consuming xanthan-enriched muffins, the subjects had lowered glucose tolerance curves, although the shape of the curves was not altered.

$$\begin{array}{c}
\beta\text{-}D\text{-Glc}p \\
1 \\
\downarrow \\
6(2) \\
\rightarrow 6)\text{-}\beta\text{-}D\text{-Glc}p\text{-}(1\rightarrow 2(6))\text{-}\beta\text{-}D\text{-Gal}p\text{-}(1\rightarrow 4)\text{-}\alpha\text{-}D\text{-Gal}p\text{-}(1\rightarrow 3)\text{-}\beta\text{-}D\text{-Gal}p\text{-}(1\rightarrow 4)\text{-}\alpha\text{-}D\text{-Glc}p\text{-}(1\rightarrow
\end{array}$$

Structure 10: kefiran from kefir grains[97]

$$\begin{array}{c}
(R)\ \text{pyruvate} \\
/\backslash \\
46 \\
\alpha\text{-}D\text{-Gal}p \\
1 \\
\downarrow \\
2 \\
\rightarrow 3)\text{-}\alpha\text{-}L\text{-Rha}p\text{-}(1\rightarrow 3)\text{-}\beta\text{-}D\text{-Glc}p\text{-}(1\rightarrow 3)\text{-}\alpha\text{-}L\text{-Rha}p\text{-}(1\rightarrow 3)\text{-}\alpha\text{-}L\text{-Rha}p\text{-}(1\rightarrow 3)\text{-}\alpha\text{-}L\text{-Rha}p\text{-}(1\rightarrow 2)\text{-}\alpha\text{-}D\text{-Glc}p\text{-}(1\rightarrow
\end{array}$$

Structure 11: EPS from *Lactobacillus rhamnosus* RW-9595M[98]

$$\begin{array}{c}
\beta\text{-}D\text{-Gal}f\text{-}(1\rightarrow 6)\text{-}\beta\text{-}D\text{-Glc}p\text{-}(1\rightarrow 6)\text{-}\beta\text{-}D\text{-Glc}p\text{NAc} \\
1 \\
\downarrow \\
3 \\
\rightarrow 4)\text{-}\alpha\text{-}D\text{-Glc}p\text{-}(1\rightarrow 4)\text{-}\beta\text{-}D\text{-Gal}p\text{-}(1\rightarrow 4)\text{-}\beta\text{-}D\text{-Glc}p\text{-}(1\rightarrow
\end{array}$$

Structure 12: EPS from *Streptococcus macedonicus* Sc136[99]

FIGURE 18.1 Structures 10 through 12.

F. OTHER USES OF EXOPOLYSACCHARIDES

Hyperuricemia and gout are caused by either overproduction or underexcretion of uric acid. Excessive intake of RNA can also lead to hyperuricemia. Using a rat model, Japanese researchers have shown that highly viscous dietary fibers, especially the EPS xanthan gum, are able to alter digestive and metabolic processes that may contribute to hyperuricemia by lowering serum and urine uric acid levels, reducing RNA digestion by RNase A, and increasing RNA excretion in feces.[133,134]

The EPS produced by *Streptococcus macedonicus* Sc136 (Figure 18.1, structure 12) has been shown to contain a trisaccharide fragment β-D-GlcpNAc-(1→3)-β-D-Galp-(1→4)-β-D-Glcp that is related to oligosaccharides found in human milk.[99] Adding such an EPS to infant formula might produce a formula that is more bifidogenic and capable of inhibiting pathogenic microorganism adhesion in the gut.

The ability of some EPSs to resist digestion has prompted research into the possible use of EPSs as coating material for drugs, nutraceutical products, and probiotic bacteria to be delivered to the colon. Gellan gum is digested by the colonic enzyme galactomannanase, and it has been shown *in vitro* that beads of gellan gum undergo initial surface erosion, followed by rapid release of interior contents at pH and galactomannanase concentrations typically found in the colon.[135] A mixture of gellan gum and xanthan gum has been used to encapsulate *Bifidobacterium infantis* to protect the live bacteria. Bacteria encapsulated in this way remained viable longer in pH 4 peptone water, in yogurt, or in simulated gastric juice.[136]

The water holding capacity of xanthan gum may contribute to its moistening and lubricating properties that has led to its use in a saliva substitute that is used by radiation patients to treat feelings of a dry mouth or xerostomia.[137]

V. CONCLUSIONS

Fermented foods are consumed around the world for practical and health reasons. From a foodscience perspective, EPSs are important because they contribute to the sensory properties of foods. As our knowledge of the fermentation process increases, it is evident that many of the microorganisms involved are producing EPSs that may be beneficial to health. So far, these complex carbohydrates are not a large part of the diet. However, as the structure and function of these EPSs become better characterized, new functional foods and nutraceuticals containing EPSs will become available to consumers.

REFERENCES

1. Looijesteijn, P.J., Trapet, L., de Vries, E., Abee, T., and Hugenholtz, J., Physiological function of exopolysaccharides produced by *Lactococcus lactis*, *Int. J. Food Microbiol.*, 64: 71–80, 2001.

2. Ruas-Madiedo, P., Hugenholtz, J., and Zoon, P., An overview of the functionality of exopolysaccharides produced by lactic acid bacteria, *Int. Dairy J.*, 12: 163–171, 2002.

3. De Vuyst, L., De Vin, F., Vaningelgem, F., and Degeest, B., Recent developments in the biosynthesis and applications of heteropolysaccharides from lactic acid bacteria, *Int. Dairy J.*, 11: 687–707, 2001.

4. Hassan, A.N., Ipsen, R., Janzen, T., and Qvist, K.B., Microstructure and rheology of yogurt made with cultures differing only in their ability to produce exopolysaccharides, *J. Dairy Sci.*, 86: 1632–1638, 2003.

5. Mozzi, F., Savoy de Giori, G., Oliver, G., and Font de Valdez, G., Effect of culture pH on the growth characteristics and polysaccharide production by *Lactobacillus casei*, *Milchwissenschaft*, 49: 667–670, 1994.

6. Rawson, H.L. and Marshall, V.M., Effect of 'ropy' strains of *Lactobacillus delbrueckii* ssp. *bulgaricus* and *Streptococcus thermophilus* on rheology of stirred yogurt, *Int. J. Food Sci. Technol.*, 32: 213–220, 1997.

7. De Vuyst, L., Zamfir, M., Mozzi, F., Adriany, T., Marshall, V., Degeest, B., and Vaningelgem, F., Exopolysaccharide-producing *Streptococcus thermophilus* strains as functional starter cultures in the production of fermented milks, *Int. Dairy J.*, 13: 707–717, 2003.

8. Ritu, R. and Gandhi, D.N., Extracellular polysaccharides from lactic acid bacteria — a review, *Ind. J. Dairy Sci.*, 57: 223–231, 2004.

9. Broadbent, J.R., McMahon, D.J., Oberg, C.J., and Welker, D.L., Use of exopolysaccharide-producing cultures to improve the functionality of low fat cheese, *Int. Dairy J.*, 11: 433–439, 2001.

10. Moreira, M., Bevilacqua, A., and de Antoni, G., Manufacture of Quartirolo cheese using exopolysaccharide-producing starter cultures, *Milchwissenschaft*, 58: 301–304, 2003.

11. Perry, D.B., McMahon, D.J., and Oberg, C.J., Manufacture of low fat Mozzarella cheese using exopolysaccharide-producing starter cultures, *J. Dairy Sci.*, 81: 563–566, 1998.

12. Sanni, A.I., Onilude, A.A., Ogunbanwo, S.T., Fadahunsi, I.F., and Afolabi, R.O., Production of exopolysaccharides by lactic acid bacteria isolated from traditional fermented foods in Nigeria, *Eur. Food Res. Technol.*, 214: 405–407, 2002.

13. Akcelik, M. and Sanlbaba, P., Characterization of an exopolysaccharide preventing phage adsorption in *Lactococcus lactis* subsp. *cremoris* MA39, *Turk J. Vet. Anim. Sci.*, 26: 1151–1156, 2002.

14. Forde, A. and Fitzgerald, G.F., Analysis of exopolysaccharide (EPS) production mediated by the bacteriophage adsorption blocking plasmid, pCI658, isolated from *Lactococcus lactis* ssp. *cremoris* HO2, *Int. Dairy J.*, 9: 465–472, 1999.

15. Kocer, E., Tukel, C., and Akcelik, M., Relationship between exopolysaccharide production and phage resistance in *Lactococcus lactis*, *Gida*, 28: 47–53, 2003.

16. Deveau, H., Van Calsteren, M.-R., and Moineau, S., Effect of exopolysaccharides on phage-host interactions in *Lactococcus lactis*, *Appl. Environ. Microbiol.*, 68: 4364–4369, 2002.

17. Hong, S.H. and Marshall, R.T., Natural exopolysaccharides enhance survival of lactic acid bacteria in frozen dairy desserts, *J. Dairy Sci.*, 84: 1367–1374, 2001.

18. Martensson, O., Oste, R., and Holst, O., Texture promoting capacity and EPS formation by lactic acid bacteria in three different oat-based non-dairy media, *Eur. Food Res. Technol.*, 214: 232–236, 2002.

19. Tieking, M., Korakli, M., Ehrmann, M.A., Ganzle, M.G., and Vogel, R.F., *In situ* production of exopolysaccharides during sourdough fermentation by cereal and intestinal isolates of lactic acid bacteria, *Appl. Environ. Microbiol.*, 69: 945–952, 2003.

20. Duggan, E. and Waghorne, E., Long-term evaluation of production protocols for stirred yogurts produced using two different cultures, *Milchwissenschaft*, 58: 52–55, 2003.

21. Martensson, O., Duenas-Chasco, M., Irastorza, A., Oste, R., and Holst, O., Comparison of growth characteristics and exopolysaccharide formation of two lactic acid bacteria strains, *Pediococcus damnosus* 2.6 and *Lactobacillus brevis* G-77, in an oat-based, nondairy medium, *Leben. Wiss. Technol.*, 36: 353–357, 2003.

22. Vaningelgem, F., Zamfir, M., Mozzi, F., Adriany, T., Vancanneyt, M., Swings, J., and de Vuyst, L., Biodiversity of exopolysaccharides produced by *Streptococcus thermophilus* strains is reflected in their production and their molecular and functional characteristics, *Appl. Environ. Microbiol.*, 70: 900–912, 2004.

23. Torino, M.I., Mozzi, F., Sesma, F., and Font de Valdez, G., Effect of stirring on growth and phospho-polysaccharide production by *Lactobacillus helveticus* ATCC 15807 in milk, *Milchwissenschaft*, 55: 204–207, 2000.

24. Shihata, A. and Shah, N.P., Influence of addition of proteolytic strains of *Lactobacillus delbrueckii* subsp. *bulgaricus* to commercial ABT starter cultures on texture of yogurt, exopolysaccharide production and survival of bacteria, *Int. Dairy J.*, 12: 765–772, 2002.

25. Giraffa, G. and Bergere, J.L., Nature du caractère épaississant de certaines souches de *Streptococcus thermophilus*: étude préliminaire, *Lait*, 67: 285–298, 1987.

26. Ruas-Madiedo, P., Alting, A.C., and Zoon, P., Effect of exopolysaccharides and proteolytic activity of *Lactococcus lactis* subsp. *cremoris* strains on the viscosity and structure of fermented milks, *Int. Dairy J.*, 15: 155–164, 2005.

27. Hassan, A.N., Frank, J.F., and Elsoda, M., Observation of bacterial exopolysaccharide in dairy products using cryo-scanning electron microscopy, *Int. Dairy J.*, 13: 755–762, 2003.

28. Laws, A.P. and Marshall V.M., The relevance of exopolysaccharide to the rheological properties in milk fermented with ropy strains of lactic acid bacteria, *Int. Dairy J.*, 11: 709–722, 2001.

29. Cerning, J., Production of exopolysaccharides by lactic acid bacteria and dairy propionibacteria, *Lait*, 75: 463–472, 1995.

30. Tallon, R., Bressollier, P., and Urdaci, M.C., Isolation and characterization of two exopolysaccharides produced by *Lactobacillus planta*rum EP56, *Res. Microbiol.*, 154: 705–712, 2003.

31. Vaningelgem, F., van der Meulen, R., Zamfir, M., Adriany, T., Laws, A.P., and De Vuyst, L., *Streptococcus thermophilus* ST 111 produces a stable high-molecular-mass exopolysaccharide in milk-based medium, *Int. Dairy J.*, 14: 857–864, 2004.

32. Petry, S., Furlan, S., Waghorne, E., Saulnier, L., Cerning, J., and Maguin, E., Comparison of the thickening properties of four *Lactobacillus delbrueckii* subsp. *bulgaricus* strains and physicochemical characterization of their exopolysaccharides, *FEMS Microbiol. Lett.*, 221: 285–291, 2003.

33. Duboc, P. and Mollet, B. Applications of exopolysaccharides in the dairy industry, *Int. Dairy J.*, 11: 759–768, 2001.

34. Korakli, M., Pavlovic, M., Ganzle, M. G., and Vogel, R.F., Exopolysaccharide and kestose production by *Lactobacillus sanfranciscensis* LTH2590, *Appl. Environ. Microbiol.*, 69: 2073–2079, 2003.

35. van den Berg, D.J.C., Robijn, G.W., Janssen, A.C., Giuseppin, M.L.F., Vreeker, R., Kamerling, J.P., Vliegenthart, J.F.G., Ledeboer, A.M., and Verrips, C.T., Production of a novel extracellular polysaccharide by *Lactobacillus sake* 0-1 and characterization of the polysaccharide, *Appl. Environ. Microbiol.*, 61: 2840–2844, 1995.

36. Bergmaier, D., Lacroix, C., Macedo, M.G., and Champagne, C.P., New method for exopolysaccharide determination in culture broth using stirred ultrafiltration cells, *Appl. Microbiol. Biotechnol.*, 57: 401–406, 2001.

37. Levander, F., Svensson, M., and Radstrom, P., Small-scale analysis of exopolysaccharides from *Streptococcus thermophilus* grown in a semi-defined medium, *BMC-Microbiol.*, 1: 23, 2001; epub 2001 Sep 26.

38. Macedo, M.G., Laporte, M,F., and Lacroix, C., Quantification of exopolysaccharide, lactic acid, and lactose concentrations in culture broth by near-infrared spectroscopy, *J. Agric. Food Chem.*, 50:1774–1779, 2002.

39. Gancel, F. and Novel, G., Exopolysaccharide production by *Streptococcus salivarius* ssp. *thermophilus* cultures. 2. Distinct modes of polymer production and degradation among clonal variants, *J. Dairy Sci.*, 77: 689–695, 1994.

40. Macura, D. and Townsley, P.M., Scandinavian ropy milk — identification and characterization of endogenus ropy lactic streptococci and their extracellular excretion, *J. Dairy Sci.*, 67: 735–744, 1984.

41. Iliev, I., Radoilska, E., Ivanova, I., and Enikova, R., Biosynthesis of exopolysaccharides by two strains of *Lactobacillus bulgaricus* in whey-based media, Mededelingen Faculteit Landbouwkundige en Toegepaste Biologische Wetenschappen, Universiteit Gent, 66: 511–516, 2001.

42. Degeest, B., Vaningelgem, F., and de Vuyst, L., Microbial physiology, fermentation kinetics, and process engineering of heteropolysaccharide production by lactic acid bacteria, *Int. Dairy J.,* 11: 678–707, 2001.

43. Cerning, J., Bouillanne, C., Landon, M., and Desmazeaud, M., Isolation and characterization of exopolysaccharides from slime-forming mesophilic lactic acid bacteria, *J. Dairy Sci.,* 75: 692–699, 1992.

44. Cerning, J., Renard, C.M., Thibault, J.F., Bouillanne, C., Landon, M., Desmazeaud, M., and Topi-sirovic, L., Carbon source requirements for exopolysaccharide production by *Lactobacillus casei* CG11 and partial structure analysis of the polymer, *Appl. Environ. Microbiol.,* 60: 3914–3919, 1994.

45. Briczinski, E.P. and Roberts, R.F., Production of an exopolysaccharide-containing whey protein concentrate by fermentation of whey, *J. Dairy Sci.,* 85: 3189–3197, 2002.

46. Gassem, M.A., Sims, K.A., and Frank, J.F., Extracellular polysaccharide production by *Lactobacillus delbrueckii* subsp. *bulgaricus* in a continuous fermentor, *Lebensm. Wiss. Technol.,* 30: 273–278, 1997.

47. Grobben, G.J., Sikkema, J., Smith, M.R., and de Bont, J.A.M., Production of extracellular polysaccharides by *Lactobacillus delbrueckii* ssp. *bulgaricus* NCFB 2772 grown in a chemically defined medium, *J. Appl. Bacteriol.,* 79: 103–107, 1995.

48. Cheirsilp, B., Shimizu, H., and Shioya, S., Modelling and optimization of environmental conditions for kefiran production by *Lactobacillus kefiranofaciens*, *Appl. Microbiol. Biotechnol.,* 57: 639–646, 2001.

49. Cheirsilp, B., Shimizu, H., and Shioya, S., Enhanced kefiran production by mixed culture of *Lactobacillus kefiranofaciens* and *Saccharomyces cerevisiae*, *J. Biotechnol.,* 100: 43–53, 2003.

50. Torino, M.I., Taranto, M.P., Sesma, F., and Font-de-Valdez, G., Heterofermentative pattern and exopolysaccharide production by *Lactobacillus helveticus* ATCC 15807 in response to environmental pH, *J. Appl. Microbiol.,* 91: 846–852, 2001.

51. Dupont, I., Roy, D., and Lapointe, G., Comparison of exopolysaccharide production by strains of *Lactobacillus rhamnosus* and *Lactobacillus paracasei* grown in chemically defined medium and milk, *J. Ind. Microbiol. Biotechnol.,* 24: 251–255, 2000.

52. Gamar-Nourani, L., Blondeau, K., and Simonet, J.M., Influence of culture conditions on exopolysaccharide production by *Lactobacillus rhamnosus* strain C83, *J. Appl. Microbiol.,* 85: 664–672, 1998.

53. Bergmaier, D., Champagne, C.P., and Lacroix, C., Exopolysaccharide production during batch cultures with free and immobilized *Lactobacillus rhamnosus* RW-9595M, *J. Appl. Microbiol.,* 95: 1049–1057, 2003.

54. Bergmaier, D., Champagne, C.P., and Lacroix, C., Growth and exopolysaccharide production during free and immobilized cell chemostat culture of *Lactobacillus rhamnosus* RW-9595M, *J. Appl. Microbiol.,* 98: 272–284, 2005.

55. Looijesteijn, P.J. and Hugenholtz, J., Uncoupling of growth and exopolysaccharide production by *Lactococcus lactis* subsp. *cremoris* NIZO B40 and optimization of its synthesis, *J. Biosci. Bioeng.,* 88: 178–182, 1999.

56. De Vuyst, L., Vanderveken, F., Van de Ven, S., and Degeest, B., Production by and isolation of exopolysaccharides from *Streptococcus thermophilus* grown in a milk medium and evidence for their growth-associated biosynthesis, *J. Appl. Microbiol.,* 84: 1059–1068, 1998.

57. Degeest, B. and De Vuyst, L., Indication that the nitrogen source influences both amount and size of exopolysaccharides produced by *Streptococcus thermophilus* LY03 and modelling of the bacterial growth and exopolysaccharide production in a complex medium, *Appl. Environ. Microbiol.,* 65: 2863–2870, 1999.

58. Mozzi, F., Savoy de Giori, G., and Font de Valdez, G., UDP-galactose 4-epimerase: a key enzyme in exopolysaccharide formation by *Lactobacillus casei* CRL 87 in controlled pH batch cultures, *J. Appl. Microbiol.,* 94: 175–183, 2003.

59. Gancel, F. and Novel, G., Exopolysaccharide production by *Streptococcus salivarius* ssp. *thermophilus* cultures. 1. Conditions of production, *J. Dairy Sci.,* 77: 684–688, 1994.

60. Pham, P.L., Dupont, I., Roy, D., Lapointe, G., and Cerning, J., Production of exopolysaccharide by *Lactobacillus rhamnosus* R and analysis of its enzymatic degradation during prolonged fermentation, *Appl. Environ. Microbiol.,* 66: 2302–2310, 2000.

61. Mozzi, F., Oliver, G., Savoy de Giori, G.S., and Font de Valdez, G., Influence of temperature on the production of exopolysaccharides by thermophilic lactic acid bacteria, *Milchwissenschaft*, 50: 80–82, 1995.

62. Gassem, M.A., Schmidt, K.A., and Frank, J.F., Exopolysaccharide production in different media by lactic acid bacteria, *Cult. Dairy Prod. J.*, 30: 18–21, 1995.

63. Gamar, L., Blondeau, K., and Simonet, J.M., Physiological approach to extracellular polysaccharide production by *Lactobacillus rhamnosus* strain C83, *J. Appl. Microbiol.*, 83: 281–287, 1997.

64. Gassem, M.A., Schmidt, K.A., and Frank, J.F., Exopolysaccharide production from whey lactose by fermentation with *Lactobacillus delbrueckii* ssp. *bulgaricus*, *J. Food Sci.*, 62: 171–173, 207, 1997.

65. Mozzi, F., Savoy de Giori, G., Oliver, G., and Font de Valdez, G., Exopolysaccharide production by *Lactobacillus casei* in milk under different growth conditions, *Milchwissenschaft*, 51: 670–673, 1996.

66. Mozzi, F., Savoy de Giori, G., Oliver, G., and Font de Valdez, G., Exopolysaccharide production by *Lactobacillus casei* under controlled pH, *Biotechnol. Lett.*, 18: 435–439, 1996.

67. Kimmel, S.A. and Roberts, R.F., Development of a growth medium suitable for exopolysaccharide production by *Lactobacillus delbrueckii* ssp. *bulgaricus* RR, *Int. J. Food Microbiol.*, 40: 87–92, 1998.

68. Christiansen, P.S., Pedersen, J.N., Edelsten, D., and Nielsen, E.W., Slime formation in whey by ropy *Lactococcus lactis* ssp. *cremoris* 322, *Milchwissenschaft*, 56: 545–549, 2001.

69. Macedo, M.G., Lacroix, C., and Champagne, C.P., Combined effects of temperature and medium composition on exopolysaccharide production by *Lactobacillus rhamnosus* RW-9595M in a whey permeate based medium, *Biotechnol. Prog.*, 18: 167–173, 2002.

70. Vaningelgem, F., Zamfir, M., Adriany, T., and De Vuyst, L., Fermentation conditions affecting the bacterial growth and exopolysaccharide production by *Streptococcus thermophilus* ST 111 in milk-based medium, *J. App. Microbiol.*, 97: 1257–1273, 2004.

71. Degeest, B., Mozzi, F., and Vuyst, L., Effect of medium composition and temperature and pH changes on exopolysaccharide yields and stability during *Streptococcus thermophilus* LY03 fermentations, *Int. J. Food Microbiol.*, 79: 161–174, 2002.

72. Chervaux, C., Ehrlich, S.D., and Maguin, E., Physiological study of *Lactobacillus delbrueckii* subsp. *bulgaricus* strains in a novel chemically defined medium, *Appl. Environ. Microbiol.*, 66: 5306–5311, 2000.

73. Grobben, G.J., Smith, M.R., Sikkema, J., and de Bont, J.A.M., Influence of fructose and glucose on the production of exopolysaccharides and the activities of enzymes involved in the sugar metabolism and the synthesis of sugar nucleotides in *Lactobacillus delbrueckii* subsp. *bulgaricus* NCFB 2772, *Appl. Microbiol. Biotechnol.*, 46: 279–284, 1996.

74. Prasher, R., Malik, R.K., and Mathur, D.K., Utilization of whey for the production of extracellular polysaccharide by a selected strain of *Lactococcus lactis*, *Microbiol. Alim. Nutr.*, 15: 79–88, 1997.

75. Hujanen, M. and Linko, Y.Y., Effect of temperature and various nitrogen sources on L-lactic acid production by *Lactobacillus casei*, *Appl. Microbiol. Biotechnol.*, 45: 307–313, 1996.

76. Gu, R.X., Liu, A.P., and Luo, C.X., A suitable culture medium for the production of exopolysaccharide by *Streptococcus salivarius* subsp. *thermophilus*, *J. Northeast Agri. Univ. English Ed.*, 7: 43–49, 2000.

77. Leroy, F., Degeest, B., and De Vuyst, L., A novel area of predictive modelling: describing the functionality of beneficial microorganisms in foods, *Int. J. Food Microbiol.*, 73: 251–259, 2002.

78. Grobben, G.J., Chin-Joe, I., Kitzen, V.A., Boels, I.C., Sikkema, J., Smith, M.R., and de Bont, J.A.M., Enhancement of exopolysaccharide production by *Lactobacillus delbrueckii* subsp. *bulgaricus* NCFB 2772 with a simplified defined medium, *App. Environ. Microbiol.*, 64: 1333–1337, 1998.

79. Grobben, G.J., Boels, I.C., Sikkema, J., Smith, M.R., and de Bont, J.A.M., Influence of ions on growth and production of exopolysaccharides by *Lactobacillus delbrueckii* subsp. *bulgaricus* NCFB 2772, *J. Dairy Res.*, 67: 131–135, 2000.

80. Macedo, M.G., Lacroix, C., Gardner, N.J., and Champagne, C.P., Effect of medium supplementation on exopolysaccharide production by *Lactobacillus rhamnosus* RW-9595M in whey permeate, *Int. Dairy J.*, 12: 419–426, 2002.

81. Mozzi, F., Savoy de Giori, G., Oliver, G., and Font de Valdez, G., Exopolysaccharide production by *Lactobacillus casei*. I. Influence of salts, *Milchwissenschaft*, 50: 186–188, 1995.

82. Mozzi, F., Savoy de Giori, G., Oliver, G., and Font de Valdez, G., Exopolysaccharide production by *Lactobacillus casei*. II. Influence of the carbon source, *Milchwissenschaft*, 50: 307–309, 1995.

83. Zisu, B. and Shah, N.P., Effects of pH, temperature, supplementation with whey protein concentrate, and adjunct cultures on the production of exopolysaccharides by *Streptococcus thermophilus* 1275, *J. Dairy Sci.*, 86: 3405–3415, 2003.

84. Frengova, G.I., Simova, E.D., Beshkova, D.M., and Simov, Z.I., Production and monomer composition of exopolysaccharides by yogurt starter cultures, *Can. J. Microbiol.*, 46: 1123–1127, 2000.

85. Cheirsilp, B., Shoji, H., Shimizu, H., and Shioya, S., Interactions between *Lactobacillus kefiranofaciens* and *Saccharomyces cerevisiae* in mixed culture for kefiran production, *J. Biosci. Bioeng.*, 96: 279–284, 2003.

86. Ruas-Madiedo, P. and de los Reyes-Gavilán, C.G., Methods for screening, isolation, and characterization of exopolysaccharides produced by lactic acid bacteria, *J. Dairy Sci.*, 88: 843–856, 2005.

87. Simova, E.D., Frengova, G.I., and Beshkova, D.M., Exopolysaccharides produced by mixed culture of yeast Rhodotorula rubra GED10 and yogurt bacteria (*Streptococcus thermophilus* 13a+*Lactobacillus bulgaricus* 2-11), *J. Appl. Microbiol.*, 97: 512–519, 2004.

88. Tetsuguchi, M., Nomura, S., Katayama, M., and Sugawa-Katayama, Y., Effects of curdlan and gellan gum on the surface structures of intestinal mucosa in rats, *J. Nutr. Sci. Vitaminol.*, 43: 515–527, 1997.

89. Lemoine, J., Chirat, F., Wieruszeski, J.-M., Strecker, G., Favre, N., and Neeser, J.-R., Structure characterization of the exocellular polysaccharides produced by *Streptococcus thermophilus* SFi39 and SFi12, *Appl. Environ. Microbiol.*, 63: 3512–3518, 1997.

90. Born, K., Langerdorff, V., and Boulenguer, P., Xanthan, in *Biopolymers,* Vol. 5: *Polysaccharides I: Polysaccharides from Procaryotes*, Vandamme, E.J., De Baets, S., and Steinbüchel, A., Eds., Wiley-VCH, Weinheim, Germany, 2002.

91. van Casteren, W.H.M., Dijkema, C., Schols, H.A., Beldman, G., and Voragen, A.G.J., Characterisation and modification of the exopolysaccharide produced by *Lactococcus lactis* subsp. *cremoris* B40, *Carbohydr. Polym.*, 37: 123–130, 1998.

92. Nakajima, H., Hirota, T., Toba, T., Itoh, T., and Adachi, S., Structure of the extracellular polysaccharide from slime-forming *Lactococcus lactis* subsp. *cremoris* SBT 0495. *Carbohydr. Res.* 224: 245–253, 1992.

93. Yamamoto, Y., Murosaki, S., Yamauchi, R., Kato, K., and Sone, Y., Structural study on an exocellular polysaccharide produced by *Lactobacillus helveticus* TY1-2, *Carbohydr. Res.*, 261: 67–78, 1994.

94. Yamamoto, Y., Nunome, T., Yamauchi, R., Kato, K., and Sone, Y., Structure of an exocellular polysaccharide of *Lactobacillus helveticus* TN-4, a spontaneous mutant strain of *Lactobacillus helveticus* TY1-2, *Carbohydr. Res.*, 275: 319–332, 1995.

95. van Casteren, W.H.M., Dijkema, C., Schols, H.A., Beldman, G., and Voragen, A.G.J., Structural characterisation and enzymic modification of the exopolysaccharide produced by *Lactococcus lactis* subsp. *cremoris* B39, *Carbohydr. Res.*, 324: 170–181, 2000.

96. van Casteren, W.H.M., de Waard, P., Dijkema, C., Schols, H.A., and Voragen, A.G.J., Structural characterisation and enzymic modification of the exopolysaccharide produced by *Lactococcus lactis* subsp. *cremoris* B891, *Carbohydr. Res.*, 327: 411–422, 2000.

97. Maeda, M., Zhu, X., Suzuki, S., Suzuki, K., and Kitamura, S., Structural characterization and biological activities of an exopolysaccharide produced by *Lactobacillus kefiranofaciens* WT-2B., *J. Agric. Food Chem.*, 52: 5533–5538, 2004.

98. Van Calsteren, M.-R., Pau-Roblot, C., Bégin, A., and Roy, D., Structure determination of the exopolysaccharide produced by *Lactococcus rhamnosus* strains RW-9595M and R, *Biochem. J.*, 363: 7–17, 2002.

99. Vincent, S.J.F., Faber, E.J., Nesser, J.-R., Stingele, F., and Kamerling, J.P., Structure and properties of the exopolysaccharide produced by *Streptococcus macedonicus* Sc136, *Glycobiology*, 11: 131–139, 2001.

100. Eastwood, M.A., Brydon, W.G., and Anderson, D.M.W. A dietary study of xanthan gum in man, *Food Addit. Contam.*, 4: 17–26, 1987.

101. Anderson, D.M.W., Brydon, W.G., and Eastwood, M.A., The dietary effects of gellan gum in humans, *Food Addit. Contam.*, 5: 237–249, 1988.

102. Ikegami, S., Tsuchihashi, F., Harada, H., Tsuchihashi, N., Nishide, E., and Innami, S., Effect of viscous indigestible polysaccharides on pancreatic-biliary secretion and digestive organs in rats, *J. Nutr.*, 120: 353–360, 1990.

103. Ruijssenaars, H.J., Stingele, F., and Hartmans, S., Biodegradability of food-associated extracellular polysaccharides, *Curr. Microbiol.*, 40: 194–199, 2000.

104. Bugaut, M. and Bentéjac, M., Biological effects of short-chain fatty acids in nonruminant mammals, *Ann. Rev. Nutr.*, 13: 217–241, 1993.

105. Korakli, M., Ganzle, M.G., and Vogel, R.F., Metabolism by bifidobacteria and lactic acid bacteria of polysaccharides from wheat and rye, and exopolysaccharides produced by *Lactobacillus sanfranciscensis*, *J. Appl. Microbiol.*, 92: 958–965, 2002.

106. Shimizu, J., Wada, M., Takita, T., and Innami, S., Curdlan and gellan gum, bacterial gel-forming polysaccharides, exhibit different effects on lipid metabolism, cecal fermentation and fecal bile acid excretion in rats, *J. Nutr. Sci. Vitaminol.*, 45: 251–262, 1999.

107. Edwards, C.A. and Eastwood, M.A., Caecal and faecal short-chain fatty acids and stool output in rats fed on diets containing non-starch polysaccharides, *Br. J. Nutr.*, 73: 773–781, 1995.

108. Sreekumar, O. and Hosono, A., The antimutagenic properties of a polysaccharide produced by *Bifidobacterium longum* and its cultured milk against some heterocyclic amines, *Can. J. Microbiol.*, 44: 1029–1036, 1998.

109. Farnworth, E.R. and Mainville, I., Kefir: a fermented milk product. In *Handbook of Fermented Functional Foods,* Farnworth, E.R. Ed., CRC Press, Boca Raton, FL, 2003, 77–111.

110. Shiomi, M., Sasaki, K., Murofushi, M., and Aibara, K., Antitumor activity in mice of orally administered polysaccharide from kefir grains, *Jpn. J. Med. Sci. Biol.*, 35: 75–80, 1982.

111. Murofushi, M., Shiomi, M., and Aibara, K., Effect of orally administered polysaccharide from kefir grain on delayed-type hypersensitivity and tumor growth in mice, *Jpn. J. Med. Sci. Biol.*, 36: 49–53, 1983.

112. Murofushi, M., Mizuguchi, J., Aibara, K., and Matuhasi, T., Immunopotentiative effect of polysaccharide from kefir grain, KGF-C, administered orally in mice, *Immunopharmacol.*, 12: 29–35, 1986.

113. Oda, M., Hasegawa, H., Komatsu, S., Kambe, M., and Tsuchiya, F., Anti-tumor polysaccharide from *Lactobacillus* sp., *Agric. Biol. Chem.*, 1623–1625, 1983.

114. Furukawa, N., Takahashi, T., and Yamanaka, Y., Effects of supernatant of Peyer's patch cell culture with kefir grain components on the mitogenic response of thymocyte and splenocyte in mice, *Anim. Sci. Technol.*, 67: 153–159, 1996.

115. Furukawa, N., Matsuoka, A., Takahashi, T., and Yamanaka, Y., Anti-metastatic effect of kefir grain components on Lewis lung carcinoma and highly metastatic B16 melanoma in mice, *J. Agric. Sci. Tokyo Nogyo Daigaku,* 45: 62–70, 2000.

116. Kitazawa, N., Yamaguchi, T., and Itoh, T., B-cell mitogenic activity of slime products produced from slime-forming, encapsulated *Lactococcus lactis* spp. *cremoris, J. Dairy Sci.*, 75: 2946–2951, 1992.

117. Kitazawa, H., Yamaguchi, T., Miura, M., Saito, T., and Itoh, T., B-cell mitogen produced by slime-forming, encapsulated *Lactococcus lactis* ssp. *cremoris* isolated from ropy sour milk, viili, *J. Dairy Sci.*, 76: 1514–1519, 1993.

118. Kitazawa, H., Itoh, T., Tomioka, Y., Mizugaki, M., and Yamaguchi, T., Induction of IFN- and IL-1 production in macrophages stimulated with phosphopolysaccharide produced by *Lactococcus lactis* ssp. *cremoris, Int. J. Food Microbiol.*, 31: 99–106, 1996.

119. Forsén, R., Heiska, E., Herva, E., and Arvilommi, H., Immunobiological effects of *Streptococcus cremoris* from cultured milk "viili"; application of human lymphocyte culture techniques, *Int. J. Food Microbiol.*, 5: 41–47, 1987.

120. Nakajima, H., Toba, T., and Toyoda, S., Enhancement of antigen-specific antibody production by extracellular slime products from slime-forming *Lactococcus lactis* subspecies *cremoris* SBT 0495 in mice, *Int. J. Food Microbiol.*, 25: 153–158, 1995.

121. Chabot, S., Yu, H.-L., de Léséleuc, L., Cloutier, D., Van Calsteren, M.-R., Lessard, M., Roy, D., Lacroix, M., and Oth, D., Exopolysaccharides from *Lactobacillus rhamnosus* RW-9595M stimulate TNF, IL-6, and IL-12 in human and mouse cultured immunocompetent cells, and IFN-γ in mouse splenocytes, *Lait*, 81: 683–697, 2001.

122. Kitazawa, H., Ishii, Y., Uemura, J., Kawai, Y., Saito, T., Kaneko, T., Noda, K., and Itoh, T., Augmentation of macrophage fractions by an extracellular phosphopolysaccharide from *Lactobacillus delbrueckii* spp. *bulgaricus, Food Microbiol.*, 17: 109–118, 2000.

123. Nishimura-Uemura, J., Kitazawa, H., Jawai, Y., Itoh, T., Oda, M., and Saito, T., Functional alteration of murine macrophages stimulated with extracellular polysaccharides from *Lactobacillus delbrueckii* ssp. *bulgaricus* OLL1073R-1, *Food Microbiol.*, 20: 267–273, 2003.

124. Kitazawa, H., Harata, T., Uemura, J., Saito, T., Kaneko, T., and Itoh, T., Phosphate group requirement for mitogenic activation of lymphocytes by an extracellular phosphopolysaccharide from *Lactobacillus delbrueckii* ssp. *bulgaricus*, *Int. J. Food Microbiol.*, 40: 169–175, 1998.

125. Soh, H.-P., Kim, C-S., and Lee, S-P., A new in vitro assay of cholesterol adsorption by food and microbial polysaccharides, *J. Med. Food*, 6: 225–230, 2003.

126. Pigeon, R.M., Cuesta, E.P., and Gilliland, S.E., Binding of free bile acids by cells of yogurt starter culture bacteria, *J. Dairy Sci.*, 85: 2705–2710, 2002.

127. Nakajima, H., Suzuki, Y., Kaizu, H., and Hirota, T., Cholesterol lowering activity of ropy fermented milk, *J. Food Sci.*, 57: 1327–1329, 1992.

128. Levrat-Verny, M.-A., Behr, S., Mustad, V., Rémésy, C., and Demigné, C., Low levels of viscous hydrocolloids lower plasma cholesterol in rats primarily by impairing cholesterol absorption, *J. Nutr.*, 130: 243–248, 2000.

129. Yomamoto, Y., Sogawa, I., Nishina, A., Saeki, S., Ichikawa, N., and Iibata, S., Improved hypolipidemic effects of xanthan gum — galactomannan mixtures in rats, *Biosci. Biotechnol. Biochem.*, 64: 2165–2171, 2000.

130. Maeda, H., Zhu, X., Omura, K., Suzuki, S., and Kitamura, S., Effects of an exopolysaccharide (kefiran) on lipids, blood pressure, blood glucose and constipation, *BioFactors*, 22: 197–200, 2004.

131. Cameron-Smith, D., Collier, G.R., and O'Dea, K., Effect of soluble dietary fibre on the viscosity of gastrointestinal contents and the acute glycaemic response in the rat, *Br. J. Nutr.*, 71: 563–571, 1994.

132. Osilesi, O., Trout, D.L., Glover, E.E., Harper, S.M., Koh, E.T., Behall, K.M., O'Dorisio, T.M., and Tartt, J., Use of xanthan gum in dietary management of diabetes mellitus, *Am. J. Clin. Nutr.*, 42: 597–603, 1985.

133. Koguchi, T., Nakajima, H., Koguchi, H., Wada, M., Yamamoto, Y., Innami, S., Maekawa, A., and Tadokoro, T., Suppressive effects of viscous dietary fiber on elevations of uric acid in serum and urine induced by dietary RNA in rats is associated with strength of viscosity, *Int. J. Vitam. Nutr. Res.*, 73: 369–376, 2003.

134. Koguchi, T., Koguchi, H., Nakajima, H., Takano, S., Yamamoto, Y., Innami, S., Maekawa, A., and Tadokoro, T., Dietary fiber suppresses elevation of uric acid and urea nitrogen concentrations in serum of rats with renal dysfunction induced by dietary adenine, *Int. J. Vitam. Nutr. Res.*, 74: 253–263, 2004.

135. Singh, B.N., Trombetta, L.D., and Kim, K.H., Biodegradation behavior of gellan gum in simulated colonic media, *Pharm. Dev. Technol.*, 9: 399–407, 2004.

136. Sun, W. and Griffiths, M.W., Survival of bifidobacteria in yogurt and simulated gastric juice following immobilization in gellan-xanthan beads, *Int. J. Food Microbiol.*, 61: 17–25, 2000.

137. Nieuw Amerongen, A.V. and Veerman, E.C.I., Current therapies for xerostomia and salivary gland hypofunction associated with cancer therapies, *Support Care Cancer*, 11: 226–231, 2003.

19 Omega-3 Fatty Acids, Tryptophan, B Vitamins, SAMe, and Hypericum in the Adjunctive Treatment of Depression

Dianne H. Volker and Jade Ng

CONTENTS

I. INTRODUCTION

Clinical depression is a unipolar mood disorder characterized by a pervasive negative mood (persisting for greater than 14 consecutive days) accompanied by a generalized loss of interests, an inability to experience pleasure, and suicidal tendencies. It is costly in terms of human suffering and health service use, and has severe implications for physical health.[1] Until recently, many individuals had limited knowledge and inaccurate beliefs about mental health problems, and people who suffer from depression were all too often stigmatized and ostracized from society.[1] Fortunately, this situation is now gradually changing as government and public health initiatives help to increase community awareness and understanding of depression, with the successful implementation of "Beyond Blue" and the "Black Dog" programs, to name a few.[2,3] The causes of depression can be biological, (including genetic and biochemical causes), and psychosocial, which involves upbringing, emotional experiences, and cultural and environmental influences, as well as interpersonal behaviors and interactions.[4]

Depression is a treatable condition, with early intervention and treatment underpinning an optimistic prognosis. William Styron observed, in the account of his own depressive episode, that "acute depression inflicts few permanent wounds."[5] The overriding concern in very severe cases is to ensure the safety of the depressed person, both from deliberate self-injury and inappropriate risk-taking behavior. Once stabilized, the main goal of management is to reverse the lowered mood, using a combination of nonpharmacological and pharmacological treatments.[4]

Psychotherapy includes such techniques as cognitive behavior therapy (CBT) and interpersonal therapy, where a person's negative thoughts, attitudes and beliefs are challenged and positively refocused.[6] Medication may prove necessary where psychotherapy alone does not elicit satisfactory results.[6] Electroconvulsive therapy (ECT), a treatment for severe refractory depression that is used only after psychotherapy and pharmacotherapy have failed over some time period, may prove necessary in the more severe forms of depression.[6]

Antidepressant drugs fall into these main groups — the tricyclic antidepressants (TCAs), monoamine oxidase inhibitors (MAOIs) and selective serotonin reuptake inhibitors (SSRIs) and serotonin and norepinephrine reuptake inhibitors (SNRIs).[7] Many studies have confirmed that these drugs are effective; however, long-term use gives rise to a number of common and unpleasant side effects, such as weight gain, gastrointestinal disturbances (xerostoma, indigestion, gastric ulceration, and constipation), blurred vision, drowsiness and dizziness.[7] An additional requirement when taking MAOIs is strict dietary restriction of foods containing high levels of tyramine. The list of tyramine-containing foods is extensive and includes many common foods, such as bananas, avocado, soy products, cheese, coffee and tea.[7,8]

Although newer antidepressant drugs such as the SSRIs and SNRIs (with fewer side effects in the short to medium term) have been developed to reduce adverse effects, there is still considerable interest, in the medical arena, to search for safe and effective alternatives.[8] This is reflected in the great deal of current research investigating the links between dietary components and the development and treatment of depression. One of the most active areas of research concerns the relationship between the omega-3 long-chain polyunsaturated fatty acids and depression and the use of omega-3 fatty acid supplements in the treatment of depression.[9,10] Other nutrients and "natural" substances identified as having potential implications in the treatment of depression are folate, tryptophan, vitamin B_6, B_{12}, S-adenosyl-L-methionine, and *Hypericum perforatum*.[11]

II. PREVALENCE

Depression is one of the most common mental health problems in the general population. The World Health Organization (WHO) estimates that major depressive disorders will become the second leading cause of disability worldwide by the year 2020, after ischemic heart disease.[12] In the report titled *The Global Burden of Disease*, Murray and Lopez comprehensively assessed the mortality and disability from all diseases, injuries and risk factors using inclusive methodological approaches.[12] The summary of this landmark study highlighted the finding that "the burden of mental illnesses, such as mood disorders, alcohol and drug dependence and schizophrenia have previously been seriously underestimated by approaches that focus on mortality, rather than morbidity and mortality."

In Australia, depression is currently the leading cause of nonfatal disability, with analysis of statistics showing that one in five Australians will develop depression at some stage in their lives. Thus, the lifetime prevalence rate is generally taken to be in the order of 10–20%.[13] However, it is necessary to note that the findings of individual studies vary considerably depending on the diagnostic tools implemented and the criteria used to define clinical depression. For example, the 2003 Australian National Survey of Mental Health and Wellbeing[14] found the current prevalence rate of depression to be 3.2%. The prevalence rate of depression for both genders, as compared to other mental health disorders in Australia, is given in Table 19.1.

TABLE 19.1
Prevalence Rates of Mental Health Disorders in Australian Adults

	Males		Females	
	%	Population Estimate	%	Population Estimate
Any depressive disorder	4.2	275,300	7.4	503,300
Any anxiety disorder	7.1	470,400	12.0	829,600
Any substance use disorder	11.1	734,300	4.5	307,500
Any mental health disorder	17.4	1,151,600	18.0	1,231,500

Source: Adapted from Weissman, M., Bland, R., Joyce, P., Newman, S., Wells, J., and Wittchen, H., Sex differences in rates of depression: cross-national perspectives, *J. Affect. Disord.* 29: 77–84, 1993.

Sequelae associated with depression include significant physical and social impairment, severe reduction in quality of life, exacerbation of coexisting illness, deliberate self-harm or suicide, premature death and overuse of health services, which all cost an estimated A\$600 million per annum.[15] Depression represents a significant disease burden in Australia, causing an average of 3.7 "healthy" life years loss to the disability.[15] The most recent Australian Burden of Disease study calculated the burden of mental disorders in Australia at 15% of the total, third in importance after heart disease and cancer, a proportion that further supports the public health importance of mental disorders.[15] Table 19.2 shows the leading causes of disease burden in Australia in 1996. According to the Australian Health Insurance Commission, 10.1 million prescriptions were written for anti-depressant medication in 2003, with the Selective Serotonin Reuptake Inhibitors (SSRIs), such as fluoxetine (Prozac) and sertraline (Zoloft), accounting for greater than half of those prescribed.[16]

TABLE 19.2
The 10 Leading Causes of Disease Burden in Australia in 1996

Disease	Disability-Adjusted Life Years[a]
Ischemic heart disease	12.4
Cerebral vascular accidents (strokes)	5.4
Chronic obstructive pulmonary disease (COPD)	3.7
Depression	3.7
Lung cancer	3.6
Dementia	3.5
Diabetes mellitus	3.0
Colorectal cancer	2.7
Asthma	2.6
Osteoarthritis	2.2

[a] Disability-adjusted life year is a measure of the years of "healthy" life lost due to premature death, illness, or injury.

Source: Adapted from Andrews, G., Sanderson, K., Slade, T., and Issakidis, C., Why does the burden of disease persist? Relating the burden of anxiety and depression to the effectiveness of treatment. *Bulletin of the World Health Organization*, 78: 446–454, 2000.

III. PATHOGENESIS

Mental illness is a multifactorial disease that can develop for many reasons. The contributing factors can be as wide ranging as organic changes in the brain, environmental influences or genetic influences.[4] Organic changes in the brain can be the result of alcohol abuse, drug induced brain damage, or altered production of neurotransmitters. Environmental influences affecting mental health can include the effects of stress, social isolation, or major life events such as divorce, bereavement or redundancy. Genetically, some individuals may be predisposed to some types of mental illness. Depression is classified as a mood disorder of dysphoric nature, characterized by hopelessness, sadness, and misery.[4]

IV. CLINICAL FEATURES

The signs of depression fall into four main groups: mood disturbances, such as overwhelming sadness or guilt; behavioral changes, such as loss of interests; altered cognition and thought processes, such as a marked lack of concentration; and physical symptoms, such as weight loss and sleep disturbances.[17] These symptoms may manifest themselves differently, depending on developmental age. For example, depressed children may regress to an earlier stage of psychological functioning (e.g., a 5-year-old reverting to thumb-sucking and baby-talk), and depressed adolescents may exhibit oppositional and conduct disorders, including aggression, compulsive lying, high-risk sexual behaviors, and truancy. Depressed middle-aged and elderly people, in contrast, are more likely to experience the physical symptoms, such as constipation and fatigue.[17]

From a nutritional point of view, depression is usually accompanied by acute anorexia. There is a loss of interest in food and the pleasure of eating, as vividly described by the American novelist William Styron in his book *Darkness Visible*, which gives an insight into his personal descent into depression — "I found myself eating only for subsistence: food, like everything else within the scope of sensation, was utterly without savour."[5] Consequently, a serious feature is weight loss greater than 5% of total body weight or 3–4 kg over the past month.[17]

V. DIAGNOSIS

A number of structured interview formats incorporating specific investigative techniques and questions have been developed to aid in the assessment of depressed people, including the Structured Clinical Interview for DSM, the Structured Clinical Assessment for Neuropsychiatry, the Composite International Diagnostic Interview and the Diagnostic Interview Schedule.[18] The severity of depression is assessed using rating scales designed for this purpose. Rating scales also serve as a tool for tracking the progress of treatment as they can be applied, with good repeatability, over the course of one or more therapies. Three of the most commonly used scales in current clinical practice are the Hamilton Depression Rating Scale, the Beck's Depression Inventory, and the Montgomery Asberg Depression Rating Scale.[18]

There is no clear division between ordinary sadness, grief, and clinical depression. Furthermore, no single diagnostic test can adequately diagnose depression and the nature of depression as a syndrome means that diagnosis is based on a group of symptoms and observable physical and mental signs that commonly occur in conjunction.[18] The only broadly identifiable distinction between generalized sadness, which is consolable and self-limiting, and depression is the prolonged period of time for which a lowered mood persists, and the incapacitating or disabling extent of the condition to the point where there is an inability to cope with the demands of everyday living.[18] The criteria for diagnosing clinical depression, according to the Fourth Edition of the Diagnostic and Statistical Manual of Mental Disorders (DSM-IV) is given in Table 19.3.[19]

TABLE 19.3
Criteria for a Major Depressive Episode (DSM-IV)

Five (5) of the Most Common Symptoms of Depression

- Depressed mood (or irritable mood in children or adolescents) most of the day, nearly every day, as indicated by either subjective report (e.g., feels sad or empty) or observation made by others (e.g., appears tearful)
- Markedly diminished interest or pleasure in all, or almost all, activities most of the day, nearly every day (as indicated by either subjective account or observation made by others)
- Significant weight loss when not dieting or weight gain (e.g., a change of more than 5% of body weight in a month), or decrease or increase in appetite nearly every day
- Feelings of worthlessness or excessive or inappropriate guilt (which may be delusional) nearly every day (not merely self-reproach or guilt about being sick)
- Recurrent thoughts about death (not just fear of dying), recurrent suicidal ideation without a specific plan, or a suicide attempt or a specific plan for committing suicide

Source: Adapted from Taskforce on DSM IV, *Diagnostic and Statistical Manual of Mental Disorders,* 4th ed., American Psychiatric Association, Washington, D.C., 2000. Copyright American Psychiatric Association 2000.

VI. RISK FACTORS

The accumulated evidence regarding the etiology of clinical depression suggests that it is a complex disorder. Reference is often made to the biopsychosocial model as an attempt to account for the interaction of biological, psychological and social factors involved in determining the liability to lifetime clinical depression. Biological factors arise from the physiology and biochemistry of body systems and function, as well as from genetic influences; psychological factors are derived from upbringing, emotional experiences and interpersonal interactions; and social factors result from a person's cultural environment and current life situation.[4,17]

A. GENDER AND BIOLOGICAL FACTORS

Knowledge of neurotransmitter function provides an understanding of the biology of depression.[20] Neurotransmitters are chemicals that are used to relay, amplify, and modulate electrical signals between neurons and other cells. They are broadly classified into small molecule transmitters or neuroactive peptides. The neurotransmitters implicated in depression and related conditions are the small molecule transmitters: dopamine, norepinephrine, epinephrine and serotonin.[20] Within cells, these transmitter molecules are usually packaged in vesicles, so that when an action potential travels to a synapse, the rapid depolarization causes calcium channels to open. Calcium then stimulates the transport of vesicles to the synaptic membrane, which then fuse, releasing the neurotransmitter. The receptor involved then determines the effect of the neurotransmitter. Imbalances of these neurotransmitters, dopamine, norepinephrine, epinephrine, and serotonin, are associated with mental illness.[21]

Dopamine, norepinephrine, and epinephrine are derived from the hydroxylation and decarboxylation of the amino acids tyrosine and phenylalanine in a common pathway consisting of several steps.[20] These neurotransmitters are then metabolized to biologically inactive products through oxidation by monoamine oxidase (MAO) and methylation by catechol-O-methyltransferase (COMT). Serotonin, 5-hydroxy tryptamine (5-HT) is released specifically by cells in the brain stem and formed by the hydroxylation and decarboxylation of tryptophan. Normally, the hydrolase is not saturated, thus an increased uptake of tryptophan in the diet can increase brain serotonin content.[21] Virtually all of the brain tryptophan is converted to serotonin. The serotonin concentration in the brain is far more sensitive to the effects of diet than any other monoamine neurotransmitter, and can be increased up to 10-fold by supplementation in laboratory animals.[22] These neurotransmitters are removed from the synaptic cleft by a reuptake mechanism that prevents the continued stimulation or inhibition of the post-synaptic neuron. Released serotonin is inactivated by MAO to form 5-hydroxyindoleacetic acid (5-HIAA).[22]

Neurotransmitters have specific actions and are often targeted by prescription drugs such as antidepressants, as well as recreational drugs. Norepinephrine is a 'feel good' neurotransmitter, its release is enhanced by amphetamines, and removal from synapse is blocked by tricyclic antidepressants and cocaine.[22] Dopamine is also a 'feel good' neurotransmitter; its release is enhanced by L-dopa and amphetamines, and reuptake is blocked by cocaine. It is deficient in Parkinson's disease and it is thought to be involved in the pathogenesis of schizophrenia. Serotonin is an inhibitory transmitter that plays a role in sleep, appetite, nausea, migraine headaches, and regulation of mood. Drugs that block its uptake (Prozac) relieve anxiety and depression. LSD also blocks serotonin activity.[22]

Antidepressants are drugs that relieve the symptoms of depression. There are three main types; tricyclics (TCAs), monoamine oxidase inhibitors (MAOIs) and reuptake inhibitors, such as selective serotonin reuptake inhibitors (SSRIs), and serotonin and norepinephrine reuptake inhibitors (SNRIs). Tricyclic antidepressants derive their name from their three ring structure. The therapeutic effects of antidepressants are believed to be related to an effect on neurotransmitters by inhibiting the monoamine transporter proteins of serotonin and norepinephrine.[22] SSRIs specifically prevent the reuptake of serotonin, which increases the level of serotonin in synapses of the brain, while SNRIs slow down the reuptake of both serotonin and norepinephrine. MAOIs block the destruction of neurotransmitters by enzymes that normally metabolize them to an inactive form. TCAs prevent the reuptake of serotonin, norepinephrine, and dopamine. The current mechanistic theory of action is that the long term effect on modification of the neurotransmitter on receptors produces the antidepressant effect, not the short term effect of a few days.[22,23]

There appears to be a strong genetic predisposition associated with the development of depression, as consistently shown in genetic epidemiological studies.[24] Thus, a positive family history is a powerful biological risk factor for depression. Five family studies of clinical depression have demonstrated its familial nature.[18] A recent meta-analysis of these studies calculated the odds ratio for this relationship to be 2.84 (95% CI, 2.31–3.49). Six twin studies have shown that genetic factors are highly significant in the development of depression, more so than individual-specific and shared environmental influences, such as general parenting style and background sociodemographic levels.[18,25] Subsequently, the concordance rate is observed to be higher in identical twins than nonidentical twins.[25]

Women are more vulnerable to mental illness at any age, with anxiety and depressive disorders predominating, although the male–female ratios change over lifespan.[26] The female brain synthesizes about 2/3 as much serotonin as the male brain.[26] Men, in contrast, are more likely to suffer from antisocial personality disorder and drug and alcohol abuse.[26] There are also gender differences in rates and expression of depression. Being female is a strong risk factor for depression, with women having twice the risk of men at any given age.[13] Women between the ages of 18–34 appear to be particularly at risk, with depression reaching a peak in young mothers. Family studies have discounted an X-chromosome linked genetic transmission of depression.[27] Research into female vulnerability show the contributing effects of marital status, work and social roles, such as lack of a confidant, the presence of young children, lower socioeconomic status and not working outside the home.[27]

Women experience their highest risk of having a depressive episode during pregnancy and following childbirth. Up to 70% of new mothers notice a transient change in their mood, usually describing themselves as being more anxious, tearful, irritable and emotional than normal, in the days following childbirth.[28] This is sometimes referred to as the "postnatal or baby blues," and this condition commonly resolves within a few days, when mothers are given appropriate support and reassurance from partners, family, and friends. Given its widespread nature, "postnatal blues" is often regarded as a normal psychological reaction to the accumulated stress associated with pregnancy and labor. This is in stark contrast to antenatal and postnatal depression, both of which require medical assessment, identification, and possible treatment. Research suggests that the incidence and prevalence of antenatal depression are similar or equivalent to those of the postnatal period, with the rate of antenatal depression showing an increase in the past decade.[29]

Two possible explanations to account for this increase have been proposed. Firstly, there is a tendency across all cultures to idealize pregnancy and as a result, the positive aspects of pregnancy are often overestimated.[3] If and when the reality differs from expectations, a sense of disillusionment is felt, which may be one contributing factor to the development of antenatal depression.[3] The second explanation concerns the rising age of first pregnancies in women in Western societies and the seemingly ambivalent approach of the "modern" women towards family planning and child-bearing, possibly driven in part by various competing career and social demands.[29] The clinical significance of antenatal depression lies in its potential to adversely affect the psychological preparation process of both mother and father-to-be in their adjustment to accommodate a new baby into their lives. Thus, individual biology and genetic inheritance are both important factors to be considered in the development of antenatal depression.[29]

Postnatal depression affects between 10–15% of women in the first 6 months following childbirth.[30] Because of its association with childbirth, it has been questioned as to whether postnatal depression is caused by hormonal changes. However, no definite link has been demonstrated with fluctuations in estrogen or progesterone levels,[31] thus the etiology of postnatal depression may have a psychosocial element as well. With regard to demographics, socially disadvantaged teenage mothers with poor social and emotional support networks appear to be at the highest risk of developing postnatal depression. Adverse childhood experiences, such as sexual abuse and/or maternal deprivation, may add to the risk. Individual personality style also has an influence, in particular anxious, neurotic and overly sensitive traits.[31] Women with previous histories of anxiety or depression are at higher risk, as are those who experienced antenatal depression.[3] Traumatic obstetric difficulties during labor and delivery, such as high-forceps delivery or emergency caesarean section, may lead to post-traumatic stress disorder, which may either resolve or evolve into postnatal depression.[3]

B. PSYCHOLOGICAL FACTORS

A person's style of thought and the way in which they interpret and react to life experiences may either protect or predispose them to mood disorders. Though clinical depression is now definitively refuted as being a "character weakness," people with certain personality traits remain more vulnerable to developing depression.[17] Two personality disturbances, which have been implicated as psychological risk factors for depression, are dependent and obsessional.[17] People with dependent personalities submit to others and appear incapable of making decisions without considerable advice and approval.[17] They transfer responsibility to others and are unable to work and live independently.[17] Consequently, they often feel anxious and frightened when alone. This fear of being abandoned, coupled with a general lack of self-esteem, may explain the higher prevalence of depression in this group.[17]

People with obsessive personalities exhibit an inflexible perfectionism, which interferes with their ability to complete everyday tasks. There is a preoccupation with rules, procedure, and order, which results in great inefficiency and a loss of pleasure in accomplishment.[6] Obsessive people often appear emotionally cold and judgmental and their need for control leads to long-term interpersonal difficulties. In addition, their required ideal standards are such that rarely do their own achievements measure up, creating much self-criticism and a gradual loss of self-confidence.[6] This type of behavior has obvious implications for the development of depression. Therefore, psychological functioning, including the complex issues of individual personality, temperament, problem-solving skills, values, and personal resilience, are etiologically significant in clinical depression.

Of particular relevance are the associations between the obsessive behaviors displayed in eating disorders and depression, as well as the link between the development of obesity and depression.[32]

The association between depressive and eating disorders has been investigated in recent years following the observation that there appeared to be a high frequency of co-occurrence, whether it is prior to, simultaneously or subsequent to development of the disorder.[33] Prevalence of depression is higher in clinical samples because of referral and other biases (e.g., Berkson's bias — people suffering from more than one disorder are more likely to present for treatment), but even community-dwelling people with eating disorders, as identified in epidemiological surveys, have elevated rates of mood disorder compared with normal controls. Current rates for comorbid depression in specific subtypes of eating disorders, including about 60% of people suffering from anorexia nervosa, have been found to experience depressive episodes, with this figure increasing up to 90% for individuals with bulimia nervosa.[34] The clinical significance of this comorbidity lies in the fact that deliberate self-harm and suicide risk may be elevated for people with concurrent eating disorders and depression. A meta-analysis of long-term outcome studies into anorexia nervosa estimated that up to half of the 5.6% mortality per decade of followup was due to suicide in anorexia nervosa and depression.[35]

The cause-and-effect relationship between eating disorders and depression is unclear. Starvation studies carried out during the Second World War provide evidence that food restriction in itself can lead to a lowering of mood.[36] Thus, there are a number of proposed theories that eating disorders may be merely an atypical presentation of an underlying depressive disorder, or that depression is a secondary mood disorder resulting from the physiological effects of food restriction and an extremely suboptimal body-weight for height.[36]

The observation that people of all ages and cultures turn to food as a source of comfort at times of emotional distress has led to the postulation of a link between depression and the development of obesity. Even though it is recognized that to an extent, this reaction is normal and may indeed be a psychological technique used to adjust to or overcome the stressor, the long-term effectiveness of employing food as a coping strategy is questioned.[37] Obesity, like depression, is the end result of interplay of many biological, psychological, and social factors. Whether overeating associated with low mood leads to obesity is controversial; however, it may certainly be a contributing factor. In terms of co-occurrence, studies have found that the prevalence of depression in obese people is two to three times higher than in the general population.[37]

C. SOCIAL FACTORS

Clinical depression is usually preceded by a greater frequency of demanding life events. Acute adverse changes in environmental and social circumstances appear to have an effect on the onset, maintenance, and relapse of depression. Grief resulting from the experience of loss, whether that is of a loved one, a job, a diminution of social status, or deterioration in health, is closely related to depression. In some cases, depression may be seen as a form of inappropriate and abnormal grief. The difference, however, lies in the observation that grief is a normal response to loss and as such is self-limiting and consolable in nature, but untreated depression persists and is unlikely to resolve independently.[17]

Chronic stressors, including long-term unemployment, marital/familial dysfunction, and caring for an ailing relative, may also precipitate or maintain a depressive episode. With regard to upbringing and childhood events, the experience of intrafamilial sexual abuse, extended parental separations, and a poorer perceived parental relationship appear to increase the risk of depression. Psychoanalytical theory advocates that as early life experiences are vital in the formation of personality, childhood psychological difficulties are closely associated with emotional disorders in later life. For example, disruptions in an infant's relationship with its mother or other primary caregiver and the prolonged or recurrent absence of a mother figure during childhood may lead to a greater vulnerability to depression in adolescence and adulthood.[18]

TABLE 19.4
Common Side Effects of Antidepressant Medication

Gastrointestinal	Cardiovascular	CNS[a]	Sexual	Anticholinergic[b]
Anorexia	Prolonged bleeding	Headache	Loss of libido	Dry mouth
Nausea and vomiting	time	Agitation, restlessness,	Impotence/erectile	Blurred vision
Weight loss or gain	Orthostatic	anxiety	difficulties	Urinary retention
Diarrhea/constipation	hypotension	Insomnia/somnolence	Ejaculatory	Delirium/dizziness
	Tachycardia	Tremor, sweating	failure/premature	
	Slowed cardiac	Muscle weakness	ejaculation	
	conduction	Fatigue	Anorgasmia	

[a] Central nervous system.

[b] Relevant to TCAs.

Source: Adapted from Bloch, S. and Singh, B., *Foundations of Clinical Psychiatry*, Melbourne University Press, Melbourne, 2000.

VII. MANAGEMENT

A. PHARMACOLOGICAL REGIMES

Many patients with depression are successfully and effectively treated with antidepressant medication. These drugs fall into three main groups: the tricyclic antidepressants (TCAs), monoamine oxidase inhibitors (MAOIs), and selective serotonin and norepinephrine reuptake inhibitors (SSRIs and SNRIs).[22] Of particular importance to this review is the mode of action of such antidepressant medications, from which stems the potential for nutritional manipulation as an adjunct to conventional drug treatment and psychotherapy. Research investigating the links between dietary components and depression explore the multiple mechanisms through which nutrients can act in similar ways to antidepressant drugs.[11]

All antidepressants act by increasing the availability of the monoamine neurotransmitters — serotonin, norepinephrine, or dopamine — at the synaptic junction. The monoamine reuptake pump terminates the action of these released neurotransmitters once the electrical impulse has been transmitted. SSRIs and SNRIs selectively and relatively powerfully block presynaptic serotonin or norepinephrine reuptake, while TCAs block the general reuptake of monoamines more weakly. MAOIs inhibit the monoamine oxidase enzyme that metabolizes the monoamine neurotransmitters, allowing for longer-lasting action of each released neurotransmitter. Antidepressant medications have a number of side effects, as shown in Table 19.4.[17] Short term use leads to an increase in neuronal firing, while longer term use leads to the down regulation of neuronal firing; for example, the use of an SSRI for 4–6 weeks is associated with the down regulation of serotonergic transmission.[22] Patients prescribed MAOIs are given strict dietary restrictions on foods, beverages and other medications containing the naturally occurring amino acid, tyramine, to reduce the risk of hypertensive crises.[4] The symptoms characteristic of this rapid rise in blood pressure are severe headache, chest pain, palpitations, neck stiffness and possible intracranial hemorrhage and death. A list of restricted foods is given in Table 19.5.[4]

B. ADJUNCTIVE NUTRITIONAL REGIMES

There has been an association between depression and nutrition since the first emergence of the study of mood disorders. In the late 19th century, Krafft-Ebing exerted great influence on the thinking about depression (then known as melancholia) with his famous work *Textbook of Psychiatry* (1879), in which the illness is described as being due to "an abnormal condition of the psychic

TABLE 19.5
Foods and Beverages Prohibited when Taking MAOIs

Foods and Beverages with a High Tyramine Content

Banana, banana-flavored desserts, banana chips

Broad bean pods

Sauerkraut

Matured and aged cheeses

Aged meat or liver products (e.g., pate, foie gras), dry sausage (e.g. salami),
  smoked or pickled fish

Soy and soy products (e.g., miso, tofu)

Yeast-based spreads (e.g., Vegemite, Marmite, Promite)

Protein shakes, red wine, beer

Source: Adapted from Garrow, J. and James, W., *Human Nutrition and Die-tetics*, 9th ed., Churchill Livingstone, London, 1993.

organ dependent upon a disturbance of nutrition."[38] This association has persisted over the centuries and is now reflected in the great deal of research investigating the links between dietary components and the development and treatment of depression. The majority of the research explores the biological changes seen in depression and the potential for nutrients to exert beneficial effects on modulating or correcting such biochemical imbalances. As the understanding of the neurobiology of depression expands, the theories relating nutrition to depression similarly increase.

There are multiple mechanisms by which nutrients can have an effect on the development, maintenance, and relapse of depression. Nutritional factors such as n-3 polyunsaturated fatty acids, n-6 to n-3 PUFA ratio, folate, tryptophan, vitamin B_6, B_{12}, S-adenosyl-L-methionine (SAMe), and *Hypericum perforatum* (St John's wort) and various cofactors in enzyme systems may influence depression by the modulation of neuronal membrane fluidity. This can cause changes in neuronal uptake and binding, action of nutrients as neurotransmitter substrates, or initiation of neurotrans-mitters in the brain and up-regulation of neurotransmitter receptors.[9,10, 23,40,41]

A review of epidemiological data suggests that there is a link between depression and fish consumption, and although it is true that correlation is not causation, there is evidence that fish and fish oils may be protective against depression. Hibbeln compared the rates of depression in nine countries to the estimated per capita fish consumption.[10] Results showed an inversely propor-tional relationship: Western countries had an annual prevalence of depression in the range of 3–6% and a low to moderate per capita fish intake of 11–32 kg, but countries with high per capita fish consumption, such as Japan at 68 kg, had a depression rate of only 0.12%. This data suggests an 84% correlation between high fish intake and low incidence of depression, and demonstrates that the risk of having depressive symptoms was significantly higher among infrequent fish-consumers, than in people who ate fish at least once per week (OR=1.31; 95 and CI, 1.10–1.56).[42] Conversely, a larger and more recent study of 29,133 Finnish men (50–69 years of age) failed to show any association between dietary intake of omega-3 fatty acids or fish consumption and lowered mood or major depressive episodes.[43]

The Inuit people of Greenland (commonly referred to as the Eskimos) are an ethnic group that has extremely high levels of fish consumption. The predominant fish species in such diets are the cold-water adapted marine animals, the fat of which is uniquely rich in the long-chain omega-3 fatty acids, eicosapentaenoic acid (EPA) and docosahexaenoic acid (DHA). In such societies, depression is virtually absent, despite the extreme climate and challenging environmental condi-tions.[44] In the book *Fats that Heal, Fats that Kill*, the author comments on the phenomenon that "the traditional Inuit did not get depressed and suicidal during winters of total darkness."[45] The results from such studies of epidemiological evidence support the observation that there exists a correlation between the levels of omega-3 fatty acids in different bodily tissues, that is the measurement of plasma phospholipids or erythrocyte membrane omega-3 content may be taken to represent omega-3 content of brain phospholipids and neuronal cell membranes.[46]

A 1995 review promotes the hypothesis that a deficiency in n-3 fatty acids is of etiological importance in the development of depression.[10] Epidemiological data show the trend in decreasing dietary n-3 fatty acids consumption and the increasing incidence of depression, both over time and between nations.[10,42] Further investigation suggests that the significance may lie in the increase in n-6 to n-3 ratio, rather than simply low omega-3 intake alone, as these two fatty acids compete in binding to enzyme systems that produce chain elongation and further desaturation. A high n-6 diet therefore prevents the incorporation of n-3 fatty acids into cell membrane phospholipids,[46] which may lead to decreased membrane fluidity and impaired cell signaling. An imbalance between omega-6 and omega-3 fatty acids intake also has harmful effects on the cardiovascular system. The predisposition of vascular cells to lipid peroxidation[47] and the reduced endogenous production of apoprotein A-I, may mean lower HDL-cholesterol levels, less reverse cholesterol transport and consequently, a higher risk of atherosclerosis.[48] The proinflammatory effects of a diet excessively high in omega-6 fatty acids have been implicated in the development of a number of joint conditions, most notably arthritis.[49]

The change in omega-6 to omega-3 fatty acid ratio of dietary intake is highlighted when comparison is made between the Paleolithic diet and the current Western ways of eating. Anthropological information suggests that the intake of omega-6 and omega-3 fatty acids during the Paleolithic era was roughly equal, whereas the present omega-6 to omega-3 fatty acid ratio in Western countries has been estimated to be between 10 and 25 to 1.[10,50] This fatty acid imbalance has been due mainly to the increase in vegetable and seed oil use, and a decrease in fish or fish oil intake. Data from the 1995 National Nutrition Survey estimates suggest that the omega-6 to omega-3 fatty acid ratio is 15 to 1 in the Australian diet, which would preclude the incorporation of omega-3 fatty acids in membrane phospholipids.[51]

Direct evidence of a role for omega-3 fatty acids in depression is provided by a number of studies, which examined the fatty acid compositions of erythrocyte membranes, serum cholesteryl esters, and phospholipids. Two major studies in this area, carried out between 1996 and 1999, found that depression is associated with significantly decreased total omega-3 fatty acids, increased monounsaturated fatty acid proportions, and increased omega-6 to omega-3 fatty acid ratio; more specifically, arachidonic acid to eicosapentaenoic acid ratio, in cholesteryl esters and phospholipids.[52,53] A supporting study, carried out in 1998, also found a significant depletion in total omega-3 fatty acids, and in particular DHA, in the erythrocyte membranes of depressed patients.[54] In 1998, the strong correlation between a low dietary intake of omega-3, omega-3 content of erythrocyte membranes, and the severity of depression was further elucidated.[55] Analyses of the results of biochemical studies suggest that omega-3 fatty acids increase CSF 5-HIAA, with resulting improvements in depressive symptoms.[56] Depressed subjects have also been found to have low CSF concentrations of serotonin, 5-hydroxytryptamine (5-HT), or have impairments in serotonin metabolism.[23]

Membrane fluidity refers to the state of the fatty acid chains comprising the lipid bilayer microstructure of cell membranes.[57] In general, an optimal state exists where the physical properties of the cell membrane are most conducive to its biological function. In neuronal membranes, this relates to a variety of functions such as the secretion of neurotransmitters, effective neurotransmitter binding and intracellular signaling, production of secondary messengers, ion channel function, receptor function, enzyme activity, and gene expression. Omega-3 fatty acids are essential components of the lipid bilayer in such membranes and a deficiency may adversely affect the signaling pathways in neurons. There is a growing body of evidence which consistently suggests that membrane lipid abnormalities occur in depression. Omega-3 fatty acids, in particular DHA, are depleted in depressed subjects.[52–55,57,58]

An analysis of recent research findings linking physical and mental illness has highlighted the cause-and-effect relationship of cardiovascular disease (CVD) and depression. A meta-analysis of 83 studies showed that depression correlated highly significantly with coronary artery disease and myocardial infarction.[59] Depression was the strongest psychological predictor of coronary heart disease (CHD). In addition, patients with lowered mood have a worse prognosis following a cardiac event.[60] Although there is a growing body of literature on the role of fish and fish oil consumption in depression (most of which report of results from epidemiological and observational studies), clinical experimental data in this area remains scarce. To date, there have been only a small number of well-designed and executed trials conducted in this area. An evaluation of the omega-3 fatty acid DHA as an alternative to pharmacological treatment of major depression involving 35 depressed subjects failed to show a significant effect of DHA monotherapy.[61] In another study, the ethyl ester of the omega-3 fatty acid EPA (E-EPA) was investigated. At a dose of 200 mg/d, and as an adjunct to usual antidepressant treatment, E-EPA reduced symptoms of depression, as measured by the 24-item Hamilton Depression Rating Scale.[62] However, whether the antidepressant effect of this specific omega-3 fatty acid can be translated to encompass the broader omega-3 family cannot be determined by this study. The dose–range response of EPA was investigated in a larger study involving 70 depressed subjects. Significant improvements in mood were observed in the intervention group receiving 100 mg of EPA, but not at higher doses.[63] The phenomenon of a "threshold" once optimal omega-3 fatty acid dose is reached is also seen in rheumatoid arthritis trials, where a higher dose of omega-3 fatty acids did not result in further improvements in end measures.[64] The final study used both EPA and DHA as an intervention, with results after the 8-week trial showing highly significant improvements in depressive symptoms.[65]

It is clear that the research area of diet and brain function is in a relatively early stage and as yet, there have been no therapeutic values defined for the optimum dose of omega-3 fatty acids for the alleviation of negative symptoms associated with depression.[66] Therefore, the safest and most sensible approach to take when considering omega-3 fatty acid supplementation may be to follow the recommendations set for optimum fatty acid intake for cardiovascular health. The American Heart Association,[67] the European Society for Cardiology,[68] the Scientific Advisory Committee on Nutrition (UK),[69] the National Health and Medical Council (NHMRC),[70] and The National Heart Foundation of Australia (NHF)[71] have all released recommendations for persons with or at risk of cardiovascular disease to increase their intake of omega-3 fatty acids.

According to a recent report released by an expert subcommittee of the International Society for the Study of Fatty Acids and Lipids (ISSFAL), an adequate linoleic acid (omega-6) intake is 2% of total energy, a healthy intake of ALA (omega-3) is 0.7% of total energy, and for cardiovascular health, a minimum intake of EPA and DHA combined is 500 mg per day.[72] The ideal omega-6 to omega-3 intake ratio is thus approximately 5 to 1. In more practical terms, the NHF recommends 2 meals of oily fish per week, not only for people with cardiovascular risk factors, but also for the general population.[73] However, it should be noted that recent studies suggest that the optimal omega-6 to omega-3 ratio may vary according to the disease and disease severity.[74] Until more extensive trials of omega-3 fatty acids and depression have been conducted, the above recommended intakes should be considered as the levels associated with a general healthy diet and/or potential supplementation.

The amino acid tryptophan is the precursor to the neurotransmitter serotonin. Many studies have demonstrated that the tryptophan availability to the brain influences the conversion to serotonin.[75] When tryptophan is administered as a supplement or is derived from a meal, it increases the amount of tryptophan available to serotonin neurons.[75] This availability can rapidly increase serotonin production to enhance serotonin release in neurons that are rapidly firing.[76] The effect of readily available tryptophan either through supplementation or meal manipulation can change sleep and mood patterns.[77,78] The effects are small compared with the effects of potent drugs that enhance serotonin function in the brain.[79] As with many dietary regimens, a dichotomous paradigm of nutritional therapy and pharmacotherapy as used in the treatment of diabetes and cardiovascular disease has much to recommend it.

Wurtman and colleagues suggests that high carbohydrate meals increase serotonin synthesis.[80] Consumption of a meal that is high in carbohydrate, branched chain amino acids, and tryptophan has a significant effect because both glucose from the carbohydrate and the branched chain amino acids (particularly leucine) increase insulin secretion.[80] Insulin facilitates the transport of branched chain amino acids into muscle cells, thereby reducing the competition for tryptophan by the large neutral amino acids for the tryptophan transporter protein to carry it across the blood–brain barrier. Drowsiness induced by increased serotonin is the common effect of a large carbohydrate meal.[80]

A number of other nutritional factors, mainly in relation to micronutrients, amino acids, and herbal remedies, have been proposed in the development, maintenance, and relapse of depression. The possibility of clinical and subclinical nutritional deficiencies in depressed patients has been raised following the suggestion that this group may have physiological requirements for certain nutrients above and beyond the recommended dietary intake (RDI). Several studies have found that there is an increased incidence of folate deficiency in psychiatric patients, especially in those with severe depression,[40] with up to one third having suboptimal folate status.[81] Whether this widespread deficiency is a result of chronic low folate intake or a compromised folate metabolism is unclear. However, one of the most common clinical features of depression is a diminished interest in food.[5] This, accompanied with a generalized lassitude and a withdrawal from social interactions, may lead to poor dietary intake and impaired nutritional status.[3] Morris and coworkers recommend that a folate supplement may be important during the year following a depressive episode.[82]

Despite an increasing body of research, the associations between B_{12}, B_6, folate, and SAMe and treatment outcomes in depressive disorders are still unsolved and much of this body of research has produced conflicting results.[83] Low concentrations of folate and B_{12} may impair methylation reactions and both nutrients are necessary for methionine synthesis and the subsequent formation of SAMe, the universal methyl donor, important in the formation of neurotransmitters and phospholipids.[83] Culturally defined dietary habits may influence the relationship between folate status and depression in different societies: a low folate level was not detected in Chinese patients or Latino men, but was found in Latino women.[84,85] Tolmunen and colleagues reported that low dietary folate and depressive symptoms are associated in middle-age Finnish men.[86] The association between folate and depression may be more prominent in elderly subjects, among whom folate deficiency has been relatively common in some studies.[87] Hintikka and colleagues demonstrated that higher B_{12} levels are significantly associated with better outcomes in young and middle aged subjects, but further studies were warranted.[88]

Because the metabolite of vitamin B_6, pyridoxal 5′-phosphate (PLP), is a coenzyme in the tryptophan–serotonin pathway, a lack of B_6 might theoretically cause depression, despite being readily available in a balanced diet[89,90] Penninx and coworkers found that individuals with a B_{12} deficiency had a 2-fold risk of severe depression.[91] Bottiglieri and colleagues reported that depressed patients had increased plasma homocysteine.[92] Low folate status was found in depressed individuals in the general population of the United States[82] and the response to antidepressants was poorer in patients with a low folate status.[93] Hvas and colleagues, in a study of an elderly population, suggest that B_6 plays a role in developing symptoms of depression with a significant association between the B_6 derivative PLP and symptoms of depression.[94] The mechanism of antidepressant effect involved in B_{12}, B_6, folate, and SAMe may well be mediated through homocysteine and/or the synthesis of monoamines in the brain.[86] The higher rates of depressive disorders in subjects with low folate and high homocysteine levels are due to differences in cardiovascular factors and physical comorbidity.[95] Serum folate is more sensitive to nutritional intake than vitamin B_{12} and folate deficiency can be a consequence of loss of appetite.[95]

The antidepressant mechanism of SAMe has not been elucidated; however it is known that SAMe exerts a stimulatory effect on monoamine metabolism and turnover.[96,97] SAMe treatment increases the concentration of 5-HIAA.[98] Two mechanisms have been proposed; the stimulatory effect on monoamine transmitters or alternatively increased or restored membrane phospholipids methylation.[83] SAMe, through its activity as a methyl donor, has the ability to increase the fluidity of cell membranes by stimulating phospholipids methylation.[99] The effect of SAMe on receptor systems is interesting because the evidence suggests that age related changes in the membrane environment may result in increased membrane viscosity and thus membrane dysfunction.[100]

St. John's wort is an herbal extract derived from the plant *Hypericum perforatum*. It has been extensively studied in Europe, particularly in Germany, where it is as commonly recommended in the treatment of depression as Prozac (fluoxetine) is in the U.S.[101] An early meta-analysis of 23 randomized control trials of the efficacy of St. John's wort in the treatment of depression indicated that there was a therapeutic benefit.[101] Of the 23 clinical trials, 20 were double-blinded in study design, and there were 1757 test subjects, with differing severities of depression. The subjects received one of the following interventions: herbal supplement of St. John's wort (dose range from 200 mg to 1800 mg per day), a traditional antidepressant drug, or a placebo, for 4 to 8 weeks. In 13 of the trials, St. John's wort resulted in a 55% alleviation of depressive symptoms, compared to 22% for placebo. The difference was less in the 3 trials comparing St. John's wort with antidepressant drugs; however, the additional advantage of a significant reduction in adverse side effects was noted. This 1996 review reported that St. John's wort was not only better tolerated than the commonly prescribed antidepressant medications; it was also more effective in the alleviation of negative symptoms associated with depression. However, the analysis of the results of two large clinical trials carried out more recently in the U.S. does not support the views expressed in the 1996 review.[102,103] Gupta and coworkers suggest that the reasons for differences in study findings are related to St John's wort interactions with prescribed medications and patients taking both should be closely monitored.[102]

VIII. CONCLUSION

The WHO estimates that major depressive disorders will become the second leading cause of morbidity world wide by the year 2020. Fortunately, depression is a treatable condition. Successful management of depression involves pharmacological and psychotherapeutic treatments. As is common today, chronic diseases such as diabetes mellitus, cardiovascular disease, and some musculoskeletal disorders have a dichotomous treatment paradigm in which nutritional regimens have an adjunctive treatment role with pharmacotherapy. There are many promising candidates for nutritional adjuvant treatment for depression; omega-3 fatty acids and the phospholipid hypothesis are the most promising. However tryptophan, vitamins B_6, B_{12}, folate, and SAMe also demonstrate promise in contribution to the phospholipid methylation hypothesis. Despite the increasing body of research, differences in dietary cultures, stages in the human life cycle and comorbidities all cloud the issues involved. Optimistically, the role of balanced nutrition should be recognized and then nutrition and specific nutrients will be used as adjuvant treatment in the maintenance of good mental health.

REFERENCES

1. Jorm, A., Korten, A., Jacomb, P., Christensen, H., Rodgers, B., and Pollitt P., Mental health literacy: a survey of the public's ability to recognise mental disorders and their beliefs about the effectiveness of treatment, *Med. J. Aust.*, 166: 182–186, 1997.
2. Ellis, P. and Smith, D., Treating depression: the beyondblue guidelines for treating depression in primary care, *Med. J. Aust.*, 176: S77–S83, 2002.

3. Black Dog Institute, www.blackdoginstitute.org.au/depression, accessed November 12, 2005.
4. Thomas, B., Mental illness, in *Manual of Dietetic Practice,* 3rd ed., Thomas, B. and British Dietetic Association, Eds., Blackwell Publishing, London, 2002.
5. Styron, W., *Darkness Visible*, Jonathon Cape, London, 1991.
6. Bloch, S. and Singh, B., *Understanding Troubled Minds: A Guide to Mental Illness and Its Treatment*, Melbourne University Press, Melbourne, 1997.
7. Garrow, J. and James, W., *Human Nutrition and Dietetics*, 9th ed., Churchill Livingstone, London, 1993.
8. Information Leaflet about Antidepressants from the Royal College of Psychiatrists, www.rcpsych.ac.uk/factsheet/pfacanti.asp, accessed November 12, 2005.
9. Timonen, M., Horrobin, D., Jokelainen, J., Laitinen, J., Herva, A, and Rasanen, P., Fish consumption and depression: the Northern Finland 1966 birth cohort study, *J. Affect. Disord.* 82: 447–452, 2004.
10. Hibbeln, J. and Salem, N., Dietary polyunsaturated fats and depression: when cholesterol does not satisfy, *Am. J. Clin. Nutr.*, 62: 1–9, 1995.
11. Baumel, S., *Dealing with Depression Naturally*, Keats, IL, 2000.
12. Murray, C. and Lopez, A., *The Global Burden of Disease Study: A Comprehensive Assessment of Mortality and Disability from Disease, Injuries, and Risk Factors in 1990 and Projected to 2020*, Harvard University Press on behalf of the World Health Organisation and the World Bank, Cambridge, MA, 1996.
13. Weissman, M., Bland, R., Joyce, P., Newman, S., Wells, J., and Wittchen, H., Sex differences in rates of depression: cross-national perspectives, *J. Affect. Disord.* 29: 77–84, 1993.
14. Wilhelm, K., Mitchell, P., Slade, T., Brownhill, S., and Andrews, G., Prevalence and correlation of DSM-IV major depression in an Australian National Survey, *J. Affect. Disord.* 75: 155–162, 2003.
15. Andrews, G., Sanderson, K., Slade, T., and Issakidis, C., Why does the burden of disease persist? Relating the burden of anxiety and depression to the effectiveness of treatment. *Bulletin of the World Health Organization*, 78: 446–454, 2000.
16. Australian Health Insurance Commission, www.hic.gov.au, Accessed August 14, 2004.
17. Bloch, S. and Singh, B., *Foundations of Clinical Psychiatry*, Melbourne University Press, Melbourne, 2000.
18. Joyce, P. and Mitchell, P., *Mood Disorders: Recognition and Treatment*, The University of New South Wales Press Ltd, Sydney, 2004.
19. Taskforce on DSM IV, *Diagnostic and Statistical Manual of Mental Disorders,* American Psychiatric Association, Washington, D.C., 2000.
20. Ganong, W., *Review of Medical Physiology,* 15th ed., Prentice Hall, Englewood Cliffs, NJ, 1991.
21. Marieb, E., *Human Anatomy and Physiology,* 6th ed., Pearson Benjamin Cummings, San Francisco, CA, 2004.
22. Information leaflet about Neurotransmitters, www.en.wikipedia.org/wiki/neurotransmitters, Accessed November 14, 2005.
23. Bottiglieri, T., Laundy, M., Crellin, R., Toone, B., Carney, M., and Reynolds, E., Homocysteine, folate, methylation, and monoamine metabolism in depression, *J. Neurol. Neurosurg. Psychiatry*, 9: 228–232, 2000.
24. Sullivan, P., Neale, M., and Kendler, K., Genetic epidemiology of major depression: review and meta-analysis., *Am. J. Psychiatry*, 157: 1552–1565, 2000.
25. Bierut, L., Heath, A., Bucholz, K., Dinwiddie, S., Madden, P., Statham, D., Dunne, M., and Martin, N., Major depressive disorder in a community-based twin sample: are there different genetic and environmental contributions for men and women? *Arch. Gen. Psychiatry*, 56: 557–563, 1999.
26. Nishizawa, S., Benkelfat, C., Young, S., Leyton, M., Mzengeza, S., de Montigny, C., and Blier, P., Differences between males and females in rates of serotonin synthesis in human brain, *Proc. Natl. Acad. Sci.* 94: 5308–5313, 1997.
27. Nolen-Hoeksema, S., Sex differences in unipolar depression: evidence and theory, *Psychol. Bull.*, 101: 256–282, 1987.
28. Pope, S., Watts, J., Evans, S., McDonald, S., and Henderson, S., An Information Paper on Postnatal Depression: A Systematic Review of Published Scientific Literature to 1999, National Health and Medical Research Council, Canberra, 2000.
29. Evans, J., Heron, J., Francomb, H., Oke, S., and Golding, J., Cohort study of depressed mood during pregnancy and after childbirth, *Br. Med. J.*, 323: 257–260, 2001.

30. O'Hara, M. and Swain, A., Rates and risks of postpartum depression — a meta-analysis, *Int. Rev. Psychiatry*, 8: 37–54, 1996.
31. Bloch, M., Schmidt, P., Danaceau, M., Murphy, J., Nieman, L., and Rubinow, D., Effects of gonadal steroids in women with a history of postpartum depression, *Am. J. Psychiatry*, 157: 924–930, 2000.
32. Dixon, J., Dixon, M., and O'Brien, P., Depression in association with severe obesity: changes with weight loss, *Arch. Intern. Med.*, 163: 2058–2065, 2003.
33. Zaider, T., Johnson, J., and Cockell, S., Psychiatric comorbidity associated with eating disorder symptomatology among adolescents in the community, *Int. J. Eating Disord.*, 28: 58–67, 2000.
34. O'Brien, K. and Vincent, N., Psychiatric comorbidity in anorexia and bulimia nervosa: nature, prevalence and causal relationships, *Clin. Psychol. Rev.*, 23: 57–74, 2003.
35. Sullivan, P., Mortality in anorexia nervosa, *Am. J. Psychiatry*, 152: 1073–1074, 1995.
36. Keys, A., Brozek, J., Honschel, A., Mickelson, O. and Taylor, H., *The Biology of Human Starvation*, University of Minnesota Press, Minneapolis, 1950.
37. International Obesity Task Force 2004, www.iotf.org, accessed August 14, 2004.
38. Wolpert, L., *Malignant Sadness*, Faber and Faber, London, 1999.
39. Fernstrom, J.D., Can nutrient supplements modify brain function? *Am. J. Clin. Nutr.*, 1: 1669S–1673S, 2000.
40. Butterweck, V., Mechanism of action of St John's Wort in depression: what is known?, *C. N. S. Drugs*, 17: 539–562, 2003.
41. Crellin, R., Bottiglieri, T., and Reynolds, E., Folates and psychiatric disorders: clinical potential, *Drugs*, 45: 623–636, 1993.
42. Tanskanen, A., Hibbeln, J., Hintikka, J., Haatainen, K., Honkalampi, K., and Viinamaki, H., Fish consumption, depression and suicidality in general population, *Arch. Gen. Psychiatry*, 8: 512–513, 2001.
43. Hakkarainen, R., Partonen, T., Haukka, J., Virtamo, J., Albanes, D., and Lonnqvist, J., Is low dietary intake of omega-3 fatty acids associated with depression? *Am. J. Psychiatry*, 161: 567–569, 2004.
44. O'Keefe, H., Jr. and Harris, W., From Inuit to implementation: omega-3 fatty acids come of age, *Mayo Clin. Proc.*, 75: 607–614, 2000.
45. Erasmus, U., *Fats That Heal, Fats That Kill*, Alive Books, Burnaby, Canada, 1993.
46. Spector, A. and Yorek, M., Membrane lipid composition and cellular function, *J. Lipid Res.*, 26: 1015–1035, 1985.
47. Alexander-North, L., North, J., Kiminyo, K., Buettner, G., and Spector, A., Polyunsaturated fatty acids increase lipid radical formation induced by oxidant stress in endothelial cells, *J. Lipid Res.*, 35: 1773–1785, 1994.
48. Shepherd, J., Patsch, J., Packard, C., Gotto, A., Jr., and Taunton, O., Dynamic properties of human high density lipoprotein apoproteins, *J. Lipid Res.*, 19: 383–389, 1978.
49. Volker, D.H., FitzGerald, P., Major, G., and Garg, M., Efficacy of fish oil concentrate in the treatment of rheumatoid arthritis, *J. Rheumatol.*, 27: 343–346, 2000.
50. Simopoulos, A., Evolutionary aspects of omega-3 fatty acids in the food supply, *Prostaglandins Leukot. Essent. Fatty Acids,* 60: 421–429, 1999.
51. Australian Bureau of Statistics, www.abs.gov.au, Accessed August 14, 2004.
52. Maes, M., Smith, R., Christophe, A. and Cosyns, P., Fatty acid composition in major depression: decreased omega-3 fractions in cholesteryl esters and increased C20: 4 n-6/C20: 5 n-3 ratio in cholesteryl esters and phospholipids, *J. Affect. Disord.* 36: 35–46, 1996.
53. Maes, M., Christophe, A., Delanghe, J., Altmura, C., Neels, H., and Meltzer, H., Lowered omega-3 polyunsaturated fatty acids in serum phospholipids and cholesteryl esters of depressed patients, *Psychiatry Res.*, 85: 275–291, 1999.
54. Peet, M., Murphy, B., Shay, J., and Horrobin, D., Depletion of omega-3 fatty acid levels in red blood cell membranes of depressive patients, *Biol. Psychiatry*, 43: 315–319, 1998.
55. Edwards, R., Peet, M., Shay, J., and Horrobin, D., Omega-3 polyunsaturated fatty acid levels in the diet and in red blood cell membranes of depressed patients, *J. Affect. Disord.*, 48: 149–155, 1998.
56. Nizzo, M., Tegros, S., Gallamini, A., Toffano, G., Polleri, A., and Massarotti, M., Brain cortex phospholipid liposome effects on CSF HVA, 5-HIAA and on prolactin and somatotropin secretion in man, *J. Neural Transm.* 43: 93–102, 1978.

57. Youdim, K., Martin, A., and Joseph, J., Essential fatty acids and the brain: possible health implications, *Int. J. Dev. Neurosci.* 18: 383–399, 2000.

58. Adams, P., Lawson, S., Sanigorski, A., and Sinclair, A., Arachidonic acid to eicosapentaenoic acid ratio in blood correlates positively with clinical symptoms of depression, *Lipids*, 31: S157–S161, 1996.

59. Booth-Kewley, S. and Friedman, H., Psychological predictors of heart disease: a quantitative review, *Psychol. Bull.*, 101: 343–362, 1987.

60. Frasure-Smith, N., Lesperance, F., and Talajic, M., Depression following myocardial infarction, impact on 6 month survival, *Am. J. Med.*, 270: 819–825, 1993.

61. Marangell, L., Martinez, J., and Zboyan, H., A double-blind, placebo-controlled study of the omega-3 fatty acid docosahexaenoic acid in the treatment of major depression, *Am. J. Psychiatry*, 160: 996–998, 2003.

62. Nemets, B., Stahl, Z., and Belmaker, R., Addition of omega-3 fatty acid to maintenance medication treatment for recurrent unipolar depressive disorder, *Am. J. Psychiatry*, 159: 477–479, 2002.

63. Peet, M. and Horrobin, D., A dose-ranging study of the effects of ethyl-eicosapentaenoate in patients with ongoing depression despite apparently adequate treatment with standard drugs, *Arch. Gen.Psychiatry*, 59: 913–919, 2002.

64. Kremer, J., Lawrence, D., Petrillo, G., Litts, L., Mullaly, P., Rynes, R., Stocker, R., Parhami, N., Greenstein, N., Fuchs, B., Mathur, A., Robinson, D., Sperling, R., and Bigaouette, J., Effects of high-dose fish-oil on rheumatoid arthritis after stopping nonsteroidal antiinflammatory drugs: clinical and immune correlates, *Arthritis Rheum.*, 38: 1107–1114, 1995.

65. Su, K., Huang, S., Chiu, C., and Shen, W., Omega-3 fatty acids in major depressive disorder: a preliminary double blind, placebo-controlled trial, *Eur. Neuropsychopharmacol.*, 13: 267–271, 2003.

66. International Society for the Study of Fatty acids and Lipids, *ISSFAL Newsletter*, 11: 27–30, 2004.

67. Kris-Etherton, P., Harris, W. and Appel, L., Fish consumption, fish oil, omega-3 fatty acids and cardiovascular disease, *Circulation*, 106: 2742–2757, 2002.

68. De Backer, G., Ambrosioni, E., Borch-Johnsen, K. et al., Third Joint Task Force of European and Other Societies on Cardiovascular Disease Prevention in Clinical Practice. European Guidelines on cardiovascular disease prevention in clinical practice: 3rd Joint Task Force of the European and other societies of cardiovascular disease prevention in clinical practice, *Eur. Heart J.*, 24: 1601–1610, 2003.

69. Scientific Advisory Committee on Nutrition, U.K., www.sacn.gov.uk/reports/, Accessed August 14, 2004.

70. National Health and Medical Research Council (NHMRC), Report of the NHMRC Working Party: The Role of Polyunsaturated Fats in the Australian Diet, A. G. P. S., Canberra, 1992.

71. National Heart Foundation of Australia, Review of the relationship between dietary fat and cardiovascular disease, *Aust. J. Nutr. Diet.*, 56: S5–S22, 1999.

72. ISSFAL Subcommittee 2004, Recommendations for intake of PUFA in healthy adults, *ISSFAL Newsletter*, 11: 12–25, 2004.

73. Bunker, S., Colquhoun, D., Esler, M., Hickie, I., Hunt, D., Jelinek, V., Oldenburg, B., Peach, H., Ruth, D., Tennant, C., and Tonkin, A., "Stress" and coronary heart disease: psychosocial factors — a National Heart Foundation of Australia position statement, *Med. J. Aust.*, 178: 272–276, 2003.

74. Simopoulos, A., The importance of the ratio of omega-6/omega-3 essential fatty acids, *Biomed. Pharmacother.*, 56: 365–379, 2002.

75. Wurtman, J., Moses, P., and Wurtman, R., Prior carbohydrate consumption affects the amount of carbohydrate that rats choose to eat, *J. Nutr.*, 113: 70–78, 1983.

76. Sharp, T., Bramwell, S., and Grahame-Smith, D., Effect of acute administration of L-tryptophan on serotoninergic neuronal activity: an in vivo microdialysis study, *Life Sci.* 1215–1223, 1992.

77. Borbely, A. and Youmbi-Balderer, G., Effects of tryptophan on human sleep, *Interdisciplinary Top. Gerontol.*, 22: 111–127, 1987.

78. Young, S. and Gauthier, S., Tryptophan availability and the control of 5-hydroxytryptamine and tryptamine synthesis in human CNS, *Adv. Exp. Med. Biol.*, 133: 211–230, 1981.

79. Lyons, P. and Truswell, A.S., Serotonin precursor influenced by type pf carbohydrate meal in healthy adults, *Am. J. Clin. Nutr.*, 47: 433–439, 1988.

80. Wurtman, R., Wurtman, J., Regan, M., McDermott. J., Tsay, R., and Breu, J., Effects of normal meals rich in carbohydrates or proteins on plasma tryptophan and tyrosine ratios, *Am. J. Clin. Nutr.*, 77: 128–132, 2003.

81. Carney, M., Chary, T., and Laundry, M., Red cell folate concentrations in psychiatric patients, *J. Affect. Disord.*, 9: 207–213, 1990.

82. Morris, M., Fava, M., Jacques, P., Selhub, J. and Rosenberg, I., Depression and folate status in the U.S. population, *Psychother. Psychosom.*, 72: 80–87, 2003.

83. Bottiglieri, T., S-Adenosyl-L-methionine (SAMe): from the bench to the bedside: molecular basis of a pleitrophic molecule, *Am. J. Clin. Nutr.*, 76: 1151S–1157S, 2002.

84. Lee, S., Wing, Y., and Tong. S., A controlled study of folate levels in Chinese inpatients with major depression in Hong Kong, *J. Affect. Disord.*, 49: 73–77, 1998.

85. Ramos, M., Allen, L., Haan, M., Green, R., and Miller, J., Plasma folate concentrations are associated with depressive symptoms in elderly Latina women despite folic acid fortification, *Am. J. Clin. Nutr.*, 80: 1024–1028, 2004.

86. Tolmunen, T., Voutilaimen, S., Hintikka, J., Rissanen, T., Tanskanen, A., Viinamak, H., Kaplan, G. and Salonen, J., Dietary folate and depressive symptoms are associated in middle-aged Finnish men, *J. Nutr.*, 133: 3233–3236, 2003.

87. Quinn, K. and Basu, T., Folate and vitamin B_{12} status of the elderly, *Eur. J. Clin. Nutr.*, 50: 340–342, 1996.

88. Hintikka, J., Tolmunen, T., Tanskanen, A., and Viinamaki, H., High vitamin B_{12} level and good treatment outcome may be associated in major depressive disorder, *B. M. C. Psychiatry*, 3: 17–22 2003.

89. Bernstein, A., Vitamin B_6 in clinical neurology, *Ann. N. Y. Acad. Sci.*, 585: 250–260, 1990.

90. Stewart, J., Harrison, W., Quitken, F., and Baker, H., Low B_6 levels in depressed outpatients, *Biol. Psychiatry*, 19: 613–616, 1984.

91. Penninx, L., Allen, R., and Stabler, S., Vitamin B_{12} deficiency and depression in physically disabled older women: Epidemiologic evidence from Women's Health and Aging Study, *Am. J. Psychiatry*, 157: 715–721, 2000.

92. Bottiglieri, T., Laundy, M., Crellin, R., Toone, B., Carney, M., and Reynolds, E., Homocysteine, folate, methylation, and monoamine metabolism in depression, *J. Neurol. Neurosurg. Psychiatry*, 69: 228–232, 2000.

93. Fava, M., Borus, J., Alpert, J., Nierenberg, A., Rosenbaun, J., and Bottiglieri, T., Folate, vitamin B_{12} and homocysteine in major depressive disorders, *Am. J. Psychiatry*, 153: 426–428, 1997.

94. Hvas, A., Juul, S., Bech, P., and Nexo, E., Vitamin B_6 level is associated with symptoms of depression, *Psychother. Psychosom.* 73: 340–343, 2004.

95. Tiemeier, H., van Tuijl, H., Hofman, A., Meijer, J., Kiliaan, A., and Breteler, M., Vitamin B_{12}, folate and homocysteine in depression: the Rotterdam Study, *Am. J. Psychiatry*, 159: 2099–2101, 2002.

96. Otero-Losado, M. and Rubio, M., Acute effects of S-Adenosyl-L-methionine on catecholaminergic central function, *Eur. J. Pharmacol.*, 163: 535–356, 1989.

97. Otero-Losado, M. and Rubio, M., Acute changes in 5HT metabolism after S-Adenosyl-L-methionine administration, *Gen. Pharmacol.*, 20: 403–406, 1989.

98. Bottiglieri, T., Laundy, M., Martin, R., Carney, M., Nissenbaum, H., Toone, B., Johnson, A., and Reynolds, E., S-Adenosyl-L-methionine influences monoamine metabolism, *Lancet,* 2: 224–234, 1984.

99. Muccioli, G., Scordamaiglia, A., and Di Carlo, R., Effect of S-Adenosyl-L-methionine on brain muscarinic receptors, *Eur. J. Pharmacol.*, 227: 293–299, 1992.

100. Kowatch, M. and Roth, G., Effect of specific membrane perturbations in alpha-adrenergic and mus-carinic-cholinergic signal transduction in rat parotid cell aggregates, *Life Sci.*, 2003–2010, 1994.

101. Linde, K., Ramerez, G., Mulrow, C.D., Pauls, A., Weidenhammer, W., and Melchart, D., St. John's Wort for depression — an overview and meta-analysis of randomised clinical trial, *Br. Med. J.*, 13: 253–258, 1996.

102. Gupta, R. and Moller, H., St. John's Wort: an option for the primary care treatment of depressive patients?, *Eur. Arch. Psychiatry Clin. Neurosci.*, 253: 140–148, 2003.

103. Bilia, A., Gallori, S., and Vincieri, F., St. John's Wort and depression: efficacy, safety and tolerability: an update, *Life Sci.*, 70: 3077–3096, 2000.

20 Protein as a Functional Food Ingredient for Weight Loss and Maintaining Body Composition

Jennifer E. Seyler, Robert E.C. Wildman, and Donald K. Layman

CONTENTS

Obesity is rapidly becoming the number one public health problem in modern societies. In the U.S., national survey data suggests that more than 60% of adults are overweight with more than half of these obese.[1,2] In 1991 only 4 out of 45 states that participated in the study had an adult obesity prevalence rate of 15–19%. In 2004, 7 states had obesity prevalence rates of 15–19%, whereas 33 states had rates between 20–24% and 9 states had rates more than 25%.[3] The increase in obesity has occurred in both sexes, in all age groups, and across all ethnic groups.[4] As of 2004, over 24% of Americans were obese.[5] Being obese or overweight can increase risks for secondary health diseases such as hypertension, dislipidemia, and diabetes.[6] Currently, the standard definition of an overweight adult is a BMI between 25–29.9 kg/m^2, whereas obesity is defined as a BMI of ≥ 30. When defining obesity as a measure of body fatness, men and women are considered obese with 25% and 33%, respectively.

The economic impact expands past health and into the pocketbooks of many Americans. Indirect and direct costs were estimated at $117 billion in 2000, with slightly more money contributing to the direct cost.[7] Direct costs refer to services that involve the treatment, prevention, or diagnosis of obesity and overweight, whereas indirect costs are associated with wages lost due to inability to work in the present and future.[7]

There are various possibilities for the cause and prevention of obesity. Although obesity may have genetic links, the epidemic increase in obesity during the past 20 years appears to stem from consistent overconsumption of calories[8,9] and chronic inactivity.[10]

I. MACRONUTRIENT LEVELS AND WEIGHT LOSS

With the prevalence of obesity and continued popularity of weight loss books, it is no surprise that most American adults claim to be "dieting."[11] So, which meal plan is best? In regard to weight loss there is a consensus that successful weight loss requires a calorie intake that is below the need for weight maintenance. However, there is continued debate over the effect of the varied macronutrient composition of a meal plan in relation to its success in weight loss.

Various researches have shown that the macronutrient composition of a calorie-controlled meal plan plays a role in the treatment of obesity.[12–14] Previously, high fat meal plans have been thought to be a fundamental cause in the development of obesity.[15] Based on this notion, weight loss recommendations included a decrease in dietary fat consumption to 60 g or less per day.[16] By default, Americans increased carbohydrate intake[17] and actually increased total energy intake.[6] The result was a reduction in body fat oxidation,[18,19] an increase in blood triglycerides,[20] and a reduction in satiety,[21] leaving many unaware of which direction to turn when it came to choosing what to eat.

The above trend led to the increasing body of evidence related to the incidence of obesity and its association with excess calories in a high carbohydrate meal plan.[22] High carbohydrate intake increases blood glucose levels and induces an elevated secretion of insulin into the blood to increase tissue uptake of glucose or decrease the amount of glucose in the blood (circulation). Increased insulin output[23] and potential postprandial hypoglycemic response may be contributing factors to excess energy consumption and positive energy balance.

Other researchers suggest a nutrition plan higher in protein as another possible weight loss approach.[24,25] Increased dietary proteins help to maintain muscle mass but do not appear to exhibit an increase in blood glucose levels as carbohydrates are known to do.[26] Meal plans high in protein and lower in carbohydrates reduce the postprandial glucose and insulin response and provide a continuous fuel supply of amino acid substrates for hepatic glucose production, which aids in stabilization of blood glucose.[27] This new research has led to rethinking the potential protein importance in the nutrition plan.

II. DISCOVERING PROTEIN

Proteins are vital to life; a fundamental component of the meal plan necessary for physical development and organ and cell functions. Proteins are labeled as macronutrients, like carbohydrates and fat. Until recently the role of specific proteins and amino acids as functional ingredients has been limited more to the weightlifting and body building communities focused on muscle development. Furthermore, protein intakes in excess of the Recommended Dietary Allowance (RDA) are often stated as potentially detrimental to renal function and bone mineralization. These concepts have been challenged and are being replaced by a new understanding of the importance of dietary protein for adult health.

Over the past decade or so, protein has emerged as a functional food ingredient for several health areas including weight loss and diabetes. The weight loss industry in the U.S. is quickly approaching 50 billion dollars in annual revenue, and it will continue to grow as the number of

TABLE 20.1
Essential and Nonessential Amino Acids

Essential Amino Acids (9)	Nonessential Amino Acids (13)
Leucine	Alanine
Isoleucine	Glutamine
Valine	Arginine
Tryptophan	Ornithine
Threonine	Glutamic acid
Lysine	Proline
Phenylalanine	Glycine
Methionine	Tyrosine
Histidine	Cysteine
	Cystine
	Serine
	Asparagine
	Aspartic acid

Source: Adapted from Rosenbloom, C., *Sports Nutrition: A Guide for the Professional Working with Active People*, 3rd ed., The American Dietetic Association, Chicago, IL, 2000.

overweight and obese individuals continues to increase.[28] Through a maze of fad diets and supplements, protein has emerged as a critical nutrient for improving body composition and a core ingredient for weight loss products. This chapter provides an overview of protein with special attention to protein levels and sources, as well as amino acids with unique metabolic roles that are particularly intriguing with regard to weight loss.

III. OVERVIEW OF PROTEIN

Protein is a general term used to refer to a diverse category of molecules that contain amino acids. Proteins can be as small as the hormone insulin, containing 51 amino acids, or as large as myosin, a structural component of muscle containing 6,100 amino acids. Whereas the body contains a large array of proteins in structures, enzymes, and hormones, each protein is constructed from just 22 individual amino acids. These 22 amino acids are assembled in different amounts and different sequences to give each protein a unique size, shape, and function.

Amino acids are categorized in two groups as shown in Table 20.1. Nine amino acids are termed *essential* or indispensable for humans because they must be present in the daily meal plan, whereas 13 amino acids are considered *nonessential* or dispensable because the body can make them in adequate qualities; they are not required in the daily meal plan.[29]

Quantity and quality of proteins differ among food sources due to the amino acid amount and types present in each protein. In general, foods from animal sources contain more protein and provide a more complete amino acid mixture than foods from plant sources (Table 20.2). A *complete protein* such as egg albumin contains adequate amounts of each of the essential amino acids in proper ratios, whereas an *incomplete protein*, such as wheat gluten does not have all the essential amino acids in adequate amounts or correct proportions.

IV. ROLES OF AMINO ACIDS AND PROTEINS

Amino acids and the resulting proteins have multiple bodily functions. The essential roles of body structure and function include serving as:

- Structures in cell membranes, muscles, and bones
- Enzymes to help regulate chemical reactions
- Antibodies for the immune system
- Hormones as regulators of metabolic processes
- Clotting factors in the blood
- Blood proteins for transporting nutrients and oxygen
- Receptors on cells
- Enzymes for digestion and absorption of food
- Unique metabolic regulators (such as leucine) in protein synthesis and arginine in nitrous oxide
- An important energy source for muscle, liver, and the intestine

Among the many diverse roles of amino acids some of the most noteworthy effects have been observed with the branched-chain amino acid (BCAA) leucine.[30,31,32] Leucine participates in numerous metabolic processes,[29] its obvious role being as an indispensable amino acid for new protein synthesis. Leucine also functions as a critical regulator of translation initiation of protein synthesis, a modulator of the insulin–PI3 kinase signal cascade, and a nitrogen donor for muscle production

TABLE 20.2
Sources of Protein by Weight

Food Item (1 oz)	Protein (g)	Leucine (g)	Lysine (g)	Isoleucine (g)	% Leucine	% BCAA
Whey, powder[a]	24.00	2.53	2.23	1.57	10.54	26.38
Soybeans, roasted	9.98	0.77	0.63	0.46	7.72	18.64
Pork, lean	8.83	0.71	0.79	0.41	8.04	21.63
Chicken, breast	8.79	0.66	0.75	0.46	7.51	21.27
Beef, lean	8.66	0.69	0.73	0.39	7.97	20.90
Tuna	8.50	0.69	0.78	0.39	8.12	21.88
Halibut	7.57	0.61	0.69	0.35	8.06	21.80
Peanut butter	7.11	0.46	0.25	0.25	6.47	13.50
Cheese, low-fat[b]	6.75	0.61	0.53	0.40	9.04	22.81
Nuts, peanut	6.71	0.43	0.24	0.23	6.41	13.41
Turkey, breast[b]	5.00	0.40	0.46	0.26	8.00	22.40
Soybean, cooked[b]	3.78	0.38	0.31	0.23	10.10	24.34
Egg	3.57	0.3	0.25	0.19	8.40	20.73
Cottage cheese, 1%	3.51	0.32	0.25	0.19	9.12	21.65
Egg whites	3.09	0.27	0.21	0.17	8.74	21.04
Hummus[b]	2.24	0.14	0.12	0.08	6.25	15.18
Bread, white	2.17	0.15	0.06	0.08	6.91	13.36
Tofu, firm	1.98	0.15	0.12	0.09	7.58	18.18
Yogurt, low-fat[b]	1.75	0.15	0.13	0.08	8.57	20.57
Black beans[b]	1.73	0.14	0.12	0.08	8.09	19.65
Milk, skim	0.96	0.09	0.07	0.04	9.38	20.83
Rice, white	0.76	0.06	0.03	0.03	7.89	15.79
Potato, baked	0.71	0.04	0.04	0.03	5.63	15.49

[a] Optimum nutrition 100% whey protein Gold Standard.

[b] USDA National Nutrient Database for Standard Reference. Release 18 (2005).

Source: ESHA Research, Professional Nutrition Analysis Software and Databases v. 9.6.1 2002–2003 ESHA Research.

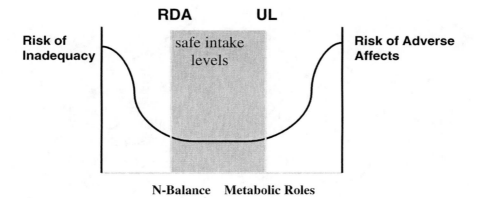

FIGURE 20.1
Figure modified from the Food and Nutrition Board, National Academies of Sciences, 1994.

of alanine and glutamine. The potential for leucine to impact protein synthesis, insulin signaling, and production of alanine and glutamine is dependent on dietary intake and increasing leucine concentration in skeletal muscle.

V. PROTEIN REQUIREMENTS

Beginning in 1943, the RDAs have been used as a standard for nutrition guidelines. These guidelines were developed as minimal standards for health policy. By definition, the RDAs are designed to be (simply) adequate for most healthy people;[33] they are intended as guidelines to prevent deficiencies. In the past decade, Americans have become increasingly dissatisfied with nutrition guidelines defined to be simply adequate. In response to these concerns, the Food and Nutrition Board (FNB) of the National Academies of Sciences developed a broader concept of nutrition intakes. In 2002, the FNB published the Dietary Reference Intakes (DRIs) for the macronutrients.

The U.S. and Canada DRIs were established as reference values, quantitative estimates of nutrient intake and a dietary planning tool for healthy people ensuring sufficient intake of essential nutrients. These references are associated with reduced risks of chronic diseases. The DRIs define safe ranges for nutrient intakes, ranging from minimum intake for the prevention of deficiencies (RDA) up to an upper limit (UL), defined as a safe intake below any adverse affects of excess intake (Figure 20.1). The DRI protein range is 0.8 g/kg up to ~2.0 g/kg, a range expressed as 10% to 35% of energy intake. It is important to recognize that the protein intake range relates to body weight and not energy intake. A dietary intake of 90 g/d (~1.1 g/kg for an 80 kg person) represents 12% of energy intake at 3000 kcal/d but 24% of energy intake at 1500 kcal/d. It is important to recognize that protein intake relates to body weight. At low energy intakes, protein might represent a higher percentage of daily energy, whereas at high energy intakes, protein may represent a lower percentage of daily intakes. This is a fundamental concept that is not adequately characterized in current health guidelines and leads to misrepresentations of nutrition plan quality.

The DRIs provide a concept of a safe range. The RDA represents the minimum level to avoid a deficiency, and the UL represents the maximum safe level to avoid toxicity. There is a need for DRIs based on metabolic outcomes, the optimum levels of amino acids for growth or metabolic outcomes, the optimum intake for individuals engaged in strength training or cardiovascular exercise such as fitness enthusiasts or competitive athletes, and the optimum protein intake to maintain muscle and bone health in the elderly.[34] Further, in a society exposed to excess energy and epidemic increases in obesity and diabetes, it is unclear if a meal plan designed to provide the minimum amount of protein to prevent a deficiency is consistent with lifelong health.

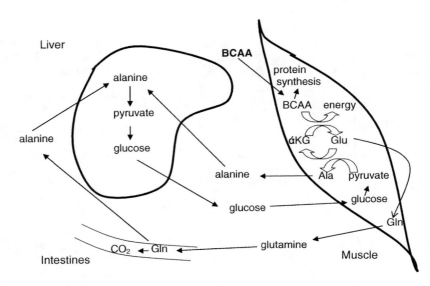

FIGURE 20.2 Metabolism of branched-chain amino acids.

VI. PROTEIN SOURCES

Within food sources, there are different dietary protein types. For example, the primary protein in bread is gluten, eggs contain albumin, and milk contains casein and whey. Many of these protein types are actually families or chemically associated protein molecules. For instance, egg albumin includes ovalbumin, ovotransferrin, ovomucoid, ovomucin, and lysozyme. Meanwhile, milk whey includes β-lactoglobulin, α-lactalbumin, immunoglobulins, bovine serum albumin, lactoferrin, and lactoperoxidase, as well as glycomacropeptide (GMP), a casein-derived protein in cheese whey. On the other hand, the principal casein fractions are α(s1) and α(s2)-caseins, β-casein, and kappa-casein.

Milk has evolved as a unique protein for mammals, partially because of its protein composition. Casein, the main protein in milk, makes up roughly 80% of total milk protein and is deemed a slow-acting protein. Because of the complex chemical nature of casein protein, digestion and absorption of its amino acids can take up to a few hours, depending on the amount consumed.[30] Therefore, casein would provide a slow, steady rise in blood levels and uptake of amino acids into circulation. Whey, on the other hand, is more readily digested, allowing for a quick increase in blood amino acid levels and an increase in protein synthesis.[35] The combination of whey and casein protein (fast- and slow-acting proteins) is believed to be beneficial during muscle recovery, especially the time that immediately follows a strength training session.

When whey protein is mentioned, the first thought that usually enters the mind is its use by body builders or athletes because of its popularity as a protein supplement. However, whey is also a major part of infant formulas because of all its nutrient value. Whey is comprised of calcium, phosphorus, lactose, water, magnesium, fat and, of course, protein.[36] What's more, whey protein is also thought to be more satisfying than casein because of the levels of circulating amino acids after a meal is consumed.[37] Whey is rich in the essential amino acids, particularly the branched-chained amino acids (BCAA), leucine, isoleucine, and valine. These amino acids are major contributors to skeletal muscle replenishment after exercise[31] or short-term periods of food restriction, such as overnight fasting. If the meal plan is adequate in leucine, then the muscles can build or maintain muscle protein. However, if the meal plan is inadequate in protein/leucine, then muscle protein synthesis is blocked, and to maintain metabolic functions, the breakdown of muscle can occur. This is one reason why whey is believed to increase muscle mass in a strength-training individual. Even though whey has many other agreed-upon benefits, the ability to increase muscle mass is still controversial.[38]

VII. PROTEIN DIGESTION AND ABSORPTION

The process of converting dietary protein into amino acids for use in the body is a complex process involving the stomach, small intestine, and liver. Although the process is complex, it is highly efficient with nearly 100% of dietary protein digested and absorbed into the intestinal cells, known as *enterocytes*. Protein digestion begins in the stomach as gastric acids denature complex protein structures, and pepsin begins to cleave protein chains. The resulting polypeptides are released into the small intestine where proteases derived from the pancreas and enterocytes continue protein digestion. Ultimately, protein digestion produces a mixture of free amino acids and di- and tri-peptides in ratios of approximately 1:1:1. These amino acid mixtures and small peptides are absorbed into the enterocytes by amino acid and peptide transporters. Once inside enterocytes, the remaining peptides are hydrolyzed to amino acids before being released into portal circulation.

Amino acids within the enterocyte can be used for intestinal enzyme synthesis, e.g., proteases, used for energy, or transported to portal blood for use by the rest of the body. Use of amino acids by the intestine varies greatly among amino acids. Dietary glutamine and glutamate are completely removed by the enterocyte as fuels; neither one of these amino acids, from a meal (or supplements), reaches the blood. In total, the enterocytes remove approximately 25% of dietary amino acids before they reach the blood and become available to other tissues.

Amino acids leave the intestine via the portal blood to the liver. The liver is the most active amino acid metabolism tissue in the body. Amino acids that reach the liver can be used for protein synthesis, an energy source, or released to the blood. Similar to the intestine, the liver removes nearly 25% of dietary amino acids for energy. Surprisingly, the primary energy sources for both the intestine and the liver are amino acids. This means that less than one-half of dietary amino acids ever reach the blood or a majority of tissues.

Although the liver and intestines use amino acids for energy, amino acids are not removed uniformly. The enterocyte is active in removing glutamine, glutamate, asparagine, and aspartate, whereas the liver is capable of metabolizing most of the remaining amino acids. The major exemptions to the intestine and liver are the BCAAs. These three amino acids are unique in that the liver lacks the necessary enzymes to metabolize them; the net result, BCAAs appear in the blood in nearly the exact amounts present in a meal.

VIII. PROTEIN TURNOVER

Amino acids enter the blood, move throughout the body, are transported into cells, and become available for synthesis of new proteins. Proteins within the body are constantly being made and destroyed (see Figure 20.3). Some proteins such as enzymes have a lifespan of only a few hours, whereas other structural proteins such as connective tissues are retained for as long as 6 months. Hence, the body has a daily need to replace most enzymes, whereas a sprained ankle may take 4 to 6 months to be completely repaired.

The process of synthesis and degradation of proteins is called *protein turnover*. Each day, the body makes and degrades over 250 g of protein. The magnitude of this turnover is surprising as few people consume more than 100 g of protein per day. The lack of direct relationship between the amount of dietary protein and the level of daily protein turnover emphasizes the difficulty in defining protein requirements.

Body protein quantity is largely determined by the balance of protein synthesis and degradation. Although the daily turnover is greater than 250 g/d, the actual potential to accumulate new proteins is very limited. During maximum growth, protein turnover is positive, i.e., synthesis is greater than

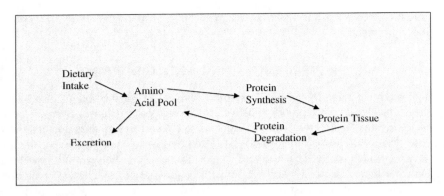

FIGURE 20.3 Protein turnover.

degradation, but the net balance is less than 10 g/d. Protein turnover balance appears to be largely regulated by protein synthesis change.

Protein synthesis is a complex process that assembles the 22 amino acids into hundreds of individual proteins. This complex process is regulated by gene expression of mRNA (the blueprints for each new protein), the availability of amino acids and energy, and regulatory proteins called initiation factors. These controls allow the body to make new proteins in the correct cells at the correct time. Review of protein synthesis is beyond the scope of this chapter; however, new research has shown an important link between insulin and leucine in regulation of protein synthesis that appears to be a key to understanding management of body weight and composition.

IX. BCAAs — SPECIFICALLY, LEUCINE AND WEIGHT LOSS

BCAAs are mainly used for protein synthesis[39] and are participants in signal transduction pathways, which may help provide the anabolic effect protein has on muscle tissue.[40] Leucine, in particular, has shown the same effects as amino acid mixtures[40] and therefore will be the focus of the BCAA section.

The BCAA leucine has multiple roles in metabolism, including being a substrate for protein synthesis,[41] a fuel for skeletal muscle,[42] and a nitrogen donor for production of alanine and glutamine in skeletal muscles.[43] These roles are dependent on the dietary intake of leucine.[41] Due to leucine metabolism, the levels consumed are relative to the levels that reach the skeletal muscle. Leucine's contribution to stimulation of protein synthesis is supported by human studies.[44]

Leucine or even a mixture of the BCAAs, can stimulate protein synthesis during energy restriction.[41] Low-calorie controlled high-protein meal plans (one providing 10 g of leucine per day equivalent to around 125 g of dietary protein per day) compared to USDA Food Guide Pyramid recommendations, showed a greater loss of weight and improved body composition (increase in body fat loss and decrease in muscle mass loss) with the high-protein meal plan. See Table 20.2 for breakdown of BCAAs in food sources.

X. PROTEIN AND GLYCEMIC CONTROL

Dietary protein plays a role in blood glucose regulation via its affects on insulin[46] and increased availability of substrates (amino acids) for gluconeogenesis.[47] Janey and colleagues[48] demonstrated that 50–80 g of glucose could be generated from 100 g of ingested protein, while Jungas and colleagues stated that the primary liver fuel source in the fasted state is amino acids.[27] Amino acids are produced by protein breakdown in the muscle. They transfer to the liver, deaminate, and become carbon skeletons for gluconeogenesis.[47] Common substrates for gluconeogenesis include alanine and glutamine, which are deaminated into pyruvate and glutamate, respectively. Gluconeogenic substrate availability is thought to be proportional to dietary amino acid consumption.[49] Therefore, an increase in dietary protein would lead to an increased availability of gluconeogenic substrates, also relative to BCAA amount. The fasted state is accompanied with a decrease in insulin and an increase in glucagon, which causes an increase in hepatic glucose production and degradation of glycogen, via a series of dephosphorylations, to produce fuel for the body.[50] Glucagon is also known to be a stimulator of gluconeogenesis.[46] With increased substrate availability and stimulation of hepatic glucose production, a moderate protein meal plan increases the role of the liver in blood glucose control.[51,52] This blood glucose control method has been used for regulation in type 2 diabetes for years.[53]

XI. ENERGY METABOLISM

Meal consumption stimulates a series of physiological and metabolic processes. When food is consumed, the metabolic state changes from a catabolic to an anabolic state, due to an increase in protein synthesis and decrease of protein breakdown.[54] Generally, during the absorptive period, there is a rise in blood glucose levels. Insulin will aid in the uptake and utilization of glucose into muscle and adipose, decrease hepatic glucose output, increase glycogen synthesis, decrease lipolysis, and decrease protein degradation. Therefore, within a few hours after a meal, dietary glucose is either stored or oxidized,[55] whereas fat is either used or stored for future use, and protein is either used for the previously mentioned functions or made into glucose and then stored as glycogen.[27]

Once the food has been absorbed, the body relies on endogenous energy sources for fuel. Maintained blood glucose levels sustain the brain and glycolytic requirement of glucose. As the exogenous supply of glucose decreases, insulin secretion follows suit, whereas glucagon secretion increases. Glucagon stimulates liver glycogenolysis to release glucose into circulation. Liver glycogen as a glucose resource will also be prolonged by tissues such as skeletal muscle, increasing the use of alternative fuel sources. The insulin level fall allows for an increase in adipose tissue lipolysis, resulting in the release of free fatty acids (FFA) into circulation. This decrease in glucose and insulin, and increase in FFA availability for fuel, is known as the glucose–fatty acid cycle or Randle cycle.[56]

When inadequate blood glucose-producing carbohydrate is consumed, blood glucose is maintained through glycogen breakdown and gluconeogenesis. Liver glycogen is the primary glycogen tissue, whereby the derived glucose can be released into the blood. However, liver glycogen is limited for adults and easily exhaustible. For instance, liver glycogen levels can be reduced to nadir levels within the first day of starvation. During semistarvation, glycogen levels are dramatically decreased, and the role of hepatic glycogenolysis in maintaining blood glucose levels is lessened in a relative manner.

Gluconeogenesis creates glucose from noncarbohydrate substrates, namely pyruvate, lactate, glycerol, alanine, and glutamine. Lactate and alanine carbons are recycled between the brain and liver or skeletal muscle and liver, respectively, and are, respectively, called the Cori and glucose–alanine cycles. The major gluconeogenic precursors are amino acids alanine and glutamine, which are derived mainly from proteolysis in skeletal muscle. This combination of actions helps maintain blood glucose levels during a fasted period.[55] Thus, dietary protein is an important fuel consideration during caloric imbalances.

XII. WEIGHT LOSS AND ENERGY INTAKE

Weight loss is often stated as a matter of simple energy economy. When calories out exceed calories in, there must be a net energy expenditure resulting in a body mass reduction. A calorie in is the cumulative amount of the calories consumed, which, by and large, are carbohydrate, protein, fat, and alcohol. On the opposite hand, daily caloric expenditure is a reflection of resting metabolism, lifestyle (daily activities), and exercise. When considering strategies for weight loss, both sides of the energy balance equation must be considered.

Increased food availability (e.g., portion sizes, buffets, convenience stores, etc.) partly explains the caloric consumption increase. In addition, public perception of calorie consumption vs. certain foods can be a contributing factor. For instance, the American Institute for Cancer Research conducted a survey to gauge public perception as to which was more important for weight management, the amount or type of food eaten.[57] Of those surveyed, 78% of the respondents said that eating certain foods was more crucial to weight management success than the actual amount of food consumed.[57]

Weight loss can be accomplished via a calorie restriction and/or an increase in caloric expenditure (exercise). Researchers have reported positive study results with prevention or treatment of adult obesity that focuses on modifying the calorie intake.[58,59] Energy restriction also reduces secondary health risks associated with obesity.[60] In support, energy restriction positively influences fasting blood glucose, hepatic glucose production, and blood insulin values with effects seen within 7–10 d of initial energy restriction.[61–63] All of these can enhance weight loss success.

Blood glucose control, in fed and fasted states, is important when maintaining and/or losing weight. As discussed above, the fed state produces a blood glucose increase which causes an increase in insulin secretion via the pancreas. Insulin causes translocation of the intracellular glucose transporters to the plasma membrane for tissue glucose uptake,[64] suppression of hepatic glucose production in the liver,[65] and synthesis of glycogen.[66] Gluconeogenic precursors (alanine, pyruvate, glutamine) are shifted toward glycogen formation,[67] and insulin manages glucose uptake.

Humans adapt to restricted energy intake using numerous mechanisms.[68] One adaptation is conservation of energy via metabolic responses.[69] An adult will adapt to energy restriction with reduced hepatic glucose production,[70,71] a decrease in basal metabolic rate, and a reduction in weight and activity.

Control of blood glucose is important as many obese people exhibit chronic hyperinsulinemia, insulin resistance, and dysfunction of oxidative and nonoxidative glucose disposal pathways. This may be a result of how the body handles consistent high carbohydrate eating patterns.[22] It is logical to ask whether the meal plan composition can influence these conditions.

XIII. PROTEIN AND WEIGHT LOSS

As previously stated, protein is used for many metabolic and physiological reasons. Generally, during a state of weight loss, there is an emphasis on a caloric intake decrease and a caloric expenditure (activity) increase. During an energy imbalance favoring weight loss, the dependence on body protein to sustain its energy needs increases. Being the largest and most accessible protein resource, muscle mass is targeted. The weight loss plan does not provide enough protein to service the anatomical and physiological needs as well as provide energy through the weight loss period. Dietary protein would need to compensate for the additional protein need in general, but also provide adequate amounts of the essential amino acids.

As discussed above, one of the adaptations to an energy restricted meal plan is a decrease in hepatic glucose production. If this continues, it can produce a drop in blood glucose levels if gluconeogenesis does not increase production of glucose for the blood. Meal plans high in protein have shown an increase in PEPCK mRNA, a key enzyme in gluconeogenesis,[72,73] which causes an increase in glucose production. This suggests that maintenance of glucose homeostasis during energy restriction may depend on meal plan composition, and provides a link between energy restriction and glucose homeostasis, which is important in obesity prevention/treatment.[21]

Modifications in energy intake, exercise, and specific macronutrient composition can decrease body weight, fasting plasma glucose, and insulin concentrations closer to homeostatic values.[60] An increase in dietary protein and a decrease in dietary carbohydrate has been shown to produce glucose homeostasis, increase lean body mass, increase fat loss, and improve blood lipid profiles.[14] These studies suggest that meal plans with a reduced amount of carbohydrates and increase in protein, can increase weight loss and loss of body fat, and reduce loss of lean tissue.[20] For instance, one study involved overweight women assigned to one of two groups: a high carbohydrate or a moderate protein meal plan for 10 weeks.[14] The higher carbohydrate group received a plan similar to the Food Guide Pyramid which had a carbohydrate-to-protein ratio of 3.5 (~68 g protein/day). The moderate protein group received a carbohydrate-to-protein ratio of ~1.4 (~125 g protein/day). Both groups lost weight, but the moderate protein group had a significantly higher loss of fat/lean tissue ratio. This meant that more fat was lost and more lean muscle mass was preserved (protein sparing) than in the high carbohydrate meal plan. The high carbohydrate group also had an increased meal insulin response and postprandial hypoglycemia when compared to the moderate protein group.

An animal model with similar meal plans, but no energy restriction, resulted in comparable glucose and insulin outcomes. Basal hepatic glucose production was greater in the moderate protein group as compared to the high carbohydrate group; increased hepatic glucose production was influenced by the increased amount of dietary protein consumed.[67] Increased hepatic glucose production has been reported to be important in blood glucose maintenance in the fasted state.[74,51] Other studies show similar beneficial results in blood lipids and body composition with dietary substitution of protein for carbohydrates.[13,19,20,40,75]

XIV. PROTEIN AND APPETITE

Appetite can be influenced by biological, environmental, and behavioral factors. The biological factor that drives an individual to consume food is hunger. A food that inhibits further consumption produces satiety and a delay in the onset of the next meal. A food that is considered to have a high level of satiety is one that produces a long period of time between feelings of hunger.

Macronutrients at equivalent calorie levels have been shown to have different satiety effects.[76,77] Higher protein intake is often thought to reduce appetite, which can lead to reduced caloric consumption. A review of energy density (calories/gram) noted a hierarchical effect on satiety in the order of protein > carbohydrates > fat.[78,79,80] Participants in one study were fed protein, carbo-hydrate, and fat contributing either 29%, 61%, and 10% of energy, respectively (higher in protein and carbohydrate), or 9%, 30%, and 61% of energy (higher in fat), respectively, both in energy balance.[81] Diet-induced thermogenesis (DIT) and satiety were higher on the high protein/carbohy-drate diet than in the high fat group. Researchers in another study fed protein, carbohydrate, and fat contributing 10%, 60%, and 30% of energy, respectively, or 30%, 40%, and 30% to healthy women in energy balance.[82] The researchers reported an increase in sleeping metabolic rate, DIT, and satiety, and a lower 24-h hunger (calorie consumption) and respiratory quotient (RQ) in the high protein group. They also found incidental relationships between satiety and ghrelin, and glucagon-like peptide 1, but only with the higher protein intake.

XV. WEIGHT LOSS AND EXERCISE

Positive study results of adult obesity prevention/treatment focus on increased exercise.[83,84] The NIH guidelines for weight management emphasize the need for both proper nutrition and increased physical activity (minimum of 30 min per day of moderate intensity for exercise 7 d a week) for weight control. During 2003, 59% of adults did not engage in vigorous leisure-time physical activity, whereas only 26% of adults engaged in vigorous leisure-time physical activity 3 or more times per week.[85]

Exercise has been projected to be important in production of weight/fat loss,[87] prevention/treat-ment of obesity,[86] maintenance of blood glucose,[88] decrease of plasma insulin concentrations,[89] and maintenance of muscle mass. Exercise is known to induce a fall in circulating insulin levels with an increase in glucose utilization and increased insulin sensitivity.[90] Paffenbarger and colleagues[91] reported epidemiological studies showing the association between decreased obesity risks when physical activity was performed. Satabin and colleagues[92] used male Wistar CF rats with a high protein diet compared to a control, high in carbohydrates. Rats were exercised on a treadmill for 60 min/d for 3 weeks. Blood glucose was measured and found to remain in homeostasis, via an increase in liver gluconeogenesis, with rats on the high protein diet.

Previous *in vitro* studies have shown an increase in insulin's action on glucose uptake when muscular contractions are present.[93] Ji and colleagues[94] showed that after 10 weeks of training there was a significant increase in gluconeogenic enzyme activity. This produced an increase in glucose production, through gluconeogensis, supporting the stabilization of blood glucose. Holm and colleagues[95] conducted a study involving obese women who exercised for 1 h at 70% of their maximal working capacity. Subjects were fasted for 16–18 h, then tested for blood values. The results showed a decrease in plasma insulin and triglycerides a few days following exercise. Rodnick and colleagues also demonstrated this in a study with rats that were exercise-trained in wheel cages for 6 weeks.[96] Results showed a significant difference in fasting serum insulin between the exercise trained group and the sedentary group, with the exercise trained group having a lower insulin value than the sedentary group. Thus, exercise appears to improve insulin sensitivity[97] leading to glucose uptake, which is further enhanced in trained skeletal muscle.[96]

XVI. PROTEIN, EXERCISE, AND WEIGHT LOSS

The debates continue on whether eating the recommend RDA for protein is adequate for a person who exercises regularly. Some[38] feel it is adequate but others[98] think it can lead to an increase in protein breakdown and decrease in protein synthesis, possibly leading to an increase in protein needs. Over time, not eating enough protein can lead to a decrease in muscle mass[99] and physical performance.[99] During exercise, the BCAA leucine is mainly used by the muscles,[100] with an increase in leucine oxidation.[101] After exercise, leucine stimulates muscle recovery.[102]

Layman and colleagues[103] conducted a 4-month, 2×2 weight loss study with adult obese (determined by BMI) women. Meal plans were either a high protein or a high carbohydrate meal plan with or without exercise. The dietary composition of the carbohydrate group consisted of 0.8 grams of protein per kilogram body weight per day (~15% of energy intake) and ~30% of energy intake from dietary fat. The dietary composition of the protein group consisted of 1.6 g of protein per kilogram body weight per day (~30% of energy intake) and ~30% of energy intake from dietary fat. The exercise treatments consisted of walking 5 d per week for 30 min per day with an additional 2-d-a-week 30-min resistance training session. The nonexercise groups followed the NIH guidelines and exercised (walked) for 30 min, 5 d a week.

The high protein meal plan with and without exercise produced greater weight loss after 16 weeks than the carbohydrate meal plan. The higher protein meal plan with exercise eliminated the most body fat. All groups lost weight on these calorie-controlled meal plans, but subjects in the protein groups lost more total weight and body fat and maintained more muscle mass than the carbohydrate groups. The protein group with exercise appeared to experience an additive effect on body composition and weight loss.[103]

XVII. CONCLUSIONS

Ongoing research will continue to support the need for customized meal plans. Weight loss methods need to be considered on an individual basis, including personal choices in lifestyle and how the meal plan will affect individual metabolic outcomes.

Nutrition plans with increased levels of the protein and the BCAA leucine, present in high levels in animal proteins, can be used to substitute for high glycemic carbohydrates and have been shown to enhance insulin sensitivity,[45] stimulate muscle protein synthesis,[102,104] reduce the role of insulin in glycemic control,[45] and stimulate the role of the liver in stabilization of blood glucose.[45] In these studies, the net effects of these changes are lower body fat, increased lean muscle mass, increased insulin sensitivity, increased hepatic gluconeogenesis, stabilization of fasting blood glucose, and reduced serum triglycerides.[14]

As previously stated, if these types of meal plans are sustainable throughout a person's lifespan, fit into a person's lifestyle, and taste good, then that person may benefit from a high-protein meal plan during weight loss. The choice is up to individual bodies.

REFERENCES

1. U.S. Department of Health and Human Services, National Center for Health Statistics, Centers for Disease Control and Prevention, Prevalence of Overweight and Obesity among Adults, Hyattsville, MD, 1999.
2. U.S. Department of Health and Human Services, National Center for Health Statistics, Centers for Disease Control and Prevention, Prevalence of Obesity among Adults Aged 20 Years and Over: U.S., 1997–2001, Hyattsville, MD, 2002.
3. U.S. Department of Health and Human Services, National Center for Health Statistics, Centers for Disease Control and Prevention, Overweight and Obesity: Obesity Trends: U.S. Obesity Trends 1985–2004, Hyattsville, MD.
4. Variyam, JN., Economic Research Service, USDA. *Food Rev.*, 25(3): 16–20, 2002.
5. U.S. Department of Health and Human Services, National Center for Health Statistics, Centers for Disease Control and Prevention, Early Release of Selected Estimates Based on Data from the January–June 2004 National Health Interview Survey (12/2004).
6. National Heart, Lung, and Blood Institute, National Institute of Diabetes and digestive and Kidney Diseases. Obesity education initiative. In *Clinical Guidelines on the Identification, Evaluation, and Treatment of Overweight and Obesity in Adults: The Evidence Report*, Bethesda, MD: National Heart, Lung and Blood Institute, in cooperation with the National Institute of Diabetes and Digestive and Kidney Diseases: 1998: 12–19, NIH publication No. 98-4083.
7. Wolf, A.M., Colditz, G.A., Current estimates of the economic cost of obesity in the U.S., *Obes Res*, 6: 97–106, 1998.
8. McCance, R.A., Widdowson, E.M., Nutrition and Growth, *Royal Society of London Proceeding*, 158: 326–337, 1962.
9. Hill, J.O., Peters, J.C., Environment Contributions to the Obesity Epidemic, *Science* 280: 1371–1374, 1998.
10. U.S. Department of Health and Human Services, Physical Activity and Health: A Report of the Surgeon General, Atlanta, GA, 1996.
11. Serdula, M.K., Mokdad, A.H., Williamson, D.F. et al., Prevalence of attempting weight loss and strategies for controlling weight, *JAMA*, 282: 1353–1358, 1999.
12. Alford, B.B., Blankenship, A.C., Hagen, R.D., The effects of variations in carbohydrate, protein, fat content of the diet upon weight loss, blood values, and nutrient intake of adult obese women, *J Am Diet Assoc*, 90: 534–540, 1990.
13. Skov, A.R., Toubro, S., Ronn, B., Holm, L., Strup, A., Randomized trial on protein vs. carbohydrate in ad libitum fat reduced diet for the treatment of diabetes, *Int J Obes*, 23: 528–536, 1999.
14. Layman, D.K., Boileau, R.A., Erickson, D.J., Painter, J.E., Shiue, H., Sather, C., Christou, D.D., A reduced ratio of dietary carbohydrate to protein improves body composition and blood lipid profiles during weight loss in adult women, *J Nutr*, 133: 411–417, 2003.
15. Tremblay, A., Differences in fat balance underlying obesity, *Int J Obes*, 19(Suppl. 7): 10S–14S, 1995.
16. *Nutrition and Your Health, Dietary Guidelines for Americans.* U.S. Department of Agriculture, Washington, D.C.: U.S. Govt. Print. Off., 1980.
17. Jahoor, R., Peters, E.J., and Wolfe, R.R., Gluconeogenic precursors supply and glucose production, *FASEB J,* 2:1215, 1988.
18. McGarry, J.D., Kuwajima, M., Newgard, C.B., Foster, D.W., From Dietary Glucose to Liver glycogen, *Annu Rev Nutr*, 7: 51–73, 1987.

19. Wolfe, R.R., Metabolic interactions between glucose and fatty acids in humans, *Am J Clin Nutr*, 67(3 Suppl.): 519S–526S, 1998.

20. Parker, B., Nokes, M., Luscombe, N., Clifton, P., Effects of a high-protein, monounsaturated fat weight loss diet on glycemic control and lipid levels in type 2 diabetes, *Diabetes Care*, 25: 425–430, 2002.

21. Ludwig, D.S., Dietary glycemic index and obesity, *J Nutr*, 130: 280S–283S, 2000.

22. Heller, R.F., Heller, R.F., Hyperinsulinemic obesity and carbohydrate addiction: the missing link is the carbohydrate frequency factor, *Med Hypothesis*, 42: 307–312, 1994.

23. Ullrich, I.H., Albrink, M.J., The effect of dietary fiber and other factors on insulin response: role in obesity, *J Environ Pathol Toxicol Oncol*, 5(6): 137–155, 1985.

24. Cohen, D., Dodds, R., Viberti, G.C., Effect of protein restriction in insulin-dependent diabetics at risk of nephropathy, *Br Med J*, 294: 795–798, 1987.

25. Seney, F.D. Jr., Wright, F.S., Dietary protein suppresses feedback control of glomerular filtration in rats, *J Clin Invest*, 75: 558–568, 1985.

26. Gannon, M.C., Nuttal, F.Q., Lane, J.T., Burmeister, L.A., Metabolic response to cottage cheese or egg white protein, with or without glucose in type 2 diabetic subjects, *Metabolism*, 41: 1137–1145, 1992.

27. Jungas, R.L., Halperin, M.L., Brosnan, F.T., Quantitative analysis of amino acid oxidation and related gluconeogenesis in humans, *Physiol Rev* 72(2): 419–448, 1992.

28. *Nutrition Business Journal*, NBJs Sport Nutrition and Weight Loss Report 2005.

29. Berdanier, C., Proteins, in *Advanced Nutrition: Macronutrients*, 2nd ed., Boca Raton, FL: CRC Press, 130–196, 2000.

30. Dangin, M. et al., The digestion rate of protein is an independent regulating factor of postprandial protein retention, *Am J Physiol Endocrinol Metab.*, 280: E340–E348, 2001.

31. Blomstrand, E., Hassmen, P., Ekblom, B., Newsholme, E.A., Administration of branched-chain amino acids during sustained exercise — effects on performance and on plasma concentration of some amino acids, *Eur J Appl Physiol*, 63: 83–88, 1991.

32. Gibson, N.R., Fereday, A., Cox, M., Halliday, D., Pacy, P.J., Millward, D.J., Influences of dietary energy and protein on leucine kinetics during feeding in healthy adults, *Am J Physiol*, 270: E282–E291, 1996.

33. *Recommended Dietary Allowance*, 10th ed., National Academy Press, Washington, DC, 1989.

34. Evans, W.J., Exercise and nutritional needs of elderly people: effects on muscle and bone, *Gerodontology*, 15: 15, 1998.

35. *Dairy Council Digest*, Health-Enhancing Properties of Dairy Ingredients, 72(2): 7–12, 2001.

36. Boire, Y. et al., Slow and fast dietary proteins differently modulate postprandial protein accretion, *Proc Natl Acad Sci USA*, 94: 14930–14935, 1997.

37. Hall, W.L., Millward, D.J., Long, S.J., Morgan, L.M., Casein and whey exert different effects on plasma amino acid profiles, gastrointestinal hormone secretion and appetite, *Br J Nutr*, 89: 239–248, 2003.

38. Rosenbloom, C., *Sports Nutrition: A Guide for the Professional Working with Active People*, 3rd ed., The American Dietetic Association, Chicago, IL, 2000.

39. Holecek, M., Sprongl, L., Tilser, I., Metabolism of branched-chain amino acids in starved rats: the role of hepatic tissue, *Physiol Res*, 50: 25–33, 2001.

40. Hutson, S.M., Harris, R.A., Leucine as a nutritional signal, *J Nutr*, 131: 839S–840S, 2001.

41. Layman, D.K., The role of leucine in weight loss diets and glucose homeostasis. symposium: dairy product components and weight reduction, *J Nutr*, 133: 261S–267S, 2003.

42. Wagenmaker, A.J.M., Muscle amino acid metabolism at rest and during exercise: role in human physiology and metabolism, *Exerc Sport Sci Rev*, 26: 287–314, 1998.

43. Ruderman, N.B., Muscle amino acid metabolism and gluconeogenesis, *Annu Rev Med*, 26: 245–258, 1975.

44. Platell, C., Kong, S.E., McCauley, R., Hall, J.C., Branched-chain amino acids, *J Gastroenterol Hepatol*, 15: 706–717, 2000.

45. Layman, D.K., Shiue, H., Sather, C., Erickson, D., Baum, J., Increased dietary protein modifies glucose and insulin homeostasis in adult women during weight loss, *J. Nutr*, 133: 405–410, 2003.

46. Muller, W.A., Foloona, G.R., Unger, R.H., The influence of the antecedent diet upon glucagon and insulin secretion, *N Engl J Med*, 285: 1450–1455, 1976.

47. Jahoor, R., Peters, E.J., Wolfe, R.R., Gluconeogenic precursors supply and glucose production, *FASEB J*, 2: 1215, 1988.

48. Janey, N.W., The metabolic relationship of the proteins to glucose, *J Biol Chem*, 20: 321–347, 1915.

49. Harper, A.E., Miller, R.H., Block K.P., Branch-chain amino acid metabolism, *Annu Rev Nutr*, 4: 409–454, 1984.

50. Hers, H.G., Van-Schaftingen, E., Fructose 2,6 bisphosphate 2 years after its discovery, *Biochem J*, 206: 1–12, 1982.

51. Katz, J., Tayek, J.A., Gluconeogenesis and the Cori cycle in 12-, 20-, and 40-h-fasted humans, *Am J Physiol*, 38: E537–E542, 1998.

52. Balasubramanyam, A., McKay, S., Nadkarni, P., Rajan, A.S., Farza, A., Paulik, V., Herd, J.A., Jahoor, F., Reeds, P.J., Ethnicity affects the postprandial regulation of glycogenolysis, *Am J Physiol Endocrinol Metab*, 40: E905–E914, 1999.

53. Mayer, J., Dietary controls of diabetes. In *Human Nutrition: Its Physiological, Medical and Social Aspects*, Charles C Thomas, Springfield, IL, 1972, pp. 525–535.

54. Millward, D.J., Fereday, A., Gibson, N.R., Pacy, P.J., Post-prandial protein metabolism, *Baillere's Clin Endocrinol Metab*, 10: 533–549, 1996.

55. Stipanuk, M.H., Regulation of fuel utilization, in *Biochemical and Physiological Aspects of Human Nutrition*, Stipanuk, M.H. (Ed.), W.B. Saunders, Philadelphia, 2000, chap. 16.

56. Randle, P.J., Garland, P.B., Hales, C.N., and Newsholme, E.A., The glucose fatty acid cycle: its role in insulin sensitivity and the metabolic disturbances of diabetes mellitus, *Lancet*, I: 785–794, 1963.

57. American Institute for Cancer Research, New Survey Shows Americans Ignore Importance of Portion Size in Managing Weight, March 24, 2000, American Institute for Cancer Research http://www.aicr.org/r032400.htm (accessed 26 July 2006).

58. Simon, E., Portillo, M., Fernandez-Quintela, A., Zulet, M., Martinez, J.A., Del Barrio, A.S., Responses to dietary macronutrient distribution of overweight rats under restricted feeding, *Ann Nutr Metab*, 46: 24–31, 2002.

59. Lean, Me.J., Han, T.S., Pravn, T., Richmond, P.R., Avenell, A., Weight loss with high and low carbohydrates 1,200 kcal diets in free living women, *Eur J Clin Nutr*, 51: 243–248, 1997.

60. Tuomilehto, J., Linstrom, J., Erikkson, J.G., Valle, T.T., Hamalainen, H., Ilane-Parikka, P., Keinanen-Kiukaanniemi, S., Laakso, M., Louheranta, A., Rastas, M., Salminen, V., Uusitupa, M., For the Finnish Diabetes Prevention Study Group: Prevention of type 2 diabetes mellitus by changes in lifestyle among subjects with impaired glucose tolerance, *N Engl J Med*, 344: 1343–1350, 2001.

61. Wing, R.R., Blair, E.H., Bononi, P., Marcus, M.D., Watanabe, R., Bergman, R.N., Caloric restriction per se is a significant factor in improvements in glycemic control and insulin sensitivity during weight loss in obese NIDDM patients, *Diabetes Care*, 17: 30–36, 1994.

62. Henry, R.R., Scheaffer, L., Olefsky, J.M., Glycemic effects of intensive caloric restriction and isocaloric refeeding in non-insulin-dependent diabetes mellitus, *J Clin Endocrinol Metab*, 61: 917–925, 1985.

63. Dhahbi, J.M., Mote, P.L., Wingo, J., Rowley, B.C., Cao, S.X., Walford, R.L., Spindler, S.R., Caloric restriction alters the feeding response of key metabolic enzyme genes, *Mech Aging Dev*, 122: 1033–1048, 2001.

64. Karnieli, E., Zarnowski, M.J., Hissin, P.J. et al., Insulin-stimulated translocation of glucose transport systems in the isolated rat adipose cell, *J Biol Chem*, 256(10): 4772–4777, 1981.

65. Sheppard, P.R., Kahn, B.B., Glucose transporters and insulin action, *N Engl J Med*, 341: 248–257, 1999.

66. Cohen, P., *In Control of Enzyme Activity*, 2nd ed., Chapman and Hall, New York, 1983, pp. 42–71.

67. Rossetti, L., Rothman, D.L., DeFronzo, R.A., Shulman, GI., Effects of dietary protein on in vivo insulin action and liver glycogen repletion, *Am J Physiol*, 257: E212–E219, 1989.

68. Mohan, P.F., Rao, B.S.N., Adaptation to underfeeding in growing rats: effect of energy restriction at two dietary protein levels on growth, feed efficiency, basal metabolism and body composition, *J Nutr*, 113: 79–85, 1983.

69. Lee, M., Lucia, S.P., Some relationships between caloric restriction and body weight in the rat. 1. Body composition, liver lipids, and organ weights, *J Nutr*, 74: 243–248, 1961.

70. Hellerstein, M.K., Letscher, A., Schwarz, J.M., Cesar, D., Shackleton, C.H., Turner, S., Nesses, R., Wu, K., Bock, S., Kaempfer, S., Measurement of hepatic Ra UDP-glucose in vivo in rats: relation to glycogen deposition and labeling patterns, *Am J Physiol*, 272: E155–E162, 1997.

71. Christiansen, M.P., Linfoot, P.A., Nesse, R.A., Hellerstein, M.K., Effect of dietary energy restriction on glucose production and substrate utilization in type 2 diabetes, *Diabetes*, 49: 1691–1699, 2000.

72. Boisjoyeux, B., Chanez, M., Azzout, B., Peret, J., Comparison between starvation and consumption of a high protein diet: plasma insulin and glucagon and hepatic activities of gluconeogenic enzymes during the first 24 h, *Diabetes Metab*, 12(1): 21–27, 1986.

73. Peret, J., Chanez, M., Cota, J., Macaire, I., Effects of quantity and quality of dietary protein and variation in certain enzyme activities on glucose metabolism in the rat, *J Nutr*, 105(12): 1525–1534, 1975.

74. Pascual, M., Jahoor, F., Reeds, P.J., Dietary glucose is extensively recycled in the splanchnic bed of fed adult mice, *J Nutr*, 127: 1480–1488, 1997.

75. Mikkelsen, P.B., Toubro, S., and Astrup, A., Effect of fat-reduced diets on 24-h energy expenditure: comparisons between animal protein, vegetable protein, and carbohydrate, *Am J Clin Nutr*, 72: 1135–1141, 2000.

76. Blundell, J.E., Lawton, J.R., Cotton, J.R., Macdiarmid, J.L., Control of human appetite: implications for the intake of dietary fat, *Annu Rev Nutr*, 16: 285–319, 1996.

77. Holt, S.H., Miller, J.C., Petocz, P., Farmakalidis, E., A satiety index of common foods, *Eur J Clin Nutr*, 49: 675–690, 1995.

78. Stubbs, J., Ferres, S., Horgan, G., Energy density of foods: effects on energy intake, *Crit Rev Food Sci Nutr*, 40: 481–515, 2000.

79. Johnstone, A.M., Stubbs, R.J., Harbron, C.G., Effect of overfeeding macronutrients on day-to-day food intake in man, *Eur J Clin Nutr*, 50: 418–430, 1996.

80. Blundell, J.E., Macdiarmid, J.I., Fat as a risk factor for overconsumption: satiation, satiety, and patterns of eating, *J Am Diet Assoc*, 97(Suppl.): S63–S69, 1997.

81. Westerterp-Plantenga, M.S., Rolland, V., Wilson, S.A., Westerterp, K.R., Satiety related to 24 h diet-induced thermogenesis during high protein/carbohydrate vs high fat diets measured in a respiration chamber, *Eur J Clin Nutr*, 53(6): 495–502, 1999.

82. Lajeune, M.P., Westerterp, K.R., Adam, T.C., Luscombe-Marsh, N.D., Westerterp-Plantenga, M.S., Ghrelin and glucagon-like peptide 1 concentrations, 24-h satiety, and energy and substrate metabolism during a high-protein diet and measured in a respiration chamber, *Am J Clin Nutr*, 83(1): 89–94. 2006.

83. Jeffery, R.W., Bjornson-Benson, W.M., Rosenthal, B.S., Linquist, R., Kurth, C.L., Johnson, S.L., Correlates of weight loss and its maintenance over two years of follow-up among middle-aged men, *Prev Med*, 13: 155–168, 1984.

84. Sherwood, N.E., Jeffery, R.W., French, S.A., Hannan, P.J., Murry, D.M., Predictors of weight gain in Pound of Prevention Study, *Int J Obes Relat Metab Disord*, 24: 395–403, 2000.

85. Summary Health Statistics for U.S. Adults: National Health Interview Survey, 2003, Table 29, U.S. Department of Health and Human Services, National Center for Health Statistics, Centers for Disease Control and Prevention, Available at http://www.cdc.gov/nchs/data/series/sr_10/sr10_225.pdf.

86. Segal, K.R. and Pi-Sunyer, F.X., Exercise and obesity, *Med Clin N Am*, 73(1), 1989.

87. Parizkova, J., Impact of age, diet and exercise on man's composition, *Ann N Y Acad. Sci*, 110: 661–674, 1963.

88. Koivisto, V., Hendler, R., Nadel, E., Felig, P., Influence of physical training on fuel-hormone response to prolonged low intensity exercise, *Metabolism* 31: 192–197, 1982.

89. Bjorntorp, P., Fahlen, M., Grimby, G., Gustafson, A., Holm, J., Renstrom, P., Schersten, T., Carbohydrate and lipid metabolism in middle-aged physically well trained men, *Metabolism*, 21: 1037–1044, 1972.

90. Wasserman, D.H., Geer, R.J., Rice, D.E., Bracy, D., Flakoll, P.J., Brown, L.L., Hill, J.O., Abumrad, N.N., Interaction of exercise and insulin action in humans, *Am J Physiol*, 260 (*Endocrinol. Metab* 23): E37–E45, 1991.

91. Paffenbarger, R.S., Hyde, R.T., Wing, A.L. et al., A natural history of athleticism and cardiovascular health, *JAMA*, 252: 491–495, 1984.

92. Satabin, P., Bois-Joyeux, B., Chanez, M., Guezennec, C.Y., Peret, J., Effects of long-term feeding of high-protein or high-fat diets on the response to exercise in the rat, *Eur J Appl Physiol*, 58: 583–590, 1989.

93. James, D.E., Kraegan, E.W., Chisholm, D.J., Muscle glucose metabolism in exercising rats: comparison with insulin stimulation, *Am J Physiol*, 248 (*Endocrinol Metab* 11): E575–E580, 1985.

94. Ji, L.L., Lennon, D.L.F., Kochan, R.G., Nagle, F.J., Hardy, H.A., Enzymatic adaptation to physical training under B-blockade in the rat: evidence of a B2-adrenergic mechanism in skeletal muscle, *J Clin Invest*, 78: 771–778, 1986.
95. Holm, G., Bjorntorp, P., Jagenburg, R., Carbohydrate, lipid, and amino acid metabolism following physical exercise in man, *J Appl Physiol: Respir Environ Exerc Physiol*, 45(1): 128–131, 1978.
96. Rodnick, K.J., Reaven, G.M., Azhar, S., Goodman, M.N., Mondon, C.E., Effects of insulin on carbohydrate and protein metabolism in voluntary running rats, *Am J Physiol*, 259 (*Endocrinol Metab* 22): E706–E714, 1990.
97. Bofardus, C., Ravussin, E., Robbins, D.C., Wolfe, R.R., Horton, E.S., Sims, E.A.H., Effects of physical training and diet therapy on carbohydrate metabolism inpatients with glucose intolerance and non-insulin-dependent diabetes mellitus, *Diabetes*, 33: 311–318, 1984.
98. Wolf, R.R., Goodenough, R.D., Wolfe, M.H., Royle, G.T., Nadel, E.R., Isotopic analysis of leucine and urea metabolism in exercising humans, *J Appl Physiol*, 52: 458–466, 1982.
99. Lemon, P.W., Is increased dietary protein necessary or beneficial for individuals with a physically active lifestyle?, *Nutr Rev*, 54: S169–S175, 1996.
100. Young, V.R., Bier, D.M., Pellet, P.L., A theoretical basis for increasing current estimates of the amino acids requirements in adult men with experimental support, *Am J Clin Nutr*, 50: 80–92, 1989.
101. Bowtell, J.L., Lesse, G.P., Smith, K., Watt, P.W., Nevill, A., Rooyackers, O., Wagenmakers, A.J., Rennie, M.J., Modulation of whole body protein metabolism, during and after exercise, by variation of dietary protein, *J Appl Physiol*, 85: 1744–1752, 1998.
102. Anthony, J.C., Anthony, T.G., Layman, D.K., Leucine supplementation enhances skeletal muscle recovery in rats following exercise, *J Nutr*, 129: 1102–1106, 1999.
103. Layman, D.K., Evans, E., Baum, J.I., Seyler, J.E., Erickson, D.J., Boileau, R.A., Dietary protein and exercise have additive effects on body composition during weight loss in adult women, *J Nutr*, 135: 1903–1910, 2005.
104. Gautsch, T.A., Anthony, J.R., Kimball, S.R., Paul, G.L., Layman, D.K., Jefferson, L.S., Eukaryotic initiation factor 4E availability regulates skeletal muscle protein synthesis during recovery from exercise, *Am J Physiol*, 274: C406–C414, 1998.

21 Nutraceuticals and Inflammation in Athletes

Brendan Plunkett, Robin Callister, and Manohar L. Garg

CONTENTS

I. INTRODUCTION

Optimal nutrition is essential for maintaining or improving athletic performance. Exercise is a catabolic state[1–3] that elicits changes in metabolic signals. Also, exercise has been shown to affect immune function, and these effects may be influenced in part by the nutritional status of the athlete.[4] Acute moderate exercise or regular moderate exercise training may stimulate the immune system whereas intense or prolonged acute exercise or exercise training may compromise immune function.[4] Exercise may also result in tissue damage. Inflammation is an important component of the tissue repair process and is observed in response to exercise as well as to other physical stressors such as trauma, surgery, and burns. Chronic inflammation, however, is likely to compromise the well-being of athletes and compromise athletic performance. Cytokines and eicosanoids are important intracellular signaling molecules involved in regulating inflammation and immune responses, and many are known to be affected by exercise.

Several dietary components have been reported to affect the inflammatory response. This review is focused on the proposed role of dietary supplementation with omega-3 fatty acids and glutamine to modify the inflammatory response to exercise. Relevant articles were obtained through searches of the Medline, Web of Science, Embase, and Cochrane Library databases in which keywords such as *glutamine, omega–3, inflammation, cytokine, eicosanoid*, and *exercise* were used.

In this review, we first summarize the known effects of exercise on inflammatory mediators. We then examine the roles of omega-3 fatty acids and glutamine, and their known effects in nonexercise models of inflammation. Finally, we review the as yet limited data on the effects of omega-3 fatty acids and glutamine on inflammatory mediators related to exercise, and conclude with speculation on the athletes most likely to benefit from omega-3 fatty acids and glutamine dietary supplements.

II. EXERCISE AND INFLAMMATORY MEDIATORS

Strenuous or prolonged endurance exercise is accompanied by increased plasma levels of cate-cholamines, leukocytosis, free fatty acids,[5] interlukin-6 (IL-6), IL-1 receptor antagonist (Ra) and TNF-α, as well as reduced plasma insulin levels,[6] which are similar to the conditions observed in sepsis or trauma.[7] Exercise affects the production of the proinflammatory cytokines IL-1β and TNF-α as well as IL-6 (Table 21.1), which has antiinflammatory as well as pro-inflammatory properties as it can inhibit the production of IL-1β and TNF-α.[8]

Although much remains to be determined regarding cytokine responses to exercise, the type, intensity, and duration of exercise performed are known to influence the production of IL-1β, IL-6, and TNF-α. The production of proinflammatory cytokines is generally increased in response to aerobic exercise in healthy trained and untrained adults. Exercise (45–100% VO$_2$max) increased plasma IL-1β concentrations up to 1 h postexercise,[9] 2 h postexercise,[10] 24 h postexercise,[11] and plasma IL-1 concentrations increased 3 min postexercise[12] in healthy trained and untrained adults. No change in postrace plasma IL-1β concentrations was reported in trained male athletes completing a marathon.[13] Plasma TNF-α concentrations are increased immediately postexercise (60–70% VO$_2$max) and up to 24 h in healthy trained and untrained adults.[6,9,14]

Plasma IL-6 concentrations are increased immediately postmarathon[6,9,13,15] up to 1 h postmarathon in trained males,[16] and up to 2 h postexercise (60–70% VO$_2$max) in healthy untrained adults,[10,11] although no change in plasma IL-6 concentration during and immediately postmarathon has been reported in trained athletes.[17]

The effects of exercise on the major antiinflammatory cytokines IL-4, IL-10 and IL-1Ra (Table 21.1) have been reported to increase, decrease, and be unaffected by exercise. Plasma IL-4 concentrations are not affected immediately postmarathon[13] or up to 1.5 hours postmarathon in trained adults.[18] Plasma IL-10 concentrations are increased immediately postmarathon in trained adults,[9,13,15,17,18] although a decrease postexercise (90% VO$_2$max) in healthy males[19] and postexercise (60% VO$_2$max) in healthy untrained adults[17] has also been reported. IL-1Ra plasma concentrations are increased immediately postmarathon,[15] up to 1 h postmarathon,[9] and up to 1.5 h postmarathon in trained adults,[6] although no significant change in plasma IL-1Ra concentration has been reported during and immediately postmarathon in trained adults.[17] Thus the specific aspects of exercise that determine the changes in the major antiinflammatory cytokines are unclear at this stage.

Eicosanoids are involved in the modulation of the intensity and duration of the inflammatory process. The two major eicosanoids that have been studied in relation to the inflammatory process are prostaglandin E$_2$ (PGE$_2$) and leukotriene B$_4$ (LTB$_4$) (Table 21.1), both of which have a number of proinflammatory properties.[20] Plasma PGE$_2$ concentrations are increased 30 min postexercise[21] and 2 h postexercise in healthy trained and untrained adults.[22] During exercise vastus lateralis interstitial fluid PGE$_2$ concentrations are increased in healthy males.[23] Also, exercise has been reported to have no affect on urinary PGE$_2$ excretion up to 4 h postexercise[24] and no affect on plasma PGE$_2$ concentrations during exercise in healthy trained and untrained adults.[25] Plasma LTB$_4$ concentrations are not significantly changed up to 1 h postexercise in elite athletes[26] and bronchoalveolar fluid LTB$_4$ concentrations are unchanged in healthy trained and untrained adults 1 h postexercise.[27] The effects of exercise on the two major eicosanoids PGE$_2$ and LTB$_4$ are unclear at present as the data available is limited, but it does suggest that PGE$_2$ concentrations are increased and LTB$_4$ concentrations are unchanged in response to exercise by healthy trained and untrained adults.

III. OMEGA-3 FATTY ACIDS

Omega-3 fatty acids are polyunsaturated fatty acids (PUFA) that cannot be synthesized by the body and have to be sourced via the diet; hence, they are termed *essential fatty acids*. Fatty acids are

TABLE 21.1

Major Inflammatory Mediators and Their Actions

Mediator	Action
IL-1	Induces fever
	Up-regulates adhesion molecule expression
	Induces acute phase protein expression
	Costimulates T cell activation
	Stimulates B cell proliferation and maturation
IL-1Ra	Competes with IL-1α and IL-1β for receptor binding
IL-2	Activates T cells
	Stimulates B cell proliferation
sIL-2R	Binds to IL-2
IL-4	Stimulates T_{H2} cell formation
	Inhibits T_{H1} cells
	Inhibits NO production
	Up-regulates B cell and macrophage MHC II expression
	Decreases IL-1β expression
	Up-regulates IL-1Ra synthesis
IL-6	Up-regulates adhesion molecule expression
	Enhances T cell proliferation
	Enhances differentiation of myeloid and B cells into plasma cells
	Induces acute phase protein expression
	Induces IL–1Ra synthesis
IL-10	Inhibits IL-1 and TNF synthesis
	Induces IL-1Ra synthesis
IL-12	Stimulates T_{H1} cell formation
TNF–α	Activates macrophages
	Up-regulates adhesion molecule expression
	Induces cytokine secretion
LTB_4	Increases endothelium permeability
	Up-regulates PMN adhesion molecule expression
	Increases PMN chemotaxis
	Stimulates neutrophil chemotaxis
	Up-regulates monocyte IL-6 expression
PGE_2	Induces fever
	Increases vascular permeability
	Inhibits lymphocyte proliferation
	Inhibits T cell and macrophage cytokine production
IFN-α	Inhibits viral replication
IFN-γ	Up-regulates macrophage activity
	Up-regulates NK cell activity
	Up-regulates expression of MHC II
	Induces NO synthase
CRP	Fixes complement and opsonisation
	Induces expression of endothelial adhesion molecules
PAF	Increases endothelium permeability
	Up-regulates PMN adhesion molecule expression

Note: T_H, T helper cell; NO, nitric oxide; MHC, major histocompatibility complex; PMN, polymorphonuclear neutrophil; NK, natural killer cell.

important in the maintenance of cell membrane structure and are key determinants of membrane bound enzyme activity and receptor expression.[28] There are three essential fatty acids: arachidonic acid (20:4n-6), α-linolenic (omega-3) (18:3n-3), and linoleic acid (18:2n-6). The main PUFA consumed is omega-6 (intake approximately 14g/d for adults) with omega-3 fatty acids contributing approximately 2g/d.[20] The typical Western diet is deficient in omega-3 fatty acids.[29] Omega-3 fatty acids can be sourced from foods such as tuna, sardines, mackerel, green vegetables, macadamia nuts, and oils such as canola, soy, and flaxseed. An inadequate intake of omega-3 fatty acids causes symptoms of hemorrhagic dermatitis, hemorrhagic folliculitis, skin atrophy, and scaly dermatitis.[30]

Omega-3 fatty acids are involved in physiologic processes such as brain and retina function, the transcriptional regulation of gene expression, and the modulation of eicosanoid action. Omega-3 fatty acids affect the inflammatory process and the immune system by affecting cell membrane fatty acid content, the production of inflammatory mediators, adhesion molecule expression, lymphocyte proliferation, antibody production, natural killer cell activity, the triggering of cell death,[31] phagocytosis, reactive oxygen species (ROS) production, leukocyte migration, and antigen presentation by macrophages.[31] Dietary supplementation of omega-3 fatty acids can be beneficial in conditions such as cardiovascular disease,[32,33] thrombotic disease,[34-36] cancer,[37-39] hypertension,[40,41] arthritis,[42-44] and asthma.[45,46]

IV. CELL MEMBRANE FATTY ACID CONTENT

The predominant mechanism by which omega-3 fatty acids may effect the inflammatory response is via eicosapentaenoic acid (EPA) replacing arachidonic acid in the cell membrane, the end product of which produces eicosanoids that are not as biologically active as those derived from arachidonic acid.[20] The predominant fatty acid present in human immune cell membranes is arachidonic acid, which is 15–25% of all phospholipids, with EPA 0.1 to 0.8% and docosahexaenoic acid (DHA) 2 to 4%.[20] EPA and DHA are metabolized from omega-3 fatty acids via chain elongation and desaturation.[47] Changes in cell membrane fatty acid composition alter the membrane fluidity and flexibility, which can affect the binding of cytokines to receptors.[48]

The eicosanoids prostaglandin (PG) and leukotriene (LT) are metabolized from arachidonic acid via the cyclooxygenase and lipoxygenase pathways. Free arachidonic acid, which is mobilized by phospholipase enzymes, acts as a substrate for cyclooxygenase and lipoxygenase to produce 2-series PG and 4-series LT. Omega-3 fatty acids, particularly EPA, that replace arachidonic acid in the cell membrane, are able to competitively inhibit the oxygenation of arachidonic acid and be metabolized via the same pathway.[49] EPA derived eicosanoids are of the 3-series and 5-series, which are not as biologically active as the 2-series and 4-series eicosanoids[20] and can even have antiinflammatory effects.[50] The role of PG and LT in the inflammatory process includes stimulating macrophages and leukocytes to begin the process of destroying invading bacteria.[51] The major proinflammatory eicosanoids studied are LTB_4 and PGE_2.[20]

V. ADHESION MOLECULES

Adhesion molecules, including selectins, vascular adhesion molecules, and intercellular adhesion molecules, are involved in mediating the initial events of the inflammatory process. Adhesion molecules direct leukocyte endothelium interactions, transendothelial migration of leukocytes, and leukocyte trafficking in general.[52] DHA incorporation into cellular lipids decreases the cytokine-induced expression of leukocyte adhesion molecules, secretion of inflammatory mediators, and leukocyte adhesion to endothelial cells.[53,54] The incubation of peripheral blood lymphocytes in EPA and DHA decreased the concentration of cell surface L-selectin.[55] Although the incubation of human umbilical vein endothelial cells with EPA or DHA did not affect adhesion molecule expression, it did suppress monocyte rolling and adherence.[56]

VI. OMEGA-3 FATTY ACIDS AND INFLAMMATORY MEDIATORS

Omega-3 fatty acid supplementation mediates its effects predominantly through altering cell membrane fatty acid content and adhesion molecule expression. Dietary supplementation decreased stimulated IL-1β, IL-1α, and TNF concentration in peripheral blood mononuclear cells (PBMC),[57] IL-1β and TNF-α concentration in blood in trained athletes,[26] and IL-1β, TNF-α, and IL-6 concentration in stimulated lymphocytes in healthy adults.[58] Supplementation decreased PGE$_2$ and LTB$_4$ concentrations in stimulated PBMC supernatant,[59] PGE$_2$ concentration in stimulated lymphocytes,[58] neutrophil LTB$_4$ concentration,[60] and plasma PGE$_2$[26,58] and LTB$_4$ concentrations in healthy adults.[26] This indicates that omega-3 fatty acids inhibit the production of the major proinflammatory cytokines (IL-1β, TNF-α, and IL-6), and eicosanoids (PGE$_2$ and LTB$_4$) in healthy adults.

No direct effects of dietary omega-3 fatty acid supplementation on exercise performance have been demonstrated. Omega-3 fatty acid supplementation does not enhance endurance exercise[61] or maximal exercise performance in trained adults.[62] Although it has been reported that supplementation plus exercise training increases VO$_2$max in sedentary adults, it was also reported that exercise alone increased VO$_2$max to a similar extent,[63] indicating that it was the exercise training and not the fatty acid supplementation that enhanced exercise performance.

VII. GLUTAMINE

Glutamine is a nonessential amino acid, which is produced endogenously and sourced like other amino acids from dietary protein. It is the most abundant amino acid present in the human body, with relatively high concentrations observed in muscle and plasma. The roles of glutamine in the body include: nitrogen transfer between organs, detoxification of ammonia, maintenance of the acid base balance during acidosis, a nitrogen precursor for purine nucleotide synthesis, a fuel for gut mucosal cells, and the regulation of protein synthesis and degradation.[64] Amino acids, principally alanine and glutamine, are the most important source of *de novo* carbon available for glucose metabolism.[65] In a healthy person, endogenous glutamine synthesis is sufficient to maintain normal immune function. Under conditions of stress, reductions in plasma glutamine concentrations can occur. It has been proposed that decreased plasma glutamine levels could be used as a possible indicator of overtraining syndrome (OS) in athletes.[1,2,66] Glutamine synthesis (Figure 21.1) occurs in the skeletal muscle, lungs, liver, brain, and adipose tissue,[1,67] with the main consumers of glutamine being the kidneys, gut, and cells of the immune system.[64] The major site of glutamine utilization is the gastrointestinal tract.[68] Under conditions such as a reduction in dietary carbohydrate, the liver can also become a consumer of glutamine.[64]

Although glucose is the main source of energy for the immune system, glutamine is important in the proliferation of immune cells,[69] cytokine production,[70,71] macrophage phagocytosis,[72] and the synthesis of DNA, RNA, and protein.[73] Glutamine affects the immune system via glutathione,[74] nitric oxide (NO),[75] and heat shock protein (HSP) expression.[76] The main site of glutamine synthesis in the body is skeletal muscle. The rate of glutamine released by muscle to plasma is affected by muscular activity,[77] and a decrease in resting plasma glutamine concentrations has been reported in overtrained endurance athletes.[78]

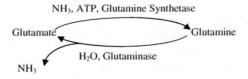

FIGURE 21.1 Glutamine synthesis and hydrolysis.

Dietary amino acids are essential precursors for the production of nitric oxide (NO) and glutathione.[79] NO is an important messenger in the signal transduction process, is involved in innate immunity as a toxic agent towards infectious organisms, is implicated as a pro- and antiinflammatory agent via its inhibitory or apoptotic effect on cells,[80] and is a mediator of sepsis.[81] Glutathione is the most important nonprotein antioxidant in immunocompetent cells. It is essential for normal cell function and replication,[82] and as a sink for ROS.[83] Glutamine can also mediate its antiinflammatory effects through HSP, which are present in cell membranes and protect the cell from proinflammatory mediators.[84] Glutamine is a known inducer of HSP70 expression, which is the major HSP.[85]

Lymphocyte activated killer cell activity is reported to be dependent on glutamine with optimal target cell lysis at glutamine concentrations of 300 μM.[86] An immunological challenge to lymphocytes and monocytes causes an increase in glutaminase activity,[87] which would increase glutamine uptake, hydrolysis (Figure 21.1) and the production of glutamate and ammonia. In incubated lymphocytes glutamine uptake is fourfold higher than glucose.[88] The depletion of glutamine decreases the mitogen-inducible proliferation of lymphocytes[89] while *in vitro* lymphocyte proliferation increases with increasing glutamine concentrations.[73] Gut function can also be disrupted by low glutamine concentrations leading to higher risks of bacterial and viral translocations.[90] A reduction in lymphocyte proliferation can also decrease the production of IL-1 and 2.[73] The optimal plasma glutamine concentration for immune cell proliferation is 300–1000 μM.[87]

Glutamine supplementation is beneficial in reducing tumor growth,[91] length of hospital stay in bone marrow patients,[92] and reducing infection rate in bone marrow transplant patients[93] and multiple trauma patients.[94] It may also be effective in decreasing overall inflammation and increasing measures of nutrition in burns patients,[95] and increasing bodyweight in HIV patients.[96] Glutamine supplementation dosages vary with the current hallmark at 0.5g/kg bodyweight.[97] Glutamine supplementation (0.57 g/kg bodyweight) has not shown any clinical toxicities or generated toxic metabolites (ammonia and glutamate),[98] which can have neurological effects.[99]

Catabolic conditions such as excessive exercise or trauma can decrease plasma glutamine concentrations while glutamine supplementation can maintain normal plasma glutamine concentrations[100–102] or even increase plasma glutamine concentrations.[87,103] Enhanced natural killer cell activity seen with glutamine supplementation can be attributed to the inhibition of PGE_2 synthesis mediated by glutathione.[83] Glutamine supplementation decreases the production of IL-6 and IL-8 in the human gut.[70]

VIII. EXERCISE AND OVERTRAINING SYNDROME

Factors such as exercise, trauma, sepsis, burns, and surgery can reduce plasma glutamine concentrations and potentially compromise the effectiveness of the immune system. Muscular activity can affect the rate of glutamine release by muscle and plasma glutamine concentrations.[77] A reduction in plasma glutamine concentrations is a potential indicator of OS. OS is often characterized by fatigue, chronic or recurrent infections, impaired immune function, and reduced exercise performance.[66] Prolonged exercise can increase plasma cortisol concentration, which stimulates protein catabolism, glutamine release, and hepatic gastrointestinal and renal gluconeogenesis.[2] A drop in the ratio of testosterone to cortisol is proposed to also be an indicator of overtraining.[90] A reduction in plasma glutamine concentration could be a result of either an increase in uptake and demand for glutamine by the tissues that are involved in the use of glutamine or a change in the transport and/or production of glutamine.

The type and duration of exercise performed has different effects on plasma glutamine concentrations. Brief high-intensity exercise has been reported to both increase plasma glutamine concentrations[104,105] and decrease plasma glutamine concentrations.[106] Prolonged endurance exercise decreases plasma glutamine concentrations.[78,107] Athletes with decreased plasma glutamine concentrations can be susceptible to upper respiratory tract infections (URTI).[108] A significant relationship between the frequency of reported URTI symptoms and a prolonged decrease in plasma glutamine concentrations has been observed in overtrained endurance athletes.[78,109] Infection rates may be higher among athletes who participate in endurance-based sports[110] or following intensified training.[111]

There is limited data available on which to evaluate the effects of dietary glutamine supplementation on exercise performance, but the current consensus is that glutamine supplementation has not been shown to enhance exercise performance.[112] Supplementation has been studied in relation to resistance training and high intensity exercise. Glutamine supplementation has no significant effect on muscle performance, body composition, or protein degradation in healthy young adults performing resistance training,[113] does not improve high-intensity exercise performance in trained males,[114] and does not improve the weight-lifting performance of resistance-trained men.[115] Glutamine plus creatine supplementation improves lean body mass and power production during multiple cycle ergometer bouts,[116] but creatine was most likely the effector as a second group of participants that received creatine supplementation minus glutamine had similar gains in lean body mass and power production.

IX. COMBINATION OF GLUTAMINE AND OMEGA-3 SUPPLEMENTATION

Glutamine and omega-3 supplementation has predominantly been studied in the form of immune-enhancing diets and immune formulas for the treatment of patients that have undergone stress such as trauma, surgery, or burns. Nutrition is one of the most important treatments for severe trauma or burns patients.[117] Immune-enhancing formulas and diets that contain glutamine, omega-3 fatty acids, nucleotides, and other amino acids such as arginine can positively modulate postsurgical immunosuppressive and inflammatory responses in patients who have undergone major operations in gastrointestinal cancer, can decrease polymorphonuclear leukocyte supernatant IL-6 and TNF-α,[118] can shorten intensive care unit stay, and can decrease C-reactive protein up to 14 d posttrauma in severe trauma and burn patients[117] and reduce infectious complications in severely injured patients.[119] It is not known what effects combinations of glutamine and omega-3 fatty acids may have on athletes, exercise performance, or exercise-related inflammatory mediators as no studies have been performed.

Athletes most likely to benefit from glutamine and omega-3 fatty acid supplementation may be those on energy restricted diets or in an immuno-compromised state. Low intakes of carbohydrate may increase the utilization of glutamine for energy (anaplerosis) and consequently compromise glutamine availability for other functions. Low intakes of protein may compromise glutamine concentrations, and low intakes of dietary fat or specifically omega-3 fatty acids may increase the risk of chronic or prolonged inflammation during stressed states. Athletes who engage in large training volumes, prolonged high intensity training, or training with a large eccentric component that increases the risk of muscle damage may also benefit. Finally, athletes in sports that have high levels of impact, such as those in the martial arts or contact sports involving tackling, are likely to experience regular inflammation-inducing body impact during training. Athletes in the martial arts in particular may benefit from glutamine and omega-3 fatty acid supplementation as they are frequently on restricted diets in order to compete in particular weight divisions.

X. SUMMARY

Exercise increases the production of the major proinflammatory cytokines IL-1β, TNF-α, and IL-6, but the effects of exercise on PGE$_2$, LTB$_4$, IL-1Ra, IL-4, and IL-10 is unclear at present. Omega-3 fatty acids have antiinflammatory properties via altering eicosanoid production and adhesion molecule expression. Glutamine supplementation can attenuate the decrease in plasma glutamine concentration that occurs under stress conditions and maintain normal immune function. Combined dietary omega-3 fatty acid and glutamine supplementation can be beneficial in reducing infection rate and decreasing the length of hospital stay in patients that have undergone stress such as trauma, surgery, and burns. Whether the beneficial effects of glutamine and omega-3 fatty acid supplementation in trauma patients are applicable to athletes undergoing stress from exercise is unclear. No research has yet been conducted on the effects of dietary omega-3 fatty acid and glutamine supplementation on the inflammatory process or exercise performance in athletes. The types of exercise training, performance, and athletes that may benefit from supplementation with omega-3 fatty acids and/or glutamine remain to be determined.

REFERENCES

1. Rowbottom, D.G., Keast, D., and Morton, A.R., The emerging role of glutamine as an indicator of exercise stress and overtraining, *Sports Med*, 21(2): 80–97, 1996.
2. Walsh, N.P. et al., Glutamine, exercise and immune function, links and possible mechanisms, *Sports Med*, 26(3): 177–91, 1998.
3. Hiscock, N. and Pedersen, B.K., Exercise-induced immunodepression-plasma glutamine is not the link, *J Appl Physiol*, 93(3): 813–22, 2002.
4. Gleeson, M., Pyne, D.B., and Callister, R., The missing links in exercise effects on mucosal immunity, *Exerc Immunol Rev*, 10: 107–28, 2004.
5. Wigernaes, I. et al., Active recovery and post-exercise white blood cell count, free fatty acids, and hormones in endurance athletes, *Eur J Appl Physiol*, 84(4): 358–66, 2001.
6. Toft, A.D. et al., N-3 polyunsaturated fatty acids do not affect cytokine response to strenuous exercise, *J Appl Physiol*, 89(6): 2401–6, 2000.
7. Pedersen, B.K. et al., The cytokine response to strenuous exercise, *Can J Physiol Pharmacol*, 76(5): 505–11, 1998.
8. Suzuki, K. et al., Systemic inflammatory response to exhaustive exercise, Cytokine kinetics, *Exerc Immunol Rev*, 8: 6–48, 2002.
9. Ostrowski, K. et al., Pro- and anti-inflammatory cytokine balance in strenuous exercise in humans, *J Physiol*, 515(Pt. 1): 287–91, 1999.
10. Haahr, P.M. et al., Effect of physical exercise on in vitro production of interleukin 1, interleukin 6, tumor necrosis factor-alpha, interleukin 2 and interferon-gamma, *Int J Sports Med*, 12(2): 223–7, 1991.
11. Moldoveanu, A.I., Shephard, R.J., and Shek, P.N., Exercise elevates plasma levels but not gene expression of IL-1beta, IL-6, and TNF-alpha in blood mononuclear cells, *J Appl Physiol*, 89(4): 1499–504, 2000.
12. Lewicki, R. et al., Effect of maximal physical exercise on T-lymphocyte subpopulations and on interleukin 1 (IL 1) and interleukin 2 (IL 2) production in vitro, *Int J Sports Med*, 9(2): 114–7, 1988.
13. Suzuki, K. et al., Circulating cytokines and hormones with immunosuppressive but neutrophil-priming potentials rise after endurance exercise in humans, *Eur J Appl Physiol*, 81(4): 281–7, 2000.
14. Kimura, H. et al., Highly sensitive determination of plasma cytokines by time-resolved fluoroimmunoassay; effect of bicycle exercise on plasma level of interleukin-1 alpha (IL-1 alpha), tumor necrosis factor alpha (TNF alpha), and interferon gamma (IFN gamma). *Anal Sci*, 17(5): 593–7, 2001.
15. Nieman, D.C. et al., Influence of vitamin C supplementation on cytokine changes following an ultramarathon, *J Interferon Cytokine Res*, 20(11): 1029–35, 2000.
16. Castell, L.M. et al., Some aspects of the acute phase response after a marathon race, and the effects of glutamine supplementation, *Eur J Appl Physiol Occup Physiol*, 75(1): 47–53, 1997.
17. Nieman, D.C. et al., Influence of vitamin C supplementation on oxidative and immune changes after an ultramarathon, *J Appl Physiol*, 92(5): 1970–7, 2002.
18. Nieman, D.C. et al., Cytokine changes after a marathon race, *J Appl Physiol*, 91(1): 109–14, 2001.
19. Brenner, I.K. et al., Impact of three different types of exercise on components of the inflammatory response, *Eur J Appl Physiol Occup Physiol*, 80(5): 452–60, 1999.
20. Calder, P.C. and Grimble, R.F., Polyunsaturated fatty acids, inflammation and immunity, *Eur J Clin Nutr*, 56(Suppl. 3): S14–9, 2002.

21. Laustiola, K. et al., Exercise-induced increase in plasma arachidonic acid and thromboxane B2 in healthy men: effect of beta-adrenergic blockade, *J Cardiovasc Pharmacol*, 6(3): 449–54, 1984.

22. Rhind, S.G. et al., Indomethacin inhibits circulating PGE2 and reverses postexercise suppression of natural killer cell activity, *Am J Physiol*, 276(5 Pt. 2): R1496–505, 1999.

23. Karamouzis, M. et al., The response of muscle interstitial prostaglandin E(2)(PGE(2)), prostacyclin I(2)(PGI(2)) and thromboxane A(2)(TXA(2)) levels during incremental dynamic exercise in humans determined by in vivo microdialysis, *Prostaglandins Leukot Essent Fatty Acids*, 64(4–5): 259–63, 2001.

24. Boger, R.H. et al., Increased prostacyclin production during exercise in untrained and trained men: effect of low-dose aspirin, *J Appl Physiol*, 78(5): 1832–8, 1995.

25. Laustiola, K. et al., The effect of pindolol on exercise-induced increase in plasma vasoactive prostanoids and catecholamines in healthy men, *Prostaglandins Leukot Med*, 20(2): 111–20, 1985.

26. Mickleborough, T.D. et al., Fish oil supplementation reduces severity of exercise-induced bronchoconstriction in elite athletes, *Am J Respir Crit Care Med*, 168(10): 1181–89, 2003.

27. Hopkins, S.R. et al., Sustained submaximal exercise does not alter the integrity of the lung blood-gas barrier in elite athletes, *J Appl Physiol*, 84(4): 1185–9, 1998.

28. Zurier, R.B., Fatty acids, inflammation and immune responses, *Prostaglandins Leukot Essent Fatty Acids*, 48(1): 57–62, 1993.

29. Simopoulos, A.P., Omega-3 fatty acids in health and disease and in growth and development, *Am J Clin Nutr*, 54(3): 438–63, 1991.

30. Bjerve, K.S. et al., Alpha-linolenic acid and long-chain omega-3 fatty acid supplementation in three patients with omega-3 fatty acid deficiency: effect on lymphocyte function, plasma and red cell lipids, and prostanoid formation, *Am J Clin Nutr*, 49(2): 290–300, 1989.

31. Pompeia, C. et al., Effect of fatty acids on leukocyte function, *Braz J Med Biol Res*, 33(11): 1255–68, 2000.

32. Stark, K.D. et al., Effect of a fish-oil concentrate on serum lipids in postmenopausal women receiving and not receiving hormone replacement therapy in a placebo-controlled, double-blind trial, *Am J Clin Nutr*, 72(2): 389–94.

33. Golay, A. et al., [The dual protective effect of fish oil in preventing coronary diseases]. *Schweiz Med Wochenschr*, 119(27–28): 965–9, 1989.

34. Iso, H. et al., Intake of fish and omega-3 fatty acids and risk of stroke in women, *JAMA*, 285(3): 304–12, 2001.

35. Mehta, J., Lawson, D., and Saldeen, T.J., Reduction in plasminogen activator inhibitor-1 (PAI-1) with omega-3 polyunsaturated fatty acid (PUFA) intake, *Am Heart J*, 116(5 Pt. 1): 1201–6, 1988.

36. Dyerberg, J. and Bang, H.O., Haemostatic function and platelet polyunsaturated fatty acids in Eskimos, *Lancet*, 2(8140): 433–5, 1979.

37. Rhodes, L.E. et al., Effect of eicosapentaenoic acid, an omega-3 polyunsaturated fatty acid, on UVR-related cancer risk in humans: an assessment of early genotoxic markers, *Carcinogenesis*, 24(5): 919–25, 2003.

38. Tevar, R. et al., Omega-3 fatty acid supplementation reduces tumor growth and vascular endothelial growth factor expression in a model of progressive non-metastasizing malignancy, *JPEN J Parenter Enteral Nutr*, 26(5): 285–9, 2002.

39. Ge, Y. et al., Effects of adenoviral gene transfer of *C. elegans* n-3 fatty acid desaturase on the lipid profile and growth of human breast cancer cells, *Anticancer Res*, 22(2A): 537–43, 2002.

40. Lungershausen, Y.K. et al., Reduction of blood pressure and plasma triglycerides by omega-3 fatty acids in treated hypertensives, *J Hypertens*, 12(9): 1041–1045, 1994.

41. Bonaa, K.H. et al., Effect of eicosapentaenoic and docosahexaenoic acids on blood pressure in hypertension: a population-based intervention trial from the Tromso study, *N Engl J Med*, 322(12): 795–801, 1990.

42. Volker, D. et al., Efficacy of fish oil concentrate in the treatment of rheumatoid arthritis, *J Rheumatol*, 27(10): 2343–6, 2000.

43. Curtis, C.L. et al., n-3 fatty acids specifically modulate catabolic factors involved in articular cartilage degradation, *J Biol Chem*, 275(2): 721–4, 2000.

44. Hughes, D.A. and Pinder, A.C., n-3 polyunsaturated fatty acids inhibit the antigen-presenting function of human monocytes, *Am J Clin Nutr*, 71(1 Suppl.): 357S–60S, 2000.

45. Nagakura, T. et al., Dietary supplementation with fish oil rich in omega-3 polyunsaturated fatty acids in children with bronchial asthma, *Eur Respir J*, 16(5): 861–5, 2000.

46. Okamoto, M. et al., Effects of dietary supplementation with n-3 fatty acids compared with n-6 fatty acids on bronchial asthma, *Intern Med*, 39(2): 107–11, 2000.

47. Nair, S.S. et al., Prevention of cardiac arrhythmia by dietary (n-3) polyunsaturated fatty acids and their mechanism of action, *J Nutr*, 127(3): 383–93, 1997.

48. Grimble, R.F. and Tappia, P.S., Modulation of pro-inflammatory cytokine biology by unsaturated fatty acids, *Z Ernahrungswiss*, 37(Suppl. 1): 57–65, 1998.

49. Mayser, P. Grimm, H., and Grimminger, F., n-3 fatty acids in psoriasis, *Br J Nutr*, 87(Suppl. 1): S77–82, 2002.

50. Foitzik, T. et al., Omega-3 fatty acid supplementation increases anti-inflammatory cytokines and attenuates systemic disease sequelae in experimental pancreatitis, *JPEN J Parenter Enteral Nutr*, 26(6): 351–6, 2002.

51. Hansen, H.S., New biological and clinical roles for the n-6 and n-3 fatty acids, *Nutr Rev*, 52(5): 162–7, 1994.

52. Grimm, H. et al., Regulatory potential of n-3 fatty acids in immunological and inflammatory processes, *Br J Nutr*, 87(Suppl. 1): S59–67, 2002.

53. De Caterina, R. et al., Omega-3 fatty acids and endothelial leukocyte adhesion molecules, *Prostaglandins Leukot Essent Fatty Acids*, 52(2–3): 191–5, 1995.

54. De Caterina, R. et al., The omega-3 fatty acid docosahexaenoate reduces cytokine-induced expression of proatherogenic and proinflammatory proteins in human endothelial cells, *Arterioscler Thromb*, 14(11): 1829–36, 1994.

55. Khalfoun, B. et al., Docosahexaenoic and eicosapentaenoic acids inhibit in vitro human lymphocyte-endothelial cell adhesion, *Transplantation*, 62(11): 1649–57, 1996.

56. Mayer, K. et al., Omega-3 fatty acids suppress monocyte adhesion to human endothelial cells: role of endothelial PAF generation, *Am J Physiol Heart Circ Physiol*, 283(2): H811–8, 2002.

57. Endres, S. et al., The effect of dietary supplementation with n-3 polyunsaturated fatty acids on the synthesis of interleukin-1 and tumor necrosis factor by mononuclear cells, *N Engl J Med*, 320(5): 265–71, 1989.

58. Meydani, S.N. et al., Effect of oral n-3 fatty acid supplementation on the immune response of young and older women, *Adv Prostaglandin Thromboxane Leukot Res*, 21A: 245–8, 1991.

59. Gallai, V. et al., Cytokine secretion and eicosanoid production in the peripheral blood mononuclear cells of MS patients undergoing dietary supplementation with n-3 polyunsaturated fatty acids, *J Neuroimmunol*, 56(2): 143–53, 1995.

60. Sperling, R.I. et al., Dietary omega-3 polyunsaturated fatty acids inhibit phosphoinositide formation and chemotaxis in neutrophils, *J Clin Invest*, 91(2): 651–60, 1993.

61. Oostenbrug, G.S. et al., Exercise performance, red blood cell deformability, and lipid peroxidation: effects of fish oil and vitamin E. *J Appl Physiol*, 83(3): 746–52, 1997.

62. Raastad, T., Hostmark, A.T. and Stromme, S.B., Omega-3 fatty acid supplementation does not improve maximal aerobic power, anaerobic threshold and running performance in well-trained soccer players, *Scand J Med Sci Sports*, 7(1): 25–31, 1997.

63. Brilla, L.R. and Landerholm, T.E., Effect of fish oil supplementation and exercise on serum lipids and aerobic fitness, *J Sports Med Phys Fitness*, 30(2): 173–80, 1990.

64. Walsh, N.P. et al., The effects of high-intensity intermittent exercise on the plasma concentrations of glutamine and organic acids, *Eur J Appl Physiol Occup Physiol*, 77(5): 434–8, 1998.

65. Garber, A.J. et al., Cyclic nucleotide regulation of glutamine metabolism in skeletal muscle, *Glutamine Metabolism in Mammalian Tissues*, Haussinger, D. and Sies, H., Eds., Berlin, 1984.

66. Rowbottom, D.G. et al., The haematological, biochemical and immunological profile of athletes suffering from the overtraining syndrome, *Eur J Appl Physiol Occup Physiol*, 70(6): 502–9, 1995.

67. Frayn, K.N. et al., Amino acid metabolism in human subcutaneous adipose tissue in vivo, *Clin Sci (Lond)*, 80(5): 471–4, 1991.

68. Elia, M. and Lunn, P.G., The use of glutamine in the treatment of gastrointestinal disorders in man. *Nutrition*, 13(7–8): 743–7, 1997.

69. Castell, L.M. and Newsholme, E.A., The effects of oral glutamine supplementation on athletes after prolonged, exhaustive exercise, *Nutrition*, 13(7–8): 738–42, 1997.

70. Coeffier, M. et al., Glutamine decreases interleukin-8 and interleukin-6 but not nitric oxide and prostaglandins e(2) production by human gut in-vitro, *Cytokine*, 18(2): 92–7, 2002.

71. Aosasa, S. et al., A clinical study of the effectiveness of oral glutamine supplementation during total parenteral nutrition: influence on mesenteric mononuclear cells, *JPEN J Parenter Enteral Nutr*, 23(5 Suppl): S41–4, 1999.

72. Newsholme, P., Why is L-glutamine metabolism important to cells of the immune system in health, postinjury, surgery or infection? *J Nutr*, 131(9 Suppl): 2515S–22S; discussion 2523S–4S, 2001.

73. Newsholme, E.A. and Calder, P.C., The proposed role of glutamine in some cells of the immune system and speculative consequences for the whole animal, *Nutrition*, 13(7–8): 728–30, 1997.

74. van Acker, B.A. et al., Glutamine: the pivot of our nitrogen economy? *JPEN J Parenter Enteral Nutr*, 23(5 Suppl): S45–8, 1999.

75. Bellows, C.F. and Jaffe, B.M., Glutamine is essential for nitric oxide synthesis by murine macrophages, *J Surg Res*, 86(2): 213–9, 1999.

76. Wischmeyer, P.E., Glutamine and heat shock protein expression, *Nutrition*, 18(3): 225–8, 2002.

77. Newsholme, E.A., Biochemical mechanisms to explain immunosuppression in well-trained and over-trained athletes, *Int J Sports Med*, 15(Suppl. 3): S142–7, 1994.

78. Parry-Billings, M. et al., Plasma amino acid concentrations in the overtraining syndrome: possible effects on the immune system, *Med Sci Sports Exerc*, 24(12): 1353–8, 1992.

79. Wu, G., Intestinal mucosal amino acid catabolism, *J Nutr*, 128(8): 1249–52, 1998.

80. Coleman, J.W., Nitric oxide in immunity and inflammation, *Int Immunopharmacol*, 1(8): 1397–406, 2001.

81. Babu, R. et al., Glutamine and glutathione counteract the inhibitory effects of mediators of sepsis in neonatal hepatocytes, *J Pediatr Surg*, 36(2): 282–6, 2001.

82. Hack, V. et al., Decreased plasma glutamine level and CD4+ T cell number in response to 8 wk of anaerobic training, *Am J Physiol*, 272(5 Pt. 1): E788–95, 1997.

83. Amores-Sanchez, M.I. and Medina, M.A., Glutamine, as a precursor of glutathione, and oxidative stress, *Mol Genet Metab*, 67(2): 100–5, 1999.

84. Oehler, R. et al., Glutamine depletion impairs cellular stress response in human leucocytes, *Br J Nutr*, 87(Suppl. 1): S17–21, 2002.

85. Hayashi, Y. et al., Preoperative glutamine administration induces heat-shock protein 70 expression and attenuates cardiopulmonary bypass-induced inflammatory response by regulating nitric oxide synthase activity, *Circulation*, 106(20): 2601–7, 2002.

86. Rohde, T. et al., Effects of glutamine on the immune system: influence of muscular exercise and HIV infection, *J Appl Physiol*, 79(1): 146–50, 1995.

87. Rohde, T., MacLean, D.A., and Pedersen, B.K., Effect of glutamine supplementation on changes in the immune system induced by repeated exercise, *Med Sci Sports Exerc*, 30(6): 856–62, 1998.

88. Newsholme, E.A., Crabtree, B., and Ardawi, M.S., Glutamine metabolism in lymphocytes: its biochemical, physiological and clinical importance, *Q J Exp Physiol*, 70(4): 473–89, 1985.

89. Roth, E., Spittler, A., and Oehler, R., Glutamine: effects on the immune system, protein balance and intestinal functions, *Wien Klin Wochenschr*, 108(21): 669–76, 1996.

90. Petibois, C. et al., Biochemical aspects of overtraining in endurance sports: a review, *Sports Med*, 32(13): 867–78, 2002.

91. Fahr, M.J. et al., Harry M. Vars Research Award. Glutamine enhances immunoregulation of tumor growth, *JPEN J Parenter Enteral Nutr*, 18(6): 471–6, 1994.

92. Schloerb, P.R. and Amare, M., Total parenteral nutrition with glutamine in bone marrow transplantation and other clinical applications (a randomized, double-blind study), *JPEN J Parenter Enteral Nutr*, 17(5): 407–13, 1993.

93. Ziegler, T.R. et al., Clinical and metabolic efficacy of glutamine-supplemented parenteral nutrition after bone marrow transplantation: a randomized, double-blind, controlled study, *Ann Intern Med*, 116(10): 821–8, 1992.

94. Houdijk, A.P. et al., Randomised trial of glutamine-enriched enteral nutrition on infectious morbidity in patients with multiple trauma, *Lancet*, 352(9130): 772–6, 1998.

95. Wischmeyer, P.E. et al., Glutamine administration reduces Gram-negative bacteremia in severely burned patients: a prospective, randomized, double-blind trial versus isonitrogenous control, *Crit Care Med*, 29(11): 2075–80, 2001.

96. Shabert, J.K. et al., Glutamine-antioxidant supplementation increases body cell mass in AIDS patients with weight loss: a randomized, double-blind controlled trial, *Nutrition*, 15(11–12): 860–4, 1999.
97. Savy, G.K., Glutamine supplementation: heal the gut, help the patient, *J Infus Nurs*, 25(1): 65–9, 2002.
98. Ziegler, T.R. et al., Safety and metabolic effects of L-glutamine administration in humans, *JPEN J Parenter Enteral Nutr*, 14(4 Suppl.): 137S–146S, 1990.
99. Garlick, P.J., Assessment of the safety of glutamine and other amino acids, *J Nutr*, 131(9 Suppl.): 2556S–61S, 2001.
100. Rohde, T. et al., Competitive sustained exercise in humans, lymphokine activated killer cell activity, and glutamine — an intervention study, *Eur J Appl Physiol Occup Physiol*, 78(5): 448–53, 1998.
101. Hiscock, N. et al., Glutamine supplementation further enhances exercise-induced plasma IL-6, *J Appl Physiol*, 95(1): 145–8, 2003.
102. Krzywkowski, K. et al., Effect of glutamine supplementation on exercise-induced changes in lymphocyte function, *Am J Physiol Cell Physiol*, 281(4): C1259–65, 2001.
103. Valencia, E., Marin, A., and Hardy, G., Impact of oral L-glutamine on glutathione, glutamine, and glutamate blood levels in volunteers, *Nutrition*, 18(5): 367–70, 2002.
104. Katz, A. et al., Muscle ammonia and amino acid metabolism during dynamic exercise in man, *Clin Physiol*, 6(4): 365–79, 1986.
105. Sewell, D.A., Gleeson, M., and Blannin, A.K., Hyperammonaemia in relation to high-intensity exercise duration in man, *Eur J Appl Physiol Occup Physiol*, 69(4): 350–4, 1994.
106. Keast, D. et al., Depression of plasma glutamine concentration after exercise stress and its possible influence on the immune system, *Med J Aust*, 162(1): 15–8, 1995.
107. Rohde, T. et al., The immune system and serum glutamine during a triathlon, *Eur J Appl Physiol Occup Physiol*, 74(5): 428–34, 1996.
108. Mackinnon, L.T., Immunity in athletes, *Int J Sports Med*, 18(Suppl. 1): S62–8, 1997.
109. Mackinnon, L.T. et al., Hormonal, immunological, and hematological responses to intensified training in elite swimmers, *Med Sci Sports Exerc*, 29(12): 1637–45, 1997.
110. Castell, L.M., Poortmans, J.R., and Newsholme, E.A., Does glutamine have a role in reducing infections in athletes? *Eur J Appl Physiol Occup Physiol*, 73(5): 488–90, 1996.
111. Mackinnon, L.T. and Hooper, S.L., Plasma glutamine and upper respiratory tract infection during intensified training in swimmers, *Med Sci Sports Exerc*, 28(3): 285–90, 1996.
112. Nieman, D.C., Immunological management of athletes: nutritional concerns, *Brain Behav Immun*, 19(5): 465, 2005.
113. Candow, D.G. et al., Effect of glutamine supplementation combined with resistance training in young adults, *Eur J Appl Physiol*, 86(2): 142–9, 2001.
114. Haub, M.D. et al., Acute L-glutamine ingestion does not improve maximal effort exercise, *J Sports Med Phys Fitness*, 38(3): 240–4, 1998.
115. Antonio, J. et al., The effects of high-dose glutamine ingestion on weightlifting performance, *J Strength Cond Res*, 16(1): 157–60, 2002.
116. Lehmkuhl, M. et al., The effects of 8 weeks of creatine monohydrate and glutamine supplementation on body composition and performance measures, *J Strength Cond Res*, 17(3): 425–38, 2003.
117. Chuntrasakul, C. et al., Comparison of an immunonutrition formula enriched arginine, glutamine and omega-3 fatty acid, with a currently high-enriched enteral nutrition for trauma patients, *J Med Assoc Thai*, 86(6): 552–61, 2003.
118. Wu, G.H., Zhang, Y.W. and Wu, Z.H., Modulation of postoperative immune and inflammatory response by immune-enhancing enteral diet in gastrointestinal cancer patients, *World J Gastroenterol*, 7(3): 357–62, 2001.
119. Kudsk, K.A. et al., A randomized trial of isonitrogenous enteral diets after severe trauma: an immune-enhancing diet reduces septic complications, *Ann Surg*, 224(4): 531–40; discussion 540–3, 1996.

22 Oxidative Stress and Antioxidant Requirements in Trained Athletes

Trent A. Watson, Robin Callister,
and Manohar L. Garg

CONTENTS

I. INTRODUCTION

Oxidative stress has been linked to the pathogenesis of many chronic diseases[1] and has demonstrated links to fatigue,[2] muscle damage[2] and reduced immune function,[3] which can all affect exercise performance. Exercise has been shown to increase oxidative stress through the increased production of reactive oxygen species (ROS).[4] Despite this increase in oxidative stress, regular exercise has well-known beneficial effects for health and exercise performance. This unique situation is often termed the *exercise–oxidative stress (EXOS) paradox*.[5] It is not known why the EXOS paradox exists, but it has been hypothesised that the capacity and adaptation of the body's antioxidant defenses may be part of the reason.[6] Ingesting a diet rich in antioxidants to defend against oxidative stress is clearly important, but many other questions remain unanswered. It is largely unknown how dietary antioxidants influence the body's oxidative balance, whether those who participate in regular exercise require antioxidants in addition to the Australian Recommended Dietary Allowances (RDIs), whether diet alone provides enough antioxidants to combat the increases in ROS production induced by exercise, or whether supplementation is required. Questions also remain as to whether dietary or supplemental antioxidants can be used to manipulate the oxidative environment into one that is favourable for health and/or enhance sporting performance.

II. OXIDATIVE STRESS

Oxidative stress is defined as an imbalance between free radical production and the antioxidant defense mechanisms of a biological organism, which results directly or indirectly in cellular damage.[7] Under normal circumstances, the body has adequate antioxidant defenses to cope with resting and significant increases in the production of free radicals. However, if the production of free radicals is excessive or if antioxidant defenses are compromised, the balance tips in favor of free radicals.[8] Free radicals then have the potential to react with and damage every component of the cell including cellular membranes (lipids), cellular enzymes (proteins), and nucleic acids DNA and RNA (nucleic acids) that can alter cellular functioning.[9]

A. FREE RADICALS

A free radical is defined as any molecule or molecular fragment that contains one or more unpaired electrons.[10] The presence of unpaired electrons makes free radicals more reactive than the corresponding nonradicals because free radicals strive to balance their unpaired electrons with electrons from other molecules. When a radical reacts with a nonradical another free radical is formed, creating a chain reaction. Depending on the free radical and the nonradical molecule involved, a chain reaction can give rise to a wide array of free radicals, which potentially could be more or less reactive than the free radical that initiated the chain reaction.[11,12]

B. REACTIVE OXYGEN SPECIES AND OXYGEN-DERIVED FREE RADICALS

Reactive oxygen species (ROS) is an umbrella term used to describe oxygen-derived free radicals and other oxygen-derived molecules (e.g., hydrogen peroxide) that have the capacity to generate highly reactive free radicals. Oxygen generally exists in its diatomic ground state (O_2), which by definition is a diradical because it has two unpaired electrons spinning parallel (i.e., they both share the same spin quantum number) to one another in separate orbitals.[6] This means that oxygen is not very reactive with nonradicals despite its strong oxidizing potential, because nonradical molecules have paired electrons spinning in opposite directions and would not fit the vacant orbital spaces of molecular oxygen, in accordance with Pauli's principle. Consequently, oxygen tends to accept one electron at a time with the potential to form highly reactive oxygen intermediates or ROS, which can potentially cause oxidative stress.[13,14] Paradoxically, oxygen has an essential role in aerobic

TABLE 22.1
Types of Reactive Oxygen Species and Related Species

Radicals		Nonradicals	
$O_2^{-\cdot}$	Superoxide	H_2O_2	Hydrogen peroxide
OH•	Hydroxyl radical	$^1O_2$	Singlet oxygen
$HO_2^{\cdot}$	Hydroperoxyl radical	HOCl	Hypochlorous acid
$NO_2^{\cdot}$	Nitrogen dioxide	$ONOO^-$	Peroxynitrite
$NO^{\cdot}$	Nitrogen oxide		

Source: Data from Noguchi, N. and Niki, E., *Chemistry of Active Oxygen Species and Antioxidants*, Boca Raton, FL: CRC Press, 1998.

metabolism oxidizing carbon- and hydrogen-rich substrates to obtain energy to maintain life. The balance between the essential role and potentially harmful effects of oxygen is commonly referred to as the *oxygen paradox*.[7]

1. Types of ROS

Examples of ROS and related species are listed in Table 22.1. The related species that are created as a result of interaction with ROS will be discussed in later sections.

C. CHARACTERISTICS OF OXIDATIVE STRESS

In biological organisms oxidative stress is characterized by cellular damage. Free radicals have the potential to react with and damage every functional component of the cell by attacking lipids (cellular membrane), proteins (structural and enzymes), and nucleic acids (DNA and RNA). Thus, oxidative stress can be characterized as lipid peroxidation, protein peroxidation, and/or nucleic acid damage. Extensive damage to any one of these components has the potential to alter cellular homeostasis or cause cell death.

D. ANTIOXIDANTS

Antioxidants are defined as molecules, present in small concentrations compared to other oxidizable biologically-relevant molecules, that prevent or reduce the extent of oxidative damage to other biologically-relevant molecules.[14] In other words, antioxidants neutralize ROS to less toxic byproducts and prevent oxidative damage. Thus, the extent of oxidative damage is determined not only by the level of free radical generation but also by the capacity of antioxidant defenses.

There is no such thing as a "universal" antioxidant.[16] A broad array of antioxidants exists endogenously and various antioxidant nutrients consumed in the diet provide additional protection against ROS. Antioxidants are divided into two broad categories: endogenous and exogenous antioxidants. Endogenous antioxidants are produced by the body and include uric acid, bilirubin, plasma proteins and the enzymes superoxide dismutase, glutathione peroxidase, and catalase. Exogenous antioxidants exist in common foods such as vegetables, legumes, nuts, seeds, grains, and fruits that are consumed in our diet, and include vitamin E, vitamin C, and carotenoids. Exogenous antioxidants can also be consumed as manufactured antioxidant supplements, and their possible merits are still largely unknown. Also, there are those antioxidants that can be produced endogenously and consumed in the diet, which include glutathione and coenzyme Q10.[14]

There are various mechanisms by which antioxidant molecules protect against oxidative damage.[17] These act to:

1. Prevent ROS formation
2. Scavenge ROS before they react with biologically-relevant molecules, either by reducing the potency of the ROS or by enhancing the resistance of the biological molecules
3. Ensure less-reactive ROS (e.g., superoxide) don't transform to more deleterious molecules (e.g., hydroxyl radical)
4. Facilitate the repair of damage caused by ROS and trigger the expression of genes encoding antioxidant enzymes
5. Provide a favorable environment for the effective functioning of antioxidants, either by recycling or acting as cofactors to other antioxidants or by binding to metal ions that are capable of generating free radicals such as Fe^{2+}

The point at which an antioxidant has its effect, and the potency of the effect, is dependent on an antioxidant's reduction potential, polarity, bioavailability and pharmacokinetics, and the synergism it has with other antioxidants. The reduction potential of antioxidants is a measure of the ability to reduce a free radical or donate an electron.[18] An antioxidant with a large negative reduction potential has greater ability to donate an electron, increasing its antioxidant ability. Polarity will determine the distribution of antioxidants in polar (aqueous) and no polar (lipid) parts of the body. For example, vitamin E is located strictly within lipid membranes, thus having minimal effect in protecting cellular components outside the membrane.[18] The bioavailability and pharmacokinetics of an antioxidant will also influence its efficiency. In other words, it first has to be absorbed through the gut and persist either unchanged or as sulfated, methylated, conjugated, or active metabolites, which continue having antioxidant effects. Antioxidants that are not absorbed may still have significant antioxidant action within the gastrointestinal tract.[18]

The efficacy of antioxidants to defend against radical species is also dependent on the synergistic interaction between antioxidants. The protection provided by the synergistic interaction between antioxidants is not yet fully understood. It is likely that the body requires a balanced presence of antioxidants to work effectively. For example, an increased carotenoid concentration may result in the formation of cation radicals at levels beyond which vitamin E and C pools can effectively regenerate, resulting in a prooxidant attack.[16] When this balance is intact, the interaction between antioxidants has been suggested to magnify antioxidant capacity and, to some extent, can compensate for antioxidant nutrients that are lacking, by substitution or regeneration, using other antioxidants that are in abundance resulting in a negligible shift in antioxidant capacity.[19, 20]

1. Enzymatic Antioxidants

Three primary antioxidant enzymes exist in the human body: (1) superoxide dismutase (SOD), (2) glutathione peroxidase (GPX), and (3) catalase (CAT). These enzymes work synergistically to neutralize ROS to generate less reactive byproducts.

2. Nonenzymatic Antioxidants

A summary of well known nonenzymatic antioxidants and their potential mode of action are presented in Table 22.2. These antioxidants also work synergistically, which serves to regenerate them following their action against ROS and/or amplify their action against ROS.

E. ANTIOXIDANTS AS PROOXIDANTS

High dose antioxidant supplements are generally perceived at worst as innocuous, which disregards Paracelsus' (1493–1541) fundamental rule of toxicology that every compound is toxic provided the dose is high enough. There are accumulating reports citing potential prooxidant effects of commonly known antioxidants including tocopherols,[21] ascorbic acid,[14] carotenoids,[22] flavanoids, [12,21] dihydrolipoic acid,[23] N-acetyl-cysteine (NAC),[24] urate,[14] and ubiquinone.[25, 26]

TABLE 22.2
Well Known Nonenzymatic Antioxidants and Their Potential Mode of Action

	Action
	Lipid Phase
Vitamin E (α-tocopherol)	Quenches singlet oxygen
	Prevents/breaks lipid peroxidation
	Stabilizes membranes
β-carotene	Quenches singlet oxygen
	Quenches superoxide radical provitamin A
Ubiquinone (coenzyme Q_{10})	Prevents lipid peroxidation
	Can spare vitamin E 2-electron reduction of ubiquinone-10
Flavonoids	Phenolic plant antioxidant
	Inhibit lipid peroxidation (*in vitro*)
	Inhibit lipoxygenase, cyclooxygenase
	Antiinflammatory agent
	Appear to have the highest antioxidant capability *in vitro*
	Aqueous Phase
Ascorbic acid	Quenches aqueous soluble radicals
	Quenches singlet oxygen
	Regenerates vitamin E to reduced form
	Possibly increases glutathione peroxidase activity in red blood cells
	Essential for certain hydroxylase enzymes
Glutathione	Scavenges singlet oxygen
	Regenerates vitamin E and C
	Scavenges hydroxyl radicals
	Removal of hydrogen peroxide (by peroxidase activity)

Antioxidants may act as prooxidants in several ways. First, the radical formed following antioxidant interaction with an ROS has the capacity to generate further oxygen radicals through interaction with cellular components. This will only occur if these antioxidant radicals are not regenerated by synergistic interaction with other antioxidants. This highlights the importance of balanced antioxidant intake and the risk relating to unbalanced antioxidant consumption. Perhaps the relatively smaller amounts of vitamin E and β-carotene provided by whole foods in combination with other antioxidants are examples of this and may explain why the diet provides health benefit, whereas supplementation of these antioxidants fails.[27,28] Second, the reducing power that allows antioxidants to scavenge ROS may also allow it to reduce transition metals, which can facilitate the formation of highly reactive free radicals. Whether these effects are relevant *in vivo* are not known. Most transitional metal ions in healthy humans are bound to transport and storage proteins and are not available to catalyse free radical reactions. Thus, it would be expected that the antioxidant properties of vitamin C would predominate over any prooxidant effects in healthy people. However, situations may occur where the concentration of free metal irons are increased such as in people with haemochromatosis, a condition characterised by iron overload, or in people who have significant tissue injury or cellular disruption that is known to release free metal ions. Childs and colleagues[24] found that participants who exercised eccentrically (known for causing muscle damage) and were supplemented with vitamin C and NAC had increased oxidative stress and cell damage above levels induced by the exercise protocol alone. Prooxidant effects have been shown to occur only *in vitro* when carotenoids are either in high concentrations or subject to high oxygen tension.[22]

The prooxidant action of antioxidants may also depend on how it is delivered to the body. For example, when taken as a supplement vitamin C is totally in the reduced form and can contribute to prooxidant activity whereas vitamin C present in food is comprised of equal portions of reduced and oxidized forms.[20] Similarly, the levels of carotenoid required to act as a prooxidant appear physiologically out of reach unless someone consumes a high supplemental dose of carotenoids in addition to the diet. The prooxidative aspects of antioxidants illustrate that much needs to be learned about the beneficial as well as the detrimental effects of antioxidants and the impact of these compounds on health and exercise performance.

F. EXERCISE-INDUCED OXIDATIVE STRESS

There is an ever-increasing body of direct and indirect evidence showing that exercise increases levels of oxidative stress in both animals and humans. There is evidence that oxidative stress is present in various pathophysiological conditions (e.g., atherosclerosis, retinopathies, muscular dystrophy, some cancers, diabetes, rhuematoid arthritis, aging, ischaemia-reperfusion injury, and Alzheimer's disease).[17] There is also evidence of an association between oxidative stress, fatigue,[29] muscle damage,[29,30] and reduced immune function,[3] all of which can adversely affect exercise performance. Despite an increase in oxidative stress due to exercise, regular exercise has well known beneficial effects for health and exercise performance. This unique situation is often termed the EXOS paradox.[5]

It must also be recognised that oxidative stress has important roles in cell maintenance and turnover, and in the body's immune system. Clanton[31] argued that oxidative stress and the oxidants generated as a result of exercise might simply be a part of the normal homeostatic environment of the cell. Thus, terming it *oxidative stress* may be inappropriate, as it is not a "stress" because it does not seriously threaten the cell's survival. Rather, the minimal alterations in the oxidative state of antioxidants and the generation of ROS and oxidized cellular molecules in response to exercise might be an important part of cell signaling, perhaps as negative-feedback signalling molecules, functioning to protect the muscle from over-stimulation and subsequent injury. Oxidants and their products may also have important roles in normal contracting myocyte to regulate Ca^{2+} metabolism, contractile behavior, or perhaps utilization and control of energy substrates.

An understanding of the mechanisms that contribute to exercise-induced oxidative stress, the associated physiological responses, and the mechanisms that defend against oxidative stress are fundamental to:

1. Gaining a greater understanding of the balance between ROS and antioxidants
2. Controlling oxidative stress-related damage and avoiding possible adverse health effects
3. Determining optimal antioxidant intakes for preventative and therapeutic purposes
4. Determining optimal exercise levels for health and exercise performance [17]

III. EVIDENCE OF OXIDATIVE STRESS IN EXERCISE

A small number of studies have measured electron spin resonance (ESR) or electron paramagnetic resonance (EPR) to provide direct evidence of increased free radical production during exercise. These numbers have remained small because of the inherent limitations with this technique and the inability to use this technique in human muscle-models.[7,13] Davies[4] found EPR signals to increase two- to threefold in rat muscle homogenates following exhaustive treadmill running, providing direct evidence of the increased generation of free radicals in exercising muscle. Jackson[32] also observed an increase (70%) in ESR signals in working vs. resting muscles in rats. In humans, venous blood ESR signals have been investigated by Ashton and coworkers[5,33] who found a three- to fivefold elevation of free radicals postexercise as compared to preexercise samples. These results clearly indicate that exercise increases free radical production within the exercising muscle and in blood post exercise. The exact nature of the free radical (i.e., oxygen-, nitrogen-, or carbon-centered) is still unclear. All of these studies, except Jackson and colleagues,[32] observed lipid peroxidation markers in conjunction with the EPR/ESR signals and found they, too, were significantly elevated following the exercise protocols, supporting the notion that the ESR/EPR signals were generated by ROS.[5]

Most studies investigating the relationship between oxidative stress and exercise have used malondialdehyde (MDA) as an indirect marker.[7] MDA concentration in animal muscle tissue immediately after exercise has been shown to be significantly increased in the majority of studies.[4,34–39] Some studies have observed no change,[38,40] but this was generally muscle-specific and was accompanied by increased MDA concentrations in other muscle types.[34,37] In many human studies plasma MDA immediately following exercise has increased.[5,20,41–49] Other studies found that MDA concentrations remain similar to resting levels,[33,44,48,50–60] and some have reported a fall in plasma MDA following exercise.[61,62] Overall, MDA as an indirect marker has shown a tendency to increase immediately after exercise in tissue and plasma in both animal and human models, suggesting that exercise increases oxidative stress; however, there are many equivocal findings. The TBARS method used to quantify MDA is often criticized because it lacks specificity, and it is believed that this has led to inconsistencies in findings and uncertainty over the relationship between oxidative stress and exercise.

Measuring F_2-Isoprostane has overcome many of the problems associated with MDA and has been recognized as the most promising biomarker for use in human trials examining oxidative stress and associated interventions (e.g., antioxidant or exercise).[63] To date, although there have been few studies investigating the effect of exercise on F_2-Isoprostane concentrations,[24,64–69] those studies have consistently indicated that high-intensity aerobic exercise increases plasma F_2-Isoprostane concentrations during and immediately postexercise.[64–68] These findings support the notion that exercise increases ROS production and oxidative stress.

IV. MECHANISMS THAT MAY INCREASE ROS PRODUCTION IN EXERCISE

A. Electron Transport Chain

The electron transport chain (ETC) is a series of enzyme complexes embedded in the inner membrane of the mitochondria and is best known for its role in generating energy for the body. Electrons are univalently passed down this chain of complexes, while protons are simultaneously moved across the mitochondrial membrane to create a proton gradient. Two terminal complexes (cytochrome oxidase and adenosine triphosphate [ATP] synthase) then catalyse reactions, oxygen (O_2) accepting four electrons to form water (Reaction 1), and the proton gradient being utilized to generate energy in the form of adenosine triphosphate (ATP).[70] The process of reducing oxygen is referred to as *aerobic metabolism* and has been calculated to account for 95 to 98% of the body's total oxygen consumption. The other fraction (2 to 5%) of oxygen is univalently reduced to form the superoxide radical, which can then go on to create the wider range of ROS.[71]

$$O_2 + e^- \rightarrow O_2^{-\bullet} + e + 2H^+ \rightarrow H_2O_2 + e^- + H^+ \rightarrow OH^\bullet + e^- + H^+ \rightarrow H_2O \qquad (22.1)$$

During exercise, energy (ATP) requirements are increased in direct proportion to the level of intensity and duration of exercise. This increases the electron flux along the ETC, thus a greater amount of oxygen is required to terminally accept electrons. It is reported that during exercise whole body O_2 consumption can increase by 10- to 15-fold, and that O_2 flux in an active muscle may increase 100-fold to 200-fold.[17] Thus, if superoxide production increases in proportion with oxygen consumption, the potential of oxidative stress is significantly increased.

There is good evidence to substantiate that ROS production occurs at rest and increases during exercise in both rodent and human models.[4,32] However, the idea that ROS production increases in direct proportion with oxygen consumption during exercise appears unlikely. Rats exposed to 100% oxygen (5 times the normal concentration at sea level) died within 72 h of exposure perhaps due to oxidative stress.[72] Exercise, however, appears protective against early death, which suggests that during exercise there are several mechanisms that protect against massive oxidative stress, such as antioxidant adaptation and/or a reduction in the number of electron leakage sites.[73]

B. XANTHINE OXIDASE

Xanthine oxidase (XO) is an enzyme that functions to clean up any nucleatide byproducts that have not been regenerated into ATP and has been proposed as a potential generator of superoxide following exercise.[74] During resting conditions 80 to 90% of XO exists in the form of xanthine dehydrogenase (XDH), which uses NAD as an electron acceptor in these oxidation reactions. During stressful metabolic events such as exercise, XDH may be converted to XO, which uses O_2 as an electron acceptor to form $O_2^{-\bullet}$.

During high-intensity exercise, XO activity, hypoxanthine, xanthine, and uric acid are increased, suggesting that the XO pathway does play a role in ROS generation during exercise.[74] The evidence that it plays a critical role in oxidant formation during exercise in humans remains unclear. Ischaemic muscle contraction, isometric exercise, sprinting, exercising in a hypoxic environment, and exercise with impaired blood flow due to vascular disease would appear the most likely exercise modalities where XO would play a significant role.[74]

C. INFLAMMATION AND IMMUNITY

The body's inflammatory response is critical in removing damaged protein and preventing bacterial and viral infection. Polymorphonuclear neutrophils, macrophages, and eosinophils are cells involved in this process, which engulf unwanted microorganisms or damaged tissue (phagocytosis) and then break down these components by generating ROS, such as $O_2^{-\bullet}$, H_2O_2, hypochlorous acid (HOCl), and HO•.[75] This process is known as the *oxidative burst*. Although this inflammatory response is considered critical to health, ROS and other oxidants generated from the inflammatory response can also cause secondary damage to functional molecules such as membrane lipids, cellular protein, and DNA.

Exercise is capable of causing muscle tissue damage, via oxidative stress or mechanical forces, which initiates an inflammatory response. This inflammatory response could be responsible for further ROS generation in exercise. However, given the time required for neutrophil infiltration, this mechanism is probably not the primary source of ROS production during short-term exercise.[74] However, it may serve as an important secondary source of ROS production during the recovery period following high intensity, long duration or eccentric exercise.[74]

There are two proposed mechanisms that induce muscle tissue damage during exercise: oxidative stress and mechanical stress (for review, see Reference 75). Oxidative-stress damage to muscle tissue arises when ROS formed from metabolic disturbances (as discussed previously in the electron transport chain and xanthine oxidase sections) exceed antioxidant defenses and attack cellular components. Mechanical muscle tissue damage is caused by, as the name suggests, shear mechanical forces produced during muscle fibre contraction. Mechanical muscle tissue damage appears more pronounced as a result of eccentric-exercise (muscle lengthening) as opposed to concentric-exercise (muscle shortening), and high-intensity exercise. The damaged cells induce an inflammatory response, and ROS are produced to eliminate and/or regenerate the damaged cell (Figure 22.1). This mechanism may be active in exercise that is highly strenuous or long lasting, where ATP is in short supply and maximal oxygen uptake is exceeded.[75]

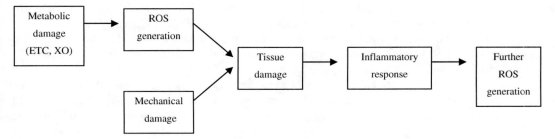

FIGURE 22.1 Inflammatory generation of oxidative stress.

D. METAL IONS

Transitional metals (iron and copper) are important constituents of numerous enzymes in the body. Transitional metals present in the body in their free ionic form have the potential to react with $O_2^{-\bullet}$ and H_2O_2 generating the highly reactive $OH^\bullet$ radical (e.g. $Fe^{2+} + O_2 \rightarrow Fe^{3+} + O_2^{-\bullet}$), which unless removed is likely to create oxidative stress.[10] Most transitional metal ions in healthy humans are bound to transport and store proteins and are not available to catalyze free radical reactions. However, during exercise, tissue injury and cellular disruption may occur, releasing free metal ions.[24]

E. PEROXISOMES

Peroxisomes are organelles located in cells that are involved in nonmitochondrial oxidation of fatty acids and D-amino acids.[74] Several enzymes catalyzing oxidation reactions within peroxisomes that generate H_2O_2 contribute to the steady-state production of ROS in normal metabolism.[14] It has also been shown that when fatty acid oxidation is elevated, H_2O_2 generation is increased.[74] During prolonged exercise fatty acid oxidation becomes a primary energy source for myocardium and skeletal muscle, thus peroxisomes may be a potential site for ROS production during exercise. Catalase is almost entirely located in peroxisomes and its activity has been suggested to act as an indirect measure of ROS production in peroxisomes. Given the equivocal findings with regard to the response of catalase to exercise and exercise training, no clear conclusions can be made of the contribution of peroxisomal ROS production during exercise.[74]

F. OTHER FACTORS

In addition to those mechanisms discussed above, various other factors can induce oxidative stress regardless of exercise. These include cigarette smoke and other air pollutants, alcohol, radiation, and medication (for review see[76]).

V. ANTIOXIDANTS AND EXERCISE

A broad array of antioxidant defense mechanisms exist endogenously and various antioxidant nutrients consumed in the diet provide protection against the production of ROS. However, the response of the body's antioxidant defenses to acute exercise and to regular exercise training remains uncertain.

Total antioxidant capacity (TAC) assays are proposed to reflect the body's overall antioxidant capacity and seem a good starting point to unravel this uncertainty. TAC has been shown to increase in response to exercise,[8,77–79] with few exceptions.[20] Exercise training studies that have measured TAC have yielded conflicting results. Brites and coworkers[80] measured plasma TAC in sportsmen, compared their levels to those of more sedentary subjects, and found resting plasma TAC to be significantly higher (25%) in athletes, indicating that exercise training increases the body's antioxidant capacity. In contrast, Bergholm and colleagues[81] trained (4×1 hr run/wk) male athletes for 3 months and observed a nonsignificant but 15% reduction in TRAP.

Three adaptive processes that increase antioxidant defenses have been identified to occur in response to acute and regular exercise, which may combat the increased production and possible accumulation of ROS. These are (1) the up-regulation of endogenously produced antioxidant enzymes, (2) the *de novo* production of endogenous antioxidant molecules glutathione and urate, and coenzyme increase, and (3) the mobilization of antioxidant vitamins from tissue stores and their transfer through the plasma to sites undergoing oxidative stress. The extent to which these adaptive mechanisms improve the body's ability to defend against oxidative stress is unknown, and the mechanisms behind these adaptive endogenous processes are not well understood.

VI. UP-REGULATION OF ENDOGENOUSLY PRODUCED ANTIOXIDANT ENZYMES

Several studies have observed acute changes in antioxidant enzyme activities.[82–85] The exact mechanism responsible for this up-regulation is unknown, but it has been suggested that the response of antioxidant enzyme activities to acute exercise is too rapid to result from new protein synthesis, although it could be due to posttranslational modifications.[82]

Those that have reviewed the effect of exercise training on endogenous antioxidant enzymes have found slightly conflicting results but have mostly come to similar conclusions (for review, see[29,71,74,86,87]). In most studies, SOD activity has been shown to increase, although a few have suggested that it remains unchanged with training. Similarly, GSHPx activity appears mostly to increase with regular exercise training. CAT was mostly found to remain unchanged but has also been found to increase and decrease as a result of exercise training. It does appear that highly oxidative tissue produces the most marked increase in antioxidant enzymes, and high-intensity and longer duration exercise is superior to low-intensity and short-duration exercise in up-regulating these enzymes, respectively.

VII. INCREASED *DE NOVO* PRODUCTION OF ENDOGENOUS ANTIOXIDANT MOLECULES

Glutathione appears to be regenerated and produced *de novo* in response to acute exercise, and exercise training has been found to improve GSH-dependent antioxidant defenses (for review, see[74,88–90]). During moderate to high intensity exercise, a substantial amount of GSH is oxidized to GSSG in skeletal muscle, the heart, and red blood cells (RBC) when defending against the increased production of ROS. However, GSH redox status (i.e., GSH:GSSG) is tightly regulated and does not alter significantly, because GSSG is quickly reduced back to GSH by glutathione reductase (GR) in the cell using NADPH as a reducing power. Furthermore, if the generation of GSSG exceeds the capacity of GR in the cell, GSSG can be redistributed from the tissue into the blood and GSH can be imported from blood into tissue via the γ-glutamyl-transpeptidase (GGT). The liver is responsible for the supply of GSH through its synthesis of GSH from endogenous or dietary amino acids *de novo* and subsequent efflux into the blood. Muscle and blood GSH content may be reduced during prolonged endurance exercise when liver GSH reserves and/or production either diminish or are overrun by GSH uptake. Exercise training in humans and animals has generally been shown to increase plasma and erythrocyte GSH and total glutathione concentrations, and to improve tolerance to exercise-induced disturbance of blood GSH.

Uric acid appears only to be elevated transiently following both endurance[8,68,91] and short-duration high-intensity exercise.[92,93] Increased plasma urate may arise from the increased demand of ATP during high-intensity exercise. ATP can be regenerated via the adenylate kinase catalyzed reaction and subsequent breakdown of nucleotide byproducts via xanthine oxidaze (already discussed in Subsection IV.B). On the other hand, although there are exceptions,[80] exercise training in the majority of studies appears to reduce both plasma urate concentrations at rest[81,94] and its increase following high intensity exercise.[93] These findings might indicate that exercise training reduces the contribution of urate to the body's antioxidant capacity; however, it might also mean that adaptation from exercise training reduces oxidant production via the xanthine oxidase pathway.

Exercise training has also been shown to increase the ubiquinone content of animal tissue, with the most marked increases occurring in highly oxidative tissue, which is consistent with the well-known mitochondria adaptation to regular exercise.[95, 96]

VIII. MOBILIZATION

Mobilization of antioxidant vitamins from tissue pools and their transfer through the plasma to sites undergoing oxidative stress is a well-established phenomenon and may serve as a mechanism to explain increases in athletes' antioxidant defenses during exercise and in response to exercise training.

Princemail and colleagues demonstrated that tocopherol is mobilized into plasma during acute exercise.[97] Erythrocyte tocopherol stores were shown not to be responsible for the elevation in plasma tocopherol because they also increased during exercise. Thus, the authors proposed that the increase may have come from either the regeneration of tocopheryl radical by vitamin C or through the mobilization of tocopherol into plasma from tissue stores and its redistribution to sites undergoing free radical attack. The later proposal seems the most likely as Gohil recently demonstrated that vitamin C could not attenuate the detrimental effects of vitamin E deficiency.[98] The most likely store of tocopherol appears to be adipose tissue.

Increases in ascorbic acid during exercise have been suggested to arise from an efflux from the adrenal glands, which has the highest concentrations of ascorbic acid in the body.[81,99] Gleeson came to this conclusion after finding that increased ascorbic acid concentrations in plasma were positively correlated with plasma cortisol in 9 men who ran a 21-km race.[99]

Contrary to findings regarding vitamin E and C, there were lower concentrations of coenzyme Q in the plasma of animals subjected to regular exercise compared to sedentary animals. The concentrations of coenzyme Q in liver and skeletal muscle mitochondria of animals exercised until exhaustion were higher than in sedentary animals, suggesting the existence of a mobilization between plasma and mitochondrial membrane for these antioxidants as a response to an oxidative attack.[100] GSH and GSSG are also known to be mobilized from blood into tissue and from the tissue into the blood when the redox balance favors the latter in the cell.

Mobilization of antioxidants is often seen as a transient event that occurs during acute exercise and returns to preexercise levels with rest.[97] However, the recurrent rise and fall of plasma levels that occurs with regular exercise training may contribute to a chronic rise of baseline plasma vitamin levels or an improvement in the ability to mobilize antioxidants, a notion that is supported by several authors.[29,80]

Although mobilization of antioxidants may occur, findings from studies that have investigated the response of circulating exogenously supplied antioxidants to acute[8,48,50,55,62,65,68,77,79,97,101–103] and regular exercise[80,81,94,100,104,105] have been equivocal. One possible explanation for these inconsistent findings regarding the mobilzation of antioxidants is the variation in the type, intensity, and duration of exercise used in studies.

IX. ANTIOXIDANT MANIPULATION, OXIDATIVE STRESS, AND EXERCISE PERFORMANCE

Even during resting conditions, the body's endogenous antioxidant defenses have been shown to be inadequate to completely defend against the body's continual ROS production.[10] Thus, with further elevations in ROS production induced by exercise, it seems reasonable to suggest that exogenous antioxidants not only have an important role in defending against oxidative stress but that those participating in regular exercise require greater amounts.

Although favorable adaptive changes occur to antioxidant defenses as a result of exercise training, people who are unaccustomed to exercise may still be at risk of oxidative stress because their antioxidant defenses have not been conditioned.[106] Athletes may also be at considerable risk, given that they are constantly pushing the barriers of exertion in an effort to maximize performance, which may also exceed adaptive antioxidant mechanisms. At the point where adaptive mechanisms can precede no further, exogenous antioxidant manipulation may be used to create a favorable oxidative environment, which may maximize health outcomes or enhance sporting performance.

X. ANTIOXIDANT DEFICIENCY AND RESTRICTION

Removing antioxidants from a diet is an effective way to establish their role in oxidative stress and exercise performance. In animal studies, antioxidant deficiencies increase oxidative stress and reduce exercise capacity.[4,74,98,107–112] There is limited evidence from human studies to support these findings because in healthy, well-fed subjects, particularly athletes, vitamin deficiencies are rare, difficult to create, and unethical to induce.

The few human studies investigating the effects of short-term restriction of dietary intakes of antioxidants and oxidative stress or performance capacity have had varying results. These studies have predominantly restricted dietary intakes of a single antioxidant such as vitamin E or vitamin C over a short time. No differences in oxidative stress levels were observed between 11 female athletes who consumed habitually a diet low in fat and vitamin E compared to controls consuming a habitual higher-fat, higher-vitamin E diet prior to undertaking a 45 min submaximal run.[113] A difference in performance capacity between the groups was not observed in this study. In contrast, a general reduction in antioxidant defenses was observed in eight healthy men after seven weeks on a vitamin C restricted diet.[114] Another study in six healthy men with a similar methodology (i.e., 6 weeks on a vitamin C restrictive diet of less than 10 mg/d), found a significant decrease in blood vitamin C concentrations, although aerobic capacity was not affected.[115]

In a recent study, 17 healthy male athletes followed a restricted fruit and vegetable diet for 2 weeks. This diet resulted in reducing a wider range of antioxidants than just a single antioxidant source. Oxidative stress was significantly increased during and following exercise in these athletes when following the restricted fruit and vegetable diet, compared to the same athletes undertaking the same exercise test consuming their habitually high antioxidant diet.[116] This study found that antioxidant intakes were reduced threefold on a restricted antioxidant diet, and the subjects' capacity to defend against the increased production of ROS during exercise was also potentially compromised. Although the level of antioxidant restriction did not induce measurable changes in exercise performance, it did increase the athlete's perception of effort. Further dietary antioxidant restriction beyond the levels used in this study may result in reduced exercise performance but has not been tested. As suggested earlier, ethical concerns associated with inducing dietary deficiency in human subjects precludes further investigation.

Animal studies confirm that antioxidant deficiencies can increase oxidative stress and impair exercise capacity, providing strong biological plausibility. However, in human studies, short-term mild-to-moderate antioxidant restriction does not induce deficiency, which may explain why similar findings have not been confirmed in humans. The limited number of studies suggests that dietary antioxidants do provide protection against the increased production of ROS during exercise, play an important role in preventing tissue damage, and provide a more favorable oxidative environment for recovery and exercise performance.

XI. DIETARY INTAKE

Various antioxidant nutrients are consumed in the diet and are believed to provide protection against the production of free radicals, while at the same time the diet provides oxidizable substrates such as PUFAs and catalytic trace metals like iron and copper.[117] Thus, food might exert positive and negative effects, depending on whether the balance of nutrients favors antioxidants or prooxidants. The antioxidant content and activity of whole food such as fruit, vegetables, nuts, and seeds is considered to play a major role in defending the body against oxidative stress[118] and its related pathological conditions.[119]

Few studies looking at exercise-induced oxidative stress have reported dietary intakes of antioxidants[20,41,55,120] or considered the role that food sources of antioxidants have on oxidative stress and antioxidant biomarkers in exercise.[55,120] Hence, the extent to which antioxidants from food sources defend against oxidative stress induced by exercise is largely unknown.

The available research suggests that athletes may require slightly higher amounts of antioxidants than the RDIs to defend against exercise-induced oxidative stress. In athletes consuming a habitually high antioxidant diet (where vitamin C intakes were at least three times the RDI), oxidative stress was not elevated at the completion of a submaximal or maximal exercise test.[153] This outcome suggests these athletes were adequately protected against exercise-induced increases in oxidative stress. Interestingly, when the same athletes switched to a restrictive antioxidant diet for 2 weeks, oxidative stress levels observed at rest were no different than when they had been on the high antioxidant diet. This suggests that at rest, even a restricted antioxidant diet was still adequate to protect against ROS; however, significant increases in oxidative stress were observed during and following the same exercise test in the athletes on the antioxidant restricted diet. This response suggests that, for the subjects in this study, the relatively "low" level of dietary antioxidants consumed over the 2 weeks (i.e., an intake that met the RDIs for vitamin C and contained similar qualities of β-carotene to nonathletes in Australia) was not sufficient to defend against the acute increase in ROS production induced by submaximal and maximal exercise.

Studies comparing athletes with sedentary subjects also indicated that athletes may require a greater antioxidant intake to maintain adequate antioxidant status. Balakrishnan et al.[105] found a reduction in circulating antioxidant levels in athletes compared to sedentary subjects, even though the athletes, antioxidant intake was much greater than that of sedentary subjects. Schroder et al.[120] also found that circulating vitamin C concentrations were reduced throughout a playing season in elite basketball, despite adequate vitamin C intakes.

XII. SUPPLEMENTATION

Antioxidant supplements have been marketed as a means for athletes to train more effectively and maximize performance, via their ability to reduce the oxidative damage induced by exercise, and to enhance recovery.

In population studies, it is well accepted that diets rich in antioxidants are cardio-protective[121] and associated with lower risk of cancer.[122] Further, populations consuming diets rich in fruit, vegetables, and whole grains (and hence antioxidants) generally have higher plasma levels of antioxidants (e.g., vitamin C and E, carotenoids, and certain flavonoids), than populations eating low intakes of these foods.[63,123] These findings led to the widespread promotion of antioxidant supplements as a preventive measure to the general population. It has, however, been argued that these results have been a misinterpretation of mistaking correlation for causation,[12] as results from meta-analyses studies of intervention trials investigating the protective effects of single-antioxidant supplements on health outcomes have not supported their widespread use.

There have been several meta-analyses on population studies aimed at determining the health outcomes of single-antioxidant supplementation trials. The first meta-analysis looked at clinical trials investigating the effect vitamin E and β-carotene supplements have on all-cause mortality and CVD.[27] β-carotene supplementation was found to cause a small but significant increase in all-cause mortality and cardiovascular death, whereas vitamin E did not provide benefit or detriment to all-cause mortality compared to controls. A second meta-analysis investigated the dose-response relationship between vitamin E and all-cause mortality and found that high dosages of vitamin E supplementation (>400IU/d for at least 1 year) increased all-cause mortality. In the dose-response analysis, all-cause mortality progressively increased as vitamin E dosage increased by more than 150IU/d. At dosages less than 150IU/d, all-cause mortality was slightly but not significantly decreased.[28] It is generally thought that high dose antioxidant supplements are perceived at worst as innocuous. In view of the findings that both β-carotene and vitamin E supplementation at high doses increase all-cause mortality, the question must be raised of the appropriateness of high-dose antioxidant supplementation in athletes.

Most studies suggest that vitamin E supplementation in animals[124–126] and humans[127–131] provides protection against exercise-induced oxidative stress and tissue damage. In animal studies vitamin E supplementation has also provided exercise performance benefits.[132,133] In human studies vitamin E has never been found to provide performance benefits,[129,131] except for one study where exercise was conducted at high altitude.[134] Although vitamin E supplementation may reduce exercise-induced oxidative stress, all of these studies have used markers of oxidative stress that have been subject to various criticisms.[7,13,14,135] A study using F_2-isoprostane, a more reliable measure of lipid peroxidation, has found that a combination of vitamin E and C reduced F_2-isoprostane following an ultra marathon, which also contributes to the weight of evidence.[64] However, another recent study that measured F_2-isoprostane found levels were elevated in athletes taking a vitamin E supplement when compared to those taking a placebo following an ultra endurance triathlon.[65] These equivocal findings highlight the uncertainty surrounding the use of vitamin E supplementation to manipulate the antioxidant–prooxidant balance in athletes.

Studies that have examined the relationship of vitamin C supplementation, oxidative stress, and exercise performance have returned equivocal findings. Most studies have shown that vitamin C supplementation has had no effect on oxidative stress and tissue damage.[20,33,49,59,103,136,137] However, some increases[138,139] and decreases[33,137] have been shown. Although vitamin C supplementation may be useful in reducing the effects of exercise-induced muscle damage, it has not been shown to improve exercise performance in rats [98] or humans [33] with adequate or even inadequate vitamin C status. There is evidence to suggest that vitamin C supplementation may even reduce exercise capacity.[112,140]

Ubiquinone supplementation in animals suppresses exercise-induced tissue damage[141] and lipid peroxidation,[142] and improves running time to exhaustion.[142] Human studies have returned equivocal results with regard to ubiquinone supplementation. Exercise-induced cell damage has been reported to increase[25] and lipid peroxidation has been reported to be elevated[143] and remain unchanged[144,145] following supplementation. Although improvement in exercise capacity following ubiquinone supplementation[146] has been reported in healthy active humans, many studies have either found no effect on exercise performance,[145,147,148] or increased perception of effort[148] and significant reductions in exercise capacity.[25,143,144] In contrast to these findings clinical studies have indicated that ubiquinone supplementation has beneficial effects on pathological conditions such as cardiomyopathies, as well as degenerative muscle and neurodegenerative diseases.[149] Each condition has displayed low tissue levels of ubiquinone, suggesting that the benefit from the uptake of dietary sources is mainly related to endogenous deficiencies.[150] Equivocal findings of the effect and uncertainty about the mechanism of action make it impossible to draw any firm conclusions about the use of ubiquinone supplementation in exercise-induced oxidative stress and exercise performance.

Selenium and riboflavin influence glutathione peroxidase (GPX) and GSSG reductase, respectively. Tissue GPX activity is sensitive to selenium status, and selenium deficiency has been shown to increase lipid peroxidation in tissue,[133] but supplementation or deficiency has not had any effect on exercise performance.[151] Glutathione ethyl esters, NAC, and α-lipoic acid have all been used to increase cysteine availability. Glutathione ethyl ester has been shown not to be effective,[74] whereas both NAC and α-lipoic acid interventions during rest and exercise have been shown to enhance cellular GSH levels and decreased GSH oxidation, which generally has resulted in no significant change in lipid peroxidation markers' response to exercise in rats[110,152,153] or humans.[42,154] The effect of glutathione altering supplementation on exercise performance has been equivocal. They have been reported to improve muscle contractile function in rabbits,[155] reduce low frequency fatigue in human leg muscle,[156] and improve endurance time to exhaustion in mice,[157,158] but have no effect on time to exhaustion in rats[110] or humans.[154,159]

In summary, the evidence suggests that the protective effect of diets rich in antioxidants is not simply attributed to antioxidants in isolation. Fruit, vegetables, and wholegrain contain other compounds that have physiological functions that are protective (e.g., phyto-oestrogens, polyphenols, flavonoids).[63] Perhaps vitamin E and β-carotene are simply markers of fruit and vegetable intakes and may not be the primary protective compounds, or more likely, antioxidant nutrients act in synergy with other antioxidants and nutrients in whole foods. It is not surprising that whole, unprocessed food appears to provide antioxidants in the right quantities and combinations to elicit health benefits. A diet that contains antioxidant nutrients in amounts that exceed RDIs as much as threefold is recommended.[153] The levels or dosage and combination of antioxidant supplements that are needed to achieve an antioxidant–prooxidant balance that is favorable for reducing or preventing oxidative stress induced by exercise is still unknown.

XIII. CONCLUSIONS

Current evidence supports the hypothesis that athletes require higher intakes than the RDIs for dietary antioxidants to defend against the increased production of ROS induced by exercise. A diet that restricted antioxidant nutrient intake to levels similar to RDIs was less capable of protecting against the exercise-induced oxidative stress. The findings highlight the importance of the intake of dietary antioxidants when protecting against exercise-induced oxidative stress. There is still uncertainty as to whether antioxidant supplementation provides benefit or harm for an athlete's health and performance. Thus, until research suggests otherwise, the most prudent recommendation regarding antioxidant therapy to optimize the body's capacity to defend against increased ROS production during exercise would be to consume a diet high in antioxidant-rich foods that exceeds the RDIs for antioxidant nutrients by as much as threefold. Antioxidant supplements may only provide beneficial effects for athletes whose long-term diet lacks fruits, vegetables, and other sources of dietary antioxidants and provides dietary antioxidants in amounts less than or equal to the RDIs.

REFERENCES

1. Schwemmer, M., Fink, B., Kockerbauer, R., and Bassenge, E., How urine analysis reflects oxidative stress — nitrotyrosine as a potential marker, *Clin. Chim. Acta* 297: 207–216, 2000.
2. Powers, S.K. and Hamilton, K., Antioxidants and exercise, *Clin. Sports. Med.* 18: 525–536, 1999.
3. Bishop, N.C., Blannin, A.K., Walsh, N.P., Robson, P.J., and Gleeson, M., Nutritional aspects of immunosuppression in athletes, *Sports Med.* 28: 151–176, 1999.
4. Davies, K.J., Quintanilha, A.T., Brooks, G.A., and Packer, L., Free radicals and tissue damage produced by exercise, *Biochem. Biophys. Res. Commun.* 107: 1198–1205, 1982.
5. Ashton, T., Rowlands, C.C., Jones, E., Young, I.S., Jackson, S.K., Davies, B., and Peters, J.R., Electron spin resonance spectroscopic detection of oxygen-centred radicals in human serum following exhaustive exercise, *Eur. J. Appl. Physiol. Occup. Physiol.* 77: 498–502, 1998.
6. Leeuwenburgh, C. and Heinecke, J.W. Oxidative stress and antioxidants in exercise, *Curr. Med. Chem.* 8: 829–838, 2001.
7. Jenkins, R.R. Exercise and oxidative stress methodology: a critique, *Am. J. Clin. Nutr.* 72: 670S–674S, 2000.
8. Liu, M.L., Bergholm, R., Makimattila, S., Lahdenpera, S., Valkonen, M., Hilden, H., Yki-Jarvinen, H., and Taskinen, M.R., A marathon run increases the susceptibility of LDL to oxidation in vitro and modifies plasma antioxidants, *Am. J. Physiol.* 276: E1083–1091, 1999.

9. Awad, J.A., Roberts, L.J., II, Burk, R.F., and Morrow, J.D., Isoprostanes — prostaglandin-like compounds formed in vivo independently of cyclooxygenase: use as clinical indicators of oxidant damage, *Gastroenterol. Clin. North. Am.* 25: 409–427, 1996.

10. Jenkins, R.R., Exercise, oxidative stress, and antioxidants: a review, *Int. J. Sport. Nutr.* 3: 356–375, 1993.

11. Babior, B.M., Phagocytes and oxidative stress, *Am. J. Med.* 109: 33–44, 2000.

12. Halliwell, B., Antioxidants: sense or speculation?, *Nutrition Today.* 29: 15(15), 1994.

13. Clarkson, P.M. and Thompson, H.S., Antioxidants: what role do they play in physical activity and health?, *Am. J. Clin. Nutr.* 72: 637S–646S, 2000.

14. Halliwell, B. and Gutteridge, J., *Free Radicals in Biology and Medicine*, Oxford: Clarendon Press, 1989.

15. Noguchi, N. and Niki, E., *Chemistry of Active Oxygen Species and Antioxidants*, Boca Raton, FL: CRC Press, 1998.

16. Young, A.J. and Lowe, G.M., Antioxidant and prooxidant properties of carotenoids, *Arch. Biochem. Biophys.* 385: 20–27, 2001.

17. Sen, C.K., Oxidants and antioxidants in exercise, *J. Appl. Physiol.* 79: 675–686, 1995.

18. Jovanovic, S.V. and Simic, M.G., Antioxidants in nutrition, *Ann. N. Y. Acad. Sci.* 899: 326–334, 2000.

19. Wayner, D.D., Burton, G.W., Ingold, K.U., Barclay, L.R., and Locke, S.J., The relative contributions of vitamin E, urate, ascorbate and proteins to the total peroxyl radical-trapping antioxidant activity of human blood plasma, *Biochim. Biophys. Acta.* 924: 408–419, 1987.

20. Alessio, H.M., Goldfarb, A.H., and Cao, G., Exercise-induced oxidative stress before and after vitamin C supplementation, *Int. J. Sport. Nutr.* 7: 1–9, 1997.

21. Bast, A. and Haenen, G.R.M.M., The toxicity of antioxidants and their metabolites, *Environ. Toxicol. Pharmacol.* 11: 251–258, 2002.

22. Krinsky, N.I., Carotenoids as antioxidants, *Nutrition* 17: 815–817, 2001.

23. Papas, A.M. *Other Antioxidants*. Boca Raton, FL: CRC Press, 1998.

24. Childs, A., Jacobs, C., Kaminski, T., Halliwell, B., and Leeuwenburgh, C., Supplementation with vitamin C and N-acetyl-cysteine increases oxidative stress in humans after an acute muscle injury induced by eccentric exercise, *Free Radic. Biol. Med.* 31: 745–753, 2001.

25. Malm, C., Svensson, M., Sjoberg, B., Ekblom, B., and Sjodin, B. Supplementation with ubiquinone-10 causes cellular damage during intense exercise, *Acta Physiol. Scand.* 157: 511–512, 1996.

26. Nohl, H., Gille, L., and Staniek, K., The biochemical, pathophysiological, and medical aspects of ubiquinone function, *Ann. N. Y. Acad. Sci.* 854: 394–409, 1998.

27. Vivekananthan, D.P., Penn, M.S., Sapp, S.K., Hsu, A., and Topol, E.J., Use of antioxidant vitamins for the prevention of cardiovascular disease: meta-analysis of randomized trials, *Lancet* 361: 2017–2023, 2003.

28. Miller, E.R., III, Pastor-Barriuso, R., Dalal, D., Riemersma, R.A., Appel, L.J., and Guallar, E., Meta-analysis: high-dosage vitamin e supplementation may increase all-cause mortality, *Ann. Intern. Med.*, 2004.

29. Powers, S.K. and Lennon, S.L., Analysis of cellular responses to free radicals: focus on exercise and skeletal muscle, *Proc. Nutr. Soc.* 58: 1025–1033, 1999.

30. Goldfarb, A.H., Nutritional antioxidants as therapeutic and preventive modalities in exercise-induced muscle damage, *Can. J. Appl. Physiol.* 24: 249–266, 1999.

31. Clanton, T.L., Zuo, L., and Klawitter, P., Oxidants and skeletal muscle function: physiologic and pathophysiologic implications, *Exp. Biol. Med.* 222: 253–262, 1999.

32. Jackson, M.J., Edwards, R.H., and Symons, M.C., Electron spin resonance studies of intact mammalian skeletal muscle, *Biochim. Biophys. Acta.* 847: 185–190, 1985.

33. Ashton, T., Young, I.S., Peters, J.R., Jones, E., Jackson, S.K., Davies, B., and Rowlands, C.C., Electron spin resonance spectroscopy, exercise, and oxidative stress: an ascorbic acid intervention study, *J. Appl. Physiol.* 87: 2032–2036, 1999.

34. Alessio, H.M. and Goldfarb, A.H., Lipid peroxidation and scavenger enzymes during exercise: adaptive response to training, *J. Appl. Physiol.* 64: 1333–1336, 1988.

35. Alessio, H.M., Goldfarb, A.H., and Cutler, R.G., MDA content increases in fast- and slow-twitch skeletal muscle with intensity of exercise in a rat, *Am. J. Physiol.* 255: C874–877, 1988.

36. Bejma, J. and Ji, L.L., Aging and acute exercise enhance free radical generation in rat skeletal muscle, *J. Appl. Physiol.* 87: 465–470, 1999.

37. Liu, J., Yeo, H.C., Overvik-Douki, E., Hagen, T., Doniger, S.J., Chu, D.W., Brooks, G.A., and Ames, B.N., Chronically and acutely exercised rats: biomarkers of oxidative stress and endogenous antioxidants, *J. Appl. Physiol.* 89: 21–28, 2000.

38. Kayatekin, B.M., Gonenc, S., Acikgoz, O., Uysal, N., and Dayi, A., Effects of sprint exercise on oxidative stress in skeletal muscle and liver, *Eur. J. Appl. Physiol.* 87: 141–144, 2002.

39. Arslan, S., Erdem, S., Kilinc, K., Sivri, A., Tan, E., and Hascelik, H.Z., Free radical changes in rat muscle tissue after exercise, *Rheumatol. Int.* 20: 109–112, 2001.

40. Caillaud, C., Py, G., Eydoux, N., Legros, P., Prefaut, C., and Mercier, J., Antioxidants and mitochondrial respiration in lung, diaphragm, and locomotor muscles: effect of exercise, *Free Radic. Biol. Med.* 26: 1292–1299, 1999.

41. Kanter, M.M., Nolte, L.A., and Holloszy, J.O., Effects of an antioxidant vitamin mixture on lipid peroxidation at rest and postexercise, *J. Appl. Physiol.* 74: 965–969, 1993.

42. Sen, C.K., Rankinen, T., Vaisanen, S., and Rauramaa, R., Oxidative stress after human exercise: effect of N-acetylcysteine supplementation, *J. Appl. Physiol.* 76: 2570–2577, 1994.

43. Laaksonen, D.E., Atalay, M., Niskanen, L., Uusitupa, M., Hanninen, O., and Sen, C.K., Increased resting and exercise-induced oxidative stress in young IDDM men, *Diabetes Care.* 19: 569–574, 1996.

44. Marzatico, F., Pansarasa, O., Bertorelli, L., Somenzini, L., and Della Valle, G., Blood free radical antioxidant enzymes and lipid peroxides following long-distance and lactacidemic performances in highly trained aerobic and sprint athletes, *J. Sports Med. Phys. Fitness.* 37: 235–239, 1997.

45. Child, R.B., Wilkinson, D.M., Fallowfield, J.L., and Donnelly, A.E., Elevated serum antioxidant capacity and plasma malondialdehyde concentration in response to a simulated half-marathon run, *Med. Sci. Sports Exerc.* 30: 1603–1607, 1998.

46. Laaksonen, D.E., Atalay, M., Niskanen, L., Uusitupa, M., Hanninen, O., and Sen, C.K., Blood glutathione homeostasis as a determinant of resting and exercise-induced oxidative stress in young men, *Redox Rep.* 4: 53–59, 1999.

47. Child, R.B., Wilkinson, D.M., and Fallowfield, J.L., Effects of a training taper on tissue damage indices, serum antioxidant capacity and half-marathon running performance, *Int. J. Sports Med.* 21: 325–331, 2000.

48. Sacheck, J.M., Milbury, P.E., Cannon, J.G., Roubenoff, R., and Blumberg, J.B., Effect of vitamin E and eccentric exercise on selected biomarkers of oxidative stress in young and elderly men, *Free Radic. Biol. Med.* 34: 1575–1588, 2003.

49. Thompson, D., Williams, C., Garcia-Roves, P., McGregor, S.J., McArdle, F., and Jackson, M.J., Post-exercise vitamin C supplementation and recovery from demanding exercise, *Eur. J. Appl. Physiol.* 89: 393–400, 2003.

50. Duthie, G.G., Robertson, J.D., Maughan, R.J., and Morrice, P.C., Blood antioxidant status and erythrocyte lipid peroxidation following distance running, *Arch. Biochem. Biophys.* 282: 78–83, 1990.

51. Niess, A.M., Hartmann, A., Grunert-Fuchs, M., Poch, B., and Speit, G., DNA damage after exhaustive treadmill running in trained and untrained men, *Int. J. Sports Med.* 17: 397–403, 1996.

52. Surmen-Gur, E., Ozturk, E., Gur, H., Punduk, Z., and Tuncel, P., Effect of vitamin E supplementation on post-exercise plasma lipid peroxidation and blood antioxidant status in smokers: with special reference to haemoconcentration effect, *Eur. J. Appl. Physiol. Occup. Physiol.* 79: 472–478, 1999.

53. Jimenez, L., Lefevre, G., Richard, R., Duvallet, A., and Rieu, M., Exercise does not induce oxidative stress in trained heart transplant recipients, *Med. Sci. Sports Exerc.* 32: 2018–2023, 2000.

54. Alessio, H.M., Hagerman, A.E., Fulkerson, B.K., Ambrose, J., Rice, R.E., and Wiley, R.L., Generation of reactive oxygen species after exhaustive aerobic and isometric exercise, *Med. Sci. Sports Exerc.* 32: 1576–1581., 2000.

55. Sacheck, J.M., Decker, E.A., and Clarkson, P.M., The effect of diet on vitamin E intake and oxidative stress in response to acute exercise in female athletes, *Eur. J. Appl. Physiol.* 83: 40–46, 2000.

56. Akova, B., Surmen-Gur, E., Gur, H., Dirican, M., Sarandol, E., and Kucukoglu, S., Exercise-induced oxidative stress and muscle performance in healthy women: role of vitamin E supplementation and endogenous oestradiol, *Eur. J. Appl. Physiol.* 84: 141–147, 2001.

57. Benitez, S., Sanchez-Quesada, J.L., Lucero, L., Arcelus, R., Ribas, V., Jorba, O., Castellvi, A., Alonso, E., Blanco-Vaca, F., and Ordonez-Llanos, J., Changes in low-density lipoprotein electronegativity and oxidizability after aerobic exercise are related to the increase in associated non-esterified fatty acids, *Atherosclerosis* 160: 223–232, 2002.

58. Lenn, J., Uhl, T., Mattacola, C., Boissonneault, G., Yates, J., Ibrahim, W., and Bruckner, G., The effects of fish oil and isoflavones on delayed onset muscle soreness, *Med. Sci. Sports Exerc.* 34: 1605–1613, 2002.

59. Dawson, B., Henry, G.J., Goodman, C., Gillam, I., Beilby, J.R., Ching, S., Fabian, V., Dasig, D., Morling, P., and Kakulus, B.A., Effect of Vitamin C and E supplementation on biochemical and ultrastructural indices of muscle damage after a 21 km run, *Int. J. Sports Med.* 23: 10–15, 2002.

60. Quindry, J.C., Stone, W. L., King, J., and Broeder, C.E., The effects of acute exercise on neutrophils and plasma oxidative stress, *Med. Sci. Sports Exerc.* 35: 1139–1145, 2003.

61. Groussard, C., Rannou-Bekono, F., Machefer, G., Chevanne, M., Vincent, S., Sergent, O., Cillard, J., and Gratas-Delamarche, A., Changes in blood lipid peroxidation markers and antioxidants after a single sprint anaerobic exercise, *Eur. J. Appl. Physiol.* 89: 14–20, 2003.

62. Rokitzki, L., Logemann, E., Sagredos, A.N., Murphy, M., Wetzel-Roth, W., and Keul, J., Lipid peroxidation and antioxidative vitamins under extreme endurance stress, *Acta Physiol. Scand.* 151: 149–158, 1994.

63. Halliwell, B., Establishing the significance and optimal intake of dietary antioxidants: the biomarker concept, *Nutr. Rev.* 57: 104–113, 1999.

64. Mastaloudis, A., Morrow, J.D., Hopkins, D.W., Devaraj, S., and Traber, M.G., Antioxidant supplementation prevents exercise-induced lipid peroxidation, but not inflammation, in ultramarathon runners, *Free Radic. Biol. Med.* 36: 1329–1341, 2004.

65. Nieman, D.C., Henson, D.A., McAnulty, S.R., McAnulty, L.S., Morrow, J.D., Ahmed, A., and Heward, C.B., Vitamin E and Immunity after the Kona Triathlon World Championship, *Med. Sci. Sports Exerc.* 36: 1328–1335, 2004.

66. Waring, W.S., Convery, A., Mishra, V., Shenkin, A., Webb, D.J., and Maxwell, S.R., Uric acid reduces exercise-induced oxidative stress in healthy adults, *Clin. Sci. (Lond).* 105: 425–430, 2003.

67. Steensberg, A., Morrow, J., Toft, A.D., Bruunsgaard, H., and Pedersen, B.K., Prolonged exercise, lymphocyte apoptosis and F2-isoprostanes, *Eur. J. Appl. Physiol.* 87: 38–42, 2002.

68. Mastaloudis, A., Leonard, S.W., and Traber, M.G., Oxidative stress in athletes during extreme endurance exercise, *Free Radic. Biol. Med.* 31: 911–922, 2001.

69. Hinchcliff, K.W., Reinhart, G.A., DiSilvestro, R., Reynolds, A., Blostein-Fujii, A., and Swenson, R.A., Oxidant stress in sled dogs subjected to repetitive endurance exercise, *Am. J. Vet. Res.* 61: 512–517, 2000.

70. Moran, L.A., Scrimgeour, K.G., Horton, H.R., Ochs, R.S., and Rawn, J.D., *Biochemistry*, 2nd ed., Englewood Cliffs: Neil Patterson Publishers, 1994.

71. Sjodin, B., Hellsten Westing, Y., and Apple, F.S., Biochemical mechanisms for oxygen free radical formation during exercise, *Sports Med.* 10: 236–254, 1990.

72. Crapo, J.D. and Tierney, D.F., Superoxide dismutase and pulmonary oxygen toxicity, *Am. J. Physiol.* 226: 1401–1407, 1974.

73. Herrero, A. and Barja, G., ADP-regulation of mitochondrial free radical production is different with complex I- or complex II-linked substrates: implications for the exercise paradox and brain hypermetabolism, *J. Bioenerg. Biomembr.* 29: 241–249, 1997.

74. Ji, L. L. Antioxidants and oxidative stress in exercise, *Proc. Soc. Exp. Biol. Med.* 222: 283–292, 1999.

75. Pyne, D.B., Exercise-induced muscle damage and inflammation: a review, *Aust. J. Sci. Med. Sport.* 26: 49–58, 1994.

76. Moller, P., Wallin, H., and Knudsen, L.E., Oxidative stress associated with exercise, psychological stress and life-style factors, *Chem. Biol. Interact.* 102: 17–36, 1996.

77. Kaikkonen, J., Kosonen, L., Nyyssonen, K., Porkkala-Sarataho, E., Salonen, R., Korpela, H., and Salonen, J.T., Effect of combined coenzyme Q10 and d-alpha-tocopheryl acetate supplementation on exercise-induced lipid peroxidation and muscular damage: a placebo-controlled double-blind study in marathon runners, *Free Radic. Res.* 29: 85–92, 1998.

78. Maxwell, S.R., Jakeman, P., Thomason, H., Leguen, C., and Thorpe, G.H., Changes in plasma antioxidant status during eccentric exercise and the effect of vitamin supplementation, *Free Radic. Res. Commun.* 19: 191–202, 1993.

79. Vasankari, T.J., Kujala, U.M., Vasankari, T.M., Vuorimaa, T., and Ahotupa, M., Increased serum and low-density-lipoprotein antioxidant potential after antioxidant supplementation in endurance athletes, *Am. J. Clin. Nutr.* 65: 1052–1056, 1997.

80. Brites, F.D., Evelson, P.A., Christiansen, M.G., Nicol, M.F., Basilico, M.J., Wikinski, R.W., and Llesuy, S.F., Soccer players under regular training show oxidative stress but an improved plasma antioxidant status, *Clin. Sci. (Lond).* 96: 381–385, 1999.

81. Bergholm, R., Makimattila, S., Valkonen, M., Liu, M.L., Lahdenpera, S., Taskinen, M.R., Sovijarvi, A., Malmberg, P., and Yki-Jarvinen, H., Intense physical training decreases circulating antioxidants and endothelium-dependent vasodilatation in vivo, *Atherosclerosis.* 145: 341–349, 1999.

82. Ji, L.L. and Fu, R., Responses of glutathione system and antioxidant enzymes to exhaustive exercise and hydroperoxide, *J. Appl. Physiol.* 72: 549–554, 1992.

83. Ji, L.L., Antioxidant enzyme response to exercise and aging, *Med. Sci. Sports Exerc.* 25: 225–231, 1993.

84. Lawler, J.M., Powers, S.K., Visser, T., Van Dijk, H., Kordus, M.J., and Ji, L.L., Acute exercise and skeletal muscle antioxidant and metabolic enzymes: effects of fiber type and age, *Am. J. Physiol.* 265: R1344–1350, 1993.

85. Lawler, J.M., Powers, S.K., Van Dijk, H., Visser, T., Kordus, M.J., and Ji, L.L., Metabolic and antioxidant enzyme activities in the diaphragm: effects of acute exercise, *Respir. Physiol.* 96: 139–149, 1994.

86. Dekkers, J.C., van Doornen, L.J., and Kemper, H.C., The role of antioxidant vitamins and enzymes in the prevention of exercise-induced muscle damage, *Sports Med.* 21: 213–238, 1996.

87. Jenkins, R.R., Free radical chemistry: relationship to exercise, *Sports Med.* 5: 156–170, 1988.

88. Sen, C.K. and Packer, L., Thiol homeostasis and supplements in physical exercise, *J. Clin. Nutr.* 72: 653S–669S, 2000.

89. Sen, C.K., Glutathione homeostasis in response to exercise training and nutritional supplements, *Mol. Cell. Biochem.* 196: 31–42, 1999.

90. Powers, S.K., Ji, L.L., and Leeuwenburgh, C., Exercise training-induced alterations in skeletal muscle antioxidant capacity: a brief review, *Med. Sci. Sports Exerc.* 31: 987–997, 1999.

91. Sutton, J.R., Toews, C.J., Ward, G.R., and Fox, I.H., Purine metabolism during strenuous muscular exercise in man, *Metabolism.* 29: 254–260, 1980.

92. Westing, Y.H., Ekblom, B., and Sjodin, B., The metabolic relation between hypoxanthine and uric acid in man following maximal short-distance running, *Acta Physiol. Scand.* 137: 341–345, 1989.

93. Svensson, M., Malm, C., Tonkonogi, M., Ekblom, B., Sjodin, B., and Sahlin, K., Effect of Q10 supplementation on tissue Q10 levels and adenine nucleotide catabolism during high-intensity exercise, *Int. J. Sport Nutr.* 9: 166–180, 1999.

94. Robertson, J.D., Maughan, R.J., Duthie, G.G., and Morrice, P.C., Increased blood antioxidant systems of runners in response to training load, *Clin. Sci. (Lond).* 80: 611–618, 1991.

95. Gohil, K., Rothfuss, L., Lang, J., and Packer, L., Effect of exercise training on tissue vitamin E and ubiquinone content, *J. Appl. Physiol.* 63: 1638–1641, 1987.

96. Beyer, R.E., Morales-Corral, P.G., Ramp, B.J., Kreitman, K.R., Falzon, M.J., Rhee, S.Y., Kuhn, T.W., Stein, M., Rosenwasser, M.J., and Cartwright, K.J., Elevation of tissue coenzyme Q (ubiquinone) and cytochrome c concentrations by endurance exercise in the rat, *Arch. Biochem. Biophys.* 234: 323–329, 1984.

97. Pincemail, J., Deby, C., Camus, G., Pirnay, F., Bouchez, R., Massaux, L., and Goutier, R., Tocopherol mobilization during intensive exercise, *Eur. J. Appl. Physiol. Occup. Physiol.* 57: 189–191, 1988.

98. Gohil, K., Packer, L., de Lumen, B., Brooks, G.A., and Terblanche, S.E., Vitamin E deficiency and vitamin C supplements: exercise and mitochondrial oxidation, *J. Appl. Physiol.* 60: 1986–1991, 1986.

99. Gleeson, M., Robertson, J.D., and Maughan, R.J., Influence of exercise on ascorbic acid status in man, *Clin. Sci. (Lond).* 73: 501–505., 1987.

100. Quiles, J.L., Huertas, J.R., Manas, M., Ochoa, J.J., Battino, M., and Mataix, J., Oxidative stress induced by exercise and dietary fat modulates the coenzyme Q and vitamin A balance between plasma and mitochondria, *Int. J. Vitam. Nutr. Res.* 69: 243–249, 1999.

101. Meydani, M., Evans, W.J., Handelman, G., Biddle, L., Fielding, R.A., Meydani, S.N., Burrill, J., Fiatarone, M.A., Blumberg, J.B., and Cannon, J.G. Protective effect of vitamin E on exercise-induced oxidative damage in young and older adults, *Am. J. Physiol.* 264: R992–998, 1993.

102. Oostenbrug, G.S., Mensink, R.P., Hardeman, M.R., De Vries, T., Brouns, F., and Hornstra, G., Exercise performance, red blood cell deformability, and lipid peroxidation: effects of fish oil and vitamin E, *J. Appl. Physiol.* 83: 746–752, 1997.

103. Thompson, D., Williams, C., Kingsley, M., Nicholas, C.W., Lakomy, H.K., McArdle, F., and Jackson, M.J., Muscle soreness and damage parameters after prolonged intermittent shuttle-running following acute vitamin C supplementation, *Int. J. Sports Med.* 22: 68–75, 2001.

104. Battino, M., Amadio, E., Oradei, A., and Littarru, G.P., Metabolic and antioxidant markers in the plasma of sportsmen from a Mediterranean town performing non-agonistic activity, *Mol. Aspects Med.* 18: S241–245, 1997.

105. Balakrishnan, S.D. and Anuradha, C.V. Exercise, depletion of antioxidants and antioxidant manipulation, *Cell. Biochem. Funct.* 16: 269–275, 1998.

106. Evans, W.J. Vitamin E, vitamin C, and exercise, *J. Clin. Nutr.* 72: 647S–652S, 2000.

107. Li, Y., Huang, T.T., Carlson, E.J., Melov, S., Ursell, P.C., Olson, J.L., Noble, L.J., Yoshimura, M.P., Berger, C., Chan, P.H. et al., Dilated cardiomyopathy and neonatal lethality in mutant mice lacking manganese superoxide dismutase, *Nat. Genet.* 11: 376–381, 1995.

108. Kondo, T., Reaume, A.G., Huang, T.T., Murakami, K., Carlson, E., Chen, S., Scott, R.W., Epstein, C.J., and Chan, P.H., Edema formation exacerbates neurological and histological outcomes after focal cerebral ischemia in CuZn-superoxide dismutase gene knockout mutant mice, *Acta Neurochir. Suppl. (Wien).* 70: 62–64, 1997.

109. Leeuwenburgh, C. and Ji, L.L., Glutathione depletion in rested and exercised mice: biochemical consequence and adaptation, *Arch. Biochem. Biophys.* 316: 941–949, 1995.

110. Sen, C.K., Atalay, M., and Hanninen, O., Exercise-induced oxidative stress: glutathione supplementation and deficiency, *J. Appl. Physiol.* 77: 2177–2187., 1994.

111. Coombes, J.S., Rowell, B., Dodd, S.L., Demirel, H.A., Naito, H., Shanely, R.A., and Powers, S.K., Effects of vitamin E deficiency on fatigue and muscle contractile properties, *Eur. J. Appl. Physiol.* 87: 272–277, 2002.

112. Packer, L., Gohil, K., deLumen, B., and Terblanche, S.E., A comparative study on the effects of ascorbic acid deficiency and supplementation on endurance and mitochondrial oxidative capacities in various tissues of the guinea pig, *Comp Biochem Physiol. B.* 83: 235–240, 1986.

113. Sacheck, J.M. and Blumberg, J.B., Role of vitamin E and oxidative stress in exercise, *Nutrition* 17: 809–814, 2001.

114. Henning, S.M., Zhang, J.Z., McKee, R.W., Swendseid, M.E., and Jacob, R.A., Glutathione blood levels and other oxidant defense indices in men fed diets low in vitamin C, *J. Nutr.* 121: 1969–1975, 1991.

115. van der Beek, E.J., van Dokkum, W., Schrijver, J., Wesstra, A., Kistemaker, C., and Hermus, R.J., Controlled vitamin C restriction and physical performance in volunteers, *J. Am. Coll. Nutr.* 9: 332–339, 1990.

116. Watson, T.A., Callister, R., Taylor, R.D., Sibbritt, D.W., MacDonald-Wicks, L.K., and Garg, M.L., Antioxidant restriction and oxidative stress in short-duration exhaustive exercise, *Med. Sci. Sports Exerc.* 37: 63–71, 2005.

117. Jacob, R.A., Evidence that diet modification reduces in vivo oxidant damage, *Nutr. Rev.* 57: 255–258, 1999.

118. Miller, E.R., III, Appel, L.J., and Risby, T.H., Effect of dietary patterns on measures of lipid peroxidation: results from a randomized clinical trial, *Circulation* 98: 2390–2395, 1998.

119. Record, I.R., Dreosti, I.E., and McInerney, J.K., Changes in plasma antioxidant status following consumption of diets high or low in fruit and vegetables or following dietary supplementation with an antioxidant mixture, *Br. J. Nutr.* 85: 459–464, 2001.

120. Schroder, H., Navarro, E., Tramullas, A., Mora, J., and Galiano, D., Nutrition antioxidant status and oxidative stress in professional basketball players: effects of a three compound antioxidative supplement, *Int. J. Sports Med.* 21: 146–150, 2000.

121. Bazzano, L.A., Serdula, M.K., and Liu, S., Dietary intake of fruits and vegetables and risk of cardiovascular disease, *Curr. Atheroscler. Rep.* 5: 492–499, 2003.

122. Block, G., Patterson, B., and Subar, A., Fruit, vegetables, and cancer prevention: a review of the epidemiological evidence, *Nutr. Cancer.* 18: 1–29, 1992.

123. Zino, S., Skeaff, M., Williams, S., and Mann, J. Randomised controlled trial of effect of fruit and vegetable consumption on plasma concentrations of lipids and antioxidants, *Br. Med. J.* 314: 1787–1791, 1997.

124. Jackson, M.J., Jones, D.A., and Edwards, R.H., Vitamin E and skeletal muscle, *Ciba. Found. Symp.* 101: 224–239, 1983.

125. Quintanilha, A.T. and Packer, L., Vitamin E, physical exercise and tissue oxidative damage, *Ciba. Found. Symp.* 101: 56–69, 1983.

126. Kumar, C.T., Reddy, V.K., Prasad, M., Thyagaraju, K., and Reddanna, P., Dietary supplementation of vitamin E protects heart tissue from exercise-induced oxidant stress, *Mol. Cell. Biochem.* 111: 109–115, 1992.

127. Sharman, I.M., Down, M.G., and Norgan, N.G., The effects of vitamin E on physiological function and athletic performance of trained swimmers, *J. Sports Med. Phys. Fitness.* 16: 215–225, 1976.

128. Dillard, C.J., Litov, R.E., Savin, W.M., Dumelin, E.E., and Tappel, A.L., Effects of exercise, vitamin E, and ozone on pulmonary function and lipid peroxidation, *J. Appl. Physiol.* 45: 927–932, 1978.

129. Sumida, S., Tanaka, K., Kitao, H., and Nakadomo, F., Exercise-induced lipid peroxidation and leakage of enzymes before and after vitamin E supplementation, *Int. J. Biochem.* 21: 835–838, 1989.

130. Meydani, M., Vitamin E requirement in relation to dietary fish oil and oxidative stress in elderly, *EXS* 62: 411–418, 1992.

131. Rokitzki, L., Logemann, E., Huber, G., Keck, E., and Keul, J., alpha-Tocopherol supplementation in racing cyclists during extreme endurance training, *Int. J. Sport Nutr.* 4: 253–264, 1994.

132. Novelli, G.P., Bracciotti, G., and Falsini, S., Spin-trappers and vitamin E prolong endurance to muscle fatigue in mice, *Free Radic. Biol. Med.* 8: 9–13, 1990.

133. Brady, P.S., Brady, L.J., and Ullrey, D.E., Selenium, vitamin E and the response to swimming stress in the rat, *J. Nutr.* 109: 1103–1109, 1979.

134. Simon-Schnass, I. and Pabst, H., Influence of vitamin E on physical performance, *Int. J. Vitam. Nutr. Res.* 58: 49–54, 1988.

135. Abuja, P.M. and Albertini, R., Methods for monitoring oxidative stress, lipid peroxidation and oxidation resistance of lipoproteins, *Clin. Chim. Acta.* 306: 1–17., 2001.

136. Thompson, D., Bailey, D.M., Hill, J., Hurst, T., Powell, J.R., and Williams, C., Prolonged vitamin C supplementation and recovery from eccentric exercise, *Eur. J. Appl. Physiol,* 2004.

137. Thompson, D., Williams, C., McGregor, S.J., Nicholas, C.W., McArdle, F., Jackson, M.J., and Powell, J.R., Prolonged vitamin C supplementation and recovery from demanding exercise, *Int. J. Sport Nutr. Exerc. Metab.* 11: 466–481, 2001.

138. Bryant, R.J., Ryder, J., Martino, P., Kim, J., and Craig, B.W., Effects of vitamin E and C supplementation either alone or in combination on exercise-induced lipid peroxidation in trained cyclists, *J. Strength Cond. Res.* 17: 792–800, 2003.

139. Vasankari, T., Kujala, U., Sarna, S., and Ahotupa, M., Effects of ascorbic acid and carbohydrate ingestion on exercise induced oxidative stress, *J. Sports Med. Phys. Fitness.* 38: 281–285, 1998.

140. Marshall, R.J., Scott, K.C., Hill, R.C., Lewis, D.D., Sundstrom, D., Jones, G.L., and Harper, J., Supplemental vitamin C appears to slow racing greyhounds, *J. Nutr.* 132: 1616S–1621S, 2002.

141. Shimomura, Y., Suzuki, M., Sugiyama, S., Hanaki, Y., and Ozawa, T., Protective effect of coenzyme Q10 on exercise-induced muscular injury, *Biochem. Biophys. Res. Commun.* 176: 349–355, 1991.

142. Faff, J. and Frankiewicz-Jozko, A., Effect of ubiquinone on exercise-induced lipid peroxidation in rat tissues, *Eur. J. Appl. Physiol. Occup. Physiol.* 75: 413–417, 1997.

143. Malm, C., Svensson, M., Ekblom, B., and Sjodin, B., Effects of ubiquinone-10 supplementation and high intensity training on physical performance in humans, *Acta Physiol. Scand.* 161: 379–384, 1997.

144. Laaksonen, R., Fogelholm, M., Himberg, J.J., Laakso, J., and Salorinne, Y., Ubiquinone supplementation and exercise capacity in trained young and older men, *Eur. J. Appl. Physiol. Occup. Physiol.* 72: 95–100, 1995.

145. Braun, B., Clarkson, P.M., Freedson, P.S., and Kohl, R.L., Effects of coenzyme Q10 supplementation on exercise performance, VO2max, and lipid peroxidation in trained cyclists, *Int. J. Sport Nutr.* 1: 353–365, 1991.

146. Ylikoski, T., Piirainen, J., Hanninen, O., and Penttinen, J., The effect of coenzyme Q10 on the exercise performance of cross-country skiers, *Mol. Aspects Med.* 18 Suppl.: S283–290, 1997.

147. Weston, S.B., Zhou, S., Weatherby, R.P., and Robson, S.J., Does exogenous coenzyme Q10 affect aerobic capacity in endurance athletes?, *Int. J. Sport Nutr.* 7: 197–206, 1997.

148. Porter, D.A., Costill, D.L., Zachwieja, J.J., Krzeminski, K., Fink, W.J., Wagner, E., and Folkers, K., The effect of oral coenzyme Q10 on the exercise tolerance of middle-aged, untrained men, *Int. J. Sports Med.* 16: 421–427, 1995.

149. Dallner, G. and Sindelar, P.J., Regulation of ubiquinone metabolism, *Free Radic. Biol. Med.* 29: 285–294, 2000.

150. Ernster, L. and Dallner, G., Biochemical, physiological and medical aspects of ubiquinone function, *Biochim. Biophys. Acta.* 1271: 195–204, 1995.

151. Tessier, F., Margaritis, I., Richard, M.J., Moynot, C., and Marconnet, P., Selenium and training effects on the glutathione system and aerobic performance, *Med. Sci. Sports Exerc.* 27: 390–396, 1995.

152. Khanna, S., Atalay, M., Laaksonen, D.E., Gul, M., Roy, S., and Sen, C.K., Alpha-lipoic acid supplementation: tissue glutathione homeostasis at rest and after exercise, *J. Appl. Physiol.* 86: 1191–1196, 1999.

153. Sastre, J., Asensi, M., Gasco, E., Pallardo, F.V., Ferrero, J.A., Furukawa, T., and Vina, J., Exhaustive physical exercise causes oxidation of glutathione status in blood: prevention by antioxidant administration, *Am. J. Physiol.* 263: R992–995, 1992.

154. Medved, I., Brown, M.J., Bjorksten, A.R., Leppik, J.A., Sostaric, S., and McKenna, M.J., N-acetylcysteine infusion alters blood redox status but not time to fatigue during intense exercise in humans, *J. Appl. Physiol.* 94: 1572–1582, 2003.

155. Shindoh, C., DiMarco, A., Thomas, A., Manubay, P., and Supinski, G., Effect of N-acetylcysteine on diaphragm fatigue, *J. Appl. Physiol.* 68: 2107–2113, 1990.

156. Reid, M.B., Stokic, D.S., Koch, S.M., Khawli, F.A., and Leis, A.A., N-acetylcysteine inhibits muscle fatigue in humans, *J. Clin. Invest.* 94: 2468–2474, 1994.

157. Novelli, G.P., Falsini, S., and Bracciotti, G., Exogenous glutathione increases endurance to muscle effort in mice, *Pharmacol Res.* 23: 149–155, 1991.

158. Leeuwenburgh, C. and Ji, L.L., Glutathione and glutathione ethyl ester supplementation of mice alter glutathione homeostasis during exercise, *J. Nutr.* 128: 2420–2426, 1998.

159. Medved, I., Brown, M.J., Bjorksten, A.R., and McKenna, M.J., Effects of intravenous N-acetylcysteine infusion on time to fatigue and potassium regulation during prolonged cycling exercise, *J. Appl. Physiol.* 96: 211–217, 2004.

23 Coenzyme Q10: A Functional Food with Immense Therapeutic Potential

Pratibha Chaturvedi, Darrell Vachon, and Najla Guthrie

CONTENTS

I. INTRODUCTION

Oxidative stress is postulated to play an important role in the tissue injury caused by ischemia and reperfusion, inflammation, aging, and various diseases (1–3FR). Furthermore, it has been suggested that oxidative stress plays a role in brain damage, because the brain, a relatively small tissue, uses 20% of all inspired oxygen (4FR), and part (about 5%) of these oxygen molecules are converted to reactive oxygen species (ROS) (5FR). Mitochondria are one of the main sources of ROS, as 95% of molecular oxygen is metabolized within mitochondria, and 2% of total oxygen is converted to ROS as byproducts even under normal conditions (6FR). Coenzyme Q (ubiquinone, CoQ) is well known as a redox carrier in the mitochondrial respiratory chain.

Coenzyme Q (CoQ) or ubiquinone (2,3,-dimethoxy-5-methyl-6-multiprenyl-1,4-benzoquinone) is a redox-active, lipophilic substance present in the hydrophobic interior of the phospholipid bilayer of virtually all cellular membranes. It consists of a quinone head attached to a chain of isoprene units numbering 9 or 10 in the various mammalian species (7FR). CoQ exists in three redox states, fully oxidized, semiquinone, and fully reduced: nevertheless, the existence of different possible levels of protonation increases the possible redox forms of the quinone ring (8FR).

Coenzyme Q plays an essential role as an electron carrier in mitochondrial oxidative phosphorylation and may have an important role as an antioxidant.[1] A role of the bulk of the CoQ in the mitochondrial membrane (as well as in other membranes) is to serve as an antioxidant in its reduced form.[2] The CoQ pool in mitochondria is partly reduced under steady-state conditions of electron transfer; $CoQH_2$ may serve as an antioxidant under oxidative stress conditions. It has also been shown that CoQ10 has a stronger antioxidant activity than CoQ9.[3]

Coenzyme Q10 (CoQ10) is known to be highly concentrated in heart muscle cells due to the high energy requirements of this cell type. For the past 14 years, the great bulk of clinical work with CoQ10 has focused on heart disease. Specifically, congestive heart failure (from a wide variety of causes) has been strongly correlated with significantly low blood and tissue levels of CoQ10.[4] CoQ10 deficiency may well be a primary etiologic factor in some types of heart muscle dysfunction although, in others, it may be a secondary phenomenon. Whether primary, secondary or both, this deficiency of CoQ10 appears to be a major treatable factor in the otherwise inexorable progression of heart failure. Internationally, there have been a number of nine placebo-controlled studies on the treatment of heart disease with CoQ10 that have confirmed the effectiveness and remarkable safety of this method of treatment.[5–13].

II. HISTORY OF CoQ10

CoQ10 was first isolated from beef heart mitochondria in 1957.[14] The same year, a compound obtained from vitamin A-deficient rat liver was defined to be the same as CoQ10[15] and named ubiquinone, meaning the ubiquitous quinone. The precise chemical structure of CoQ10: 2,3 dimethoxy-5 methyl-6 decaprenyl benzoquinone, was determined in 1958 (Figure 23.1). In the mid-1960s, coenzyme Q7 (a related compound) was used for the first time in the treatment of congestive heart failure in humans. In 1966, Mellors and Tappel showed that reduced CoQ6 was an effective antioxidant.[16,17] In 1972 it was reported that there is a deficiency of CoQ10 in human heart disease.[18] By the mid-1970s, pure CoQ10 in sufficient quantities for larger clinical trials was being produced in Japan. Peter Mitchell received the Nobel Prize in 1978 for his contribution to the understanding of biological energy transfer through the formulation of the chemiosmotic theory, which includes the vital protonmotive role of CoQ10 in energy transfer systems.[1,19–21]

In the early 1980s, there were a number of clinical trials with CoQ10. These resulted in part from the availability of pure CoQ10 in large quantities from pharmaceutical companies in Japan and from the capacity to directly measure CoQ10 in blood and tissue by high performance liquid chromatography. Lars Ernster of Sweden enlarged upon CoQ10's importance as an antioxidant and free radical scavenger.[2] Professor Karl Folkers went on to receive the Priestly Medal from the American Chemical Society in 1986 and the National Medal of Science from President Bush in 1990 for his work with CoQ10 and other vitamins.

III. CoQ10 DEFICIENCY

Significantly decreased levels of CoQ10 have been reported in a wide variety of diseases in both animal and human studies. CoQ10 deficiency may be caused by insufficient dietary availability, impairment in its biosynthesis, excessive utilization by the body, or any combination of the three. Decreased dietary intake is presumed in chronic malnutrition and cachexia.[3]

The main source of CoQ10 in humans is biosynthesis. The biosynthesis of CoQ10 is a complex process and requires at least seven vitamins (vitamin B_2 [riboflavin], vitamin B_3 [niacinamide], vitamin B_6, folic acid, vitamin B_{12}, vitamin C, and pantothenic acid) and several trace elements. Suboptimal nutrient intake of these leads to subsequent secondary impairment in CoQ10 biosynthesis.

HMG-CoA reductase inhibitors used to treat high blood cholesterol levels by blocking cholesterol biosynthesis also block CoQ10 biosynthesis due to the partially shared biosynthetic pathway of CoQ10 and cholesterol leading to CoQ10 deficiency.[4] The lowering of CoQ10 can have a significantly harmful effect in patients with cardiovascular diseases (CVD); however, this can be controlled by oral supplementation.[5]

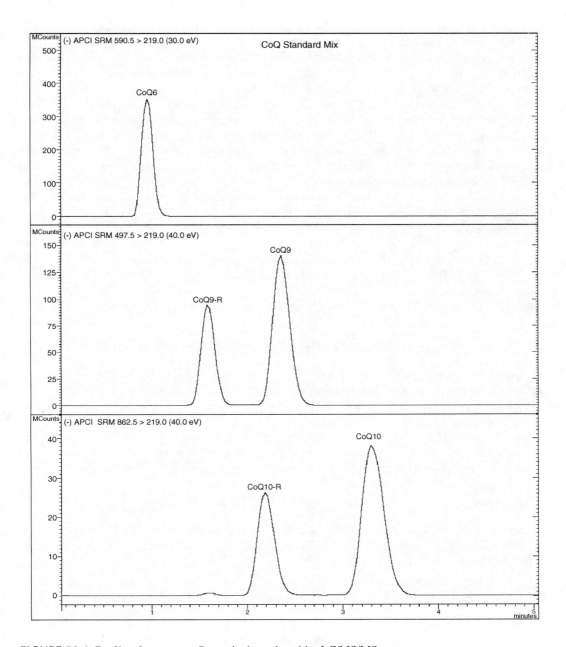

FIGURE 23.1 Profile of coenzyme Q standards analyzed by LC/MS/MS.

IV. TREATMENT OF HEART DISEASE WITH CoQ10

As previously stated, CoQ10 is highly concentrated in heart muscle cells due to the high energy requirements of these cells. Congestive heart failure (from a wide variety of causes) has been strongly correlated with significantly low blood and tissue levels of CoQ10.[6,7]

There have been a number of placebo-controlled studies on the treatment of heart disease with CoQ10: two in Japan, two in the U.S., two in Italy, two in Germany, and one in Sweden.[8–13,23,24] These studies have confirmed the effectiveness of CoQ10 as well as its remarkable safety. There have been 8 international symposia on the biomedical and clinical aspects of CoQ10 from 1976 through 1993.[25-32] These 8 symposia included over 300 papers presented by approximately 200 different physicians and scientists from 18 different countries. The majority of these scientific papers were from Japan (34%), the U.S. (26%), and Italy (20%) and the remaining 20% were from Sweden, Denmark, Germany, the United Kingdom, Belgium, Australia, Austria, France, India, Korea, The Netherlands, Poland, Switzerland, U.S.S.R., and Finland. The majority of the clinical studies concerned the treatment of heart disease and were remarkably consistent in their conclusions, namely, that treatment with CoQ10 significantly improved heart muscle function while producing no adverse effects or drug interactions. The efficacy and safety of CoQ10 in the treatment of congestive heart failure, whether related to primary cardiomyopathies or secondary forms of heart failure, has now been well established.[33-41]

It is important to note that in all of the above clinical trials, CoQ10 was used in addition to traditional medical treatments, not to their exclusion. In one study by Langsjoen and colleagues, of 109 patients with essential hypertension, 51% were able to stop between one and three antihypertensive drugs at an average of 4.4 months after starting CoQ10 treatment, whereas the overall New York Heart Association (NYHA) functional class improved significantly from a mean of 2.40 to 1.36.[42] In another study, there was a gradual and sustained decrease in dosage or discontinuation of concomitant cardiovascular drug therapy.[37] Out of 424 patients with cardiovascular disease, 43% were able to stop between one and three cardiovascular drugs with CoQ10 therapy.

V. METHODS FOR DETECTION OF CoQ10

As the deficiency of CoQ10 has been related to a number of diseases, the testing of its serum levels will become a norm in the near future. A number of laboratories have described methods for detection of CoQ10. Some of these methods use HPLC in conjunction with fluorescence detector and others have used UV detection. However, if this testing has to become a part of routine examinations, then there will be a need for a high throughput screening assay to measure serum CoQ10 levels. A method for the detection of CoQ in biological fluids as well as in tissue homogenates has been developed by the laboratory at KGK Synergize, Inc.

A. MATERIALS

Coenzyme Q6, Q9, Q10, and sodium borohydride were purchased from Sigma Aldrich. All solvents were HPLC grade and purchased from Fisher Scientific. Water was purified through a Millipore Milli-Q system.

B. INSTRUMENTS AND EQUIPMENT

The analysis was conducted on a Varian LC/MS/MS system consisting of two model 210 pumps, a model 410 refrigerated auto sampler, and model 1200L quadrupole MS/MS. The column used was a Varian 4.6×30 mm Pursuit 3 µm C18 with a Varian Metaguard 4.6 mm Pursuit 3 µm C18 guard column. The mobile phase was a 20:80 mixture of 2-propanol and methanol at a flow rate of 1 ml/min with run times at 5 min. CoQ was detected by MS/MS using the APCI interface in negative mode with a corona current of 5.0 µA and a shield voltage of 600 V. The capillary CID was set at −70 V and detector at 1900 V. The manifold temperature was 42°C and API housing temperature at 57°C with air used as the nebulizing gas at 40 psi. The nitrogen drying gas was set at 25 psi at a temperature of 275°C and the auxiliary gas at 17 psi at 550°C. All quantification was done using the 219.0 m/z fragment ions with argon as the collision gas. Collision energies were set at 40 V for all ions except for CoQ6, which was set at 30 V. All data were processed using the Varian Saturn LC/MS Workstation software.

C. STANDARDS PREPARATION

Stock solutions were made for CoQ6, CoQ9, and CoQ10 at 0.2 mg/ml in iso-octane and stored at –80°C. A 2 ng/µl standard mix solution was made by combining 100 µl of each stock solution and diluting to 10 ml with 1-propanol. A CoQ6 internal standard solution of 1 ng/µl was made by diluting 50 µl of stock to 10.0 ml with 1-propanol. A reduced standard mix solution was prepared according to Tang and colleagues[43] with some modifications. 50 µl each of CoQ9 and CoQ10 stock solution were combined in a 16 ml glass centrifuge tube with a teflon-lined cap. The solutions were evaporated to dryness under nitrogen at room temperature and then redissolved in 1 ml of reagent alcohol. 50 µl of freshly prepared 0.05M sodium borohydride in water was added, the tube vortex-mixed for 1 min, and then placed in the dark for 30 min. 10 ml of hexane and 3 ml of water were added and the contents vortex-mixed for 1 min before centrifuging at 500 × g for 5 min. The bottom aqueous layer was carefully removed with a Pasteur pipette and discarded. This procedure was repeated twice more with 3 ml of water before evaporating the hexane layer to dryness under nitrogen at room temperature. Redissolving the residue in 5.0 ml of 1-propanol, which was previously purged with nitrogen and degassed under vacuum in a sonicating water bath, made a 2 ng/µl standard mix solution. Aliquots were transferred to 1 ml vials and immediately stored at 80°C until analysis. All other standard solutions could be stored at –20°C, protected from light, for up to 2 months. Immediately before analysis an aliquot of the reduced standard mix solution was quantified for oxidized CoQ9 and CoQ10. 500 µl of reduced and 500 µl of oxidized standard mix solution were mixed together to make a 1 ng/µl complete standard mix solution. A calibration curve was constructed by injecting 10 µl of 0.01, 0.1, and 1.0 ng/µl of the complete standard mix solution in triplicate. The actual concentrations were adjusted accordingly, based on the amount of oxidized CoQ present in the reduced standard mix solution. CoQ6 was added to each sample as an internal standard and quantified to compensate for any loss during sample processing or due to ion suppression during analysis.

D. SAMPLE PREPARATION AND ANALYSIS

Samples were quickly processed in batches of 24 or less under reduced light and transferred in amber vials to the refrigerated auto sampler set at 4°C for immediate analysis. Methanol and 1-propanol were purged of air by bubbling nitrogen gas through them for at least 10 minutes before being placed in a sonicating water bath under vacuum. The bottles were sealed and placed in ice before use. Serum or plasma was quickly thawed and 50 µl pipetted into a 1.5 ml micro centrifuge tube with 50 µl of methanol, 50 µl of CoQ6 internal standard solution and 1 ml of 1-propanol. The tubes were capped and vortex-mixed at high speed for 30 sec before being centrifuged at 10,000 × g for 5 min; 1 ml of supernatant was transferred to a new tube along with 300 µl of methanol. The tube was mixed and an aliquot transferred to an auto sampler vial for analysis. 10 µl of each sample was injected in triplicate.

Tissues were individually dissected and flash frozen in <5 min to minimize the oxidation of ubiquinol. Specimens were maintained at –80°C until analysis. The method for preparation of tissue homogenates was adapted from Tang and colleagues.[43] Briefly, pieces of tissue were accurately weighed in the frozen state and subsequently homogenized with 100 µl of ubiquinone-6 solution and 2 ml of cold 1-propanol in a Tissue Homogenizer on ice bath. To the homogenized mixture, 100 µl of cold water was added and mixed on a vortex for 20s. The mixture was then transferred to a capped polypropylene tube and centrifuged at 10,000 rpm for 5 min. The clear supernatant was immediately filtered through a disposable filter (0.1 µm) into an auto-sampler vial and injected directly onto the HPLC system.

E. ANALYSIS

The amount of CoQ10 present in the sample was quantified based on peak area as compared to the calibration curve. Using a multiplier of 29.9 in the sample table gave results in µg/ml serum

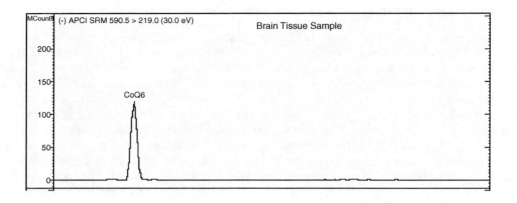

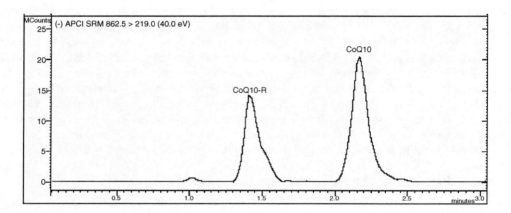

FIGURE 23.2 Detection of CoQ10 using LC/MS/MS in brain samples.

or plasma, which could be divided directly by the result for the CoQ6 internal standard to give the corrected value. The chromatograms of standards and samples are presented in Figure 23.1 to Figure 23.4. The sensitivity of detection using this method is ~10 pg/ml. The recovery of the sample was calculated to be >89% by this method.

VI. CONCLUSION

Cardiovascular diseases (CVD) and Type II diabetes are two of the major diseases affecting the developed world. Functional foods are fast becoming the choice of prevention and control of a number of diseases including CVD and Type II diabetes. A number of studies have already investigated and reported the positive effects of CoQ10 in CVD. CoQ10 deficiency has been related to the development of CVD; therefore, measuring CoQ10 levels should provide a marker for identifying people with an increased risk for developing CVD and other chronic diseases. The technique described here offers a sensitive and reproducible method for detection of CoQ10 for diagnostic purposes.

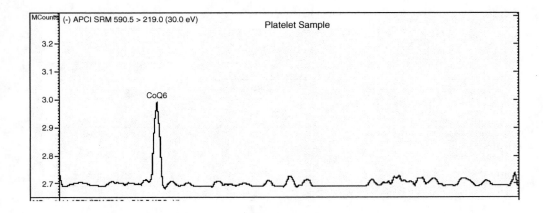

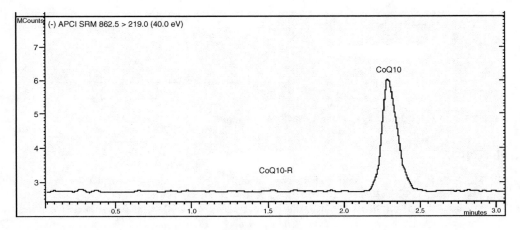

FIGURE 23.3 Detection of CoQ10 using LC/MS/MS in platelet samples.

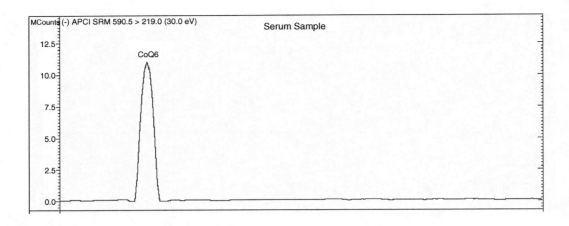

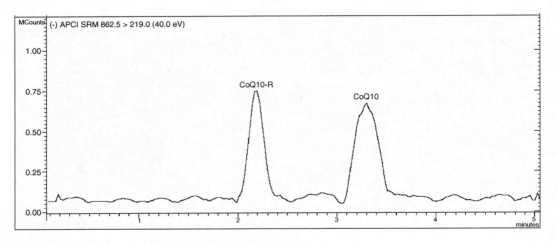

FIGURE 23.4 Detection of CoQ10 using LC/MS/MS in serum samples.

REFERENCES

1. Mitchell, P. Kelin's respiratory chain concept and its chemiosmotic consequences. *Science*, 206, 1148–1159, 1979.
2. Ernster, L. Facts and ideas about the function of coenzyme Q10 in the Mitochondria. Folkers, K., Yamamura, Y., Eds., *Biomedical and Clinical Aspects of Coenzyme Q*. Elsevier, Amsterdam, 1977, pp. 15–18.
3. Littarru, G.P., Lippa, S., Oradei, A., Fiorni, R.M., and Mazzanti, L. Metabolic and diagnostic implications of blood CoQ10 levels. Folkers, K., Yamagami, T., and Littarru, G.P., Eds., *Biomedical and Clinical Aspects of Coenzyme Q,* Vol. 6. Elsevier, Amsterdam, 1991, pp. 167–178.
4. Ghirlanda, G., Oradei, A., Manto, A., Lippa, S., Uccioli, L., Caputo, S., Greco, A.V., and Littarru, G.P. Evidence of plasma CoQ10 — lowering effect by HMG-CoA reductase inhibitors: a double blind, placebo-controlled study. *Clin. Pharmacol. J.* 33(3), 226–229, 1993.
5. Folkers, K., Langsjoen, Per.H., Willis, R., Richardson, P., Xia, L., Ye, C., and Tamagawa, H. Lovastatin decreases coenzyme Q levels in humans. *Proc. Natl. Acad Sci.* 87, 8931–8934, 1990.
6. Folkers, K., Vadhanavikit, S., and Mortensen, S.A. Biochemical rationale and myocardial tissue data on the effective therapy of cardiomyopathy with coenzyme Q10. *Proc. Natl. Acad. Sci. U.S.A.* 82(3), 901–904, 1985.
7. Mortensen, S.A., Vadhanavikit, S., and Folkers, K. Deficiency of coenzyme Q10 in myocardial failure. *Drugs Exp. Clin. Res.* X(7), 497–502, 1984.

8. Hiasa, Y., Ishida, T., Maeda, T., Iwanc, K., Aihara, T., and Mori, H. Effects of coenzyme Q10 on exercise tolerance in patients with stable angina pectoris. Folkers, K., Yamamura, Y., Eds., *Biomedical and Clinical Aspects of Coenzyme Q*, Vol. 4. Elsevier, Amsterdam, 1984, pp. 291–301.

9. Kamikawa, T., Kobayashi, A., Yamashita, T., Hayashi, H., and Yamazaki, N. Effects of coenzyme Q10 on exercise tolerance in chronic stable angina pectoris. *Am. J. Cardiol.* 56: 247–251, 1985.

10. Langsjoen, Per.H., Vadhanavikit, S., and Folkers K. Response of patients in classes III and IV of cardiomyopathy to therapy in a blind and crossover trial with coenzyme Q10. *Proc. Natl. Acad. Sci. U.S.A.* 82, 4240–4244, 1985.

11. Judy, W.V., Hall, J.H., Toth, P.D., and Folkers, K. Double blind-double crossover study of coenzyme Q10 in heart failure. Folkers, K., Yamamura, Y., Eds., *Biomedical and Clinical Aspects of Coenzyme Q*, Vol. 5. Elsevier, Amsterdam, 1986, pp. 315–323.

12. Rossi, E., Lombardo, A., Testa, M., Lippa, S., Oradei, A., Littarru, G.P., Lucente, M. Coppola, E., and Manzoli, U. Coenzyme Q10 in ischaemic cardiopathy. Folkers, K., Yamagami, T., Littarru, G.P., Eds., *Biomedical and Clinical Aspects of Coenzyme Q*, Vol. 6. Elsevier, Amsterdam, 1991, pp. 321–326.

13. Morisco, C., Trimarco, B., and Condorelli, M. Effect of coenzyme Q10 therapy in patients with congestive heart failure: A long-term multicenter randomized study. In *Seventh International Symposium on Biomedical and Clinical Aspects of Coenzyme Q*, Folkers, K., Mortensen, S.A., Littarru, G.P., Yamagami, T., Lenaz, G., Eds. *The Clinical Investigator*, 71: S34–S136, 1993.

14. Crane, F.L., Hatefi, Y., Lester, R.I., and Widmer, C. Isolation of a quinone from beef heart mitochondria. *Biochim. Biophys. Acta*, 25, 220–221, 1957.

15. Morton, R.A., Wilson, G.M., Lowe, J.S., and Leat, W.M.F. Ubiquinone. *Chem. Ind.*, 1649, 1957.

16. Mellors, A. and Tappel, A.L. Quinones and quinols as inhibitors of lipid peroxidation. *Lipids*, 1, 282–284, 1966.

17. Mellors A. and Tappel A.L. The inhibition of mitochondrial peroxidation by ubiquinone and ubiquinol. *J. Biol. Chem.*, 241, 4353–4356, 1966.

18. Littarru, G.P., Ho, L., and Folkers K. Deficiency of Coenzyme Q10 in human heart disease: Part I and II. *Int. J. Vit. Nutr. Res.*, 42(2), 291; 42(3): 413, 1972.

19. Mitchell, P. Possible molecular mechanisms of the protonmotive function of cytochrome systems. *J. Theor. Biol.*, 62, 327–367, 1976.

20. Mitchell, P. The vital protonmotive role of coenzyme Q. Folkers, K., Littarru, G.P., Yamagami, T., Eds., *Biomedical and Clinical Aspects of Coenzyme Q*, Vol. 6. Elsevier, Amsterdam, 1991, pp. 3–10.

21. Mitchell, P. Respiratory chain systems in theory and practice. Kim C.H. et al., Eds, *Advances in Membrane Biochemistry and Bioenergetics*. Plenum Press, New York, 1988, pp. 25–52.

22. Schneeberger, W., Muller-Steinwachs, J., Anda, L.P., Fuchs, W., Zilliken, F., Lyson, K., Muratsu, K., and Folkers, K. A clinical double blind and crossover trial with coenzyme Q10 on patients with cardiac disease. Folkers K., Yamamura Y., Eds., *Biomedical and Clinical Aspects of Coenzyme Q*, Vol. 5. Elsevier, Amsterdam, 1986, pp. 325–333.

23. Schardt, F., Welzel, D., Schiess, W., and Toda, K. Effect of coenzyme Q10 on ischaemia-induced ST-segment depression: a double blind, placebo-controlled crossover study. Folkers K., Yamagami T., Littarru G.P., Eds., *Biomedical and Clinical Aspects of Coenzyme Q*, Vol. 6. Elsevier, Amsterdam, 1991, pp. 385–403.

24. Swedberg, K., Hoffman-Berg, C., Rehnqvist, N., and Astrom, H. Coenzyme Q10 as an adjunctive in treatment of congestive heart failure. *64th Scientific Sessions American Heart Association*, Abstract 774–6, 1991.

25. Folkers, K. and Yamamura, Y., Eds. *Biomedical and Clinical Aspects of Coenzyme Q*. Elsevier, Amsterdam, 1977, pp. 1–315.

26. Yamamura, Y., Folkers, K., and Ito, Y., Eds. *Biomedical and Clinical Aspects of Coenzyme Q*, Vol. 2. Elsevier, Amsterdam, 1980, pp. 1–456.

27. Folkers, K. and Yamamura, Y., Eds. *Biomedical and Clinical Aspects of Coenzyme Q*, Vol. 3. Elsevier, Amsterdam, 1981, pp. 1–414.

28. Folkers, K. and Yamamura, Y., Eds., *Biomedical and Clinical Aspects of Coenzyme Q*, Vol. 4. Elsevier, Amsterdam, 1983, pp. 1–432.

29. Folkers, K. and Yamamura, Y., Eds. *Biomedical and Clinical Aspects of Coenzyme Q*, Vol. 5. Elsevier, Amsterdam, 1986, pp 1–410.

30. Folkers, K., Yamagami, T., and Littarru, G.P., Eds. *Biomedical and Clinical Aspects of Coenzyme Q*, Vol. 6. Elsevier, Amsterdam, 1991, pp. 1–555.

31. *Seventh International Symposium on Biomedical and Clinical Aspects of Coenzyme Q*. Folkers, K., Mortensen, S.A., Littarru, G.P., Yamagami, T., and Lenaz, G., Eds. *The Clinical Investigator*, Supplement to Vol.71/Issue 8, S51–S177, 1993.

32. *Eighth International Symposium on Biomedical and Clinical Aspects of Coenzyme Q*. Littarru, G.P., Battino, M., Folkers, K., Eds. *Mol. Aspects Med.* 15(Suppl.), S1–S294, 1994.

33. Mortensen, S.A., Vadhanavikit, S., and Folkers, K. Deficiency of coenzyme Q10 in myocardial failure. *Drugs Exp. Clin. Res.* X(7), 497–502, 1984.

34. Mortensen, S.A., Vadhanavikit, S., Baandrup, U., and Folkers, K. Long term coenzyme Q10 therapy: a major advance in the management of resistant myocardial failure. *Drugs Exp. Clin. Res.*, 11(8), 581–593, 1985.

35. Langsjoen, P.H., Folkers, K., Lyson, K., Muratsu, K., Lyson, T., and Langsjoen, P.H. Effective and safe therapy with coenzyme Q10 for cardiomyopathy. *Klin. Wochenschr.* 66: 583–593, 1988.

36. Langsjoen, P.H., Langsjoen, P.H., and Folkers, K. Long term efficacy and safety of coenzyme Q10 therapy for idiopathic dilated cardiomyopathy. *Am. J. Cardiol.*, 65, 521–523, 1990.

37. Mortensen, S.A., Vadhanavikit, S., Muratsu, K., and Folkers, K. Coenzyme Q10: Clinical benefits with biochemical correlates suggesting a scientific breakthrough in the management of chronic heart failure. *Int. J. Tissue React.*, 12(3), 155–162, 1990.

38. Ursini, T., Gambini, C., Paciaroni, E., and Littarru, G.P. Coenzyme Q10 treatment of heart failure in the elderly: preliminary results. Folkers K., Yamagami T., and Littarru G.P., Eds., *Biomedical and Clinical Aspects of Coenzyme Q*, Vol. 6. Elsevier, Amsterdam, 1991, pp. 473–480.

39. Poggesi, L., Galanti, G., Comeglio, M., Toncelli, L., and Vinci, M. Effect of coenzyme Q10 on left ventricular function in patients with dilative cardiomyopathy. *Curr. Ther. Res.* 49: 878–886, 1991.

40. Langsjoen, H.A., Langsjoen, P.H., Langsjoen, P.H., Willis, R., and Folkers, K. Usefulness of coenzyme Q10 in clinical cardiology: a long-term study. In *Eighth International Symposium on Biomedical and Clinical Aspects of Coenzyme Q*. Littarru, G.P., Battino, M., Folkers, K., Eds. *Mol. Aspects Med.* 15(Suppl.), S165–S175, 1990.

41. Baggio, E., Gandini, R., Plancher, A.C., Passeri, M., and Carmosino, G. Italian multicenter study on safety and efficacy of coenzyme Q10 adjunctive therapy in heart failure. In *Eighth International Symposium on Biomedical and Clinical Aspects of Coenzyme Q*. Littarru, G.P., Battino, M., Folkers, K., Eds. *Mol. Aspects Med.* 15(Suppl.), S287–S294, 1994.

42. Langsjoen, P.H., Langsjoen, P.H., Willis, R., Folkers, K. Treatment of essential hypertension with coenzyme Q10. In *Eighth International Symposium on Biomedical and Clinical Aspects of Coenzyme Q*. Littarru, G.P., Battino, M., Folkers, K., Eds. *Mol. Aspects Med.* 15(Suppl.), S287–S294, 1994.

43. Tang, P.H., Miles, M.V., Miles, L., et al. Measurement of reduced and oxidized coenzyme Q_9 and coenzyme Q_{10} levels in mouse tissues by HPLC with coulometric detection. *Clin. Chim. Acta* 341: 173–184, 2004.

24 Coffee as a Functional Beverage

Lem Taylor and Jose Antonio

CONTENTS

I. INTRODUCTION

Caffeine is the most commonly consumed drug in the world, and has been used for centuries for a variety of reasons. Caffeine is a common substance in the diets of a variety of individuals ranging from athletes to elderly. Today, caffeine can be found in numerous products such as sports gels, energy drinks, and alcoholic beverages.[1]

Coffee is likely to be the primary delivery system for caffeine today. For most people, caffeine and coffee are synonymous, but these two should not be thought of as the same. There are other ingredients in coffee besides caffeine that exert a biological effect. Caffeine can have many effects in the body, but typically caffeine is thought of as a way to boost a person's energy level on both a psychomotor level (i.e., awareness) as well as a physiological level (i.e., energy), which is clearly a role that caffeine can play.[2] These two factors alone are probably the sole reason that many people consume coffee as part of their daily ritual, and this aspect of coffee consumption is very important.

The following chapter will discuss the background on coffee and its role as a functional food. This discussion will include types of coffee, the ingredients in coffee, the effects of coffee on energy metabolism, and its role as a drink that can enhance various aspects of health and possibly prevent or reduce the risk of some diseases The effects of caffeine on various diseases and health conditions needs to be discussed due to the fact that caffeine is the active ingredient in coffee in most preparations.

TABLE 24.1
Typical Caffeine Content of Several
Coffee Products

Double espresso (2oz)	55–100 mg
Drip brewed coffee (8 oz)	80–130 mg
Instant coffee (8 oz)	70–95 mg
Decaf coffee (8 oz)	1–5 mg
Tea, black (8 oz)	45 mg
Tea, green (8 oz)	20–30 mg
Tea, white (8 oz)	15 mg
Ben and Jerry's Coffee Fudge Frozen Yogurt (8 oz)	85 mg

II. INTRODUCTION TO COFFEE AND CAFFEINE

The popularity of coffee has increased dramatically over the last decade. Drinking coffee is a ritual that suits a variety of situations, from jump-starting your day to an aspect of social engagement. Traditionally, caffeine is typically associated with coffee consumption, and this is probably the most popular form of caffeine in the U.S. today. There are many different types of coffee, and they usually differ on factors such as taste or flavor, type of preparation, and the caffeine content of various types. Obviously, the brand of the product and the flavor usually has something to do with the content of caffeine, but most caffeine in food products typically contains chocolate or a coffee flavoring. Caffeine content can range from a couple of milligrams in an ounce of milk chocolate to ~115 mg in 12 oz of a Red Bull energy drink.

The most popular form of caffeine ingestion is via coffee, and the content typically depends on the method and duration of brewing; caffeine concentrations can range from 65 mg in 7 oz of instant coffee to 175 mg in 7 oz of drip-brewed coffee. Table 24.1 gives a comprehensive list of the caffeine contents of various consumer products.

III. DOSES OF CAFFEINE

The caffeine content of coffee is one of its important aspects for many people when they drink coffee. Caffeine is a derivative of methlyxanthine and is found in numerous consumer products in the U.S.[3] The following section will address the topic of caffeine doses, particularly the doses used in research settings and/or the doses that are allowed to be used by athletes before "caffeine doping" is reached. All of these factors are important in considering how much caffeine one should ingest for both optimal performance and safety.

Whether you are drinking coffee or tea, or taking caffeine pills, the amount of caffeine that an individual consumes is important to consider. Research has focused on varying levels of caffeine ingestion to determine optimal doses for different situations. In research trials, the most commonly used dose of caffeine is approximately 6 mg/kg of body weight, and this dose has been shown to give improved endurance exercise capacity and performance.[3–6] Other doses have been used as well in research trials, with increases in performance still evident. Doses as low as 1.3–1.9 mg/kg of body weight have been reported to increase performance,[6] and these findings support other evidence that caffeine can have an ergogenic effect at intakes as low as 1–3 mg/kg of body weight.[7–9] On the other hand, doses as high as 9 mg/kg of body weight have been used in research, but it is still debated whether the ergogenic effects are additive at higher doses.[4,5]

Caffeine is not banned or restricted by the IOC.

IV. COFFEE AND CAFFEINE IN WEIGHT LOSS AND ENERGY EXPENDITURE

Like other stimulants, caffeine has been advertised and sold as a way to stimulate energy expenditure and weight loss. This potential effect on weight management is important to coffee's role as a functional food. The fact that coffee is consumed by so many people and can be a potent dose of caffeine could indicate that daily coffee consumption can be important in augmenting energy expenditure and, as a corollary, weight loss.

As discussed with caffeine's role as an ergogenic aid in endurance exercise, caffeine can stimulate both lipolysis and energy expenditure.[11] Many studies have been performed on the results of caffeine ingestion, with some examining caffeine alone, whereas others have examined caffeine combined with various herbal and vitamin products like ephedra, green tea extracts, calcium, tyrosine, chromium picolinate, capsaicin, garcinia cambogia, etc. Caffeine has even been examined when combined with another popular stimulant in the U.S., cigarette smoking, in which caffeine was suggested to increase energy expenditure in an additive manner from the smoking stimulant.[12] The method of administration has varied from coffee and/or tea ingestion to administering caffeine-containing pills. The following section will discuss the pertinent research involving caffeine's and possibly coffee's effect on energy expenditure as well as possible weight loss that could result from this decreased energy state.

Some of the original work on caffeine and energy expenditure came out of the *American Journal of Clinical Nutrition* in the late 1980s. Initial findings suggested that a single dose of 100 mg of caffeine had a significant effect on the resting metabolic rate (increase of 3–4% over 150 min) in a variety of populations. These findings lead the authors to suggest that caffeine can have a significant effect on energy balance at a commonly consumed dose and possibly have positive effects in the treatment of obesity.[13] Subsequent studies confirmed these findings, with one study reporting that caffeine ingestion increased energy expenditure by 7%, while also lowering plasma insulin and norepinephrine levels and increasing the appearance of free fatty acids in the blood.[14] Koot and Deurenberg reported similar findings of a 7% increase in energy expenditure for 3 h following ingestion of 200 mg of caffeine, which was administered as coffee.[15] Clearly, older studies have shown caffeine to have an effect on the metabolic rate of humans, and recent research has continued to back this notion.

More recent research on the effects of caffeine continues to support its role in increasing energy expenditure. As mentioned earlier, caffeine is now being combined with a variety of products to promote a thermogenic effect. One example in the literature used the combination of capsaicin, catechins, caffeine, tyrosine, and calcium. This study reported an increase in energy expenditure of 2% over a 7-d period when these products were ingested as bioactive food products.[16] Another recent study that looked at caffeine alone found an increase in energy expenditure of 13%, with doubling of lipid turnover. These researchers concluded that the effects of caffeine alter energy expenditure and are mediated via the sympathetic nervous system. Furthermore, they explain the lipid mobilization action of caffeine in two ways: increased mobilization alone is insufficient to drive oxidation, or large increments in lipid turnover can result in an increase in lipid oxidation.[11]

Clearly, caffeine does play a role in metabolism and energy expenditure. One can debate how much caffeine is necessary and the optimal time to consume it. One solution to this is to incorporate it into products that consumers use daily or at least regularly. Even coffee, which is consumed many times a day by millions of people, has now been modified by adding some of these products, plus additional caffeine. These products do have some credibility, and early research has found some functional coffee beverages (i.e., JavaFit Diet Plus) to have significant effects on energy expenditure, body weight, and fat loss when compared to regular caffeinated coffee (Experimental Biology Meeting, 2006; Ron Mendel, Ph.D., personal communication). It has yet to be determined whether or not caffeine and the many products that contain significant amounts of it have long-term effects on energy balance. Despite this, the role of coffee as a functional food is intriguing because of the popularity of consumption on a broad scale.

V. EFFECTS OF COFFEE (CAFFEINE) IN THE BRAIN AND BODY

Caffeine and caffeinated coffee can have a stimulatory effect on mental performance. This effect of consuming caffeine has been well documented. One study in particular suggested that consuming caffeinated beverages can maintain both cognitive and psychomotor performance throughout the day.[17] Because coffee is a caffeinated beverage, these beneficial effects could be associated with daily coffee consumption. In fact, additional research has focused specifically on the effects of caffeinated vs. decaffeinated coffee on various cognitive function variables. The results of this study suggest that lifetime and current consumption of caffeinated coffee may be associated with better cognitive performance among women, especially in elderly populations.[18]

VI. EXERCISE PERFORMANCE WITH COFFEE AND CAFFEINE CONSUMPTION

As we have discussed, caffeine is a popular drug all over the world as well as a frequently used ergogenic aid among athletes. There is substantial research that supports the fact that caffeine consumption can have beneficial effects on exercise performance. However, research that utilizes coffee as the means of caffeine administration is sparse. The following section will discuss the evidence to support caffeine's role in exercise performance.

Caffeine has been shown to improve performance and increase endurance during prolonged exercise, and in smaller amounts in shorter-term endurance performance.[4, 19] This enhanced performance in endurance exercise is typically not associated with elevations in VO_2 max and/or any parameters related to it, but it could allow an individual to compete at a higher power output or give the ability to train longer.[20] Other reported benefits include a reduction in perceived leg pain induced by exercise[21] and improved psychomotor performance (reaction time) during exercise.[2] Improved concentration, improved cognitive performance after exercise,[22] a reduction or delay in fatigue,[23] and enhancement in alertness,[19] have also been reported. The benefits of caffeine consumption are clear. The evidence supporting a functional role for coffee consumption on exercise performance is discussed next.

The research on coffee and caffeine intake on exercise performance began in the 1970s and is still being conducted today. One classic study was performed by Costill and colleagues to determine the effects of caffeine ingestion on performance during prolonged exercise.[24] This study utilized cycle ergometry at 80% of VO2 max until exhaustion following the consumption of either decaffeinated or regular coffee (330 mg of caffeine) to determine the physiological effects of caffeine. The results found that the caffeine group exercised longer (90.2 min) than the decaffeinated group (75.5 min), and the caffeine group also showed an enhanced fat-burning effect. In addition, the caffeine group also reported a lower rating of perceived exertion (RPE) during the exhaustive exercise bout.[24] Other studies have showed similar results when coffee was used as the means of caffeine administration. A more recent study determined that various forms of caffeine ingestion all resulted in significant increases in time-to-exhaustion exercise when compared to placebo groups. Furthermore, this study demonstrated that prior coffee consumption did not decrease the ergogenic effect of anhydrous caffeine ingestion on exercise performance.[25]

In addition to these ergogenic effects, caffeine has not been associated with any negative effects on exercise performance including rehydration status, ion imbalance, or any other negative effects on exercise performance.[1,26] Caffeine consumption stimulates a mild diuresis similar to water, but there is no evidence that the fluid–electrolyte imbalance is negatively affected on exercise performance. In fact, caffeine consumption doses ranging from 100–680 mg of caffeine have rarely affected the differences in urine output when compared to placebo. The effect on fluid–electrolyte imbalance is also affected by caffeine tolerance, and the chance of affecting it is reduced in individuals that regularly consume caffeine. Overall, whether it is coffee or another caffeine containing product, individuals who consume caffeine in moderation and maintain a typical diet will not incur any detrimental fluid–electrolyte imbalances.[27]

Despite all of these reported benefits, the mechanism of action for the respective effects is still unclear. Traditionally, the benefits on endurance exercise were associated with increased free fatty acid oxidation[24,28] and subsequent sparing of muscle glycogen.[29,30] These effects of caffeine ingestion are most likely due to the competitive antagonism of adenosine receptors at physiological concentrations.[31] Despite the findings of these studies, many other studies disagree with the mechanism of action in which caffeine is exhibiting these effects.[7,32] The primary argument in these studies is that performance enhancement has been shown to occur without changes in catecholamine or FFA/glycerol concentrations during exercise.[7] Together, these findings suggest that caffeine has an effect at the level of the skeletal muscle, which could be the result of the ergogenic effect.[7,32]

Recent studies are in agreement with the notion that the effect of caffeine is mediated at the skeletal muscle level. One study found that anaerobic exercise performance was increased following caffeine ingestion resulting from stimulation of the skeletal muscle by caffeine.[33] Other studies have suggested that caffeine has an effect on calcium release via the ryanodine receptor,[34] and this release was not a result of adenosine antagonism.[35] In addition, studies have found that caffeine ingestion can potentiate submaximal skeletal muscle contractile force,[3,36] thus eliciting an ergogenic effect. The most recent study exhibiting these findings found that caffeine ingestion of 6 mg/kg of body weight potentiated contraction force during low frequency stimulation.[3] These authors suggested that, in view of the known effects of caffeine on the ryanodine receptor, these data are consistent in demonstrating that caffeine can potentiate calcium release from the SR and further suggest that caffeine's ergogenic effects are at least partly mediated by direct effects at the skeletal muscle level.[3,7] In addition, the researchers suggest that since caffeine ingestion has no effect on MVC, high-frequency stimulation is consistent with the fact that caffeine has lesser to no effects on maximal strength and high-intensity exercises,[3] as has traditionally been thought to be the case.

Another possible mechanism that may partially explain caffeine's ergogenic effects involves its relationship to RPE and perceived pain. Research has suggested that caffeine ingestion increased high-intensity cycling performance; the authors reported that the reduction in RPE as well as an elevation in blood lactate concentration could be the reason for the ergogenic effect.[37] A meta-analysis on caffeine ingestion and RPE levels also suggests that caffeine reduces RPE levels during exercise, thus eliciting an important ergogenic effect.[38] These studies agree with a previously cited report that caffeine ingestion significantly reduced leg muscle pain ratings during moderate intensity cycling exercise. The researchers suggested that caffeine's hypoalgesic properties could play a role in improving exercise performance.[21] Although they are not the same, RPE and perceived leg pain could be associated with one another, thus suggesting that the decreased RPE and/or perceived pain resulting from caffeine ingestion could be one factor in the ergogenic effects of endurance exercise performance.[21,37,38]

In conclusion, despite the fact that the mechanism of action is somewhat still debated, caffeine consumption can result in improved exercise performance on a variety of levels. Caffeine is the most commonly consumed drug in the world, and athletes frequently use it as an ergogenic aid. Caffeine consumption improves performance and endurance during prolonged, exhaustive exercise and, to a lesser degree, caffeine enhances short-term, high-intensity athletic performance. In addition, caffeine improves concentration, reduces fatigue, and adds to alertness; all of these factors can improve performance in different events. Habitual intake does not diminish caffeine's ergogenic properties. Caffeine is safe and does not cause significant dehydration or electrolyte imbalance during exercise. The role of coffee ingestion has also been shown to be an effective way of administrating caffeine as an ergogenic aid, thus substantiating coffee's role as a functional food.

VII. HEALTH RELATED ISSUES IN COFFEE CONSUMPTION

Based on the fact that billions of individuals worldwide drink coffee, it could be assumed that if there were negative side effects to drinking coffee, the problems would be manifest in large populations of coffee consumers; however, there is no evidence that such harm occurs. In fact, there is data to suggest that coffee consumption may indeed confer numerous health benefits.

A. BLOOD PRESSURE

One very important marker of health that affects millions of people across the world is blood pressure. The role of coffee consumption and its effects on blood pressure has been studied, and these studies have shown consistent results. One large scale study examined over 3000 Japanese males who were 48–56 years old and were undergoing preretirement health screenings. These individuals completed self-administered questionnaires to determine average coffee intake over the past year. The significant findings of this study revealed that regular coffee drinkers had lower blood pressure than individuals who did not consume coffee. In addition, this effect was demonstrated at all levels of alcohol consumption, cigarette smoking, obesity, and glucose intolerance. Thus, the major conclusions of this study suggest that habitual coffee consumption does not have adverse effects on blood pressure, and drinking coffee does have significant beneficial effects on the blood pressure levels in this population.[39] Other studies examining the relationship between coffee consumption and blood pressure have found similar results. One study examined over a thousand adults during health checkups and revealed that coffee consumption had no significant effects on blood pressure in these individuals or on total or HDL blood cholesterol levels. In addition, these findings revealed a negative correlation between coffee consumption and serum triglycerides in these individuals. These findings further support the beneficial effects of coffee consumption in these populations and show that drinking coffee does not adversely affect these cardiovascular risk factors in adults.[40] Despite these positive findings, it is important to note that individuals who currently have high blood pressure should be more cautious with coffee drinking and should probably consult a physician before drinking coffee on a regular basis. This suggestion is supported by research that indicates that reducing or restricting coffee intake may have a beneficial effect on controlling high blood pressure in some populations.[41,42] Overall, habitual coffee consumption does not seem to lead to negative effects on blood pressure unless there is a preexisting problem with high blood pressure. In addition, moderate coffee consumption may have a beneficial effect on blood pressure levels.

B. CARDIOVASCULAR DISEASE

One of the most significant health issues over the last 30 years has been the prevalence of cardiovascular disease. Over the last decade or so, a false impression has risen around the relationship between coffee consumption and an increased risk of heart problems. However, coffee consumption not only does not increase the risk, but as we will discuss later, it also has beneficial effects on some of the contributing factors that result in cardiovascular disease, like Type 2 diabetes and hypertension. In fact, a recent prospective study does not support the hypothesis that moderate caffeine (from coffee) consumption significantly increases the risk of coronary heart disease.[43]

Other studies have examined the relationship between coffee consumption and various aspects of cardiovascular disease, some of which will be discussed next. One of these studies was performed on over 85,000 middle-aged registered nurses in the U.S. It examined the 10-year incidence of coronary heart disease (CHD) and found no association with caffeine intake from all sources and CHD. In addition, there was no association between CHD and decaffeinated coffee consumption in this population.[44] A more recent study conducted in hospitalized patients who had confirmed acute myocardial infarction (heart attack) found that coffee consumption was not associated with the overall rate of death in these individuals.[45]

Additional research has supported the idea that coffee consumption does not increase one's risk for cardiovascular disease. These studies report consistent findings, such as no significant effect of coffee consumption on general mortality and/or cardiovascular disease-associated mortality in men. A lower rate of general mortality was associated with coffee consumption in women.[46] The risk of occurrence for a nonfatal heart attack is not associated with coffee consumption in men, and all-cause mortality rate was decreased by increasing coffee consumption in women.[47] Thus, the evidence seems to support the understanding that moderate coffee consumption does not increase an individual's risk for developing cardiovascular disease. In addition, there is some evidence to suggest that moderate consumption may have some beneficial effects as well, thus providing evidence to support the role of coffee as a functional food.

C. DIABETES

There is a plethora of fairly recent research to support the inverse relationship between coffee consumption and Type 2 diabetes.[48–57] The following section will discuss some of the more relevant examples of the research examining the association with drinking coffee and Type 2 diabetes.

One general consensus reached in examining the relationship between coffee and Type 2 diabetes is that coffee drinking is associated with a higher insulin sensitivity and a lower risk of Type 2 diabetes.[49,53,55,57,58] This is important due to the fact that Type 2 diabetes is a disease that is characterized by a severe reduction in insulin sensitivity, thus leading to adverse metabolic affects on the body. One study demonstrating the evidence to support this was conducted in about 8,000 healthy individuals aged 35–56 years, who were administered questionnaires to obtain information regarding coffee consumption as well as other general factors. The overall findings of this study demonstrated that high coffee consumption (5 cups per day) was inversely associated with insulin resistance, thus promoting a positive effect on insulin metabolism.[48] Other studies have confirmed these findings and have suggested that coffee consumption of up to 6 cups a day (but no more than 6 cups) has beneficial effects on preventing the occurrence of Type 2 diabetes.[53] Further support from the Nurses' Health Study and Health Professionals' Followup Study that examined approximately 42,000 men and 84,000 women found another inverse association between coffee intake and Type 2 diabetes, following the adjustment for age, body mass index, and other risk factors. Additional findings from this study found that total caffeine intake from all sources was associated with a significantly lower risk for diabetes in men and women.[55]

Thus, the evidence is clear and in some cases overwhelming, that drinking moderate to high amounts (4–6 cups per day) of coffee has a protective effect on the development of Type 2 diabetes in men and women. The implication of reducing the risk of diabetes affects not only the individual, but also clearly our society and economy, due to the substantial costs related to treating this disease. Diabetes is the fifth leading cause of death by disease in the U.S.,[59] and its incidence will probably continue to rise in the future. Knowing what we now know about the protective effects coffee can have on this disease, it is clear that this fact alone should justify a role for coffee as a functional food.

D. CANCER

One of the most recent studies examining coffee consumption and cancer was conducted on pre-and-postmenopausal women to explore the relationship between coffee consumption and breast cancer. According to this, regular coffee consumption does display a protective effect against breast cancer in premenopausal women, but there was no association discovered between coffee, black tea, and/or decaffeinated coffee consumption and breast cancer in postmenopausal women.[60] Another study conducted in Swedish women found similar findings and suggested that drinking coffee, tea, and caffeine was not associated with the incidence of breast cancer in this population.[61] Breast cancer is not the only form that has been studied in regards to coffee consumption and risk of disease. Other research has suggested that drinking regular coffee (i.e., not decaf) may decrease the risk of developing oral/pharyngeal and esophageal cancer,[62] bladder, colon and rectal cancer,[63] epithelial ovarian cancer,[64] and liver cancer in men and women.[65] Caffeinated beverages have no effect on the risk of thyroid cancer,[66] and coffee intake has been shown to have no association with the risk of pancreatic cancer.[67] As you can see, the evidence is pretty clear that frequent coffee consumption does not increase the risk for developing cancer and in some cases coffee intake is associated with having a preventive effect (see Table 24.2).

To summarize, it is clear that coffee and caffeine consumption have been studied in various aspects of health and disease. Some of the more prevalent diseases in our country were discussed in the text. Coffee has been studied in other aspects of health and disease as well (Table 24.2). Despite traditional beliefs, it is now becoming apparent that both occasional and habitual coffee drinking, which is accompanied by caffeine consumption, does not have a negative affect on health. Furthermore, drinking coffee does seem to have beneficial effects on one's health, and not all of these are contributed by caffeine. Taken together, these data provide further evidence to support the role of coffee as a functional food.

VIII. CONCLUSION AND CLOSING REMARKS

This chapter has discussed the various aspects of coffee consumption in both acute and chronic instances. Coffee is one of the most popular beverages in the world and is consumed by millions of people every day. Coffee's most intriguing and studied ingredient is caffeine. Both coffee and caffeine have been studied in a variety of situations, from psychomotor effects to performance enhancement effects in exercise, to drinking coffee to prevent a number of diseases. As this chapter has demonstrated, coffee consumption is not dangerous by any means and in most cases can have a multitude of beneficial effects. Traditionally, these beneficial effects have been attributed to the caffeine content of coffee, but we now know that this is not the case in every situation, and the additional ingredients of coffee may also provide beneficial effects. In most cases, a functional food has a special effect on a particular population, but it is clear that the benefits of drinking coffee cover a wide spectrum of the population, and the benefits are not defined in isolated situations. The role that coffee consumption has in preventing some of the most devastating and prevalent diseases should justify the classification of coffee as a functional beverage.

TABLE 24.2

Coffee and Caffeine Consumption and Health

Author	Type of Study	Population	Observations of Study
Ruhl et al. (2005)	Cohort	Individuals at high risk for liver damage	Coffee and caffeine consumption were associated with lower risk of elevated ALT activity
Sudano et al. (2005)	Review	Coffee drinkers	Coffee consumption is not associated with cardiovascular health hazards and may have beneficial effects on cardiovascular health
Dorea et al. (2005)	Review	Coffee drinkers	Many studies report the beneficial effects of habitual coffee drinking on several aspects of health; coffee impacts a large population and provides a wide spectrum of health benefits
Sudano et al. (2005)	Experimental, placebo-controlled	Habitual and nonhabitual coffee drinkers	Nonhabitual coffee drinkers experience enhanced cardiovascular response to mental stress; habitual coffee drinkers experience a blunted response; ingredients other than caffeine in coffee are partly responsible in stimulating the cardiovascular system
Nawrot et al. (2003)	Review	Healthy adults	Moderate daily caffeine intakes up to 400 mg per day are not associated with adverse health effects in healthy adults; children and women of reproductive age may require modified caffeine intakes for safety
Leviton et al. (2002)	Review	Women of reproductive age	There is inadequate evidence to conclude that caffeine consumption increases risk for reproductive adversity
Baker et al. (2006)	Case-control	Pre- and post-menopausal women	Regular coffee consumption is associated with a decreased risk of breast cancer in premenopausal women; risk of breast cancer is not associated with coffee, black tea, and/or decaf coffee in postmenopausal women
Ranheim et al. (2005)	Review	Coffee drinkers	Moderate daily filtered coffee consumption is not associated with cardiovascular events; coffee has significant antioxidant capabilities and may be inversely related to risk of Type 2 diabetes
Karlson et al. (2003)	Prospective study	Women	There is minimal evidence to support an association between coffee, decaf coffee, or tea consumption and the risk for developing rheumatoid arthritis in women
Van Dam et al. (2005)	Review	Coffee drinkers	Although the mechanism of action is not known, habitual coffee consumption is associated with substantially lower risk of Type 2 diabetes
Jordan et al. (2004)	Case-control	Women with epithelial ovarian cancer	Increased coffee consumption was associated with lower risk of ovarian cancer; association not due to caffeine, but due to other components in coffee
Keemola et al. (2000)	Cross-sectional survey	20,000+ Finnish men and women	Drinking coffee does not result in increased risk for coronary heart disease and/or death

Continued.

TABLE 24.2 *(Continued)*
Coffee and Caffeine Consumption and Health

Author	Type of Study	Population	Observations of Study
Salvaggio et al. (1990)	Experimental	9,600 men and women age 18–65	Individuals who drink coffee have lower blood pressure levels than non coffee drinkers; blood pressure was highest in nondrinkers among men
Mukamal et al. (2004)	Cohort study	Individuals with past heart attack	Coffee consumption has no association with postinfarction mortality
Tavani et al. (2003)	Case-control	Case and controls of cancer patients in hospital	Coffee may decrease risk of oral and/or pharyngeal and esophageal cancer but tea and decaf coffee consumption show no association with these cancers
Mack et al. (2003)	Review	Men and women with and without thyroid cancer	Thyroid cancer has no association with consumption of coffee and/or tea in men and women
Salazar-Martinez et al. (2004)	Prospective cohort	42,000 healthy men and 84,00 healthy women	Long-term coffee consumption is associated with lower risk for Type 2 diabetes

REFERENCES

1. Graham, T.E. Caffeine and exercise: metabolism, endurance and performance. *Sports Med.* 2001; 31: 785–807.
2. Kruk, B., Chmura, J., Krzeminski, K. et al. Influence of caffeine, cold and exercise on multiple choice reaction time. *Psychopharmacology (Berl).* 2001; 157: 197–201.
3. Tarnopolsky, M., Cupido, C. Caffeine potentiates low frequency skeletal muscle force in habitual and nonhabitual caffeine consumers. *J Appl Physiol.* 2000; 89: 1719–1724.
4. Bruce, C.R., Anderson, M.E., Fraser, S.F. et al. Enhancement of 2000 meter rowing performance after caffeine ingestion. *Med Sci Sports Exerc.* 2000; 32: 1958–1963.
5. Anderson, M.E., Bruce, C.R., Fraser, S.F. et al. Improved 2000 meter rowing performance in competitive oarswomen after caffeine ingestion. *Int J Sport Nutr Exerc Metab.* 2000; 10: 464–475.
6. Cox, G.R., Desbrow, B., Montgomery, P.G. et al. Effect of different protocols of caffeine intake on metabolism and endurance performance. *J Appl Physiol.* 2002; 93: 990–999.
7. Graham, T.E., Spriet, L.L. Metabolic, catecholamine, and exercise performance responses to various doses of caffeine. *J Appl Physiol.* 1995; 78: 867–874.
8. Kovacs, E.M., Stegen, J.H.C.H., Brouns, F. Effect of caffeinated drinks on substrate metabolism, caffeine excretion, and performance. *J Appl Physiol.* 1998; 85: 709–715.
9. Pasman, W.J., van Baak, M.A., Jeukendrup, A.E., de Haan, A. The effect of different dosages of caffeine on endurance performance time. *Int J Sports Med.* 1995; 16: 225–230.
10. Graham, T.E., Spriet, L.L. Performance and metabolic responses to a high caffeine dose during prolonged exercise. *J Appl Physiol.* 1991; 71: 2292–2298.
11. Acheson, K.J., Gremaud, G., Meirim, I. et al. Metabolic effects of caffeine in humans: lipid oxidation or futile cycling? *Am J Clin Nutr.* 2004; 79: 40–46.
12. Collins, L.C., Cornelius, M.F., Vogel, R.L., Walker, J.F., Stamford, B.A. Effect of caffeine and/or cigarette smoking on resting energy expenditure. *Int J Obes Relat Metab Disord.* 1994; 18: 551–556.
13. Dulloo, A.G., Geissler, C.A., Horton, T., Collins, A., Miller, D.S. Normal caffeine consumption: Influence on thermogenesis and daily energy expenditure in lean and post obese human volunteers. *Am J Clin Nutr.* 1989; 49: 44–50.
14. Poehlman, E.T., LaChance, P., Tremblay, A. et al. The effect of prior exercise and caffeine ingestion on metabolic rate and hormones in young adult males. *Can J Physiol Pharmacol.* 1989; 67: 10–16.

15. Koot, P., Deurenberg, P. Comparison of changes in energy expenditure and body temperatures after caffeine consumption. *Ann Nutr Metab.* 1995; 39: 135–142.

16. Belza, A., Jessen, A.B. Bioactive food stimulants of sympathetic activity: effect on 24-h energy expenditure and fat oxidation. *Eur J Clin Nutr.* 2005; 59: 733–741.

17. Hindmarch, I., Rigney, U., Stanley, N., Quinlan, P., Rycroft, J., Lane, J. A naturalistic investigation of the effects of day-long consumption of tea, coffee and water on alertness, sleep onset and sleep quality. *Psychopharmacology (Berl).* 2000; 149: 203–216.

18. Johnson-Kozlow, M., Kritz-Silverstein, D., Barrett-Connor, E., Morton, D. Coffee consumption and cognitive function among older adults. *Am J Epidemiol.* 2002; 156: 842–850.

19. Paluska, S.A. Caffeine and exercise. *Curr Sports Med Rep.* 2003; 2: 213–219.

20. Graham, T.E. Caffeine, coffee and ephedrine: Impact on exercise performance and metabolism. *Can J Appl Physiol.* 2001; 26(Suppl.): S103–19.

21. Motl, R.W., O'Connor, P.J., Dishman, R.K. Effect of caffeine on perceptions of leg muscle pain during moderate intensity cycling exercise. *J Pain.* 2003; 4: 316–321.

22. Hogervorst, E., Riedel, W.J., Kovacs, E., Brouns, F., Jolles, J. Caffeine improves cognitive performance after strenuous physical exercise. *Int J Sports Med.* 1999; 20: 354–361.

23. Applegate, E. Effective nutritional ergogenic aids. *Int J Sport Nutr.* 1999; 9: 229–239.

24. Costill, D.L., Dalsky, G.P., Fink, W.J. Effects of caffeine ingestion on metabolism and exercise performance. *Med Sci Sports* 1978; 10: 155–158.

25. McLellan, T.M., Bell, D.G. The impact of prior coffee consumption on the subsequent ergogenic effect of anhydrous caffeine. *Int J Sport Nutr Exerc Metab.* 2004; 14: 698–708.

26. Fiala, K.A., Casa, D.J., Roti, M.W. Rehydration with a caffeinated beverage during the nonexercise periods of three consecutive days of twice-a-day practices. *Int J Sport Nutr Exerc Metab.* 2004; 14: 419–429.

27. Armstrong, L.E. Caffeine, body fluid — electrolyte balance, and exercise performance. *Int J Sport Nutr Exerc Metab.* 2002; 12: 189–206.

28. Ryu, S., Choi, S.K., Joung, S.S. et al. Caffeine as a lipolytic food component increases endurance performance in rats and athletes. *J Nutr Sci Vitaminol (Tokyo).* 2001; 47: 139–146.

29. Erickson, M.A., Schwarzkopf, R.J., McKenzie, R.D. Effects of caffeine, fructose, and glucose ingestion on muscle glycogen utilization during exercise. *Med Sci Sports Exerc.* 1987; 19: 579–583.

30. Spriet, L.L., MacLean, D.A., Dyck, D.J., Hultman, E., Cederblad, G., Graham, T.E. Caffeine ingestion and muscle metabolism during prolonged exercise in humans. *Am J Physiol.* 1992; 262: E891–8.

31. Holtzman, S.G., Mante, S., Minneman, K.P. Role of adenosine receptors in caffeine tolerance. *J Pharmacol Exp Ther.* 1991; 256: 62–68.

32. Mohr, T., Van Soeren, M., Graham, T.E., Kjaer, M. Caffeine ingestion and metabolic responses of tetraplegic humans during electrical cycling. *J Appl Physiol.* 1998; 85: 979–985.

33. Bell, D.G., Jacobs, I., Ellerington, K. Effect of caffeine and ephedrine ingestion on anaerobic exercise performance. *Med Sci Sports Exerc.* 2001; 33: 1399–1403.

34. Penner, R., Neher, E., Takeshima, H., Nishimura, S., Numa, S. Functional expression of the calcium release channel from skeletal muscle ryanodine receptor cDNA. *FEBS Lett.* 1989; 259: 217–221.

35. Fryer, M.W., Neering, I.R. Actions of caffeine on fast- and slow-twitch muscles of the rat. *J Physiol.* 1989; 416: 435–454.

36. Lopes, J.M., Aubier, M., Jardim, J., Aranda, J.V., Macklem, P.T. Effect of caffeine on skeletal muscle function before and after fatigue. *J Appl Physiol.* 1983; 54: 1303–1305.

37. Doherty, M., Smith, P., Hughes, M., Davison, R. Caffeine lowers perceptual response and increases power output during high-intensity cycling. *J Sports Sci.* 2004; 22: 637–643.

38. Doherty, M., Smith, P.M.. Effects of caffeine ingestion on rating of perceived exertion during and after exercise: a meta-analysis. *Scand J Med Sci Sports.* 2005; 15: 69–78.

39. Wakabayashi, K., Kono, S., Shinchi, K. et al. Habitual coffee consumption and blood pressure: a study of self-defense officials in Japan. *Eur J Epidemiol.* 1998; 14: 669–673.

40. Lancaster, T., Muir, J., Silagy, C. The effects of coffee on serum lipids and blood pressure in a U.K. population. *J R Soc Med.* 1994; 87: 506–507.

41. Rakic, V., Burke, V., Beilin, L.J. Effects of coffee on ambulatory blood pressure in older men and women: a randomized controlled trial. *Hypertension.* 1999; 33: 869–873.

42. Hakim, A.A., Ross, G.W., Curb, J.D. et al. Coffee consumption in hypertensive men in older middle-age and the risk of stroke: the Honolulu heart program. *J Clin Epidemiol*. 1998; 51: 487–494.

43. Gensini, G.F., Conti, A.A. Does coffee consumption represent a coronary risk factor? *Recent Prog Med*. 2004; 95: 563–565.

44. Willett, W.C., Stampfer, M.J., Manson, J.E. et al. Coffee consumption and coronary heart disease in women: a ten-year followup. *JAMA* 1996; 275: 458–462.

45. Mukamal, K.J., Maclure, M., Muller, J.E., Sherwood, J.B., Mittleman, M.A. Caffeinated coffee consumption and mortality after acute myocardial infarction. *Am Heart J*. 2004; 147: 999–1004.

46. Jazbec, A., Simic, D., Corovic, N., Durakovic, Z., Pavlovic, M. Impact of coffee and other selected factors on general mortality and mortality due to cardiovascular disease in Croatia. *J Health Popul Nutr*. 2003; 21: 332–340.

47. Kleemola, P., Jousilahti, P., Pietinen, P., Vartiainen, E., Tuomilehto, J. Coffee consumption and the risk of coronary heart disease and death. *Arch Intern Med*. 2000; 160: 3393–3400.

48. Agardh, E.E., Carlsson, S., Ahlbom, A. et al. Coffee consumption, Type 2 diabetes and impaired glucose tolerance in Swedish men and women. *J Intern Med*. 2004; 255: 645–652.

49. Carlsson, S., Hammar, N., Grill, V., Kaprio, J. Coffee consumption and risk of Type 2 diabetes in Finnish twins. *Int J Epidemiol*. 2004; 33: 616–617.

50. Gerber, D.A. Coffee consumption and Type 2 diabetes mellitus. *Ann Intern Med*. 2004; 141: 323, author reply 323–4.

51. Glaser, J.H., Glaser, S.K. Coffee consumption and Type 2 diabetes mellitus. *Ann Intern Med*. 2004; 141: 323; author reply 323–4.

52. Louria, D.B. Coffee consumption and Type 2 diabetes mellitus. *Ann Intern Med*. 2004; 141: 321, author reply 323–4.

53. Rosengren, A., Dotevall, A., Wilhelmsen, L., Thelle, D., Johansson, S. Coffee and incidence of diabetes in Swedish women: A prospective 18-year follow-up study. *J Intern Med*. 2004; 255: 89–95.

54. Ranheim, T., Halvorsen, B. Coffee consumption and human health — beneficial or detrimental? Mechanisms for effects of coffee consumption on different risk factors for cardiovascular disease and Type 2 diabetes mellitus. *Mol Nutr Food Res*. 2005; 49: 274–284.

55. Salazar-Martinez, E., Willett, W.C., Ascherio, A. et al. Coffee consumption and risk for Type 2 diabetes mellitus. *Ann Intern Med*. 2004; 140: 1–8.

56. Soriguer, F., Rojo-Martinez, G., de Antonio, I.E. Coffee consumption and Type 2 diabetes mellitus. *Ann Intern Med*. 2004; 141: 321–3, author reply 323–4.

57. Tuomilehto, J., Hu, G., Bidel, S., Lindstrom, J., Jousilahti, P. Coffee consumption and risk of Type 2 diabetes mellitus among middle-aged Finnish men and women. *JAMA* 2004; 291: 1213–1219.

58. van Dam, R.M., Pasman, W.J., Verhoef, P. Effects of coffee consumption on fasting blood glucose and insulin concentrations: Randomized controlled trials in healthy volunteers. *Diabetes Care*. 2004; 27: 2990–2992.

59. Hogan, P., Dall, T., Nikolov, P., American Diabetes Association. Economic costs of diabetes in the U.S. in 2002. *Diabetes Care*. 2003; 26: 917–932.

60. Baker, J.A., Beehler, G.P., Sawant, A.C., Jayaprakash, V., McCann, S.E., Moysich, K.B. Consumption of coffee, but not black tea, is associated with decreased risk of premenopausal breast cancer. *J Nutr*. 2006; 136: 166–171.

61. Michels, K.B., Holmberg, L., Bergkvist, L., Wolk, A. Coffee, tea, and caffeine consumption and breast cancer incidence in a cohort of Swedish women. *Ann Epidemiol*. 2002; 12: 21–26.

62. Tavani, A., Bertuzzi, M., Talamini, R. et al. Coffee and tea intake and risk of oral, pharyngeal and esophageal cancer. *Oral Oncol*. 2003; 39: 695–700.

63. Woolcott, C.G., King, W.D., Marrett, L.D. Coffee and tea consumption and cancers of the bladder, colon and rectum. *Eur J Cancer Prev*. 2002; 11: 137–145.

64. Jordan, S.J., Purdie, D.M., Green, A.C., Webb, P.M. Coffee, tea and caffeine and risk of epithelial ovarian cancer. *Cancer Causes Control*. 2004; 15: 359–365.

65. Kurozawa, Y., Ogimoto, I., Shibata, A. et al. Dietary habits and risk of death due to hepatocellular carcinoma in a large scale cohort study in Japan — Univariate analysis of JACC study data. *Kurume Med J*. 2004; 51: 141–149.

66. Mack, W.J., Preston-Martin, S., Dal Maso, L. et al. A pooled analysis of case-control studies of thyroid cancer: cigarette smoking and consumption of alcohol, coffee, and tea. *Cancer Causes Control.* 2003; 14: 773–785.

67. Michaud, D.S., Giovannucci, E., Willett, W.C., Colditz, G.A., Fuchs, C.S. Coffee and alcohol consumption and the risk of pancreatic cancer in two prospective United States cohorts. *Cancer Epidemiol Biomarkers Prev.* 2001; 10: 429–437.

25 Nutraceutical Stability Concerns and Shelf Life Testing

Leonard N. Bell

CONTENTS

I. INTRODUCTION

The acceptability of a food product is achieved by its quality and nutritional content being maintained from the time of processing through distribution and storage to the final consumption of the product. Although the food and pharmaceutical industries have guidelines for determining product stability and insuring label claims, such is often not the case with nutraceutical products. However, nutraceuticals are subjected to the same types of quality losses during storage as food and pharmaceutical products. To maintain consumer acceptance and avoid possible governmental action, nutraceuticals should be evaluated for stability, including determination of product shelf life and insuring accurate label claims. The physiological benefits of nutraceuticals are achieved only if (1) the product is consumed and (2) the bioactive substance is present at the required concentration. If either of these conditions is not met due to a product quality change during storage, the nutraceutical or functional food loses its beneficial effect.

Shelf life is defined as the length of time after processing that a product remains acceptable to the consumer from a quality or safety perspective. A product can lose shelf life in several ways. Microbial growth in a product can decrease sensory acceptability via spoilage (e.g., the proliferation of lactic acid bacteria in milk) or cause a health risk (e.g., *Listeria* in luncheon meat). Physical changes, such as hardening of dried fruit and softening of crunchy cereals, are other mechanisms of shelf life loss. Finally, chemical reactions can occur during processing and storage, resulting in quality changes such as unacceptable color development, nutrient loss, and flavor modification.

The Food and Drug Administration (FDA) regulates food and pharmaceutical products with respect to nutritional and potency values placed on labels; these values can decrease over time due to deteriorative chemical reactions. A nonfortified food product such as pure orange juice is expected to contain at least 80% of the label value for a listed nutrient (e.g., vitamin C), whereas fortified foods, such as orange juice with added calcium, must contain 100% of the label value for the fortified nutrient, in this case calcium.[1] If the nutrient degrades over time and the amount of the nutrient falls below that required, based on the food type and label value, the product is considered misbranded by the Food, Drug, and Cosmetic Act and becomes illegal.[1] For pharmaceutical products, the expiration date is determined by the intersection of two lines: 90% of the label potency value and the lower 95% confidence limit of concentration decrease as a function of time.[2-4] Labeling issues with nutraceuticals and dietary supplements are less clear because little is known about their chemical stability, and for some products, the active ingredient has not been identified. Regulation of products is quite limited and was not helped by the passage of the Dietary Supplement Health and Education Act (DSHEA) in 1994.[5-6] However, some nutraceuticals are in the form of a "food" and as such are subject to the same regulations as traditional foods, which is one reason understanding stability issues associated with the product is important.

Nutraceuticals and functional foods include a vast array of different product types, containing a variety of different biologically active chemical compounds. Some of these compounds include isoflavones, flavonoids, carotenoids, bioactive peptides, and vitamins. Nutraceuticals can exist as dry powders, intermediate moisture products (e.g., bars), and beverages. Some type of food processing (e.g., mixing, heating, drying) is required to prepare the aforementioned product types. Nutraceutical producers need to know how much biologically active ingredient must be consumed to obtain the desired physiological effect, and compare this value to the amount of the ingredient remaining in the product after processing, distribution, and storage. Dry powders are often stored for over a year; however, the consumer may or may not be obtaining the desired nutraceutical "dose" from this product. For example, the ginsenoside contents in ginseng preparations were found to vary from close to 0 to as high as 9%.[6-7] Whereas some of the product inconsistency is due to variations of species, maturity, and plant source (e.g., root vs. leaf),[8] the potential for degradative reactions persist and product stability should be evaluated.

To address the issues raised previously, stability testing needs to be performed on the product. The first step of the process is to identify the bioactive substance in the nutraceutical. Coffee contains hundreds of chemical compounds, but caffeine is the well-known bioactive compound, providing the stimulatory effect. Similarly, hypericin is the active substance found in St. John's wort.[9-10] After the bioactive compound has been identified, an accurate and precise analytical method for its determination is required to measure its concentration as a function of time under different conditions, including temperature, moisture, oxygen, and added ingredients. After the concentration of the active compound is measured over time, the data undergoes kinetic modeling, and shelf life predictions can be made for conditions typical of product distribution and storage. The basic aspects of stability testing are presented subsequently.

II. KINETIC MODELING OF CHEMICAL REACTIONS

Assuming the biologically active substance has been identified and a precise analytical method for its detection developed, the first step of shelf life testing is to collect concentration data as a function of time at a constant temperature. The greater the number of data points along with the greater extent of concentration change, the more statistically valid the mathematical modeling becomes.[11] It is most desirable to have at least 13 data points and to collect data past a 50% decrease in ingredient concentration because this allows for reasonable confidence limits to be calculated.[12] However, typically 10 data points are equally effective with only a slight increase in the confidence limits as compared to 13 data points. Once the number of data points is reduced below 8, the confidence limits become significantly larger and shelf life predictions become increasingly error prone.

Chemical reactions consist of reactants being converted into products as outlined below.

$$aA \rightarrow bB \qquad\qquad (25.1)$$

The loss of reactant A or the accumulation of product B results in the product losing shelf life. The elementary reaction above proceeds at a specific rate (concentration change vs. time, $-d[A]/dt$); the rate expression is defined as:

$$-d[A]/(a)dt = +d[B]/(b)dt = k[A]^a = k[B]^b \qquad (25.2)$$

where $[A]$ and $[B]$ are concentrations of reactant and product, respectively; a and b are molecularities of the compounds; and k is the rate constant.[13] The molecularity represents the true number of molecules involved in the reaction as determined from its mechanism; thus, for complex chemical reactions, the true rate expression cannot be determined from the overall reaction pathway.[13] Rate constants depend upon temperature, and their determination is central for shelf life predictions.

In complex food and pharmaceutical systems, many variables influence chemical reactions, and the overall pathway for a given reaction is frequently written as:

$$\text{reactant(s)} \rightarrow \text{product(s)} \qquad (25.3)$$

where the true reaction mechanism is generally ignored. For this type of reaction, the rate expression for reactant loss is written as:

$$-d[A]/dt = k_{obs}[A]^n \qquad (25.4)$$

where $-d[A]/dt$ is the concentration change over time, $[A]$ is the reactant concentration, k_{obs} is the observed or apparent rate constant, and n is the reaction order. As mentioned, for many chemical reactions in foods and pharmaceuticals, n is not the true reaction order as determined from physical chemistry, but is the pseudo-order of the reaction.

The reaction order can be determined from several techniques, as discussed in physical chemistry textbooks.[13] Other methods can also be found in the literature.[14–15] Because shelf life predictions are most effective with linear models, simple mathematical techniques consistent with reaction kinetic concepts are frequently employed to linearize the quality loss data. For food systems, most data can be fit to either pseudo-zero-order or pseudo-first-order kinetic models.[12] By performing a linear regression on the reactant concentration as a function of time ($n = 0$ for pseudo-zero-order) and the natural log of reactant concentration as a function of time ($n = 1$ for pseudo-first-order), the more appropriate order can be selected by evaluating the coefficient of determination (r^2). If an adequate number of data points has been collected past a concentration change of 50%, then the data having the highest r^2 value is usually the best pseudo-order for modeling quality loss associated with the change in reactant or product concentration.[12] Figure 25.1 shows an example of determining the pseudo-order for aspartame degradation using previously collected data,[16] where the data is plotted as both pseudo-zero-order and pseudo-first-order. As shown in this figure, the pseudo-first-order model provides the better linear fit and would be used to calculate the rate constant. A discussion of different pseudo-order kinetic models for calculating rate constants follows subsequently. Again, the determination of rate constants under different conditions is a critical component of shelf life studies.

The pseudo-zero-order kinetic equation ($n = 0$) for reactant loss takes the form of:

$$-d[A]/dt = k_{obs}[A]^0 = k_{obs} \qquad (25.5)$$

To model product formation, the negative sign in front of $-d[A]/dt$ is simply changed to a positive sign, $+d[A]/dt$. Upon integration of Equation 25.5, the following expression is derived:

$$[A] = [A]_0 - k_{obs}t \qquad (25.6)$$

where $[A]_0$ is the initial reactant concentration and $[A]$ is the concentration at time, t. The pseudo-zero-order rate constant, k_{obs}, is determined from the linear slope of a pseudo-zero-order kinetic

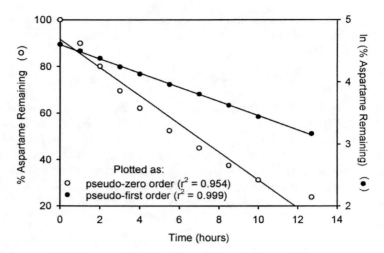

FIGURE 25.1 Aspartame degradation in 0.1 M phosphate buffer at pH 7 and 25°C plotted as pseudo-zero-order and pseudo-first-order kinetic models. (Data from Bell, L.N. *Aspartame Degradation Kinetics in Low and Intermediate Moisture Food Systems*, M.S. thesis. University of Minnesota, St. Paul, MN, 1989.)

plot, where reactant concentration, $[A]$, is plotted as a function of time. Figure 25.2 shows a general example of the pseudo-zero-order kinetic plot. The time to reach 50% of the initial reactant concentration is known as the half-life. The half-life, $t_{1/2}$, of a pseudo-zero-order reaction is calculated using the following equation:

$$t_{1/2} = [A]_0/2k_{obs} \qquad (25.7)$$

and is identified in Figure 25.2. The value of the half-life is dependent upon the initial reactant concentration. The formation of brown pigmentation from the nonenzymatic browning reaction is commonly modeled using pseudo-zero-order kinetics.[17-19]

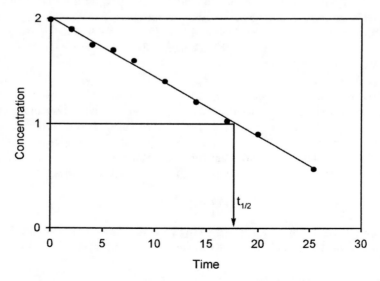

FIGURE 25.2 General example of a pseudo-zero-order kinetic plot. Slope equals pseudo-zero-order rate constant. The half-life, $t_{1/2}$, of the reaction is identified.

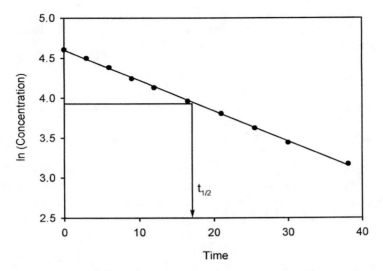

FIGURE 25.3 General example of a pseudo-first-order kinetic plot. Slope equals pseudo-first-order rate constant. The half-life, $t_{1/2}$, of the reaction is identified.

The pseudo-first-order kinetic equation ($n = 1$) for reactant loss takes the form of:

$$-d[A]/dt = k_{obs}[A]^1 = k_{obs}[A] \tag{25.8}$$

Again, to model product formation, the negative sign in Equation 25.8 is replaced with a positive sign. Integrating Equation 25.8, the following expression is derived:

$$\ln[A] = \ln[A]_0 - k_{obs}t \tag{25.9}$$

which can be rearranged into:

$$\ln([A]/[A]_0) = -k_{obs}t \tag{25.10}$$

where $[A]_0$ is the initial reactant concentration, $[A]$ is the concentration at time, t, and $[A]/[A]_0$ is the ratio (i.e., percent) of the reactant remaining at time, t. The pseudo-first-order rate constant, k_{obs}, is determined from the linear slope of a pseudo-first-order kinetic plot, where the natural log of reactant concentration is plotted as a function of time. If log base ten is used instead of the natural log, the slope needs to be multiplied by 2.303 to obtain the rate constant. Figure 25.3 shows a general example of the pseudo-first-order plot. The half-life, $t_{1/2}$, of a pseudo-first-order reaction is calculated as follows:

$$t_{1/2} = 0.693/k_{obs} \tag{25.11}$$

The value of the half-life is independent of the initial reactant concentration for pseudo-first-order reactions, unlike pseudo-zero-order reactions. The time corresponding to the half-life is also indicated in Figure 25.3; note that the y-axis values of 4.605 and 3.91 represent the natural log of 100% and 50% of the initial reactant concentration, respectively. In addition to aspartame degradation,[16,20–22] pseudo-first-order kinetics have been used to model riboflavin degradation,[23] thiamin degradation,[23–24] vitamin C degradation,[25–26] enzymatic activity loss,[27] and soy isoflavone loss.[28–29]

Pseudo-zero- and pseudo-first-order kinetics do not always adequately model quality loss data. When two compounds react to form a product, second-order kinetics are often more appropriate to use. For the reaction,

$$A + B \rightarrow \text{product(s)} \tag{25.12}$$

the rate equation for the loss of reactant A or B via a second-order reaction has the following form:

$$-d[A]/dt = -d[B]/dt = k_{obs}[A][B] \tag{25.13}$$

assuming one molecule of A reacts with one molecule of B. In Equation 25.13, [A] and [B] represent the concentrations of the reactants and k_{obs} is the second-order rate constant. If the initial concentrations of A and B are equal, Equation 25.13 can be integrated and rearranged to yield the following expression:

$$1/[A] - 1/[A]_0 = k_{obs}t \tag{25.14}$$

where $[A]_0$ is the initial reactant concentration and $[A]$ is the reactant concentration at time, t. A plot of $1/[A]$ as a function of time yields a straight line whose slope is equal to the second-order rate constant. A more detailed discussion of second-order kinetics, including kinetic modeling when the initial reactant concentrations are not equal, can be found in physical chemistry textbooks.[13] The most common food related reaction that follows this type of kinetics is reactant loss associated with the Maillard reaction.[18–19] The Maillard reaction begins with an amine (e.g., an amino acid or peptide) reacting with a carbonyl (e.g., monosaccharides), ultimately leading to the destruction of both the sugar and amino acid.

Some reactions may not follow pseudo-zero, pseudo-first, or second-order kinetics. Lipid oxidation, for example, has its own unique kinetic models.[30–31] Therefore, the scientific literature should be consulted to determine what types of kinetic models have been used successfully for a particular reaction as part of a shelf life study.

A. EFFECT OF TEMPERATURE ON STABILITY

Temperature has a dramatic effect on the rates of chemical reactions. The primary effect of temperature is on the rate constant, although other more subtle effects also exist (e.g., changes in water activity, melting of lipids, glass–rubber transitions). Product deterioration increases as temperature increases, which is the rationale for storing food and pharmaceutical products under refrigerated conditions. By determining the effect of temperature on a chemical reaction's rate constant, predictions can be made as to rates at other temperatures. To evaluate this temperature effect, the pseudo-order rate constant should be determined at a minimum of three temperatures, but preferably four or five to increase the confidence of the predictions.[12]

The effect of temperature on chemical reactions occurring in food and pharmaceutical products generally follows the Arrhenius relationship:

$$k_{obs} = (A)\exp(-E_a/RT) \tag{25.15}$$

where A is the preexponential factor, E_a is the Arrhenius activation energy, R is the ideal gas constant, and T is temperature in Kelvin.[13] Using the value of 8.314 J/(mol K) for the ideal gas constant, the activation energy is in units of J/mol. If the ideal gas constant is taken as 1.987 cal/(mol K), the activation energy has units of cal/mol. A plot of the natural log of the pseudo-order rate constant, $\ln(k_{obs})$, as a function of the reciprocal of absolute temperature, $1/T$, yields a straight line, as shown in Figure 25.4 for vitamin C degradation.[25] The slope and intercept of the line equal $-E_a/R$ and

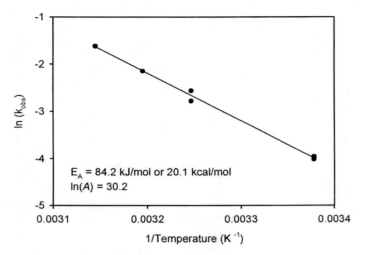

FIGURE 25.4 Arrhenius plot for vitamin C degradation in a model system at water activity 0.32. (Data from Lee, S.H. and Labuza, T.P. Destruction of ascorbic acid as a function of water activity. *J. Food Sci.,* 40: 370–373, 1975.)

ln(*A*), respectively. Using this information, pseudo-order rate constants at any other temperature can be calculated. However, the confidence of the prediction depends upon the quality of the kinetic data, the number of temperatures used to obtain the activation energy, and the distance from the experimental temperatures one is trying to predict. Labuza and Kamman have discussed aspects for optimizing the confidence of temperature extrapolations using the Arrhenius equation.[12]

Another approach for modeling the temperature effect on chemical reactions is by calculating Q_{10} values.[12] The ratio of the rate constant at one temperature to the rate constant at 10°C lower is one definition of Q_{10}. Another definition of Q_{10} is the ratio of the shelf life at one temperature to the shelf life at a temperature 10°C higher. To determine the Q_{10} value, a shelf life plot is constructed, where the natural log of shelf life (or half-life) is plotted as a function of temperature in degrees Celsius. The absolute value of the slope, b, from this plot is used to calculate the Q_{10} value, as shown below:

$$Q_{10} = \exp(10|b|) \tag{25.16}$$

A shelf life plot of the vitamin C degradation data[25] appears in Figure 25.5. The Q_{10} value of 2.96, as determined from the slope of Figure 25.5, means that the stability of vitamin C at 25°C is approximately three times less than that at 15°C. Similarly, the Q_{10} value for thiamin degradation was calculated to be 3.3 from previously published stability data.[24] Using this Q_{10} value for thiamin degradation, an 80-d shelf life at 20°C will be shortened to 38 d by increasing the temperature only 5°C to 25°C.

The relationship between the Q_{10} value and Arrhenius activation energy is shown in the following equation.[12]

$$\ln(Q_{10}) = 10E_a/RT(T + 10) \tag{25.17}$$

This equation also shows that the Q_{10} is dependent upon temperature, and as such, extrapolations are valid only over a narrow temperature range (i.e., <25°C). The Arrhenius activation energy is not temperature dependent and should therefore be used when trying to extrapolate kinetic data over larger temperature ranges. However, in both cases the assumption is made that no physical changes of the product (i.e., lipid melting, glass transition) occur over the extrapolated temperature range.

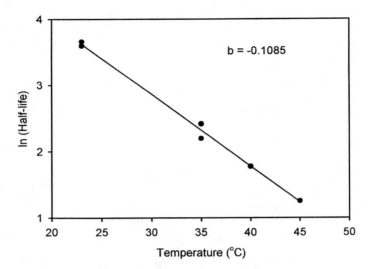

FIGURE 25.5 Shelf life plot for vitamin C degradation in a model system at water activity 0.32. (Data from Lee, S.H. and Labuza, T.P. Destruction of ascorbic acid as a function of water activity. *J. Food Sci.*, 40: 370–373, 1975.)

Temperature abuse is frequently the major factor limiting product shelf life. A prime example is outdoor storage displays of aspartame-sweetened beverages by mini-markets; these canned products sit in the hot summer sun for long periods of time before purchase. The temperature abuse these products experience enhances aspartame degradation, decreasing product sweetness and acceptability. The same situation exists for products stored in hot automobile trunks and garages. Similarly, the degradation of genistin, an isoflavone in soy milk, depends upon the storage temperature. Genistin has a half-life of over 20 months at 25°C, but at 37°C (abuse conditions) its half-life is reduced to 6 months.[28] Establishing quality control procedures during processing and distribution can help reduce excessive temperature exposure of the product. Refrigeration, though a more expensive option, can substantially extend product shelf life. Dates and handling instructions on product labels can be used to help educate consumers about the consequences of temperature abuse. One approach for indicating more accurately the thermal history of a product is by the use of time temperature indicators (TTIs). TTIs are small tags that provide a visual indication as to the net temperature exposure of a product and may improve the accuracy of shelf life dating. Concepts associated with the use of TTIs have been discussed in the literature.[32–35] Controlling temperature abuse is the primary way to increase the shelf life of nutraceuticals and functional foods and to improve the accuracy of their nutritional labeling.

B. EFFECT OF MOISTURE ON STABILITY

The importance of moisture content and water activity has long been recognized with respect to the evaluation of product stability and prediction of shelf life, especially for dry powders and intermediate moisture foods.[36–38] Food stability generally correlates better with water activity than moisture content.[39] Water activity (a_w), which is related to the chemical potential of water, can be defined as:

$$a_W = p/p_o \tag{25.18}$$

where p is the partial pressure of water in a product at a given temperature, and p_o is the partial pressure of pure water at that same temperature.[37,39] Water activity values range from 0 at dryness

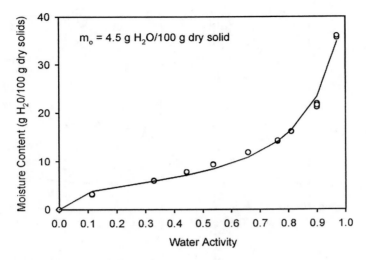

FIGURE 25.6 Moisture sorption isotherm for oat fiber at 25°C.

to 1 for pure water. Water activity is the governing force that dictates moisture transfer between a product and the environment until equilibrium is obtained.[40]

The relationship between water activity and equilibrium moisture content of a substance is shown via moisture sorption isotherms,[40] such as that shown in Figure 25.6. One of the more frequently utilized mathematical models of moisture sorption data is the GAB equation, which can be written as:

$$m = m_o k C a_W / [(1 - k a_W)(1 - k a_W + k C a_W)] \tag{25.19}$$

where m is the moisture content, m_o is the monolayer moisture content, and k and C are constants representing the thermodynamics of multilayer moisture adsorption.[40–41] Nonlinear regression of the moisture sorption data yields values for m_o, k, and C. Of interest is the value of m_o because many chemical reactions occur only minimally at and below this moisture content.[37,40,41] Chemical stability of solids generally decreases as water activity increases above m_o due to an increase in reactant mobility.[37,40] A stability minimum often exists at an intermediate water activity. At water activities above this minimum, stability may increase due to reactant dilution reducing the probability of molecular collision and subsequent reactivity.[37,40] Figure 25.7 shows the effect of water activity on aspartame shelf life,[21,42] where the shelf life is defined as the time to reach 20% of the initial aspartame concentration. The shelf life minimum is at a water activity of approximately 0.8 for aspartame at pH 5 and 30°C.

From the monolayer to the stability minimum, a plot of the log base ten of the shelf life as a function of water activity often yields a straight line.[40] From the absolute value of the slope, B, the Q_A value can be calculated using the following equation:

$$Q_A = 10^{0.1|B|} \tag{25.20}$$

Similar to the Q_{10} value discussed previously, the Q_A is the ratio of the shelf life at one water activity to the shelf life at a water activity of 0.1 units higher. This expression can be used to predict the shelf life at different water activities within the linear range. A Q_A plot of the aspartame degradation data[21,42] is shown in Figure 25.8. From this plot, a Q_A of 1.54 was determined, meaning that if the product has a 0.1 unit increase in water activity, the shelf life decreases a factor of 1.54. The Q_A values for the degradation of various vitamins (i.e., riboflavin, thiamin, ascorbic acid) were similar, ranging from 1.3–1.7 as calculated from previously published kinetic data.[23,25]

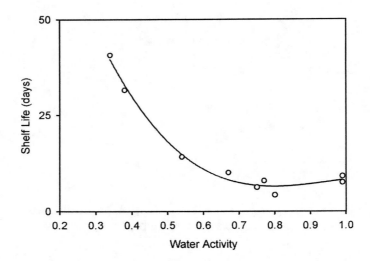

FIGURE 25.7 Shelf life of aspartame at pH 5 and 30°C as a function of water activity. (Data from Bell, L.N. and Labuza, T.P. Aspartame degradation kinetics as affected by pH in intermediate and low moisture food systems. *J. Food Sci.,* 56: 17–20, 1991; Bell, L.N. *Investigations Regarding the Definition and Meaning of pH in Reduced-Moisture Model Food Systems.* Ph.D. dissertation. University of Minnesota, St. Paul, MN, 1992.)

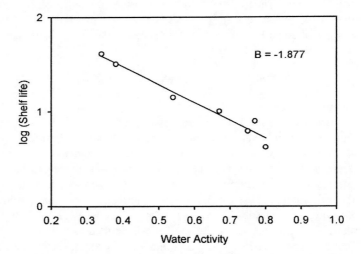

FIGURE 25.8 Q_A plot for aspartame shelf life at pH 5 and 30°C. (Data from Bell, L.N. and Labuza, T.P. Aspartame degradation kinetics as affected by pH in intermediate and low moisture food systems. *J. Food Sci.,* 56: 17–20, 1991; and Bell, L.N. *Investigations Regarding the Definition and Meaning of pH in Reduced-Moisture Model Food Systems.* Ph.D. dissertation. University of Minnesota, St. Paul, MN, 1992.)

An additional factor to consider is that in sealed packages, temperature influences the water activity of the food product. From moisture sorption data collected at different temperatures, the Clausius–Clapeyron equation, shown below, can be used to predict the water activity at a constant moisture content for the new temperature.[40–41]

$$\ln(a_{w2}/a_{w1}) = -(Q_S/R)(1/T_2 - 1/T_1) \qquad (25.21)$$

In the above equation, Q_S is the excess heat of sorption, and R is the ideal gas constant.[40–41] A plot of the natural log of water activity as a function of reciprocal temperature in Kelvin yields a straight line, from which the water activity at other temperatures can be extrapolated.[40–41] Accurate shelf life predictions require knowledge of the true water activity at the actual product storage temperature, which may be different from the experimental temperature conditions.

Another issue associated with moisture is its ability to plasticize amorphous solids; aspects of this phenomenon are presented in detail by Roos.[43] Briefly, the conversion of a rigid glassy amorphous solid into a softer more viscoelastic rubbery solid is known as the glass transition. This conversion is promoted by either increasing temperature or adsorbing moisture. The glass-to-rubber transition can promote unwanted crystallization of sugars, softening of crispy bakery products, and clumping of powders, making such products unacceptable. In addition to physical changes, the glass transition may impact chemical stability. Much research is continuing in this area to more clearly elucidate potential effects. Nevertheless, the glass transition can cause a product to become unacceptable such that the product is not consumed. As mentioned earlier, physiological effects of nutraceuticals are only achieved if the product is consumed.

As discussed, moisture transfer within a product or between the product and the exterior environment can lead to a loss of shelf life. Moisture gain can cause enhanced chemical reactivity as well as undesirable physical changes (stickiness, loss of crispness). Thus, the selection of packaging to reduce moisture gain (or loss) is important for maximizing nutraceutical stability. Understanding moisture sorption isotherms allows for proper package selection and the ultimate control of moisture transfer.[40] The use of anticaking agents, such as calcium silicate, can help reduce undesirable clumping of powders, whereas the use of humectants (e.g., glycerol, sucrose, salt) can reduce water activity.[40] Handling instructions can also help by informing consumers of the importance of properly resealing packages of partially consumed nutraceutical products. Controlling undesirable effects associated with moisture is the second approach toward improving nutraceutical stability.

C. Effect of Oxygen on Stability

Several nutraceutical ingredients are sensitive to oxygen. Polyunsaturated fatty acids, β-carotene, and vitamin C are all subject to enhanced degradation due to oxidation.[44] For example, water containing vitamin C and 5 ppm copper at pH 3.2 and 30°C lost 30% more vitamin C when shaken for 30 min (oxygen incorporated) as compared to unshaken solutions.[45] Lipid oxidation is also affected by the amount of available oxygen, as shown by the following expression for the oxidation rate, R:

$$1/R = (1/k_1)\{1 + ([O_2]/k_2)\} \tag{25.22}$$

where k_1 and k_2 are rate constants and $[O_2]$ is the oxygen concentration.[30] At low oxygen concentrations, the oxidation rate increases linearly with increasing oxygen concentration. Above a critical oxygen concentration, the rate becomes independent of oxygen concentration. More information on the kinetics of lipid oxidation can be found elsewhere.[30–31]

If oxygen-sensitive substances exist in the nutraceutical, selection of oxygen impermeable packaging can help extend product shelf life. Encapsulating these ingredients to shield them from oxygen may also limit oxidation. In addition, the use of antioxidants can be beneficial for extending product quality. For example, the stability of lycopene in tomato oleoresins was improved by incorporating antioxidants.[46] Packets of iron enclosed in the product's package also keep the oxygen content low; the iron reacts with oxygen to form iron oxide (i.e., rust). By removing oxygen from the package, these oxygen scavengers help prevent undesirable oxidation during product storage.[47]

D. Effects of Ingredients on Stability

Nutraceuticals and functional foods contain more than just the bioactive ingredient in the formulation. These products often contain amines (e.g., amino acids, proteins), carbonyls (e.g., sugars, flavors), minerals, and buffer salts, among other substances. These substances can have dramatic effects on the chemical stability and ultimate acceptability of the nutraceutical.

Amines and carbonyls react via the Maillard reaction to cause flavor modification, amino acid destruction, and brown discoloration. If the bioactive substances in nutraceuticals contain amine or carbonyl groups, the possibility exists for them to degrade via the Maillard reaction. Tagatose is an alternative nondigestible sweetener that has been shown to behave as a prebiotic by stimulating butyrate production and selecting favorable bacteria in the colon.[48–49] However, tagatose can react with amines in nutraceutical products during processing and storage, causing a loss of tagatose and a reduction of the prebiotic effect. Even without loss of the bioactive substance, other quality changes (e.g., browning, off-flavors) that reduce the likelihood of consuming the nutraceutical result in the consumer not obtaining the expected physiological effect from the product. Potential reactivity between the active nutraceutical substance and other ingredients in the formulation must therefore be evaluated.

The presence of minerals, either intentionally added or naturally occurring, can also influence product stability. Lipid oxidation is catalyzed by the presence of minerals (e.g., iron, copper), which results in potent off-flavors and aromas.[30–31] A small amount of such oxidation can result in an unacceptable product. Similarly, vitamin C degradation is also catalyzed by metal ions. For example, as the concentration of copper increased in water, the amount of vitamin C remaining dramatically decreased.[45] Thus, fortifying a nutraceutical with both vitamin C and a mineral, such as iron, can lead to enhanced vitamin C degradation and nutritional labels that are no longer in accordance with federal regulations.

Buffer salts are often added to foods for controlling the pH; however, these can also have significant effects on chemical reactivity. Phosphate buffer enhances the degradation of aspartame as compared to citrate buffer, and the effect increases as the buffer concentration increases.[50] Phosphate buffer was also shown to increase the loss of glycine and extent of browning associated with the Maillard reaction.[51] Figure 25.9 shows the relative effects of pH and buffer type on the shelf life of thiamin-containing solutions; at pH 5, thiamin is more stable in phosphate buffer, whereas at pH 7 thiamin is more stable in citrate buffer.[52] Thiamin loss also increases as buffer concentration increases.[52] Thus, the selection of buffer type and concentration can have serious implications for nutraceutical product stability.

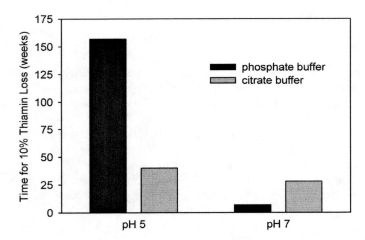

FIGURE 25.9 Effect of buffer type and pH on the stability of thiamin in 0.02 M buffer solutions at 25°C. (Data from Pachapurkar, D. and Bell, L.N. Kinetics of thiamin degradation in solutions under ambient storage conditions. *J. Food Sci.,* 70(7): C423–C426, 2005.)

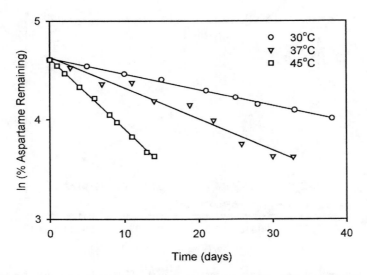

FIGURE 25.10 Pseudo-first-order kinetic plots of aspartame degradation in 0.1 M phosphate buffer at pH 3 and various temperatures. (Data from Bell, L.N., *Aspartame Degradation Kinetics in Low and Intermediate Moisture Food Systems*. Master's thesis. University of Minnesota, St. Paul, MN, 1989.)

III. ACCELERATED SHELF LIFE TESTING

Although it is desirable to investigate chemical stability in a system at conditions as close to those of the commercial product as possible, often the time constraints of product development require the use of accelerated shelf life testing for predicting product stability. Accelerated shelf life testing utilizes extreme conditions to enhance shelf life loss followed by an extrapolation to normal conditions. The extreme conditions may include high temperatures and/or high water activities. The benefit of this protocol is that answers come faster, saving time and money, but at the risk of some errors.

The best way to understand accelerated shelf life testing and shelf life prediction in general is to discuss two examples. The first example is aspartame degradation in 0.1 M phosphate buffer at pH 3, where the data was collected from 30–45°C.[16] Figure 25.10 shows the degradation data, modeled using pseudo-first-order kinetics. At least 9 data points were collected past 50% degradation. The slopes of these plots are the pseudo-first-order rate constants. Figure 25.11 shows the Arrhenius plot of the aspartame kinetic data from which pseudo-first-order rate constants at any other temperature can be mathematically extrapolated. At 25°C, the extrapolated rate constant of 0.00924 d^{-1} was found to be the same as that determined experimentally (0.0089–0.0011 d^{-1}).[50] For refrigerated storage at 4°C, the extrapolated rate constant is 0.000802 d^{-1}. If one assumes an initial aspartame concentration of 600 ppm and that the product remains acceptable to a final concentration of 500 ppm, then the shelf life, t, at 4°C is calculated using the pseudo-first-order kinetic model (Equation 25.10) as shown below:

$$\ln(500/600) = -(0.000802 \text{ d}^{-1})(t) \tag{25.23}$$

Equation 25.23 yields a shelf life of 7.5 months, which would require too long to determine experimentally for most businesses.

The second example uses aspartame degradation data from 0.01 M phosphate buffer at pH 7, but collected from 70–100°C.[22] Using the Arrhenius relationship (Equation 25.15), the pseudo-first-order rate constant for aspartame degradation at 25°C was calculated to be 0.042 h^{-1}. The experimentally determined rate constant (0.014 h^{-1})[50] is much lower than that predicted using the high

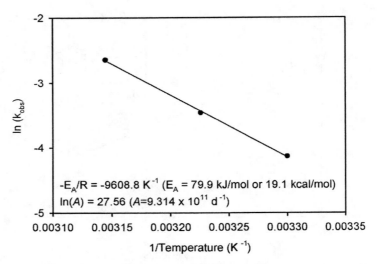

FIGURE 25.11 Arrhenius plot of aspartame degradation in 0.1 M phosphate buffer at pH 3. (Data from Bell, L.N., *Aspartame Degradation Kinetics in Low and Intermediate Moisture Food Systems*.   Master's   thesis. University of Minnesota, St. Paul, MN, 1989.)

temperature data. This result means that the true shelf life is three times longer than that predicted by accelerated shelf life testing. In this case, product would be assumed to have deteriorated three times sooner than it really would, resulting in acceptable product being discarded. The opposite effect is possible as well, where the shelf life is shorter than expected. These are two potential problems associated with accelerated shelf life testing.

The under- and overprediction of shelf life, as demonstrated previously, can be attributed in part to changes in water activity, pH, and reactant solubility as a function of temperature. In addition, thermal transitions (e.g., glass transitions and lipid melting) can impact predictions from high to low temperatures. Another limitation of accelerated shelf life testing is a substance that degrades by different mechanisms at different temperatures. Genistin degradation had different activation energies depending upon the temperature range over which the reaction was studied; the authors suggested that differing reaction mechanisms may explain these differences.[28] Extrapolating between the different temperature ranges would lead to errors in shelf life predictions.

An additional problem associated with accelerated shelf life testing is caused by competing chemical reactions. The activation energies of various chemical reaction types differ. Thus, two reactions with different activation energies will each predominate over a different temperature range. A critical crossover temperature exists as shown in Figure 25.12. Below this temperature (30°C), reaction 1 predominates and is responsible for shelf life loss; however, above this temperature reaction 2 predominates. For example, oxidation of polyunsaturated fatty acids may be the major mode of product deterioration at one temperature, whereas vitamin degradation predominates at another temperature. The possibility of multiple modes of nutraceutical deterioration needs to be recognized before using accelerated shelf life testing. The critical reaction responsible for loss of shelf life under typical storage conditions should be identified and utilized during the shelf life test. Thus, while accelerated shelf life testing has its advantages, the potential errors need to be recognized. Other aspects of accelerated shelf life testing are discussed by Labuza and Schmidl.[53]

IV. FINAL THOUGHTS

Shelf life testing is an important aspect of nutraceutical product development. The consumer demands a quality product and that is possible only by optimizing the product shelf life. If the

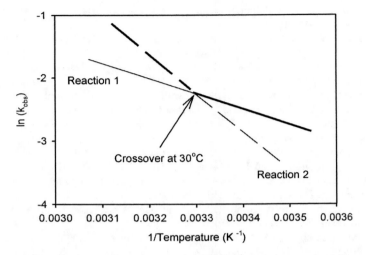

FIGURE 25.12 Arrhenius plot of two reactions occurring simultaneously in a nutraceutical. (The bold lines represent the region where each reaction predominates.)

biological activity or sensory attributes deteriorate, the product has failed to meet consumer expectations. Other implications associated with stability issues include failure of the product to meet label claims, which is a violation of federal law. Optimizing stability requires, at the very least, the ability to control temperature abuse and moisture transfer. Solutions for each of these have been presented. By using a well-designed experimental plan and appropriate kinetic modeling, accurate shelf life predictions can be made, benefiting both the company and the consumer.

REFERENCES

1. U.S. Code of Federal Regulations. Title 21, Part 101, Section 9, April 1999.
2. Carstensen, J.T. *Drug Stability Principles and Practices.* Marcel Dekker, New York, 1990.
3. Shultz, R.C. Proposed FDA guideline for stability testing. In *Stability Testing of Drug Products.* Grimm, W., Ed., Wissenschaftliche Verlagsgesellschaft mbH, Stuttgart, Germany, 1987.
4. Bolton, S. *Pharmaceutical Statistics: Practical and Clinical Applications,* 2nd ed. Marcel Dekker, New York, 1990.
5. Camire, M.E. and Kantor, M.A. Dietary supplements: nutritional and legal considerations. *Food Technol.,* 53(7): 87–96, 1999.
6. Anonymous. Herbal Roulette. *Consumer Rep.,* 60(11): 698–705, 1995.
7. Cui, J., Garle, M., Eneroth, P., and Bjorkhem, I. What do commercial ginseng preparations contain? *Lancet,* 344: 134, 1994.
8. Li, T.S.C. and Wang, L.C.H. Physiological components and health effects of ginseng, *Echinacea,* and sea buckthorn. In *Functional Foods: Biochemical and Processing Aspects.* Mazza, G., Ed., Technomic Publishing, Lancaster, PA, 1998.
9. Bennett, Jr., D.A., Phun, L., Polk, J.F., Voglino, S.A., Zlotnik, V., and Raffa, R.B. Neuropharmacology of St. John's wort (Hypericum). *Ann. Pharmacother.* 32: 1201–1208, 1998.
10. Miller, A.L. St. John's wort (*Hypericum perforatum*): clinical effects on depression and other conditions. *Altern. Med. Rev.,* 3: 18–26, 1998.
11. Benson, S.W. *The Foundations of Chemical Kinetics.* McGraw-Hill, New York, 1960.
12. Labuza, T.P. and Kamman, J.F. Reaction kinetics and accelerated tests simulation as a function of temperature. In *Computer-Aided Techniques in Food Technology.* Saguy, I., Ed., Marcel Dekker, New York, 1983.
13. Levine, I.N. *Physical Chemistry,* 3rd ed. McGraw-Hill, New York, 1988.

14. Saguy, I. and Karel, M. Modeling of quality deterioration during food processing and storage. *Food Technol.*, 34(2): 78–85, 1980.

15. Bates, D.M. and Watts, D.G. *Nonlinear Regression Analysis and Its Applications.* John Wiley & Sons, New York, 1988.

16. Bell, L.N. *Aspartame Degradation Kinetics in Low and Intermediate Moisture Food Systems.* M.S. thesis. University of Minnesota, St. Paul, MN, 1989.

17. Warmbier, H.C., Schnickels, R.A., and Labuza, T.P. Nonenzymatic browning kinetics in an intermediate moisture model system: effect of glucose to lysine ratio. *J. Food Sci.*, 41: 981–983, 1976.

18. Baisier, W.M. and Labuza, T.P. Maillard browning kinetics in a liquid model system. *J. Agric. Food Chem.*, 40: 707–713, 1992.

19. Bell, L.N., Touma, D.E., White, K.L., and Chen, Y.H. Glycine loss and Maillard browning as related to the glass transition in a model food system. *J. Food Sci.*, 63: 625–628, 1998.

20. Prudel, M. and Davidkova, E. Stability of -L-aspartyl-L-phenylalanine methyl ester hydrochloride in aqueous solutions. *Die Nahrung*, 25: 193–199, 1981.

21. Bell, L.N. and Labuza, T.P. Aspartame degradation kinetics as affected by pH in intermediate and low moisture food systems. *J. Food Sci.*, 56: 17–20, 1991.

22. Tsoubeli, M. and Labuza, T.P. Accelerated kinetic study of aspartame degradation in the neutral pH range. *J. Food Sci.*, 56: 1671–1675, 1991.

23. Dennison, D., Kirk, J., Bach, J., Kokoczka, P., and Heldman, D. Storage stability of thiamin and riboflavin in a dehydrated food system. *J. Food Proc. Preserv.*, 1: 43–54, 1977.

24. Arabshahi, A. and Lund, D.B. Thiamin stability in simulated intermediate moisture food. *J. Food Sci.*, 53: 199–203, 1988.

25. Lee, S.H. and Labuza, T.P. Destruction of ascorbic acid as a function of water activity. *J. Food Sci.*, 40: 370–373, 1975.

26. Kirk, J., Dennison, D., Kokoczka, P., and Heldman, D. Degradation of ascorbic acid in a dehydrated food system. *J. Food Sci.*, 42: 1274–1279, 1977.

27. Chen, Y.H., Aull, J.L., and Bell, L.N. Invertase storage stability and sucrose hydrolysis in solids as affected by water activity and glass transition. *J. Agric. Food Chem.*, 47: 504–509, 1999.

28. Eisen, B., Ungar, Y., and Shimoni, E. Stability of isoflavones in soy milk stored at elevated and ambient temperatures. *J. Agric. Food Chem.*, 51: 2212–2215, 2003.

29. Shimoni, E. Stability and shelf life of bioactive compounds during food processing and storage: soy isoflavones. *J. Food Sci.*, 69(6): R160–R166, 2004.

30. Labuza, T.P. Kinetics of lipid oxidation in foods. *CRC Crit. Rev. Food Technol.*, 2: 355–405, 1971.

31. Karel, M. Kinetics of lipid oxidation. In *Physical Chemistry of Foods.* Schwartzberg, H.G. and Hartel, R.W., Eds., Marcel Dekker, New York, 1992.

32. Taoukis, P.S. and Labuza, T.P. Applicability of time-temperature indicators as shelf life monitors of food products. *J. Food Sci.*, 54: 783–788, 1989.

33. Taoukis, P.S. and Labuza, T.P. Reliability of time-temperature indicators as food quality monitors under nonisothermal conditions. *J. Food Sci.*, 54: 789–792, 1989.

34. Sherlock, M., Fu, B., Taoukis, P.S., and Labuza, T.P. A systematic evaluation of time-temperature indicators for use as consumer tags. *J. Food Protect.*, 54: 885–889, 1991.

35. Taoukis, P.S., Labuza, T.P., and Francis, R.C. Time-temperature indicators as food quality monitors. In *Food Packaging Technology.* Henyon, D., Ed., American Society for Testing and Materials, Philadelphia, PA, 1991.

36. Duckworth, R.B., Ed. *Water Relations of Foods.* Academic Press, New York, 1975.

37. Labuza, T.P. The effect of water activity on reaction kinetics of food deterioration. *Food Technol.*, 34(4): 36–41 and 59, 1980.

38. Rockland, L.B. and Stewart, G.F., Eds. *Water Activity: Influences on Food Quality.* Academic Press, New York, 1981.

39. Karel, M. Recent research and development in the field of low-moisture and intermediate-moisture foods. *CRC Crit. Rev. Food Technol.*, 3: 329–373, 1973.

40. Bell, L.N. and Labuza, T.P. *Moisture Sorption: Practical Aspects of Isotherm Measurement and Use.* 2nd ed. AACC Press, St. Paul, MN, 2000.

41. Labuza, T.P., Kaanane, A., and Chen, J.Y. Effect of temperature on the moisture sorption isotherms and water activity shift of two dehydrated foods. *J. Food Sci.*, 50: 385–391, 1985.

42. Bell, L.N. *Investigations Regarding the Definition and Meaning of pH in Reduced-Moisture Model Food Systems.* Ph.D. dissertation. University of Minnesota, St. Paul, MN, 1992.

43. Roos, Y.H. *Phase Transitions in Foods.* Academic Press, San Diego, CA, 1995.

44. Fennema, O.R., Ed. *Food Chemistry,* 3rd ed. Marcel Dekker, New York, 1996.

45. Hsieh, Y.P. and Harris, N.D. Oxidation of ascorbic acid in copper-catalyzed sucrose solutions. *J. Food Sci.*, 52: 1384–1386, 1987.

46. Hackett, M.M., Lee, J.H., Francis, D., and Schwartz, S.J. Thermal stability and isomerization of lycopene in tomato oleoresins from different varieties. *J. Food Sci.*, 69(7): C536–C541, 2004.

47. Labuza, T.P. An introduction to active packaging for foods. *Food Technol.*, 50(4): 68 and 70–71, 1996.

48. Bertelsen, H., Jensen, B.B., and Buemann, B. D-Tagatose — a novel low-calorie bulk sweetener with prebiotic properties. *World Rev. Nutr. Diet.*, 85: 98-109, 1999.

49. Levin, G.V. Tagatose, the new GRAS sweetener and health product. *J. Med. Food*, 5: 23–36, 2002.

50. Bell, L.N. and Wetzel, C.R. Aspartame degradation in solution as impacted by buffer type and concentration. *J. Agric. Food Chem.*, 43: 2608–2612, 1995.

51. Bell, L.N. Maillard reaction as influenced by buffer type and concentration. *Food Chem.*, 59: 143–147, 1997.

52. Pachapurkar, D. and Bell, L.N. Kinetics of thiamin degradation in solutions under ambient storage conditions. *J. Food Sci.*, 70(7): C423–C426, 2005.

53. Labuza, T.P. and Schmidl, M.K. Accelerated shelf-life testing of foods. *Food Technol.*, 39(9): 57–62, 64 and 134, 1985.

26 Nutraceutical and Functional Food Application to Nonalcoholic Steatohepatitis

Dianne H. Volker and Diah Yunianingtias

CONTENTS

I. INTRODUCTION

Nonalcoholic steatohepatitis (NASH) is a condition characterized by liver injury, resembling alcoholic hepatitis, in the absence of significance alcohol consumption.[1–24] Although data regarding NASH prevalence is still scarce, it is thought that NASH prevalence has been increasing along with the trend of increasing risk factors.[1] *Syndrome X* and *metabolic syndrome* are the terms used to denote the cluster of abnormalities — insulin resistance, obesity, type II diabetes mellitus, hypertension, and hyperlipidemia — that are associated with NASH risk factors.[3,4] NASH is a part of the liver disorder known as nonalcoholic fatty liver disorder (NAFLD), which ranges from simple steatosis and nonalcoholic steatohepatitis (NASH) to fibrosis and cirrhosis.[5] Liver biopsy is the only way to distinguish NASH from the liver disorders within the NAFLD spectrum.[12] NASH may be asymptomatic for a long period of time; however, recent evidence has shown that NASH may develop into advanced liver disease (fibrosis, cirrhosis).[25–27] Despite the fact that there is no evidence-based treatment for NASH yet, an appropriate intervention is needed among people with high risk factors to prevent disease progression.[25] There has not been any large-scale randomized clinical trial for NASH treatment to date.[7] Key management for NASH is to treat related conditions.[28-32] Some studies have shown that NASH management involving nutritional aspects such as gradual weight loss and nutritional supplements of long chain fatty acids and antioxidants may provide beneficial results for the NASH patient.[32-48] Currently in Australia, recruitment of subjects in a longitudinal study is underway at Westmead Hospital, Royal Prince Alfred Hospital (RPAH), and the Western Sydney Division of General Practice, to examine the nutritional aspects of NASH treatment.

A. CONCEPTS AND ISSUES

In 1980, Ludwig and colleagues introduced the acronym NASH for the first time to describe liver injury in the absence of significant alcohol consumption. NASH is similar to alcoholic hepatitis.[1] NAFLD is a term used to refer to conditions ranging from simple steatosis and NASH to fibrosis and cirrhosis.[1-11] Thus, NASH is a stage of advanced disease within the NAFLD category.[24]

B. PATHOGENESIS

Pathogenesis of NASH is increasingly important in view of its relationship with NASH management.[3] Other important factors with regard to NASH pathogenesis are conditions associated with NASH, which have become more prevalent in the last two decades. Some evidence has shown that NASH may progress to advanced liver disease.[25-27] Day proposed the "two hits" concept for NASH pathogenesis in 2002.[7,21] This concept suggests a close relationship between obesity, insulin resistance, hyperlipidemia, and NASH. The "first hit" is the result of the development of steatosis, which sensitizes the liver to a "second hit" from further oxidative stress. The presence of factors associated with Syndrome X, such as obesity and insulin resistance, may increase the degree of steatosis and thus the progression of fibrosis.[7,21] Elevated insulin levels promote lipolysis, which leads to free fatty acid transported to the liver. Increasing free fatty acid supply results in fat in the form of triglycerides accumulating in the liver.[49-51] Oxidative stress in the "second hit" triggers the development of conditions, which range from simple steatosis to NASH and advanced liver disease.[21] Fatty acid oxidation produces oxidative stress. As shown in Figure 26.1, free fatty acids in the liver, which are metabolized within hepatic mitochondria, activate reactive oxygen species (ROS).[16,17,26]

Lipid peroxidation induced by ROS activation releases tumor necrosis factor alpha (TNF-α) as a consequence. A study by Crespo and colleagues has demonstrated that the degree of NASH severity is equal to the serum TNF-α.[18] Oxidative stress activates hepatic stellate cells, thus creating extracellullar matrix proteins, which are then responsible for liver fibrosis.[14-21]

II. DIAGNOSIS OF NASH

Most patients (45–100%) with NASH develop no specific symptoms.[5] Hepatomegaly is present in 75% of the patients. Although NASH is often diagnosed coincidentally, abnormal levels of serum transaminase lead to a NASH diagnosis.[3,12,14,16,17,25-37] In 65–90% of the cases, a ratio of less than one of the aspartate aminotransferase (AST)/alanine aminotransferase (ALT) helps to differentiate between NASH and alcoholic hepatitis.[49-52] A personal history, including alcohol consumption and all underlying conditions related to NASH should be investigated initially. Ultrasound and computer tomographic scans are only able to show hepatic steatosis. Liver biopsy is the only way to diagnose NASH accurately.[53-55] As NASH is thought to be responsible for two-thirds of cryptogenic cirrhosis, there is some evidence that NASH may progress to liver cancer.[56] Hepatocellular carcinoma (HCC) usually develops in the cirrhotic liver, and any form of cirrhosis predisposes to HCC, although the relative risk varies between causative factors.[57] The relative risk is highest for hepatitis B, hemochromatosis, and hepatitis C, and at an intermediate level for alcohol and metabolic related diseases.[56] Diagnostic tests become very important tools in gathering prognostic information for an early intervention to be made.[56] Liver biopsy is required for a diagnosis of NASH, in the presence

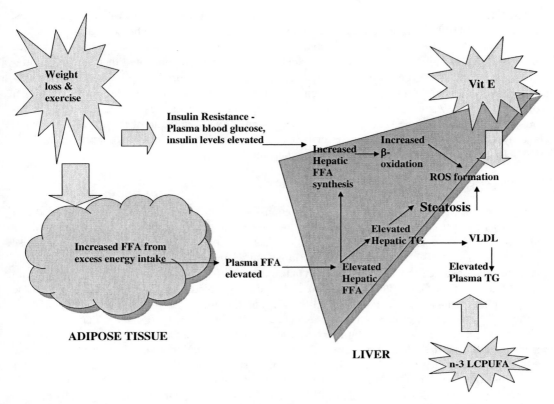

FIGURE 26.1 Pathogenesis of NASH and treatment impacts: Insulin resistance increases triglyceride (TG) lipolysis and inhibits esterification of free fatty acids (FFA) in adipose tissue. This causes plasma FFA to increase, which are then taken up by the liver. Hepatic TG synthesis is increased by the increased FFA flux. The FFA flux causes the β-oxidation pathway to convert excess FFA to TG where they are stored, leading to steatosis. Steatosis is the initial incident necessary in the development of liver cell damage in NASH. The second hit develops when reactive oxygen species (ROS) develop as a product of β-oxidation. Lifestyle and nutritional strategies of weight loss diets coupled with increased exercise and supplements of n-3 LCPUFA and vitamin E demonstrate where this cycle of damage may be interrupted.

of chronic elevation of serum transaminase and the other NASH risk factors.[52–54] Ratziu and colleagues performed an evaluation by giving one score for each variable proposed; body mass index (weight in kilograms divided by height in metres squared) (BMI > 28 kg/m^2 or age > 50 years, ALT level (twice the normal level), and triglycerides > 1.7 mmol/L).[52] Existence of more than one factor indicates a risk of liver fibrosis.[52,53] A study by Marchesini and colleagues demonstrated that the relationship between obesity, type II diabetes mellitus, and advancing age was associated with the increased development of liver fibrosis.[3] Thus, individuals with abnormal liver enzyme test results and a combination of risk factors should endeavor to modify lifestyle factors for 3–6 months. If this strategy is unsuccessful, a liver biopsy should be performed to determine the extent of the diagnosis of NASH.[54]

A. RISK FACTORS

NAFLD has been closely related to insulin resistance syndrome. Currently, NAFLD is a common condition; however, in the near future an increased incidence of NASH can be expected. Some recent studies suggest that NAFLD maybe responsible for approximately 80% of the cases of abnormal persistence of liver enzymes. In the majority of cases NAFLD is a benign condition, and it has little chance of progression to advanced liver disease. However, in 20 to 30% of the cases, this entity (NAFLD), which ranges from simple steatosis to NASH, to fibroses, to cirrhosis, can develop into NASH.[3–10,13–17,19–22,47–63] A study of NASH patients has shown that insulin resistance is present in a high proportion of NASH patients.[58–69] Evidence demonstrated that high concentrations of insulin levels could cause a blockage in the mitochondrial fatty-acid oxidation pathway.[5,7,9,11,22] This might also cause high concentrations of intracellular fatty acids that may trigger oxidative stress.[7] Another study proposed that cryptogenic cirrhosis may be the result of "burnt-out NASH."[21] This is more likely because NASH is closely associated to obesity, type II diabetes, and hyperlipidaemia.[14] Clearly, NASH cannot be categorized as a primary liver disease, because NASH is part of a multifactorial metabolic syndrome.[69]

B. OVERWEIGHT AND OBESITY

Body mass index calculated as weight in kilograms/height in metres^2 (BMI) is a strong predictor of fibrosis in overweight patients. In a series of case studies, approximately 40% of the subjects were found to be obese or overweight (Table 26.1). The overall prevalence of NASH in obese patients (using autopsy data) was at least six times more frequent than in lean individuals.[53] Other data has demonstrated that NASH occurs in approximately 15–20% of obese people.[2] The International Obesity Task Force (2000) proposed a classification standard for Asian adults in which the overweight classification was a BMI of 23 to 24.9, and the obese classification was a BMI of ≥ 25 kg/m^2.[20,55] Some ethnic groups have been associated with higher insulin resistance due to increased visceral adiposity.[9,20] The greater fat mass releases substances such as TNF-α, leptin, and free fatty acids, which eventually lead to insulin resistance.[18] Fat accumulation within hepatocytes occurs as a result of insulin resistance; liver cells are then more susceptible to the "second hit."[7,21] The other concerns about NASH in the obese are the increased risk of developing cryptogenic cirrhosis. This is shown in Table 26.2 and Table 26.3. A study conducted by Browning and colleagues from 1990 to 2001, using 41 subjects, reports that cryptogenic cirrhosis was found in 46% of obese subjects.[11] This study was consistent with the results from two previous studies investigating the cause of cryptogenic cirrhosis conducted by Poonawala and colleagues[25] and Caldwell and colleagues.[26] They

TABLE 26.1
Risk Factor Association in NASH/NAFLD

Ref. No.	Study	(N)	Type of Study	Obesity (%)	Diabetes (%)	Hyperlipidemia (%)
1	Ludwig et al. (1980)	20	Retrospective review	90	25	67
26	Caldwell et al. (1999)	50	Retrospective review	64	42	n/a
53	Wanless et al. (1990)	351	Case series[a]	18.5	n/a	n/a
58	Diehl et al. (1988)	39	Retrospective review	71	55	n/a
59	Powell et al. (1990)	42	Prospective review	93	36	81
60	Bacon et al.(1994)	33	Retrospective review	39	21	21
61	Pinto et al. (1994)	32	Retrospective review	47	34	28
62	Laurin et al. (1996)	40	Intervention study	70	28	n/a
63	Knobler et al. (1999)	48	Prospective review	64	44	73
64	Sorrentino et al. (2004)	58	Retrospective review	100	93.1	77.5

Note: n/a = not applicable.

[a] Autopsy.

Source: Adapted from Youssef, W.I. and McCullough, A.J., Steatohepatitis in obese individuals, *Best Pract Res Clin Gastroenterol.*, 16: 733–747, 2002.

TABLE 26.2
NASH Incident in Obese Patients

Ref. No.	Study	Obese Patients(n)	Mean BMI (kg/m2)	Type of Study	NASH (%)
29	Dixon et al. (2004)	36	n/a	Retrospective study	64
30	Spaulding et al. (2003)	48[a]	51	Retrospective study	56
65	Silverman et al. (1990)	100	n/a	Retrospective study	66
66	Luyckx et al. (1998)	528[b]	43 ± 7	Retrospective study	10
67	Marceau et al. (1999)	551[c]	47 ± 9	Retrospective study	24
68	Ratziu et al. (2000)	93	29.1	Retrospective study	30
69	Dixon et al. (2001)	105[d]	n/a	Retrospective study	26

Note: n/a = not applicable.

[a] Patients underwent bariatric surgery.
[b] Patients underwent biliopancreatic diversion for severe obesity.
[c] Patients underwent liver biopsy in obesity surgery.
[d] Patients underwent Roux-en-Y gastric bypass for morbid obesity.

TABLE 26.3
Incidence of Cryptogenic Cirrhosis in Metabolic Syndrome Patients

Ref. No.	Study	(n)	Type of Study	T2 Diabetes Mellitus (%)	Obesity (%)	Morbid Obesity (%)	Obesity + Diabetes (%)	Hyperlipidemia (%)
11	Browning et al. (2004)	41	Retrospective review	53	46	n/a	68	n/a
25	Poonawala et al. (2000)	49	Retrospective review	47	47	22	23	21
26	Caldwell et al. (1999)	70	Retrospective review	53	47	n/a	n/a	n/a

Note: n/a = not applicable.

found that obesity was present in 47% and 73%, respectively, of their subjects. Furthermore, Ratziu and colleagues investigated survival, liver failure, and HCC incidence in obesity-related cryptogenic cirrhosis, which revealed that the short-term survival rate was less in people with obesity-related cryptogenic cirrhosis, when compared with hepatitis-C-related cirrhosis (Table 26.3).[57]

C. TYPE II DIABETES MELLITUS

Type II diabetes mellitus is a condition that has been closely linked with NASH, especially in obese patients. Obesity is an independent risk factor for NASH.[25,49,64–70] Marchesini and coworkers demonstrated that people with type II diabetes have a two- to threefold higher risk of developing NASH.[49] Dixon and colleagues investigated the relationship of insulin resistance in 26 NASH patients.[69] Results of this study revealed that some of the subjects were diabetic after several normal fasting blood glucose levels. A similar mechanism was evident in obese people in which the cytokine TNF-α played an important role in the mechanism of the development of insulin resistance in people with type II diabetes mellitus.[18] A study conducted by Silverman and colleagues demonstrated that increasing liver pathology was found to correlate with the subject's glycemic state.[65]

Marceau and colleagues verified the results of the Silverman et al. study, in that people with impaired glucose tolerance or diabetes were seven times more likely to develop fibrosis.[67] A study conducted in India recently reported that the duration of diabetes plays an important role in NASH progression; this was mainly due to prolonged insulin resistance and fatty oxidation abnormalities.[68] Further, a large cohort in the Verona study demonstrated that liver cirrhosis was the second most frequent cause of death in people with type II diabetes mellitus.[70] Poonawala and colleagues found crypto-genic cirrhosis occurred in 47% of subjects with type II diabetes.[25] Hence, it is very important for people with NASH to undergo a glucose challenge test to exclude diabetes diagnosis, because diabetes often occurs asymptomatically in NASH patients, and this may worsen the liver prognosis. Weight loss is the most effective treatment strategy to date.[28,29]

D. HYPERLIPIDEMIA

Hyperlipidemia (hypertriglyceridemia, hypercholesterolemia) as a cause of insulin resistance is often evident in patients with NAFLD and NASH.[17] Diehl and colleagues found that one fifth of NASH and NAFLD patients developed hyperlipidemia.[58] Another study reported that hyperlipi-demia occurred in 21–83% of NASH patients.[25] However, compared to hypercholesterolemia, hypertriglyceridemia is thought to increase the risk of development of fatty liver.[28] Te Sligte and colleagues summarized some factors that may contribute to fat accumulation in NASH patients;[19] high intake of saturated fatty acids and cholesterol results in increasing plasma triglycerides and free fatty acids. The diminishing insulin sensitivity suppresses lipolysis and increases hyperinsuline-mia and TNF-α release.[19]

E. OTHER CONDITIONS ASSOCIATED WITH NASH

Although insulin resistance is strongly associated with NASH, there are some other conditions that also relate to NASH. These conditions vary from surgical procedures such as jejunoileal bypass and intestinal resection, to rapid weight loss, drugs, total parenteral nutrition (TPN), and metabolic disorders.[52,71–73]

F. PROGNOSIS

It is obvious that NASH may progress to advanced liver disease, especially in those individuals who carry a predisposing factor.[71] One retrospective study demonstrated that 25% of patients with NASH die from a liver-related cause.[73] Furthermore, Hui and colleagues found that people with NASH had similar health risks to those with untreated chronic hepatitis C (HCV). Liver failure is the main cause of morbidity and mortality in cirrhosis associated with NASH in Australia, and the cumulative probability of overall survival was 95, 90, and 84% in 1, 3, and 10 years, respectively.[73] Furthermore, Chitturi and coworkers found that patients with NASH have similar health risks to those with untreated HCV.[20] Dutta and colleagues observed in Australia a 2% annual incidence of HCC in patients over 40 years of age with HCV. Malnourished patients with a previous exposure to HBV have the highest risk of developing HCC.[74] Two Japanese studies reported HCC incidence in NASH patients as sufficiently common to warrant screening.[75,76]

III. COMPLEMENTARY THERAPIES IN THE TREATMENT OF NASH

At present there are no evidence-based guidelines that can be used in NASH treatment.[47,63–69] Although a number of drugs have been used in clinical trials, and several have been used in practice for NASH treatment, the best practice evidence remains to be elucidated.[33,61] The management of NASH currently is more focused on the underlying disease. Lifestyle and nutrition intervention, which promote gradual weight loss; dietary supplementation in the form of long-chain polyunsaturated fatty acids (with proven ability to reduce hyperlipidemia risk), and antioxidant supplements may be beneficial.[28–48] Improvement is evident not only in liver function tests but also confirmed through further examination using ultrasound or CT scan and histological findings in a follow-up liver biopsy.[34,44,46,47] It appears that nutritional interventions assist in treatment of NASH and help to control predisposing factors or putative underlying diseases.[30–37] However, literature research has revealed that studies of nutritional intervention in NASH patients are still very limited, and these strategies are yet to be incorporated into clinical practice. It is hoped that the study to commence at Westmead, RPAH, and Western Division of General Practice will clarify this situation. Fortunately, a system of staging and grading of histological changes has been developed to identify the changes that take place in the development of NASH.[77,78] Ratziu and coworkers developed a clinicobiological score combining BMI, age, ALT, and triglyceride levels to improve the selection process of patients for liver biopsy.[52]

A. Lifestyle Intervention: Weight Loss

A number of studies have demonstrated that weight loss improves NASH and, to date, this is considered to be current best practice,[28–37] although no randomized controlled trial has been conducted with regard to weight loss. Eleven studies used weight loss in NASH and NAFLD treatment with different approaches to weight loss, such as diet restriction, combination between diet restriction and exercise, gastric banding, and drugs.[28–37,63] The measurement outcomes that demonstrated significant improvements after weight loss are serum transaminase and the reduction of the degree of steatosis. Limitations found in the studies overall were the lack of liver histology as only three studies performed liver biopsies,[33,35,36] and one study used CT-scan to measure the degree of steatosis.[31] These studies did demonstrate a reduction in the degree of fibrosis. Hickman and coworkers demonstrated in the HCV setting that weight loss was associated with a decrease in fibrous scores and a reduction in activated stellate cells.[37] Liver histology outcomes are necessary in these studies to establish the degree of weight loss needed to bring liver back to normal, and none of the studies offered this information. One study conducted by Andersen and colleagues reported that rapid weight loss in people with severe fatty liver would exacerbate the degree of fibrosis and inflammation.[79] Therefore, gradual weight loss is recommended as a treatment in NASH patients, particularly those who are 30% overweight. Weight reduction around 500g–1 kg per week appears to be considered safe and effective.[47,48,79,80]

B. Physical Activity

Physical activity was found to be beneficial in improving hepatic steatosis lipid profile, and in reducing adipose tissue fat accumulation. A study conducted by Gauthier and colleagues in hepatic steatosis-induced rats suggested that eight weeks of physical training provided significant improvement in plasma concentrations of triacylglycerol in comparison with rats fed a high fat diet with sedentary activity levels.[81] Furthermore, the active rats had lower nonesterified fatty acids (NEFA), diminished insulin concentrations, and lower plasma leptin compared to the other rats with sedentary activity.[81] Two studies conducted in Japan using a combination of diet restriction and exercise produced a more beneficial effect using this strategy.[34,35] A study by Ueno and colleagues demonstrated that energy restriction (25–30 kcal/kg IBW/day) combined with exercise each day for 3 months would improve NASH patients' status.[34] This finding was confirmed with a measurement of some parameters such as BMI, liver function test, blood glucose level, total cholesterol along with histological data from liver biopsy (degree of steatosis). A study by Hickman and colleagues conducted over 12 months supported the Ueno findings that improvement was achieved in biochemical and histological data after following a restricted diet and exercise program (Table 26.4).[36]

TABLE 26.4
Weight Loss and NASH Treatment

Ref. No.	Study	(n)	Duration	Control	Intervention Type	Outcome Measurement	Results
29	Dixon et al. (2004)	36	9–51 months	No control	Gastric band	1. Wt, BMI, Wt:H ratio 2. Lipid profile (TC, fasting TG, HDL, LDL) HbA1c, insulin sensitivity, HOMA%	All parameters demonstrated an improvement after weight loss
31	Nomura et al. (1987)	24	3 months	No control	Low calorie diet (25–30 cal × IBW in kg/day)	1. Laboratory tests of serum glutamic-pyruvate transaminase 2. Body weight 3. CT attenuation value of 4 liver segments.	1. SGPT value was reduced 61%, body weight was reduced 5.7%, and increasing CT number of attenuation up to 13.9%.
32	Park et al. (1995)	25	1 year	No weight reduction	1. Low calorie diet (25–30 cal/kg IBW/day) 2. Low impact aerobic exercise	1. Liver function tests (AST,ALT) 2. TC	Significant decrease of liver function tests and total cholesterol in "weight reduction" group while there was a significant increase of liver function tests and total cholesterol in "non-weight reduction" group.
34	Ueno et al. (1997)	25	3 months	No treatment	1. Low energy diet (25 cal/kg IBW/day) 2. Exercise: walking and jogging	1. Blood biochemistry 2. BMI 3. Liver biopsy	Significant reduction of blood biochemistry values, BMI, and degree of steatosis in treatment group (except TG slightly decreased).
35	Okita et al. (2001)	28	24 weeks	Nonobese healthy adults	Moderate energy restriction (25kcal/kg of IBW) and diet rich in fish, green vegetables, and low in meat were recommended	1. BMI, body fat ratio, Waist circumference 2. LFT (AST,ALT) 3. TG	Treated group had significant reduction in BMI, waist circumference, AST, and ALT level. No significant change in male body fat ratio and tryacylglycerol level.

#	Author	n	Duration	Control	Intervention	Measures	Results
36	Hickman et al. (2004)	14	15 months	Steatosis from HCV	1. 3 months: dietitian/wk 2. 1 year: dietitian/month 3. Exercise: 150 min/week aerobic	1. BMI 2. LFT 3. Fasting BGL & HOMA	Weight loss in both subjects and controls. Pts with HCV lower decrease in fasting insulin compared with non-HCV. ALT improved in both groups at 3 and 15 months. Liver biopsy (n = 14) improved steatosis Stage of fibrosis (n = 7) improved
38	Kral et al. (2004)	68 9	44 months and 101 months	No control	Biliopancreatic diversion surgery	1. BMI & Wt 2. LFT 3. Fasting BGL 4. Lipid profile 5. Liver biopsy (n=104)	There were significant improvements in TC & TG levels (P < 0.01) as well as weight reduction in short and long term follow up for all patients, severe fibrosis decreased (n = 28)
63	Knobler et al. (1999)	48	24 months	No control	1. Diet intervention 2. Those who failed diet intervention were given lipid lowering drugs	1. LFT 2. Weight 3. Lipid profile	LFTs were improved in 96% of patients, weight loss was achieved in 79% of patients (mean loss 3.7 kg) Fasting BGL decreased. Lipid profiles decreased

Note: ALT: alanine aminotransferase; AST: aspartate aminotransferase; BGL: blood glucose level; HCV: hepatitis C virus; HDL: high-density lipoprotein; HOMA: homeostasis model assessment; IBW: ideal body weight; LDL: low-density lipoprotein; LFT: liver function tests; Lipid profile: total cholesterol, high-density lipoprotein, low density lipoprotein, triglyceride levels, SGPT: serum glutamic-pyruvic transaminase; TC: total cholesterol; TG: triglycerides; W:H: waist–hip ratio; HbA1c: glycosylated haemoglobin A1c test.

C. NUTRITIONAL ASPECTS OF TREATMENT OF NASH:
OMEGA-3 FATTY ACIDS

Supplementation with n-3 long chain polyunsaturated fatty acids (n-3 LCPUFA) suggests some promising results: however, it is not currently recommended as best practice. Gradual weight loss, although requiring more clinical trials, is considered in the literature as best practice.[28,29,36,37] Six studies investigated the association between omega-3 supplementation and the reduction of risk factors for NASH. Three studies each were conducted in animals[39-41] and in humans.[35,82,83] The majority of the studies examined the antiobesity effect of omega-3 supplementation through different aspects. Browning and colleagues investigated the antiobesity related effect of omega-3 supplementation (1.3 g EPA and 2.9 g DHA) in two groups of women with different inflammatory status (measured by sialic acid).[82] The results demonstrated that the group with the higher inflammatory status had a significant improvement in insulin sensitivity. One study conducted in humans compared the effect of omega-3 fatty acids with Atorvastatin and Orlistat.[83] Although the Orlistat group demonstrated a greater improvement in steatosis when compared to other groups, omega-3 fatty acids proved to be more effective in reducing AST. Furthermore, this study demonstrated that the omega-3 group had the highest reduction in triglyceride levels. In the three animal studies,[39-41] two were controlled, suggesting that fish oil administration would suppress sterol element regulatory binding protein-1 (SREBP-1), which is predominantly located in liver. SREBP-1 is responsible for the regulation of synthesis and storage of triglycerides in the liver. Disruption in mature SREBP-1 could improve hepatic steatosis. Although significant reduction of AST and ALT levels was not observed in these studies, one study decreased levels of triglycerides and postprandial blood glucose.[40] Promising data from clinical and animal studies without histological endpoints can be misleading. Hatzitolios et al. (2004)[83] demonstrated that n-3 LCPUFA supplementation reduced triglyceride levels; however, given the mechanism of the development of triglyceridemia in NASH patients, the significance of this effect is not yet clear (Table 26.5).[52,60,83] Clearly, further well-designed and executed studies are necessary to elucidate the mechanisms involved, so that n-3 LCPUFA can be included in clinical practice treatments of NASH patients.

D. ANTIOXIDANTS

Antioxidant therapy is not recommended as part of clinical practice, even though the research appears to be promising. At present there is a lack of strong evidence to support the supplementation of vitamin E to boost serum antioxidant levels in NASH patients. This therapy is based on the fact that oxidative stress is one of the most important factors in the promotion of NASH pathogenesis.[41] Four studies varying in length from 12 weeks to 12 months investigated the therapeutic use of vitamins in the treatment of NASH patients (Table 26.6). Lavine demonstrated in a pilot study of children less than 16 years of age that supplementation with vitamin E (400 to 1200 IU/d) resulted in the normalization of ALT.[43] In a 12-month pilot study, NASH patients receiving dietary advice for 6 months, and vitamin E supplementation for 12 months, at a rate of 300 mg/d, improved histologically.[44] In a 6-month prospective, double blind study, 45 patients were randomized to receive 1000 IU/d of vitamin E and 1000 mg/d of vitamin C or placebo together with dietary counseling and a low fat diet. There was a statistically significant improvement in fibrous score ($P = 0.002$), but not inflammation.[45] Kugelmas and colleagues conducted a pilot study of 16 NASH patients, in which the effect of a low fat diet and aerobic exercise with or without 800 IU of vitamin E daily on cytokine and liver enzyme levels was investigated.[46] Lifestyle modifications were associated with improvement in cholesterol and liver enzyme status. Cytokines were not decreased significantly with weight loss in either the supplemented or the unsupplemented groups. It is clear that a larger, multicenter, longer-term antioxidant supplementation study is warranted.

TABLE 26.5
N-3 PUFA in Relation to Risk Factors Reduction

Ref. No.	Study	Animal Type	Type of Study	Time	Control	Intervention	Outcome Measurement	Result
39	Nakatani et al. (2003)	Mice	Intervention study	1–13 weeks	No control	Mice in seven groups with different amount of fish oils. Group 1 was given 0% fish oil and then fish oil concentrations were increased incrementally 10% for each subsequent group.	Body weight, parametrial WAT, SREBP-1 expressions	Reduction in weight and parametrial WAT were observed in mice fed with 40-60% energy from fish oil in comparison with 0% energy from fish oil after 1 and 13 weeks. Liver weight was significantly increased in 20% energy fish oil and above gps. Liver damage accompanied with increasing AST or ALT was not observed in 60% energy fish oil group.
40	Sekiya et al. (2003)	ob/ob mice	Intervention study	7 d	1. HC fat-free diet supplemented with 15% triolein 2. 15% triolein and 5% EPA ethyl ester	20% fish oil	Liver lipid content (TG), SREBP-1 expression, ALT IRS-2 analysis	Mice fed fish oil showed reduction in mature SREBP-1 up to 3x compared with those fed with HC diet, while mice fed with oleat did not show any reduction of mature SREBP-1. TG levels decreased significantly in mice fed HC diet and mice fed with fish oil. No significant difference for ALT levels in each group, but elevated ALT level was decreased in test group.
41	Levy et al. (2004)	F344 rats	Intervention	4 weeks	1. HC, low fat (5.1% energy) 2. Lard (45% energy)	Rats fed 45% energy from omega PUFA	1. Body weight and body fat 2. PP lipid profile 3. BGL 4. QUICKI 5. mRNA of PPAR-α 6. SREBP-1	FO fed rats ingested more energy in first 3 wks with less weight gain. TG levels lower in FO rats. PP-BGL and PP insulin levels lower in FO rats, insulin sensitivity higher. Fasting SREBP was similar in all groups, PP-SREBP was 5x HC rats, 3 x lard rats and no increase in FO rats.

Continued.

TABLE 26.5 *(Continued)*
N-3 PUFA in Relation to Risk Factors Reduction

Ref. No.	Study	Animal Type	Type of Study	Time	Control	Intervention	Outcome Measurement	Result
34	Okita et al. (2001)	14	Intervention study	8 weeks (short term) 24 weeks (long term)	No control	Diet modification (low energy) with high omega PUFA	1. BMI 2. Waist circumference 3. LFT 4. Leucocytes and PG	LFT decreased significantly after 8 & 24 wks. Positive correlation between ALT level and Omega-3 PUFA (P < 0.05)
82	Browning (2003)	63 in 2 groups based on sialic acid content.	Controlled intervention study	12 weeks each treatment with 4 week washout	Placebo: 5 capsules/day 2.8 g LA and 1.4 g oleic	1.3g EPA and 2.9g DHA	GTT	Improvement in insulin sensitivity noted in pts with higher sialic acid receiving n-3 PUFA (P < 0.05)
83	Hatzitolios et al. (2004)	88	Intervention study	24 wks	1. Atorvastatin 2. Orlistat	Omega-3 PUFA 5 mL/d	1. BMI 2. LFTs 3. Lipid Profile 4. Ultrasound	AST decreased significantly in all groups. Hierarchy of AST reduction was Orlistat, omega-3 and Atorvastatin group. Omega-3 group had greatest reduction in TG compared to other groups and Orlistat group demonstrated greater improvement in ultrasound results.

Note: ALT: alanine aminotransferase; AST: aspartate aminotransferase; BGL: blood glucose level; BMI: body mass index; DHA: docosahexaenoic acid; EPA: eicosapentaenoic acid; GTT: glucose tolerance test; HC: high carbohydrate; HDL: high-density lipoprotein; IRS: insulin receptor substrate; LDL: low density lipoprotein; LFT: liver function tests; LDL: low density lipoprotein; PG: prostaglandins; PP: postprandial; PPAR: peroxisome proliferator-activated receptor; PUFA: polyunsaturated fatty acids; QUICKI: Quantitative Insulin Check Index; SREBP: sterol regulatory element binding protein; TC: total cholesterol; TG: triglycerides; WAT: white adipose tissue.

TABLE 26.6
Antioxidants and NASH

Ref. No.	Study	Animal Type	Type of Study	Time	Control	Intervention	Outcome Measurement	Result
43	Lavine et al. (2000)	11	Open-label pilot study	4–10 months	No control	Vitamin.E 400 and 1200 IU/d	1. BMI 2. LFTs	After treatment LFTs were reduced to normal level from 2.3 times and 3.9 times upper normal value before the treatment. No significant different found in BMI.
44	Hasegawa et al. (2001)	12NASH 10NAFLD	Pilot study	1 year	No control	Dietary therapy (30 kcal/kg BW) for 6 months, and Vitamin E 300 mg/d for 12 months	1. BW 2. Lipid profile 3. LFTs 4. Liver biopsy only in NASH group	In all groups body weight was reduced significantly. LFT tests were reduced in both groups but NASH patients had nonsignificant reduction. After alpha tocopherol administration. LFTs in NASH patients had further significant reduction (appr. 79%), 9 patients underwent liver biopsy, 5 demonstrated improvements in fibrosis and inflammation.
45	Harrison et al. (2003)	45	Prosp, double blind, and, placebo-controlled	6 months	Placebo	Vitamin E 1000 IU + Vitamin C 1000 mg	1. BMI 2. LFT 3. Liver biopsy	No clinically significant difference in BMI for each group after treatment. ALT level was improved in placebo group. Improvement of fibrosis in 47.8% of subjects from test group.
46	Kugelmas et al. (2003)	16 NASH	Pilot study	12 wks	No control	Vit E 800 IU/d and diet as American Heart Association recommendation.	1. BW 2. BMI 3. LFT 4. Lipid profile 5. Liver histology 6. Ultrasound	All parameters were decreased significantly in the test group. AST decreased by week 6 and remained on the same level up to week 12.

Note: ALT: alanine aminotransferase; AST: aspartate aminotransferase; BMI: body mass index; BW: body weight; HDL: high-density lipoprotein; lipid profile: total cholesterol, high-density lipoprotein, low density lipoprotein, triglyceride levels; LFT: liver function tests; LDL: low density lipoprotein; TC: total cholesterol; TG: triglycerides.

IV. IS THERE A LIVER CLEANSING DIET?

There is no liver cleansing diet to improve liver function.[84] Liver function can be impaired by nutritional deficiencies, and excess energy intake can lead to an accumulation of fat in the liver, causing hepatic steatosis. Liver function cannot be altered by diet, and there are not any nutrients that can restore metabolic balance to a diseased liver. The biological functions that underpin liver disease are inflammation and cell necrosis, apoptosis, proliferation, and fibrosis. These functions are not influenced by diet.[56] If a patient has an energy intake in excess of needs and has hepatic steatosis, then a low-fat, weight-reducing dietary intake combined with lifestyle changes to increase energy output can reduce the amount of fat accumulated in the liver.[5,48] This reduction of accumulated fat in the liver can reduce liver injury and improve liver function test results.[34,36]

V. CONCLUSION

There is a need to develop a better understanding of the pathogenesis and natural history of NASH. Many patients do not progress to advanced liver disease; however, it would be of benefit to clinicians to be able to identify the subset of patients who are at risk of this progression. Treatment has been focused on the management of risk factors such as obesity, type II diabetes mellitus, and hyperlipidemia. NASH associated with obesity may be resolved by gradual weight loss, although some results are not consistent. Control of glucose and lipid levels is an appropriate strategy, but this does not always reverse the condition. Some medications have the potential to benefit patients as do nutritional supplements; however, dose responses remain to be elucidated. Thus, further research involving well-reasoned study design is needed to develop a wider range of treatment strategies to benefit NASH patients.

REFERENCES

1. Ludwig, J., Viggiano, T.R., McGill, D.B., and Oh, B.J., Nonalcoholic steatohepatitis: Mayo clinic experiences with a hitherto unnamed disease, *Mayo Clin. Proc.*, 55: 434–438, 1980.
2. Marchesini, G., Marzocchi, R., Agostini, F., and Bugianesi, E., Nonalcoholic liver disease and the metabolic syndrome, *Curr. Opin. Lipidol.*, 16: 421–427, 2005.
3. Marchesini, G., Bugianesi, E., Forlani, G., Marzocchi, R., Zannoni, C., Vanni, E., Manini, R., Rizzetto, M., and Melchionda, N., Nonalcoholic steatohepatitis in patients cared for in metabolic units. *Diabetes Res. Clin. Pract.*, 63: 143–151, 2004.
4. Villanova, N., Moscatiello, S., Ramilli, S., Bugianesi, E., Magalotti, D., Vanni, E., Zoli, M., and Marchesini, G., Endothelial dysfunction and cardiovascular risk profile in nonalcoholic fatty liver disease, *Hepatology*, 42: 473–480, 2005.
5. Adams, L., Angulo, P., and Lindor, K., Nonalcoholic liver disease, *Can. Med. Assoc. J.*, 172: 899–905, 2005.
6. Mehta, K., Van Thiel, D.H., Shah, N., and Mobarhan, S., Nonalcoholic fatty liver disease: pathogenesis and the role of antioxidants. *Nutr. Rev.*, 60: 289–93, 2002.
7. Day, C.P., Nonalcoholic steatohepatitis (NASH): where are we now and where are we going? *Gut*, 50: 585–588, 2002.
8. Neuschwander-Tetri, B.A., Fatty liver and nonalcoholic steatohepatitis, *Clin. Cornerstone*, 3: 47–57, 2001.
9. Farrel, G.C., Nonalcoholic steatohepatitis: what is it, and why is it important in the Asia–Pacific region? *J. Gastroenterol. Hepatol.*, 18: 124–138, 2003.
10. Brunt, E., Brent, M., Neuschwander-Tetri, M., Oliver, D., Wehmeier, K., and Bacon, B., Nonalcoholic Steatohepatitis: Histologic features and clinical correlations with 30 blinded biopsy specimens, *Hum. Pathol.*, 35: 1070–1082, 2004.

11. Browning, J.D., Kumar, S.K., Saboorian, M.H., and Thiele, D.L., Ethnic differences in the prevalence of cryptogenic cirrhosis, *Am. J. Gastroenterol.*, 99: 292–298, 2004.
12. Skelly, M., James, P., and Ryder, S. Findings on liver biopsy to investigate abnormal liver function tests in the absence of diagnostic serology, *J. Hepatol.*, 35: 195–199, 2001.
13. James, O. and Day, C., Nonalcoholic steatohepatitis: another disease of affluence, *Lancet*, 353: 1634–1636, 1999.
14. Sanyal, A. Campbell-Sargent, C., Mirshahi, F., Rizzo, W., Contos, M., Sterling, R., Luketic, V., Shiffman, M., and Clore, J., Nonalcoholic steatohepatitis: Association of insulin resistance and mitochondrial abnormalities, *Gastroenterology*, 120: 1183–1192, 2001.
15. Burt, A.D., Mutton, A., and Day, C.P., Diagnosis and interpretation of steatosis and steatohepatitis, *Semin. Diagn. Pathol.*, 15: 246–258, 1998.
16. Medina, J., Fernandez-Salazar, L.I., Garcia-Buey, L., and Moreno-Otero, R., Approach to the pathogenesis and treatment of nonalcoholic steatohepatitis. *Diabetes Care*, 27: 2057–2066, 2004.
17. Marchesini, G., Brizi, M., Bainchi, G., Tomasetti, S., Bugianesi, E., Lenzi, M., McCullough, A.J., Natale, S., Forlani, G., and Melchoinda, N., Nonalcoholic fatty liver disease: a feature of the metabolic syndrome, *Diabetes*, 50: 1844–1850, 2001.
18. Crespo, J., Cayon, A., Fernandez-Gil, P., Hernandez-Guerra, M., Mayorga, M., Dominguez-Diez, A., Fernandez-Escalante, J., and Pons-Romero, F., Gene expression of tumor necrosis factor and TNF-receptors P 55 and P 75 in nonalcoholic steatohepatitis patients, *Hepatology*, 34: 1158–1163, 2001.
19. Te Sligte, K., Bourass, I., Sels, J., Driessen, A., Stockbrugger, R.W. and Koek, G.H., Nonalcoholic steatohepatitis: review of growing medical problem. *Eur. J. Intern. Med.*, 5: 10–21, 2004.
20. Chitturi, S., Farrell, G.C., and George, J., Nonalcoholic steatohepatitis in the Asia–Pacific region: future shock? *J. Gastroenterol. Hepatol.*, 19: 368–374, 2004.
21. Day, C.P., Pathogenesis of steatohepatititis, *Best. Pract. Res. Clin. Gastroenterol.*, 16: 663–678, 2002.
22. Harrison, S.A., Kadakia, S., Lang, K.A., and Schenker, S., Nonalcoholic steatohepatitis: what we know in the new millennium, *Am. J. Gastroenterol.*, 97: 2714–2724, 2002.
23. Clouston, A.D. and Powell, E.E., Nonalcoholic fatty liver disease: is all the fat bad? *Intern. Med. J.*, 34: 187–191, 2004.
24. Abdelmalek, M., Ludwig, J., and Lindor, K., Two cases from the spectrum of nonalcoholic steatohepatitis, *J. Clin. Gastroenterol.*, 20: 127–130, 1995.
25. Poonawala, A, Nair, S.P., and Thuluvath, P.S., Prevalence of obesity and diabetes in patients with cryptogenic cirrhosis: a case control study, *Hepatology*, 32: 689–692, 2000.
26. Caldwell, S.H. Oelsner, D.H., Iezzoni, J.C., Hespenheide, E.H., Battle, E.H., and Driscoll, C.J., Cryptogenic cirrhosis: clinical characterization and risk factors for underlying disease, *Hepatology* 29: 664–669, 1999.
27. Sreekumar, R., Rosado, B., Rasmussen, D., and Charlton, M. Hepatic gene expression in histologically progressive NASH, *Hepatology*, 38: 244–251, 2003.
28. Dixon, J.B. and O'Brien, P.E., Lipid profile in the severely obese: changes with weight loss after lap-band surgery, *Obes. Res.*, 10: 903–190, 2002.
29. Dixon, J.B., Bhathal, P.S., Hughes, N.R., and O' Brien, P.E., Nonalcoholic fatty liver disease: Improvement in liver histological analysis with weight loss, *Hepatology*, 39: 1647–1654, 2004.
30. Spaulding, L., Trainer, T., and Janiec, D., Prevalence of nonalcoholic steatohepatitis in morbidly obese subjects undergoing gastric bypass, *Obes. Surg.*, 13: 347–349, 2003.
31. Nomura, F., Ohnishi, K., Ochiai, T., and Okuda, K., Obesity-related nonalcoholic fatty liver: CT features and follow up studies after low calorie diet, *Radiology*, 162: 845–847, 1987.
32. Park, H.S., Kim, M.W., and Shin, E.S., Effect of weight control on hepatic abnormalities in obese patients with fatty liver, *J. Korean Med. Sci.*, 10: 414–421, 1995.
33. DeMeo, M., Mobarhan, S., Mikolaitis, S., and Kazi N., Three cases of comprehensive dietary therapy and pharmacotherapy of patients with complex obesity related disease. *Nutr. Rev.*, 55: 297–302, 1997.
34. Ueno, T., Sugawara, H., Sujaku, K., Hashimoto, O., Riko, T., Tamaki, S., Torimura, T., Inuzuka, S., Sata, M., and Tanikawa, K., Therapeutic effects of restricted diet and exercise in obese patients with fatty liver, *J. Hepatol.*, 27: 103–107, 1997.
35. Okita, M., Hayashi, M., Sasagawa, T., Takagi, K., Suzuki, K., Kinoyama, S., Ito, T., and Yamada, G., Effect of a moderately energy restricted diet on obese patients with fatty liver, *Nutrition*, 17: 542–547, 2001.

36. Hickman, I.J., Jonsson, J.R., Prins, J.B., Ash, S., Purdie, D.M., Clouston, A.D., and Powell, E.E., Modest weight loss and physical activity in overweight patients with chronic liver disease results in sustained improvement in alanine aminotransferase, fasting insulin, and quality of life, *Gut*, 53: 413–419, 2004.

37. Hickman, I.J., Clouston, A.D., Macdonald, G.A., Purdie, D.M., Prins, J.B., Ash, S., Jonsson, J.R., and Powell, E.E., Effect of weight reduction on liver histology and biochemistry in patients with chronic hepatitis C. *Gut*, 51: 89–94, 2002.

38. Kral, J.G., Thung, S.N., Biron, S., Hould, F.S., Lebel, S., Marceau, S., Simard, S., and Marceau, P., Effects of surgical treatment of the metabolic syndrome on liver fibrosis and cirrhosis, *Surgery*, 135: 48–58, 2004.

39. Nakatani, T., Kim, H.J., Kaburagi, Y., Yasuda, K., and Ezaki, O., A low fish oil feeding inhibits SREBP-1 proteolytic cascade, while a high fish oil feeding decreases SREBP-1 in mice liver: relationship to antiobesity, *J. Lipid. Res.*, 44: 369–379, 2003.

40. Sekiya, M., Yahagi, N., Matsuzka, T., Najima, Y., Nakakuki, M., Nagai, R., Ishibashi, S., Osagu, J., Yamada, N., and Shimano, H., Polyunsaturated fatty acids ameliorate hepatic steatosis in obese mice SREBP-1 suppression, *Hepatology*, 38: 1529–1539, 2003.

41. Levy, J.R., Clore, J.N., and Stevens, W., Dietary n-3 polyunsaturated fatty acids decreased hepatic triglycerides in Fischer 344 rats, *Hepatology*, 39: 608–616, 2004.

42. Chan, A.C., Partners in defense, vitamin E and vitamin C, *Can. J. Physiol. Pharmacol.*, 71: 725–731, 1993.

43. Lavine, J.E., Vitamin E treatment of nonalcoholic steatohepatitis in children: a pilot study, *J. Pediatr.*, 136: 734–738, 2000.

44. Hasegawa, T., Yoneda, M., Nakamura, K., Makino, I., and Terano, A., Plasma transforming growth factor-1 level and efficacy of alpha-tocopherol in patients with nonalcoholic steatohepatitis: a pilot study, *Aliment. Pharmacol. Ther.*, 15: 1667–1672, 2001.

45. Harrison, S.A., Torgerson, S., Hayashi, P., Ward, J., and Schenker, S., Vitamin E and vitamin C treatment improves fibrosis in patients with nonalcoholic steatohepatitis, *Am. J. Gastroenterol.*, 98: 2485–2490, 2003.

46. Kugelmas, M., Hill, D.B., Vivia, B., Marsano, L., and McClain, C.J., Cytokines and NASH: A pilot study of the effects of lifestyle modification and vitamin E, *Hepatology*, 38: 413–419, 2003.

47. Youssef, W.I. and McCullough, A.J., Steatohepatitis in obese individuals, *Best Pract. Res. Clin. Gastroenterol.*, 16: 733–747, 2002.

48. Patrick, L., Nonalcoholic fatty liver disease: Relationship to insulin sensitivity and oxidative stress. Treatment approaches using vitamin E, magnesium, and betaine, *Altern. Med. Rev.*, 7: 276–290, 2002.

49. Marchesini, G., Brizi, M., Morselli-Labate, A.M., Bianchi, G., Bugianesi, E., McCullough, A.J., Forlani, G., and Melchionda, N., Association of nonalcoholic fatty liver disease with insulin resistance, *Am. J. Med.*, 107: 450–455, 1999.

50. Younossi, Z., Gramlich, T., Matteoni, C., Boparai, N., and McCullough, A.J., Nonalcoholic fatty liver disease in patients with type 2 diabetes, *Clin. Gastroenterol. Hepatol.*, 2: 262–265, 2004.

51. Charlton, M., Kasparova, P., Weston, S., Lindor, K., Maor-Kendler, Y., Wiesner, R.H., Rosen, C.B., and Batts, K.P., Frequency of nonalcoholic steatohepatitis as a cause of advanced liver disease, *Liver Transpl.*, 7: 608–614, 2001.

52. Ratziu, V., Giral, P., Charlotte, F., Bruckert, E., Thibault, V., Theodorou, I., Khalil, L., Turpin, G., Opolon, P., and Poynard, T., Liver Fibrosis in overweight patients, *Gastroenterology*, 118: 1117–1123, 2000.

53. Wanless, I.R. and Lentz J.S., Fatty liver hepatitis (steatohepatitis) and obesity: an autopsy study with analysis of risk factors, *Hepatology*, 12: 1106–1110, 1990.

54. Laurin, J., Motion — All patients with NASH need to have a liver biopsy: arguments against the motion, *Can. J. Gastroenterol.*, 16: 722–726, 2002.

55. International Obesity Task Force/World Health Organization, The Asia-Pacific perspective: redefining obesity and its treatment, *Health Communications Australia*, Sydney, Australia, 2000.

56. Farrell, G.C., *Hepatitis C, Other Liver Disorders and Liver Health: A Practical Guide*, MacLennan and Petty, Sydney; Australia. 2002.

57. Ratziu, V., Bonyhay, L., Di Martino, V., Charlotte, F., Cavallaro, L., Sayegh, M., Giral, P., Grimaldi, A., Opolon, P., and Poynard, T., Survival, liver failure and hepatocellullar carcinoma I obesity-related cryptogenic cirrhosis, *Hepatology*, 35: 1485–1493, 2002.

58. Diehl, A.M., Goodman, Z., and Ishak, K.G., Alcohol-like liver disease in nonalcoholics. A clinical and histologic comparison with alcohol induced liver injury, *Gastroenterology*, 95: 1056–1062, 1988.

59. Powell, E.E., Cooksley, W.G., Hanson, R., Searle, J., Halliday, J.W., and Powell L.W., The natural history of nonalcoholic steatohepatitis: a follow up study of 42 patients for up to 21 years, *Hepatology*, 11: 74–80, 1990.

60. Bacon, B.R., Farahvash, M.J., Janney, C.G., and Neuschwander-Teri, B.A., Nonalcoholic steatohepatitis: An expanded clinical entity, *Gastroenterology*, 107: 1103–1109, 1994.

61. Pinto, H.C., Baptista, A., Camilo, M.E., Valente, A., Saragoca, A., and De Moura, M.C., Nonalcoholic steatohepatitis: Clinicopathological comparison with alcoholic hepatitis in ambulatory and hospitalized patients, *Dig. Dis. Sci.*, 41: 172–179, 1996.

62. Laurin, J., Lindor, K.D., Crippin, J.S., Gossard, A., Gregory, G.J., Ludwig, J., Rakela, J., and McGill, D.B., Ursudeoxycholic acid or clofibrate in the treatment of non-alcohol-induced steatohepatitis: a pilot study, *Hepatology*, 23: 1464–1467, 1996.

63. Knobler, H., Schattner, A., Zhornicki, T., Malnick, S.D.H., Keter, D., Sokolouskaya, N., Lurie, Y., and Bass, D., Fatty liver: An additional and treatable feature of the insulin resistance syndrome, *Q. J. Med.* 92: 73–79, 1999.

64. Sorrentino, P., Tarantino, G., Conca, P., Perrella, A., Terracciano, M.L., Vecchione, R., Garcuilo, G., Gennarelli, N., and Lobello, R., Silent nonalcoholic fatty liver disease: a clinical histological study, *J. Hepatol.*, 41: 751–757, 2004.

65. Silverman, J.F., O'Brien, K.F., Long, S., Leggett, N., Khazanie, P.G., Pories, W.J., Norris, H.T., and Caro J.F., Liver pathology in morbidly obese patients with and without diabetes, *Am. J. Gastroenterol.*, 85: 1349–1355, 1990.

66. Luyckx, F.H., Desaive, C., Thiry, A., Dewe, W., Scheen, A.J., Gielen, J.E., and Lefebvre, P.J., Liver abnormalities in severely obese subjects: effect of drastic weight loss after gastroplasty, *Int. J. Obes. Relat. Metab. Disord.*, 22: 222–226, 1998.

67. Marceau, P., Biron, S., Hould, F.S., Marceau, S., Simard, S., Thung, S.N., and Kral, J.G., Liver pathology and the metabolic syndrome X in severe obesity, *J. Clin. Endocrinol. Metab.*, 84: 1513–1517, 1999.

68. Ratziu, V., Giral, P., Charlotte, F., Bruckert, E., Thibault, V., Theodorou, I., Khalil, L., Turpin, G., Opolon, P., and Poynard, T., Liver fibrosis in overweight patients, *Gastroenterology*, 118: 1117–1123, 2000.

69. Dixon, J.B., Bhatal, P.S., and O' Brien, P.E., Nonalcoholic fatty liver disease: predictors of nonalcoholic steatohepatitis and liver fibrosis in the severely obese, *Gastroenterology*, 121: 91–100, 2001.

70. de Marco, R., Locatelli, F., Zoppini, G., Verlato, G., Bonora, E., and Muggeo, M., Cause-specific mortality in type 2 Diabetes: the Verona study, *Diabetes Care*, 22: 756–761, 1999.

71. Allard, J.P., Other disease associations with nonalcoholic fatty liver disease (NAFLD), *Best Pract. Res. Clin. Gastroenterol.*, 16: 783–795, 2002.

72. Day, C.P., NASH-related liver failure: One hit too many? *Am. J. Gastroenterol.*, 97: 1872–1874, 2002.

73. Hui, J.M., Kench, J.G., Chitturi, S., Sud, A., Farrell, G.C., Byth, K., Hall, P., Khan, M., and George, J., Long-term outcomes of cirrhosis in nonalcoholic steatohepatitis compared with hepatitis C, *Hepatology*, 38: 420–427, 2003.

74. Dutta, U., Byth, K., Kench, J., Khan, M., Coverdale, S., Weltman, M., Lin, R., Liddle, C., and Farrell, G.C., Risk factors for development of hepatocellular carcinoma among Australians with hepatitis C: a case control study, *Aust. N. Z. J. Med.*, 29: 300–307, 1999.

75. Shimada, M., Hashimoto, E., Taniai, M., Hasegawa, K., Okuda, H., Hyashi, N., Takasaki, K., and Ludwig, J., Hepatocellular carcinoma in patients with nonalcoholic steatohepatitis, *J. Hepatol.*, 37: 154–160, 2002.

76. Zen, Y., Katayanagi, K., Tsuneyama, K., Harada, K., Araki, I., and Nakanuma, Y., Hepatocelullar carcinoma arising in nonalcoholic steatohepatitis, *Pathol. Int.*, 51: 127–131, 2001.

77. Brunt, E., Janney, C., Di Bisceglie, A., Neuschwander-Tetri, B., and Bacon, B., Nonalcoholic steatohepatitis: a proposal for grading and staging the histological lesions, *Am. J. Gastroenterol.*, 94: 2467–2474, 1999.

78. Kliener, D., Brunt, E., Van Natta, M., Behling, C., Contos, M., Cummings, O., Ferrell, L., Liu, Y., Torbenson, M., Unalp-Arida, A., Yeh, M., McCullough, A., and Sanyal, A., Nonalcoholic Steatohepatitis Clinical Research Network. Design and validation of a histological scoring system for nonalcoholic fatty liver disease, *Hepatology*, 41: 1313–1321, 2005.

79. Andersen, T., Gluud, C., Franzmann, M.B., and Christoffersen, P., Hepatic effects of dietary weight loss in morbidly obese subjects, *J. Hepatol.*, 12: 224–249, 1991.

80. Angulo, P. and Lindor, K.D., Treatment of nonalcoholic steatohepatitis, *Best Pract. Res. Clin. Gastroenterol.*, 16: 797–810, 2002.

81. Gauthier, M.-S., Couturier, K., Charbonneau, A., and Lavoie, J.M., Effects of introducing physical training in the course of a 16-week high-fat diet regimen on hepatic steatosis, adipose tissue, fat accumulation, and plasma lipid profile, *Int. J. Obes.*, 28: 1064–1071, 2004.

82. Browning, L.M., N-3 Polyunsaturated fatty acids, inflammation and obesity-related disease, *Proc. Nutr. Soc.*, 62: 447–453, 2003.

83. Hatzitolios, A., Savapoulos, C., Lazaraki, G., Sidiropoulos, I., Haritani, P., Lefkopoulos, A., Karagiannopoulou, G., Tzioufa, V., and Dimitros, K., Efficacy of omega-3 fatty acids, atorvastatin and orlistatin in non-alcoholic fatty liver disease in dyslipidemia, *Indian J. Gastroenterol.*, 23: 131–134, 2004.

84. Cabot, S., *The Liver Cleansing Diet,* Women's Health Advisory Service, Cobbitty, Australia, 1999.

27 Marketing and Regulatory Issues for Functional Foods and Nutraceuticals

Nancy M. Childs

CONTENTS

I. INTRODUCTION

During the 1990s functional foods and nutraceuticals emerged as the dominant trend for the food industry, both in the U.S. and internationally. The concept of foods that could provide health-enhancing and disease-preventing properties was embraced by a growing number of consumers, increasingly documented by nutritionists and scientists, and legally endorsed by public policy and legislative mandates for food and dietary supplement labeling. These developments spawned considerable corporate attention across several industries, from agriculture, biotechnology, and life science-based concerns that grow and develop the raw commodities to nutritional, food, and pharmaceutical manufacturers that design new products.[1–3] Bringing these newly developed and newly positioned products to the consumer was the challenge and the value-added opportunity pursued by these industries.

Whereas consumer interest in the category continued to grow, 1999 emerged as a year with strong market gains for foods using Nutrition Labeling and Education Act (NLEA)–approved health claims and nutrient content claims as part of their marketing message. Product successes of note included the volume gains reported by Quaker Oats in its third quarter financial report featuring 7% gains for oatmeal for the summer quarter, a traditional down-period for hot cereal consumption. Ready-to-eat cereals increased 5% in volume for the period.[4] General Mills, in its mid-year report, highlighted 13% volume gains for Cheerios, using the oat bran and then the whole-grain health claim. Other General Mills whole-grain cereals received similar double-digit volume gains in a food category dependent on population increase (0.6%) for category growth.[5] Campbell Soup Company reported impressive success with their V8 Splash line, rich in antioxidants, which exceeded expected market growth and surpassed its category parent V8 vegetable juice.[6]

After a bellwether year of consumer response to products repositioned to market their functional advantages, the nascent market continued evolving in the new millennium. Advances in nutrition science discovery and documentation accelerated in university laboratories with both private and public sector funds. Early in the new decade the Office of Dietary Supplements at the National Institutes of Health (NIH) and U.S. Department of Agriculture (USDA) funded a variety of research projects and established numerous university research centers to address the science needed for U.S. Food and Drug Administration (FDA) review and approval of health claims on food labels. Table 27.1 presents a list of the NIH multiyear, multimillion-dollar-funded botanical research centers. The advances in scientific documentation coincided with legal challenges to the regulatory structure and science criteria. Prompted by case law, the FDA went through a series of positions to establish criteria for review and approval of "Qualified Health Claims" on food labels. At mid-decade the process is still evolving.[7] By 2003, the attention on obesity as an epidemic reached

---

TABLE 27.1
NIH Funded Botanical Research Centers 1999–2005

UCLA Center for Dietary Supplements Research

University of Illinois at Chicago: NIH Center for Dietary Supplements Research in Women's Health

The Arizona Center for Phytomedicine Research at Tucson

Purdue University and the University of Alabama at Birmingham Botanicals Research Center for Age Related Diseases

University of Missouri Center for Phytonutrient and Phytochemical Studies

University of Iowa and Iowa State University Center for Dietary Supplement Research/Botanical Supplements Research Center

The Pennington Botanical Research Center: Metabolic Syndrome (with Rutgers University)

The Wake Forest and Brigham and Women's Center for Dietary Lipids

MSKCC Center for Botanical Immunomodulators (Memorial Sloan-Kettering Cancer Center)

Source: Compiled from NIH and Office of Dietary Supplements Web sites.

critical proportions and received priority in food policy discussions. This further fueled consumer and food development interests in foods for health with benefits that could be claimed on the food label. Release of the revised and repositioned "My Pyramid" food dietary guidance in 2005 continued the attention on food for health for consumers and food marketers.

Careful attention to regulatory issues and insightful thought on communication of meaningful messages on product benefits to consumers are required for the marketing and positioning of products with health claims in the functional food area. Regulations control the language and scientific benefit that may be conveyed on the product label, in the marketing literature, and in the product advertising. Consumers, however, are often more persuaded by nuance, association, and promises of well-being than by scientific statements and numerical documentation.

II. EVOLUTION OF A MARKETING ENVIRONMENT FOR FUNCTIONAL FOODS AND NUTRACEUTICALS

From the 1970s onwards, food has taken on major connotations of being "good for you" or "bad for you," the latter types of foods, such as saturated fats and sodium, to be avoided or ingested in moderation. The good-for-you foods increasingly include foods and food components shown to lower the risk of cancer, heart disease, and other chronic diseases of aging. Since then, numerous studies and research reports have been published documenting the association between diet and health. In response, public health goals were reoriented from prevention of diseases associated with nutritional deficiencies to an emphasis on nutrition for decreasing risks for chronic disease. Early attention focused on preventing, among others, coronary heart disease, stroke, high blood pressure, cancer, diabetes, obesity, osteoporosis, dental diseases, and diverticulum disease, as pursued in the Surgeon General's landmark document on nutrition and health published in 1988.[8]

During the first Bush administration two major initiatives dominated consumer nutrition policy. The FDA, acting under Congress's directive, wrote new regulations governing health claims on food labels. The Nutrition Labeling and Education Act (NLEA) of 1990 was implemented in 1993. With the assumption that the food label is a primary nutrition education vehicle for the consumer, the NLEA carefully restricted what can be claimed on the label as well as what nutritional information must be disclosed.

The second parallel consumer nutrition education thrust involved the redefinition and reissue of the USDA Five Food Groups from 1979 as the initially controversial Food Guide Pyramid released in 1992. The new Food Guide Pyramid recommended the number of servings for six food groups. This initiative was refined and reintroduced in 2005 as My Pyramid.

In this environment emphasizing the role of diet in preventing disease and in promoting good health, a marketing, consumer, and regulatory crisis began to surface. A market for products with food components that prevent disease and prolong good health was created by consumer interest and education in such products. This was accompanied by publicized technological advances and scientific studies isolating food components such as antioxidants and carotenoids whose presence in food delivers these prophylactic benefits. These products are referred to by many terms such as *nutraceuticals, functional foods, designer foods*, and other labels from the corporate and scientific community. Interested consumers seek and respond to marketing claims that identify and elaborate on these components. Such claims, particularly as presented on the product label, created a growing dilemma to the FDA in the mid- and late-1980s.[9–11]

III. REGULATORY BACKGROUND

Since 1973, FDA regulations have stated that a food whose labeling represents that the food is adequate or effective in the "prevention, cure, mitigation, or treatment of any disease or symptom" is deemed "misbranded." These regulations were amended in 1993 to exempt FDA-approved health claims (21 C.F.R. 101.9(i)(1)(1992 ed.; recodified and extended in new NLEA regulations at 21 C.F.R. 101.9(k)(1), 58 Fed. Regis. 2533, January 23, 1993).

A. APPEARANCE OF PERMISSIVE HEALTH CLAIMS ON FOOD PRODUCTS

Contrary to the strict pre-1993 provisions, in the mid-1980s the FDA pursued a policy of selective nonenforcement, permitting an acceleration of explicit health-related and disease-related claims on food products that the FDA felt were justified and benefited the public health. The frequently cited "watershed" was the 1984 promotion of All Bran cereal by Kellogg's Company with labels that explicitly claimed preventive benefits of fiber with respect to cancer: "... eating the right foods may reduce your risk of some kinds of cancer ... eat high fiber foods ... bran cereals are one of the best sources of fiber."[12–14]

This promotion was jointly conducted with the National Cancer Institute (NCI) which, in the 1980s and 1990s, was ahead of other government agencies in promoting to the consumer the use of diet and, specifically, foods rich in certain nutrient properties. The NCI launched the well publicized Designer Foods Program specifically to address and document the role of these phytochemicals in cancer prevention.[15]

Other permitted claims in the late 1980s included claims concerning lowered blood serum cholesterol and the reduced risk of chronic heart disease for oat-based breakfast cereals and other products containing oat bran; claims that calcium helps reduce the risk of osteoporosis promoted on dairy products and dietary supplements; and vegetable oil products posting a variety of claims from "cholesterol-free" to "better for your heart than ... " to specific claims regarding "lower blood serum cholesterol" and "reduced risk of chronic heart disease." By 1990, it was reported that "... 40 percent of all new food products introduced in the first half of 1989 bore general and specific health claims."[16]

Besides the exploding number and variety of health claims promoted by food marketers — which the FDA chose to ignore, thereby informally condoning them — the FDA also officially exempted several food categories from drug status and accountability while permitting explicit health and disease-related labeling claims. These food product categories included "medical foods," "hypoallergenic" foods, diabetic foods, sugarless foods that "will not promote tooth decay," and foods that are qualified for special dietary uses (21 C.F.R.).[17]

B. REACTION AND INSTITUTION OF THE NLEA

The incipient loss of control by the FDA with its official and unofficial exemptions encouraged a flood of health claims from entrepreneurial marketers and created a consumer marketplace rife with confusion and skepticism. Adding to the loss of control and embarrassment on the FDA level was the ambitious behavior of several state attorney generals who very publicly invoked their authority in this arena, on behalf of consumer protection, opposing fraudulent and misleading food labeling claims and seizing the products.[18–20]

An early attempt to regulate this type of imitative and ambitious marketing behavior was an FDA proposal in 1987. This set of permissive guidelines never took effect and ultimately was replaced by the restrictive 1990 NLEA proposals. The strict separation of definition of food and drug returned. A food product could make a health- or disease-related claim "only if (FDA) determines, based on the totality of publicly available scientific evidence (including the evidence from well designed studies ...) that there is significant scientific agreement, among experts ... that the claim is supported by such evidence" (21 U.S.C. 343(r)(3)(B)).

Though the overall regulations were quite stringent, more restrictive, more inclusive, and set high standards for qualification, the FDA did address and rule on ten claims that the agency examined for authorization. The authorized claims were approved for use as generic health claims on foods that qualified. Table 27.2 lists the originally approved health claims under the NLEA. The

TABLE 27.2
Health Claims That Meet Significant Scientific Agreement (SSA) Receiving Approval under NLEA

Seven Health Claims Receiving Original Approval under NLEA

Calcium and osteoporosis
Sodium and hypertension
Dietary lipids (fat) and cancer
Dietary saturated fat and cholesterol and risk of coronary heart disease
Fiber-containing grain products, fruits and vegetables, and cancer
Fruits, vegetables, and grain products that contain fiber, particularly soluble fiber, and risk of coronary heart disease
Fruits and vegetables and cancer

Additional Health Claims Receiving FDA Approval under NLEA

Folic acid and neural tube defects
Dietary noncarcinogenic carbohydrate sweeteners and dental caries
Dietary soluble fiber from certain foods (such as that found in whole oats and psyllium seed husk) and risk of coronary heart disease
Soy protein and risk of coronary heart disease
Stanols/sterols and risk of coronary heart disease

Source: From FDA Web site: Label Claims — Health Claims that Meet Significant Scientific Agreement (SSA), Updated June 9, 2004, www.cfsan.fda.gov/~dms/lab-ssa.html.

FDA also established a definition for the term healthy for use in food labeling. To be labeled as healthy, food must meet the definition of "low" for fat and saturated fat, must contain cholesterol and sodium below disclosure levels prescribed in FDA regulations, and must comply with all applicable rules concerning specific nutrient content claims on the label (21 C.F.R. 101.65(d)(2), 58 Fed. Regis. 2944).

This select and limited approach permitted access to generic health claims in the food situations that qualify under the authorized categories listed in Table 27.2. Any health claim that was not explicitly approved for use in food labeling by an FDA regulation was deemed to be forbidden from use in food labeling.[21]

The implementation of the NLEA in 1993 quickly prompted concerns of ambitious enforcement from the FDA. In hindsight, two results are easily documented. Industry's adherence to the new legislation dramatically reduced the number of claims used in food product advertising (Figure 27.1). The concerns of the dietary supplement industry that the FDA would aggressively apply the new regulations to their growing industry prompted separate legislation in the area. The quick and unanticipated passage of the Dietary Supplement Health and Education Act (DSHEA) in 1994 created a separate set of label criteria for the ancillary dietary supplement industry that was distinct from the regulations required on food labels. It also created a separate and distinct regulatory category for dietary supplements with separate marketing standards for label claims and advertising statements.

C. UTILIZATION OF THE FDA MODERNIZATION ACT TO ESTABLISH HEALTH CLAIMS

The regulated market for health claims on foods and claims on dietary supplements continued to evolve in the late 1990s as claims were approved and challenged, and as various legal precedents occurred in this area. The Food and Drug Modernization Act (FDAMA) of 1997 permitted the consideration of authoritative statements as a source for health claims on foods. This led to the approval of the whole-grain health claim addressing the risk of heart disease and cancer, as cited in a National Academy of Science report on diet and health. This report also sourced the potassium

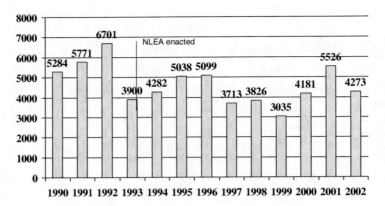

FIGURE 27.1 Use of nutrition messages on food labels 1990–2003: nutrient content — structure/function — health claim.

TABLE 27.3
Label Claims Receiving FDA Approval under the FDA Modernization Act of 1997 (FDAMA)

Potassium and the risk of high blood pressure and stroke
Whole grain foods and the risk of heart disease and certain cancers
Nutrient content claim for choline

Source: From FDA Web site: Label Claims — FDA Modernization Act of 1977 (FDAMA) Claims, updated June 9, 2004, www.cfsan. fda.gov/~dms/labfdama.html.

---

and risk of high blood pressure and stroke claim. A report of the Food and Nutrition Board of the Institutes of Medicine provided documentation to permit the institution of a nutrient content claim for choline. These are included in Table 27.3.

D. PURSUIT OF QUALIFIED HEALTH CLAIMS FOR FOOD PRODUCTS

Legal developments during 1999 triggered a significant revamping of FDA claim regulation, which is still evolving at mid-decade. The new qualified health claim criteria is still under review, and expands the possibility that manufacturers may be able to bring more "emerging" science to the label as they present their data in unbiased terms. The qualified health claim format permits discussion of a nutrient–disease connection in qualified terms, depending on the FDA's assessment of the strength of the relationship based on the presented dossier of research. This is a complex and lengthy assessment that includes multiple considerations. These include the number of studies, study type and size, strength of study findings, relevancy of the studies to the intended claim statement and target population, and consistency of findings across studies.[22] Table 27.4 lists the qualified health claims permitted for use by mid-decade.

E. ISSUES AND IMPLICATIONS FOR INVESTMENT

An applicant has two key concerns when approaching the FDA regulatory environment in pursuit of claim approval. These are the amount of documentation and time required for approval, and the type of claim and the structure of the communications message permitted. For a health claim to be approved on a food product, the claim must be submitted to the FDA with scientific documentation. All materials enter the public domain. After lengthy review and public comment, the claim

TABLE 27.4
FDA Permitted Qualified Health Claims with Qualifying Language

Selenium and cancer — *some scientific evidence suggests...evidence is limited and not conclusive*

Antioxidant vitamins and cancer — *some scientific evidence suggests...evidence is limited but not conclusive*

Nuts and heart disease — *scientific evidence suggests but does not prove...*

Walnuts and heart disease – *supportive but not conclusive research shows....*

Omega-3 fatty acids and coronary heart disease — *supportive but not conclusive research shows...*

B vitamins and vascular disease — *evidence in support of the above claim is inconclusive*

Monounsaturated fatty acids from olive oil and coronary heart disease — *limited and not conclusive evidence suggests...*

Soy-derived phosphatidylserine and cognitive dysfunction and dementia — *very limited and preliminary scientific research suggests...FDA concludes that there is little scientific evidence supporting the claim*

Source: From FDA Web site: Summary of Qualified Health Claims Permitted, updated August 4, 2005, www.cfsan.fda.gov/~dms/qhc-sum.html.

may receive generic approval for use by all products that meet the qualification of the claim. It remains a concern for the existing qualified health claim protocol that the time necessary for review and approval, the presentation of data in the public domain, and the generic availability of the resulting claim will deter private investment in documenting and developing products with functional advantages for health. Without access to patents or proprietary claims, the research incentives lie within the public domain, through university funded centers as listed in Table 27.1. Private sector situations that benefit under the existing generic claim protocol include agricultural co-ops and ingredient suppliers who can either patent or brand their functional ingredient in a way that grants them some advantage in order to provide a return on their investment in research to document the functional ingredient.

F. FUTURE ISSUES: NUTRIGENOMICS AND FOOD NANOTECHNOLOGY

The development and commercialization of next generation functional foods and nutraceuticals will be influenced by the fields of genomics and nanotechnology. There is a growing understanding that certain food components activate genetic based responses in body cells and that these responses vary on an individual level. With broader access to DNA typing and gene testing it is expected that individually customized diets can be prescribed to prevent disease when susceptibility is identified on an individual cellular level. Called *nutrigenomics,* this nascent field holds promise for customized preventive healthcare. Nanotechnology application in food delivery also promises a high tech patentable research field that can enhance and deliver functional benefits in food forms through microencapsulation and nanoprocessing, among other applications. Difficulties in extracting, standardizing, and delivering benefits in the botanical arena may be ameliorated through advances in food nanotechnology.

Both fields are aggressively pursuing intellectual property protection, though policy makers are uncertain how to regulate these processes and products. There also is preliminary debate on whether proprietary discovery will impede new product development and dissemination of healthier foods on the widest level in the future.

IV. INTRODUCTION TO CONSUMER MARKETING ISSUES FOR NUTRACEUTICALS AND FUNCTIONAL FOODS

Nutraceutical and functional food consumers tend to be female, middle-aged, affluent, and more educated than the average consumer. They represent a desirable marketing segment that is less price sensitive and more proactive regarding pursuit of good health. They segment into numerous

---

TABLE 27.5
Lessons Learned for Marketing Functional Foods

Good taste necessary
Brand name should connect to functional advantage without compromising taste assurance
Consumer education required
Consumer confused by information overload and contradiction in media
Avoid complicated claims referencing numbers or unfamiliar food components
Competitive set determined by health issue, not product category
Nonverbal messages are important: satisfied users
Suggest usage occasion and product substitution
Avoid negative or scare-tactic advertising
Functional foods serve niche markets
Recognize and exploit corporate heritage in specific product categories
Provide assurances for dosage and standardized product
Use packaging to imply dosage and penetrate multiple channels for convenient access

---

lifestyle and behavior groups, and have concerns across a number of chronic disease states. They represent a quintessential target market.

Marketing issues can be divided between general factors promoting marketing success, as listed in Table 27.5, and specific factors for product positioning on a whole health continuum. General factors, or lessons learned for marketing foods utilizing health claims, are discussed in the following sections.

A. Good Taste Necessary

Most successful new food products in the late 1990s demonstrated three criteria: taste, convenience, and nutritional advantage. Taste remains paramount of the three and is the dictating factor for repeat purchase. Although nutrition or convenience may generate trial purchase, neither will sustain repeat purchase without good taste. Not only should nutraceutical products provide good taste, they must promise good taste in their advertising and reinforce the consumer's curiosity for good taste. This is critically important for new products without benefit of a familiar brand heritage.

B. Brand Name Connects to Functional Advantage

The brand name of the product should connect to the health benefit of the product and offer insight into the unique functional value of the food, as well as not connote a taste concern. An exception would be a preexisting product like oatmeal repositioned for its functional health value, where the preexisting brand equity is retained. The early psyllium cereals demonstrated the communication strength of the more straightforward Heartwise brand offered by Kellogg's vs. the more vague implications of General Mill's Benefit brand moniker. Again, the Nabisco Brand NutraJoint product communicated with consumers but the recent Kellogg's psyllium line Ensemble did not equate the beneficial purpose of the product. Tropicana has succeeded in communicating their functional orange juice line, first under the banner Pure Premium Plus and later Essentials, with identification of the specific functional ingredient(s) and purpose. This was dramatically successful with their Healthy Kids introduction based on a nutrient bundle adding health benefits specific to children's nutrition needs and dietary deficiencies.

C. Consumer Education Required

The more specific the nutrient and its benefit, the more consumer education on the disease state and health condition that is needed. Cardiovascular disease, cancer, and osteoporosis seem to be reasonably well communicated health concerns, but many of the more specific health issues are not. Complementarily, the consumers have varying levels of understanding of the benefits of the nutrients. Popular antioxidant vitamins are readily accepted for their health value, whereas newer antioxidants such as lycopene and xianthan are less familiar and not readily identified with the health condition they sustain. Levels of consumer education appear to follow public health campaigns, and to the degree that approved health claims receive rapid exposure in the commercial and public health media, consumers quickly appreciate new nutrient benefits.

D. Avoid Information Overload

Consumers do not easily process complicated quantitative messages regarding nutritional benefit, and do not readily understand comparative mathematical relationships as validation of nutrient benefit. Although such information may be provided on the label and in the marketing literature for the product, it should not be the essence of the positioning and advertising of the product. Such information is useful for the medical audience and the informed consumer and its presence provides value for these purposes.

E. Competitive Set Determined by Health Issue

One of the most repeated fundamental marketing errors that has occurred with functional foods and nutraceuticals is the inclination to address the product category competitive set and not the substitutive competitive set defined by the health condition. Cholesterol-lowering foods, whether oatmeal, soy, or stanol ester spreads, are in direct competition with ethical drug products for this purpose and provoke strong competitive response from the pharmaceutical industry. These defensive responses are addressed to both the consumer and the medical community. Food manufacturers rarely anticipate this out-of-category — indeed, out-of-industry — counter response.

F. Importance of Nonverbal Messages

The use of nonverbal messages is an important method for communicating good taste, quality assurance, and functionality. Product functionality can be connoted in a number of ways by showing active, satisfied users. Taste assurance is conveyed with satisfied users enjoying the product. Nonverbal messages also can be used to suggest target market consumers, product quality, and to provide a "natural" halo for the product with visuals of fields, growing plants, plant botanical graphics, or other reassuring images.

G. Usage Occasion

The sight of satisfied users and the presence of the product consumed in a usage occasion environment is reassuring and provides context to the consumer. Usage occasion is an important factor as it suggests to the consumer the method for incorporating the product into a daily routine, thereby meeting dosage demands. It also suggests product substitution possibilities, which increase likelihood of product adoption.

H. Avoid Negative Advertising

Advertising focusing on the fear of the disease and a message addressing the loss of health has not resonated with consumers so far. Consumers are wary of avoidance messages, and are more favorable and receptive to messages of "more" and "better" and general promises of good health. Functional foods are excellent sources of "better" and "good-for-you" product messages and are easily positioned to emphasize their positive advantage. This good health approach also is less challenging to the regulatory structure.

I. NICHE MARKETS

Almost by definition, as bioactive ingredients are better understood, they are promoted for specific use by specific populations and represent niche market opportunities. As the category matures, competition increases, and the medical community becomes more interested in products, the niche market specificity will become more important. These specifics are necessary to communicate product differentiation, superiority, and credibility.

J. EXPLOIT CORPORATE HERITAGE

Many food and pharmaceutical companies hold enviable brand equity positions, such as Quaker Oats Oatmeal mentioned earlier, and enjoy corporate images of trust and expertise with the consumer. McNeil Consumer Health holds such a trust with the consumer as does Kellogg's with its healthy fiber cereal dominance. Kellogg's Heartwise cereal was able to secure ready consumer acceptance as a high-fiber cereal because of the Kellogg's heritage in the category. For General Mills' Cheerios brand and Tropicana's Pure Premium Plus and Essentials line, the existing equity of taste and quality were powerful foundations for their transformations to functional food positionings. The existence of a product line or portfolio allows the nutrition message and health claim to be directed at one product in the line, but the health "halo" covers the entire line, even the items that are sugar frosted, marketed to children, or otherwise inappropriately positioned to be consonant with targeted health claim marketing.

K. DOSAGE AND STANDARDIZATION

As the category for functional foods continues to mature, the regulatory environment, the educated consumer, and the medical community will be asking for levels of bioactive presence to fulfill efficacious dosage levels. Standardized product will be an important factor for assessing product quality, and perhaps to meet required product certification in the future.

L. PACKAGING

Use of individual serve packaging suggests dosage, and delivery of multipacks in sleeves can suggest and monitor weekly usage. Individual serve also offers the opportunity to market the product in multiple outlets including vending, convenience store, and food service formats, which are popular functional food channels in Japan and Europe. Individual serve packaging is particularly popular with beverage and bar product forms. For products to convey functionality, they are better presented in smaller portions. They are not meant to be refreshing beverages or meal substitutes. Lower caloric content also increases the likelihood that the products can be incorporated into a daily diet without major impact on preexisting dietary habits.

V. POTENTIAL PRODUCT POSITIONING

Consumers interested in functional foods and nutraceuticals have four categories of product function that are desired. These are therapy, prevention, performance, and particularly in the U.S., weight loss. The therapy, prevention, and performance categories have varying foci, depending on the respondent's sex and age.

Consumer studies repeatedly indicate there are segments in the population that have attitudes and lifestyles more consonant with the concept of foods for health. Typically, consumer research can segment about 40 million consumers who are "health active," meaning they act today to ensure good health when older, are concerned about family nutrition, regularly eat fruit, accept medications, and exercise twice a week. In addition, research recognizes a somewhat similar group of consumers, titled "health aware," who are like the former "active" group except they do not exercise twice a week. This group, also comprising consumers over age 18, is estimated to include 13 million consumers. These are sizable consumer markets.[23]

Of notable interest is that these "health active" and "health aware" consumers also differ from the remaining "health uninvolved" population of 137 million people by virtue of their advanced interest in the continuum of food–nutrition–health. They are far more likely to have moved farther along the continuum to food–nutrition–health–wellness–well-being. Their concept of health has a totality about it that is likely to encompass community, self-enhancement, religion, personalization, rituals, and the environment. These factors can be addressed as physical, emotional, spiritual, social, and financial dimensions. Not surprisingly, people who are willing to believe what they do and eat today may potentially impact their health far in the future have some distinguishing beliefs that can become the foundation for functional food positionings, advertising messages, promotional opportunities, and product ingredients.

A. PHYSICAL COMPONENTS

Functional food and nutraceutical positionings, regardless of product function or product form, exist along each of the five dimensions identified in the following sections. The physical dimension is the most obvious and is clustered around an attention to nutrition, exercise, and medicine. Functional foods can be positioned along a continuum of nutrition to medicine depending on their scientific credibility and purpose for therapy, prevention, or performance. Any products that complement or enhance the healthy benefits of physical exercise offer strong positioning opportunity.

B. EMOTIONAL COMPONENTS

The emotional component involves the needs for nurturing, self-knowledge, and stress management. Functional food and nutraceutical positioning is compatible with a need for nurturing one's own health as well as that of one's family. The woman's proclivity for functional food products encourages her, as primary shopper, to respond to a positioning that nurtures and protects her family. This consumer's interest in self-knowledge, which will include genome vulnerabilities and environmental exposure, as well as the individual's need for stress management, will heighten consumer interest in products, particularly customized products that address these concerns. Self-knowledge and customized/personalized/individualized products offer a potentially powerful match. Test kits and other measurements and "surrogate markers" or biomarkers (such as cholesterol for cardiovascular disease) become valuable vehicles for recognizing individual needs for protection, restoration or enhancement of performance, and recovery. These vehicles will document the need for a specific disease-associated functional food, and thereby encourage its use.

C. WELL-BEING COMPONENTS

The consumer's dimension of well-being, or spirituality, encompasses meditation, prayer, energy, and nature. The two latter components directly relate to the performance purpose of functional foods (energy) and to the desirability of natural ingredients for such products (nature). The term *natural* takes on many dimensions of purity from the desirable organic stricture to being naturally sourced, or simply being plant derived rather than a laboratory-sourced synthetic substitute. Consumers' first preference, by a wide margin, is to obtain nutraceutical substances through consumption of fruits and vegetables. This underscores their desire for familiar and natural sources for these active ingredients. Natural connotations can be conjured from the product name, label graphics, and advertising setting. In Japan, where the culture harmonizes rather than separates food and health, the FOSHU (Foods for Specified Health Use) products are required to be of natural origin.

D. SOCIAL COMPONENTS

The social component includes three factors of large and familiar promise for functional food positioning. These are family, community, and philanthropy. The first two provide reasons as well as occasions for functional food consumption. So long as nutraceuticals remain a functional food — an edible or drinkable product — they have the potential to be a part of the most social and most routine parts of our lives, namely, daily sustenance. The philanthropy connection is an important insight for marketers as it indicates that relationship marketing should be a powerful tool. Tying products in with preexisting disease foundations and fund-raisers, such as the breast cancer annual "Run for the Cure" event, should carry strong credibility to these consumers. Foundation endorsements, seals of approval, and spokespeople offer potential marketing and positioning tactics. Many may offer opportunities for exclusivity, which could become a powerful product point of differentiation in an arena of generic claims.

E. FINANCIAL COMPONENTS

The fifth dimension is financial, and it clusters into four drivers: concerns and preparations for comfort, for retirement, for maintaining independence from one's children, and for contingency planning. Though obviously no functional food is a financial investment instrument, brand positionings, nonverbal advertising messages, and promotions that focus on the enjoyment and attainment of these goals give a credible context and purpose for preventive functional food products. This is evident in the advertising campaigns for Quaker Oats Oatmeal using the health claim language in a venue of active seniors enjoying breakfast on the golf course; Tropicana Pure Premium Plus presenting active seniors hiking under the headline, "Leave the Grandkids in the Dust" and inclusion of the health claim; and in Ensure's active senior advertising. Ensure's campaigns have focused on two of the above elements: elder parent and grown child enjoying the product together and toasting "to our health," and implicit independence. More recently, a campaign of active seniors was introduced, again emphasizing the comfort and fun opportunities offered by healthy retirement.

VI. SUMMARY

In summary, product positioning potential is multidimensional for a segment of consumers of proclaimed belief in functional food and nutraceutical products. This target market responds to product purpose for prevention, therapy, and performance. They have specific disease states that concern them, in an individualized manner, for which they are receptive to seeking prevention and therapy products. Such disease concerns include heart disease, cancers, Alzheimer's, and others. As well as the segments of product purpose and target disease, described above, there are product positionings and advertising messages, verbal and nonverbal, which carry particular credibility and immediacy to these consumers. These tend to cluster into the five areas elaborated above, which include physical, emotional, spiritual, social, and financial components. Each offers numerous product "hooks" for catching consumer interest with a credible and identifiable message. Without offering specific direction for product function, form, or targeted disease state, these components offer marketing context for product positionings, insight for product names, label design, advertising campaigns, promotions, co-marketing, spokespeople, endorsing organizations, and other marketing tactics. Even though regulation does not permit proprietary health claims, powerful marketing relationships can be structured in an exclusive manner. This is a familiar aspect of sports drink marketing, a performance product category.

VII. CONCLUSION

Nutraceuticals and functional foods are clearly poised as a 21st-century industry. They promise value-added opportunities in the food industry and new market opportunities for the pharmaceutical industry. They offer advances in public health as health claim marketing messages empower consumers to select healthier food choices. Regulatory issues are complex and have evolved in a politically driven fashion with three major legislative efforts transpiring in the 1990s (NLEA, DSHEA, and FDAMA) and several legal decisions impacting regulatory interpretation and application via case law in the present decade.

The regulatory activity defines the marketing parameters for the product label, which is one of the marketing venues. Several suggestions are given for savvy marketing of functional food products. Elaboration on product positionings are offered, acknowledging that consumer receptivity often hinges on perceptions of quality, taste, acceptability, and well-being, rather than stated specifics of product potency and clinical benefit.

REFERENCES

1. Childs, N.M., Marketing functional foods: what have we learned? An examination of the Benefit and Heartwise introductions as cholesterol reducing RTE cereals, *J. Med. Foods*, 2(1): 11–19, 1999.
2. Childs, N.M., The functional food consumer: who is she and what does she want? Implications for product development and positioning, in *New Technologies for Healthy Foods and Nutraceuticals*, Yalpani, M., Ed., ATL Press, Chicago, IL, 1997.
3. Childs, N., Nutraceutical industry trends, *J. Nutraceut. Funct. Med. Foods*, 2(1), 53–85, 1999.
4. Quaker Oats Company, Third Quarter 1999 Financial Report, Chicago, IL, 1999.
5. General Mills Company, 1999 Midyear Financial Report, Minneapolis, MN, 1999.
6. Thompson, S., Campbell adds punch to growing V8 Splash, *Advertising Age,* November 15, 1999.
7. Walsh, E.M., Lietzan, E.K., and Hutt, P.B., The importance of the court decision in *Pearson v. Shalala* to the marketing of conventional food and dietary supplements in the U.S., in *Regulation of Functional Foods and Nutraceuticals*, Hasler, C. Ed., Blackwell Publishing, Ames, IA, 2005, pp. 109–136.
8. The Surgeon General's Report on Nutrition and Health, U.S. Department of Health and Human Services, Washington, D.C., 1988, p. 78.
9. Erickson, J.L. and Dognoli, J., Healthy food pace quickens, leaving regulatory forces behind, *Advertising Age*, 60(41), September 25, 1989, 3, 92.
10. Hutt, P.B., FDA regulation of product claims in food labeling, *J. Public Policy Market*, 12(1), 132–134, 1993.
11. McNamara, S.H., FDA's Rules on Health Claims for Foods — Including the New 1993 Regulations Issued under the Nutrition Labeling and Education Act (NLEA), Hyman, Phelps, and McNamara, Washington, D.C., January 1993.
12. Calfee, J.E. and Pappalardo, J.K., Public policy issues in health claims for foods, *J. Public Policy Market*, 10(1), 33–53, 1991.
13. Anon., *Develop and Market Nutrient Fortified Foods,* Institute for International Research, Orlando, FL, December 1991.
14. Anon., *Yankelovich Health Monitor,* 1995.
15. Sherman, C., Meals that heal, *Health*, March 1991, 69+.
16. McNamara, S.H., op. cit.
17. Ibid.
18. Carey, J., Snap, Crackle, Stop — States Crack Down on Misleading Food Claims, *Business Week*, September 25, 1989, 42+.
19. Lawrence, J., Texas Notches a Win Over Kellogg, *Advertising Age*, April 8, 1991, 6.
20. Leisse, J., Grocery Marketing: Health Claims — the Legacy of Benefit, *Advertising Age*, 61(19), May 7, 1990. S1, S18.
21. Golodner, L.F., Healthy confusion for consumers, *J. Public Policy Market*, 12(1): 130–132, 1993.
22. FDA Center for Food Safety and Nutrition Food Label Guide, http://www.cfsan.fda.gov/~dms/hclmgui4.html, July 10, 2003, accessed August 2005.
23. Anon, *Yankelovich Health Monitor,* 1995.

28 Obesity Policy: Opportunities for Functional Food Market Growth*

Nancy M. Childs

CONTENTS

A confluence of public events on a global scale have placed obesity front and center of food policy and corporate strategy. It has generated innumerable conferences and an entire low carb food frenzy in the short run. But its real promise is in the long-term, proven product development of foods that are demonstrated to functionally impact obesity: functional foods for obesity. Such documented products may have a double reward — eligibility for qualified health claims and possible reimbursement under Medicare as a disease treatment. They also offer laudable product franchises that provide a "healthy" balance to food company product portfolios, thereby limiting corporate liability on both legal and stock valuation fronts. Opportunities abound for ingredients and well formulated products that provide both taste and convenience with their functionality: products that carefully document and demonstrate their ability to aid weight loss and prevent weight gain.

I. EMERGENCE OF OBESITY AS MAJOR PUBLIC HEALTH ISSUE

Surgeon General David Satcher issued the formal "Call to Action to Prevent and Decrease Obesity in 2001." The lawsuits against McDonalds followed in 2002, generating tremendous media attention if not legal respect. The World Health Organization declared obesity a global epidemic in March 2003 and followed it up with bold recommendations in 2004. April 2003 witnessed the J.P. Morgan equities report, which ranked public food company product portfolios based on the volume of their products which were high in fat and calories, thereby contributing to obesity. This tied corporate stock valuation to anticipated liability risk and profit erosion from over-reliance on high-calorie foods. Later in the summer of 2003, Department of Health and Human Services Secretary Tommy Thompson announced his Obesity Roundtables, which began a well publicized and high level

---

* This chapter is expanded from the article "Obesity Policy Promises a Functional Food Feast," published in the *Nutrition Business Journal* Vol. IX (7/8) and from the IFT Annual Meeting 2005 presentation, "Obesity and Marketing Opportunities for Functional Ingredients," delivered in New Orleans in July 2005.

stakeholder dialogue on the topic. He also instructed the Surgeon General, Center for Disease Control, NIH, and the FDA to address the obesity epidemic with high priority. In 2003 and 2004 numerous state legislatures took up the obesity charge with a variety of bills to tax high caloric foods and beverages or restrict sales venues for such products. In the summer of 2004 Medicare formally declared obesity an illness with eligibility for reimbursement of medically documented products and treatments for seniors. In late 2004 the National Academies of Science instituted a national working committee on Food Marketing: Diets of Children and Youth and in 2005 published *Preventing Childhood Obesity: Health in the Balance.* Later that summer the FTC and DHHS held the public forum Perspectives on Marketing, Self-Regulation and Childhood Obesity. Public policy focused especially on the marketing of foods to children as a component of childhood obesity and, by extension, as a factor in the population's obesity epidemic.

The FDA has proposed label changes that rationalize portion size to package size and alter the Nutrition Facts Panel to emphasize calories as percent of daily total. They are giving early consideration to the possible addition of symbols on the label translating calories to physical energy expenditure. Also, they are implementing a qualified health claim policy that allows a reference to the health value of foods or ingredients provided the label carries a qualified health claim denoting the level of science and certainty behind the claim as rated by the FDA. They are proposing standardized qualified language for potentially four differentiated levels of qualified health claims for use on the food label. The vocabulary differentiates the FDA's acceptance of the documented science for the claim based on number of studies, rigor of study design, and consonance of study findings. These are the operating models until FDA sponsored consumer research is evaluated on the claims' differing language and their receptivity and viability with consumers. This consumer research will explore communication issues with consumers regarding the differing claim levels, and the research findings will impact decisions regarding the final qualified health claim format for implementation. Qualified health claims represent an evolving policy area within the FDA.

Qualified health claims provide potential communication opportunities for many functional food bioactives; they are also available for use with obesity related products. The high priority given to weight loss efforts in the public health arena suggests that the FDA would give such products timely and thorough scrutiny, in the hope of seeing genuine weight loss products entering the market with the ability to communicate their message to consumers.

II. INGREDIENTS WITH FUNCTIONAL POTENTIAL TO MITIGATE OBESITY

Obesity has been addressed by a threefold product development approach.

A. LESS IS MORE

A straightforward reduction of undesirable ingredients, such as sugars, fats, and, most recently, carbohydrates, associated with weight gain, would reduce weight. Such products had peaked rapidly in 2004 with enormous product reformulation to create low carbohydrate products and brands, overwhelming the consumer with lower carbohydrate product alternatives. By 2005 interest in these products and in a serious low carbohydrate diet had waned. Weight management formulation then shifted to embracing new and versatile sugar alternatives.

B. MORE IS LESS

A plethora of new ingredients are being developed and touted to bulk up foods to achieve a low caloric density. These can be as simple as adding more water, air, or fruits and vegetables to formulations. Whipped versions of yogurts and desserts permit lower caloric density of favorite products with desired taste and mouthfeel.

New novel oils and fats such as diacylglycerol (*Enova* by ADM Kao LLC) and structured triglycerides (*Benefat* by Danisco), sugar substitutes, flours and fibers (*Raftiline* inulin by Orafti and *Oliggo-Fiber* from Cargill) can be formulated into products to achieve a lower calorie product. Additional products, which extend products without adding excessive calories, include starch blockers, flaxseed, and soy (*Solae* from DuPont Protein Technologies and USDA's *Soytrim*), among other possibilities.

C. FUNCTIONAL INGREDIENTS

These show real potential for actively assisting weight management. Both Generally Recognized as Safe (GRAS) status and qualified health claim approval are actively being sought for several of these products. All such products would need an ongoing research program demonstrating efficacy for FDA review. Potential products range the full spectrum, from familiar ingredients with new weight management evidence such as has been found concerning calcium, to more tentative and novel products under review.

Functional food candidates in this group, as highlighted by the Institute of Food Technologists' (IFT) *Food Technology Journal* in March 2003, include leptin, chromium, soy and whey proteins, L-carnitine, conjugated linoleic acid, and other products. Fibers such as barley or oat derived beta-glucan (*Maltrim* and *Nutrim* by VanDrunen Farms; *OatVantage* by Nurture, Inc.) may aid satiety and maintain blood glucose levels for weight management. Specialty corn-derived starches (*Novelose* by National Starch and Chemical Co.) may lower glycemic responses. Extensive work with flax lignans suggests health functionality with many cofactors for obesity as licensed by ADM. Whey proteins (such as *Grande Ultra* by Grande Custom Ingredients Group) may suppress appetite, and dairy products are showing a multifaceted functionality for weight loss (including *TruCal* by Glanbia and efforts by Dairy Management Inc.). Conjugated linoleic acid (*Xenadrine* by Cytodyne Technologies or *Clarinol* by Loders Croklaan Lipid Nutrition) may accelerate fat breakdown and increase lean body mass. New functional fibers that manage sugar levels to assist weight loss include fenugreek (*FenuLife* by Acatris, Inc., and *Fenupure* by Adumin Food Ingredients) and polydextrose (*Litesse* by Danisco). Chitosan polysaccharide fibers inhibit fat digestion (*ChitoClear* from Primex BioChemicals). Chromium and chromium picolinate are long associated with weight management potential (*ChroMax* by Nutrition 21 and *CarnoChrome* by FutureCeuticals). L-Carnitine is another ingredient associated with weight control through energy. Other novel products include cocoa extract (*Chocamine* from NatTrop) and hydroxycitric acid to suppress appetite; betaine, a component of sugar beets, improving fat metabolism; 4-hydrosyisoleucine (*Promilin* from Technical Sourcing International), DHEA (*7-Keta* by Humanetics Corp.) and forskolin root extract.

Although these ingredients are identified for their potential promise in assisting weight loss and weight management, they need adequate science and GRAS status for consideration for FDA qualified health claim approval. Additionally they would need substantial medical substantiation such as clinical trials for possible qualification for Medicare reimbursement. This list, by no means complete, indicates the impressive potential for functional food opportunities to address obesity. Most encouraging is the number of trademarked and branded ingredients, which suggest an ingredient supplier may be interested in sharing the scientific effort to document the functional value of the bioactive.

As shown in Figure 28.1, the obesity market opportunities are large and growing, and exhibit various intersections between traditional diet foods, growing healthy food markets, expanding functional food markets and the diminishing low carb category. This permits entry opportunity for various types of products for weight loss and weight management and a broad spectrum of marketing and positioning opportunities for these products. This creates a continuum of differentiated product space both with and without reliance on an approved qualified health claim.

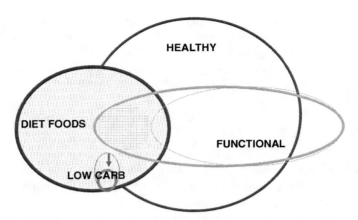

FIGURE 28.1 Market opportunity space for functional obesity products. (Developed by N. Childs, 2004.)

III. STRATEGIES FOR QUALIFIED HEALTH CLAIM USE

Qualified health claims remain generic in their application. Unless the ingredient supplier demonstrates a purported health value from a proprietarily derived ingredient, the qualified claim would have application to all similar products. Even if an ingredient is proprietary and is permitted a qualified health claim, the claim would be generically available to all food products that used the ingredient. This situation creates a dichotomized set of opportunities in the marketplace.

The value and appropriateness of qualified health claim use becomes dependent on the product's positioning in the marketplace and whether the claim is fundamental to authenticating the position or is a value-added enhancement to a position that is not primarily based on health benefit. In this case it provides a "health halo" to the product via its presence in the formulation: the actual use of the qualified health claim is not central to the positioning. For science-based positions for health specific states the qualified health claim is essential and meets the needs of consumers seeking information for specific product needs. Also, past research shows that the less familiar the bioactive, the larger the role for the qualified health claim. For Health Reward and Authenticated for General Health product positionings, the claim can be useful but not to the same degree as a science based health specific position. Figure 28.2 presents the positioning continuums in a matrix format.

IV. FUNCTIONAL FOODS AND OBESITY

Attention to obesity creates market opportunity to identify and develop promising functional ingredients to help reduce and manage weight. Documented science leading to a qualified health claim lends the necessary credence to the new ingredients. The functional food category expects 6 to 7% annual growth through the decade. This category appears as a sustainable and appropriate long term market category and important source for functional food growth. Genuine functional foods for weight loss and maintenance should be rewarded with an enormous market response. Consumer interest in obesity fighting products will not wane, and consumer patterns of faddish over-response should remain the norm. Demographics for the consumers targeted for obesity functional foods should increase in size as the American baby boom generation continues to avalanche into middle age with its spreading waistline.

The obesity foods category will continue to evolve from the deliberate *less is more* approach, to the more technically driven *more is less* capability to substitute new products for former fattier or sweeter components. Lastly the novelty and technical accomplishments of the *functional food ingredients* category offer the larger opportunity — for possible proprietary positions and for aiding consumers in obtaining a healthier diet and lifestyle. The category should remain lucrative and

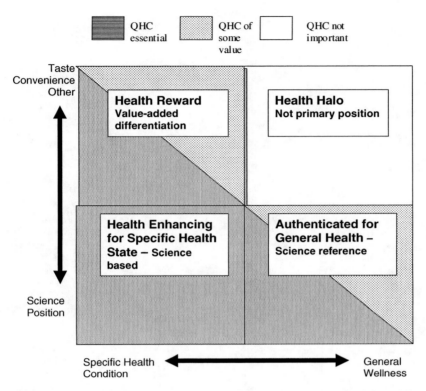

FIGURE 28.2 Advantage of qualified health claims by type of functional food positioning. (Developed by N. Childs, 2004.)

sensitive to products that provide scientific documentation rather than reliance on anecdotal endorsements too often associated with economic fraud. The abundance of branded functional ingredient products already in the market bodes well for developing a successful obesity targeted functional food category based on scientific documentation.

REFERENCES

Childs, N., Obesity and marketing opportunities for functional ingredients, IFT Annual Meeting and Food Expo Technical Program, 75:July 20, 2005.

Childs, N., Obesity policy promises a functional food feast, *Nutrition Business Journal*, Vol. IX (7/8), 15, 34–35: July–August 2004.

Food and Drug Administration Center for Food Safety and Applied Nutrition, Guidance for Industry and FDA: Interim evidence-based ranking system for scientific data, (Washington D.C.: July 10, 2003), August 2005, http://www.cfsan.fda.gov/~dms/hclmgui4.html.

Food and Drug Administration Center for Food Safety and Applied Nutrition, Food Labeling and Nutrition, Label claims: qualified health claims, (Washington D.C.: August 9, 2005) August 2005, http://www.cfsan.fda.gov/~dms/lab-qhc.html#archive.

Kaplan, J., Liverman, C., and Kraak, V., Eds., *Preventing Childhood Obesity: Health in the Balance*, National Academies Press, Washington, D.C., 2005.

Nutrition Business Journal, NBJ's Healthy and Functional Foods Report 2004, Penta Media, San Diego, 2004.

Pszaczola, D., Putting weight management ingredients on the scale, *Food Technology*, 57(3): 42–57, 2003.

Index

A

Absorption, *see specific nutraceuticals*
Accelerated solvent extraction (ACE), isoflavone analysis, 32
Acetoxypinoresinol, 300
Acetylated isoflavones, 25–31, 33–34
Acetyl coenzyme A (CoA), 9, 10, 14
N-Acetyl-cysteine, 424, 425
Activity, physical, *see* Exercise/physical activity
Actonel (risedronate), 251
Acupuncture, osteoarthritis management, 200, 204, 206, 207
Acyl carrier protein (ACP), 19
Adenosine, 6
S-Adenosyl-L-methionine (SAMe), 374, 385–386
Adhesion molecules, 412–413
Adiponectin, 159, 291
Adverse effects
    conjugated linoleic acids (CLA), 291
    omega-3 fish oils, 149
    polyphenols from grape wine and tea, 117–118
Aerobic metabolism, reactive oxygen species production in exercise, 427
Aging
    Alzheimer's disease, 319, 322
    isoflavone health benefits, 38
    and lycopene bioavailability, 60
Aglycone, polyphenol, 24, 108
Ajoene, 7, 77
Alanine, 395
Albumin, flavonoid polyphenol binding, 108–109
Alcaligenes faecalis var. *myxogenes*, 360
Alendronate (Fosamax), 251
Allergens, herbal ingredient issues, 272
Allicin, 5; *see also* Sulfur (allyl sulfur/organosulfur) compounds
Allilin, 77
Allilumin, 78
Allyl sulfur (organosulfur) compounds, *see* Sulfur (allyl sulfur/organosulfur) compounds
Alzheimer's disease, 319, 322
Amino acid-based nutraceuticals
    chemical classification, 9, 20
    fermentation systems, 4
Amino acids
    capsaicinoids, 182
    catecholamines, 377
    essential and nonessential, 393
    leucine and weight loss, 398
    phenolic compounds, 14
    role of, 393–395
Animal feed supplements, 336

Animal models, 7, 62–63
Animal trials, 65
Antagonisms, unknowns, 7
Antheraxanthin, 177
Anthocyanates, 6
Anthocyanins/anthocyanidins, 14, 15, 17
    chemical classification, 9, 14
    glycoside derivatives, 14
    grapes, 104
    phenolic compounds and, 14
Antibacterial/antimicrobial properties, 7
    functional foods, 270, 279
    garlic, 76, 78–79
Anticancer/antitumor effects, 7; *see also* Cancer/antitumor effects
Antihypercholesterolemic properties, 7; *see also* Cholesterol levels; Lipids, blood
Antihypertensive properties, 7; *see also* Cardiovascular disease/cardiovascular system effects; Hypertension
Antiinflammatory activity, 7; *see also* Inflammation/inflammatory mediators/antiinflammatory activity
Antioxidants, *see* Oxidative stress/reactive oxygen species/antioxidants
Apios, 6
Apocarotenal, 13
Apogenin glycosides, 106
Apoproteins, lipid, 145–146, 147, 148–149
Apoptosis, 288
Appetite, proteins and, 401
Arabicans, 16
Arachidonic acid pathway, *see* Inflammation/inflammatory mediators/antiinflammatory activity
Arctostaphylos uva-ursi (bearberry), 270
Arginine, 20
Arthritis, *see* Osteoarthritis; Rheumatoid arthritis
Asian populations
    calcium homeostasis, 253–254
    osteoporosis, 247, 249, 250
    prospective studies, bone mineral density, 255, 256
Astaxanthin, 12
Asthma, 117
Astragalus, 277
Atherosclerosis, *see also* Cardiovascular disease/cardiovascular system effects
    garlic, 89
    lycopene and, 67
    polyphenols from grape wine and tea and
        cholesterol and lipid effects, 110
        epidemiology, 109–110
        etiology, 110

523

H

M

Q